Writing High-Quality Medical Publications

A User's Manual

Writing High-Quality Medical Publications

A User's Manual

Stephen W. Gutkin

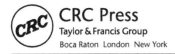

CRC Press
Taylor & Francis Group
Boca Raton London New York

CRC Press is an imprint of the
Taylor & Francis Group, an **informa** business

"Words are, of course, the most powerful drug used by mankind."

Rudyard Kipling

Contents

Preface

It's like my whole world is coming undone, but when I write, my pencil is a needle and thread, and I'm stitching the scraps back together.

Anita de la Torre
in *Before We Were Free* by Julia Alvarez[1]

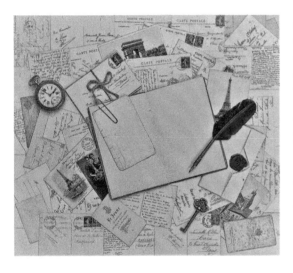

Despite eclectic interests, medical writers share unstinting affinities for science and letters. In my case, the "letters" first included telegrams and postcards. One of my earliest memories involves sorting through a box of scrupulously handwritten letters franked from exotic locales. My father, his mentor Norman Lasker, MD, and their co-workers had published a paper (on plasma renin activity in end-stage renal disease) in a peer-reviewed medical journal.[2] Intrigued researchers from around the globe were posting my dad concerning the study's merits, limitations, and implications.

The experience left a lasting impression on an intellectually curious 8-year-old. By publishing an article in a medical journal, one connects to a larger intellectual community—clinicians and other scientists eager to test, challenge, corroborate, and/or apply one's findings in new ways. So enthralled was I with the process that, not too long after reading the postcards, I began to hector my father (likely *ad nauseam* and *ad infinitum* from his perspective!) to "Do the paper!"

Approximately 50 years on, I have done more than 200 of my own papers. For over 23 years, iterations of the "Gutkin Manual" served as a standard operating procedure and style guide for my medical communications company, which collaborated with more than 500 investigators from São Paulo to Shanghai and 5 of the Top 15 global life sciences companies.

Because we were routinely tasked with ambitious publication plans that depended on high first-journal target acceptance rates, we needed a reliable guide to optimize both quality and efficiency. With the help of versions of this manual, approximately 70% of our submitted manuscripts were accepted by peer-reviewed journals of our first choice. My sincere hope is that the "Gutkin Manual" will help you to be equally successful (if not more so!).

BETWEEN YOU AND ME

Each of us is born without a user's manual. If fortunate, we learn about ourselves from a few special people in our lives: parents, teachers, clergy, friends, peers, and/or spouses, partners, and other loved ones. For those who are embarking on or seeking to build a career in medical writing, editing, and editorial management, I intend this book to accentuate your natural gifts; teach you pivotal principles of data analysis and reporting; and optimize your experiences as both scientists and communicators.

CONCLUSIONS

Gratitude is the memory of the heart.

Jean-Baptiste Massieu

Having begun this Preface on a personal note, I will now conclude on another. In short, I am at a far intellectual and spiritual, as well as chronological, remove from the callow youth who sorted through his father's box of postcards. I am indebted to so many brilliant, patient, thoughtful, gracious, kind, empathetic, and loving individuals in my life.

With Terry Jacobson, MD, professor of medicine at Emory University School of Medicine and attending internist at Grady Memorial Hospital (Atlanta), I have cherished the process of "gap analysis" to identify and meet educational needs of practitioners. Over 22 years, we asked ourselves, "Do we have a paper here? If so, what types of readers would be interested in reviewing the findings and conclusions?" We have successfully navigated this process scores of times, culminating in widely cited reviews in *Mayo Clinic Proceedings*, as well as papers in other highly discerning and prestigious publications, such as *Annals of Internal Medicine* and *Journal of the American Medical Association*.

I am also grateful to the following mentors, collaborators, and supervisors of my work:

- Denise F. Bottiglieri, PhD, a leader in medical communications who guided me to write clearly and concisely, clarifying complex scientific findings and principles without unduly simplifying ("pablumizing"; her term) them;
- Beth Weinberg, RPh, Jeffrey Emmick, MD, and Gordon M. Berry, Jr., for appreciating and nurturing my abilities as a writer;
- Charles M. Beasley, Jr., MD, who inculcated in me the proper orientation of clinical trials and

reports around efficacy, safety, and tolerability outcome measures ("Endpoints, endpoints, endpoints!"); and
- Evo Alemao, MS, RPh, who introduced me to contemporary methodologies of health economics and outcomes research.

My niece Silissa Kenney acquainted me with conventions of the publishing world. Other stalwarts in my life include Andus Baker and Rowan Murphy; Giovanna and Edward Kinahan; Suzanne Carpenter and Peter Lehman; Michael and Beth Davis; Maryclaire and Jesse Garrett; Jeff, Lisa, and Barbara Girion; John and Sandy Lehr; Richard Malen; Sydney Nathans; and Marc Rubinstein.

Dave and Julie Collins rolled up their sleeves to help me in my business and, far more importantly, introduced me to my wife. Also steadfast in their love and support of this endeavor (and every other that I have undertaken) are members of my family: my son Leland, as well as my mother, Barbara; brother, Bruce; and his family, Georgia, Henry, Marni, and Teddy Gutkin. I am also deeply grateful to my aforementioned father, Michael, as well as Gloria and Peter Gutkin; on my wife's side of the family, to Donna Hryb, Andrea House, and Alyce, Clare, and William Kenney.

I am also indebted to Terri Metules not only for envisioning the potential value of this manuscript to medical researchers and communicators but also for her indefatigable efforts to help me realize this vision. (My editorial *confrères* Sara Glickstein Bar Z'eev, PhD, and Lauren Baker, PhD, ELS, also envisaged a larger readership for our style manual.) Terri also introduced me to Jonathan Belsey, MD (JB Medical Ltd., Sudbury, Suffolk, UK; http://www.jbmedical.com/), who provided expert biostatistical review and consultation.

Finally, I will now violate a cardinal tenet of this volume by "saving the best for last," rather than "leading with the news." This book would simply not be possible without the inspiration, dedication, support, and both nurturing and mobilizing effects of my wife, Priscilla K. Gutkin. I am privileged to be married to my best friend, who has the most beautiful and giving heart of anyone I have ever known. With the publication of this work, I have now put more than 700,000 words into print, but no two ever came close to "I do." Although we met through our work in medical communications, I will close this tribute in the parlance of garage and estate sales, of which she has long been a habitué. Priscilla, I am forever grateful that you brought home this curious gewgaw (that would be me) from a nest of *tchotchkes* and treasures.

Midland Park
New Jersey

REFERENCES

1. Alvarez J. *Before We Were Free*. New York: Delacorte Press; 2007.
2. Gutkin M, Levinson GE, King AS, Lasker N. Plasma renin activity in end-stage kidney disease. *Circulation* 1969;40:563–74.

Author

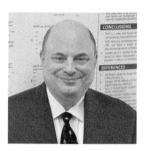

Stephen W. Gutkin is a medical communications professional who has 30 years of experience in medical writing, editing, editorial management, and publication planning and execution. A coauthor of 14 papers in peer-reviewed journals, Mr. Gutkin served as President of Rete Biomedical Communications Corp. for 23 years, during which the organization consulted widely with industry and academia. A *summa cum laude* graduate of Duke University, he served as arts critic for the *Brooklyn Paper*; research scientist for a toxicology laboratory that also assayed psychiatric biomarkers; and as copy chief and medical writer with McGraw-Hill Healthcare (New York). He has delivered invited lectures on medical writing at Johnson & Johnson and the Center for Business Intelligence (now CBINET). Mr. Gutkin is a member of the American Association for the Advancement of Science, American Medical Writers Association, International Society for Medical Publication Professionals™, International Society for Pharmacoeconomics and Outcomes Research, and The Phi Beta Kappa. He resides in Midland Park, New Jersey, with his wife, son, and colorful pet menagerie.

Acknowledgments: Image Credits

written by Dr. John Dolan. Available at: http://blog.sepscience.com/separationscience/hplc-solutions-4-the-importance-of-signal-to-noise. Reprinted with permission of LC Resources. Last accessed January 12, 2018.)

Page 131: Caravaggio, The Incredulity of Doubting Thomas. (Image available at: https://en.wikipedia.org/wiki/File:Caravaggio_-_The_Incredulity_of_Saint_Thomas.jpg. Last accessed January 11, 2018.)

Page 151: Asian Palm Civet (*Paradoxurus hermaphroditus*) pictured at the Khao Yai National Park, Thailand. (Image available at: https://en.wikipedia.org/wiki/Asian_palm_civet#/media/File:Common_Palm_Civet_(Paradoxurus_hermaphroditus)_(7781509830).jpg. Last accessed January 12, 2018.)

Principles and examples of quality in medical communications

CHAPTER OBJECTIVES

The aims of this chapter are to:

- Consider reasons why manuscripts are rejected and approaches to promote acceptance.
- Understand unique challenges confronted by medical writers.
- Review principles of ethical medical communications.
- Characterize requirements of fair balance and ways to satisfy them.
- Survey major pillars of manuscript quality, including the "ity"s: brevity, clarity, variety, and fidelity (internal and external).

1.1 GET YOUR PAPER PUBLISHED— ON THE FIRST ATTEMPT!

The pivotal data have been locked and "cleaned." The findings are promising. Treatment with an investigational product improved three coprimary outcome measures: physiologic variables associated with both longevity and well-being compared to placebo (+ usual care [UC]) in a randomized double-blind controlled trial (RCT). Treatment effects were both statistically and clinically significant; changes from baseline on the three endpoints exceeded thresholds for minimum clinically important differences (MCIDs). Findings from this government- and industry-supported phase 3 trial involving 1,124 patients with a debilitating, suboptimally managed chronic disorder have been reported in a poster at a major scientific congress, generating "buzz" in both the medical and lay communities. Physicians, their patients, and patient advocacy groups eagerly await the full report of the findings concerning what may prove to be a "best-in-class" medication.

Now it's up to you, the medical writer (MW).* Your mission? Draft, edit, and support submission of the study's report. Get it published in the highest-impact, PubMed/MEDLINE–indexed, peer-reviewed journal (PRJ) of first choice, ideally one with open access and other reader and author amenities.

Fait accompli? Au contraire!

Approximately 1.4 million articles are published annually in PRJs.[1] Given a modest, "back-of-napkin" estimate of a 50% rejection rate, this translates to nearly 3 million manuscripts undertaken each year, often without a clear path to publication.

How will your article stand out? Is it likely to be published at all?

A review published in the *British Medical Journal* found that less than half (294 [46%] of 635) of reports of US government-funded clinical trials were published in MEDLINE–indexed PRJs within 2.5 years after study completion. Results from 203 (32%) studies remained unpublished as the interval after study completion approached 5 (median = 4.25) years.[2] These studies had been registered on https://www.clinicaltrials.gov in accordance with §801 of the US Food and Drug Administration Amendments Act (FDAAA) of 2007.

Not only is the likelihood of publication of RCT reports in indexed PRJs within nearly 3 years equivalent to "the play of chance," so is the probability that a study will be cited more than a handful of times each year. Examining peer-reviewed cardiovascular journals from 1997 to 2007, Ranasinghe's group found that the number of submitted articles increased by about 57%, and the number of journals by 75%, including 164,377 articles published in 222 journals. Yet 46% of these published papers were cited no more than 5 times in 5 years, and almost 16% were never cited.[3]

This textbook offers proven, time-tested strategies and tactics based on my 23 years of success in seeing approximately 200 manuscripts published in leading PRJs: mainly journals of the authors' first choice. Most of this chapter will consider principles (and examples) of quality in medical writing (Figure 1.1).

1.2 COMMON REASONS WHY PAPERS ARE REJECTED AND STRATEGIES TO PROMOTE ACCEPTANCE

Over the last decade, new PRJs have proliferated across most medical specialties. As the number of manuscript submissions has mushroomed, so have rejections and retractions. Professional misconduct leading to retraction has ranged from fabricated data and even "fake subjects" to redundant publications and frank plagiarism.[4–8] Although we don't know for sure if the pressure to "publish, or perish" played a role in the rise of retractions and poorly or rarely cited publications, we do know that having a professional MW handle a paper reduces the risk of rejection and ethical misconduct.[9,10]

Why, then, would a paper supported by a MW be rejected?

A common reason for rejection is that the submission is not sufficiently original and/or not within the publication's Aims and Scope (posted on journal websites); most of the PRJ's readers would likely not be interested in reading the paper. Some journals publish only reports of systematic reviews, meta-analyses, and RCTs but not manuscripts reporting data from subgroup analyses, open-label studies, or observational research. To avoid this problem, always review the journal's Aims and Scope, Author Guidelines, and online content.

---

* For the purposes of this textbook, the term "medical writer" (MW) signifies anyone who reports findings in peer-reviewed journals.

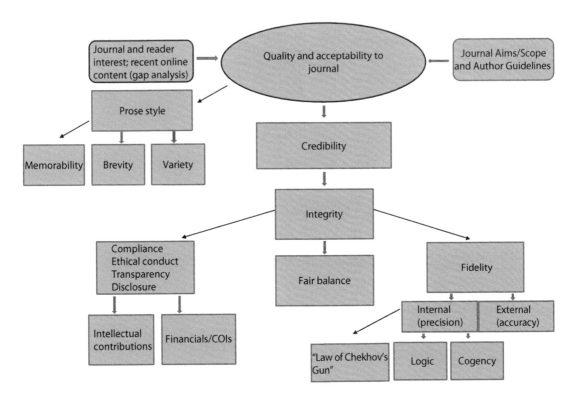

Figure 1.1 Principles of quality and manuscript acceptability in overview.
Abbreviation: COIs, conflicts of interests.

Reviewing recent online content can also help you to rule out another major reason why a manuscript is rejected. If the target journal is about to publish, or has recently published, a similar manuscript, the PRJ may reject because of redundancy. The most direct and effective way to limit this problem is to contact the PRJ's editorial office and submit a blinded abstract in order to preview/gauge journal interest and hence prevent a *prima facie* rejection (i.e., presubmission inquiry).

Even if a PRJ has recently published an article similar to your manuscript, the journal might consider a study report on a similar topic if it adds a new dimension to the existing literature. Such a manuscript might report findings from a study that involves a larger or more diverse sample population or that adds a statistical refinement such as propensity score matching to an observational study paradigm. Examine any journal advertisements about future planned content because your manuscript might fit within an upcoming special issue.

Other reasons for rejection are more basic but no less influential.[11] Was a sample size calculation

performed to ensure adequate statistical power? For inferential statistics, were null hypotheses, two-tailed α values, and other basic statistical parameters explicitly stated? Did the design of an observational study seek to control for potential biases and confounding on unmeasured variables? Were study strengths and limitations delineated in the Discussion?

What about prose style? Did many sentences "bury" key data at the end of complex sentences after numerous subordinate clauses (hypotaxis), parentheticals (or 1/M dashes), and "respectively" constructions? Were most sentences longer than 20 to 25 words (my own guide for a recommended upper limit)? At minimum, did the authors run a grammar- and spell-check and, ideally, share the manuscript with a qualified and credentialed (e.g., ELS*) editor? Did the authors reread the paper, in part to discern any medical misspellings that might "fly under the radar" of spell-check software packages? Examples include "myocardial infraction"; "trail" for "trial" (and vice versa); "complaint" for "compliant" (and vice versa); and "dairy" for "diary" (and vice versa).

---

* Editor in the Life Sciences.

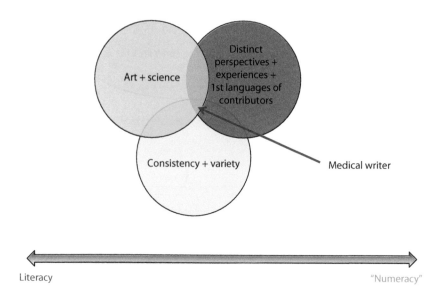

Figure 1.2 The unique challenges of medical writing.

1.3 UNIQUE CHALLENGES FOR MEDICAL WRITERS

Our work is both an art and a science (Figure 1.2). Requirements for consistent logic and prose vie with the need not only to engage readers but to sustain their interest and propel them through the essay, via sentence variety. To these diverse challenges, MWs bring unique skills and experiences. To borrow and modify a term from best-selling author John Allen Paulos,[12] MWs need to have adequate prowess in both "numeracy" (Paulos's term was "innumeracy") and literacy.

Construed broadly, the term "medical writer" is something of a misnomer: it only begins to capture our many professional roles. We are often expected to manage writing projects, and/or support or even steward and "drive" them, from investigator meeting, to the all-important kickoff meeting or teleconference (KOMT; see Chapter 2), to journal submission and peer review, to approved galley pages. We often "think like doctors and argue like lawyers," mounting compelling cases to publish our work by adducing the highest-quality and most appropriate

evidence (Figure 1.3). Similar to the proceedings of a grand jury to determine if there is sufficient evidence for a trial, so-called "gap analysis" in scientific research, communications, and publication planning helps to determine if a study and its report are warranted to address a clinical or other challenge and meet educational needs of prospective readers.

1.4 PRINCIPLES AND EXAMPLES OF ETHICAL MEDICAL COMMUNICATIONS

1.4.1 Fair balance (the foremost principle of quality) is the coin of our realm

Industry-supported publication plans and marketing objectives are never completely realized. Values of shares in life sciences companies (LSCs) rise and fall. Yet the words we commit to print are eternal—digitized for ready consumption, including, increasingly, by open access to global readers in the medical and lay communities.

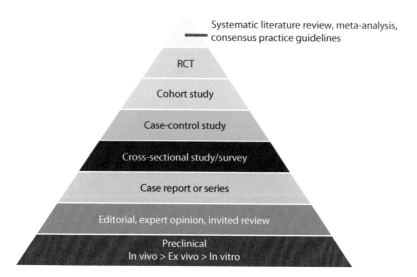

Systematic literature review, meta-analysis,
consensus practice guidelines

RCT

Cohort study

Case-control study

Cross-sectional study/survey

Case report or series

Editorial, expert opinion, invited review

Preclinical
In vivo > Ex vivo > In vitro

Figure 1.3 Traditional hierarchy of biomedical evidence (evidence pyramid). Added to the conventional top level of systematic reviews and meta-analyses (Level 1) are consensus practice guidelines. Also introduced is a bottom evidence level (8) of preclinical data.
Abbreviation: RCT, randomized controlled trial.

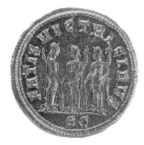

The lasting meaning of our work must be predicated on objective scientific evidence: how effectively and safely medications and other technologies restore homeostatic mechanisms (i.e., surrogate physiologic endpoints) and, ideally, augment longevity and disease-free survival (i.e., "hard" clinical endpoints). Treatment benchmarks relate to pharmacokinetics, pharmacodynamics, efficacy, safety, tolerability, patient-reported outcomes (PROs) such as health-related quality of life (HRQOL), health resource utilization, and costs. Different stakeholders have distinct perspectives and needs for such data. I refer to them as "The 4 'P's": physician (provider), patient, payer, and policymaker.

Our readers include physicians seeking to chart new diagnostic and therapeutic pathways. Our pivotal role is to inform clinical decision making via critical thinking. Hallmarks include methodical, thoughtful, and objective analyses and reporting. Medical writers light potentially divergent paths, elucidating benefit: risk profiles of different diagnostic and treatment modalities. We must provide a balanced literature perspective on these choices, evaluating widely representative databases of published reports without "cherry picking" studies and associated publications (e.g., editorials) that explicitly advance our own argument over others. Fair balance emerges when content is enriched by context, which in turn reflects multiple perspectives.

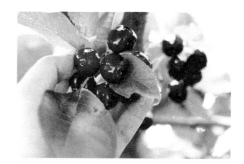

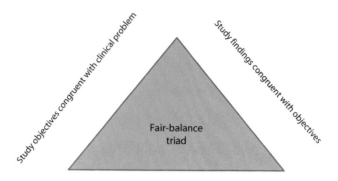

Figure 1.4 Fair-balance triad in medical publications.

Striving to disclose both potential strengths and limitations of study designs is not only ethical but scientifically sound and consistent with acceptance of manuscripts by PRJs of first choice. Achieving fair balance requires that research objectives and hypotheses are congruent with clinical problems and realities; findings are within the purview set forth by the Methods section; and the Discussion, and especially Conclusions, are commensurate with study findings reported in the Results section (Figure 1.4).

1.4.2 Fair balance culminates an open, free, and two-way (or "multi-way") collaboration

To achieve fair balance in communications, MWs need to contemplate, learn, and "own" the potentially disparate perspectives and agendas of different authors (Figure 1.5). Not only do MWs "vet and fret" every citation, every significant figure, every comma; we also need to "see the bigger picture," balancing and otherwise reconciling the distinct and often competing perspectives and interests of participants on research and publication teams. Diplomacy may be required to craft sentences that inform readers' practices yet are also mutually agreeable to key opinion leaders (KOLs), their institutions, sponsors, regulatory and other agencies, as well as professional and patient-advocacy societies (Figure 1.5).

We share a manuscript with an editor to fact check it and ensure "external fidelity" (see below), or accuracy compared to study data and published references. In addition to fact checking, what about "theory checking?" Take, for instance, a study of a medication being investigated to reduce behavioral disturbances in patients with schizophrenia that reveals very infrequent, potential psychotomimetic adverse effects (e.g., hallucinations). Although the incidence of the adverse event might be small, a caveat about this potentially distressing pharmacodynamic effect may need to be included as a limitation in the Discussion section of a study report.

As proactively as possible, we need to identify potential philosophical "seams in teams" that might rend the fabric of a writing project. One example from my own practice involved an LSC that invited a dyed-in-the-wool clinician from the Cleveland Clinic to coauthor an observational study with a paucity of high-quality patient-level data. In many cases, we rely on the corresponding author (CA) to modulate (if not resolve) such conflicts. To support these processes, the Good Publication Practice (GPP3) 2015 panel advocated that authors of a paper proactively "establish a process based on honest scientific debate" to reconcile differences among authors' perspectives on, and inferences about, study data.[13]

One example of a balanced scientific collaboration is the Investigator-Initiated Study. In this paradigm, you may be able to help a group of KOLs

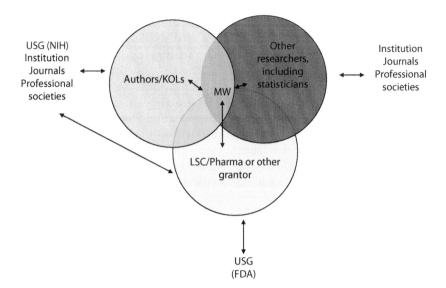

Figure 1.5 Varied perspectives of research and publication teams and associated entities. The medical writer is often situated in the central overlapping segment of the Venn diagram and is hence at the fulcrum of creative, intellectual, and even philosophical tensions.
Abbreviations: FDA, Food and Drug Administration; KOL, key opinion leader; LSC, life sciences company; MW, medical writer; NIH, National Institutes of Health; USG, United States government.

and other researchers to propose a trial to a sponsor concerning a research question that your team can uniquely address.

1.4.3 Fair balance in the planning process

In many cases of industry-supported studies, MWs receive a clinical study report (CSR) from the study sponsor as a starting point. The CSR is a pivotal resource as you write your manuscript. It is often a "living document," showing updates reflecting study amendments and introducing methods to adjust or control for certain statistical anomalies (e.g., protocol violations, data outliers). CSRs can run to thousands of pages, including individual patient adverse-event listings (e.g., every laboratory parameter for every visit by every patient!).

Though indispensable, the CSR represents the LSC's particular view of a disease state and its management. To balance this perspective, spend time reading widely (including disease management guidelines and high-quality review articles), as well as speaking with the CA and other scientists on the research and publication teams.

1.4.4 Fair balance by study report section

1.4.4.1 FAIR-BALANCED INTRODUCTION

One simple step to achieve fair balance that is consistent with the "messiness" and "heterogeneity" of patient care is to include introductory statements such as, "Some[1-8] (but not all[9]) studies have determined that active treatment is superior to placebo in improving surrogate endpoints." This sentence is preferable to one, which, though arguably "neater," is in the province of cherry picking and arguably not fair balanced: "Studies[1-8] have determined that active treatment is superior to placebo in improving surrogate endpoints." This sentence leaves out the study whose findings contradict the summary statement. Systematic literature review (SLR) and meta-analysis reports published by the Cochrane Collaboration are most helpful in appreciating the full literature landscape in a balanced way that eschews cherry picking.

In my practice, the most effective introductory statistics on disease dimensions are prevalence percentages (usually point prevalence but also sometimes lifetime prevalence) and incidence rates. Ranking data, rather than simply reporting large numbers, evidences higher-level critical analysis and overall thought compared to mindlessly regurgitating less memorable statistics. For example, which introductory fact will you remember more easily and longer: that "stroke is a leading cause of adult disability and the fifth-ranked cause of death in the United States," or that "about 800,000 Americans suffer strokes, which are fatal in 129,000 patients, annually?" To remain fair balanced, avoid patient advocacy statistics such as, "Every 30 seconds, a patient experiences a diaphragmatic spasm (i.e., hiccup)." Such "factoids" tend to shed more heat (emotionality) than light (intellect) on a particular disease state and its epidemiology.

Potential disparities between findings from RCTs and observational studies are common examples of "evidentiary incongruity" that MWs should attempt to address when preparing a fair-balanced Introduction. Berger and co-workers on a best-practices panel of the International Society for Pharmacoeconomics and Outcomes Research (ISPOR) addressed this issue effectively.[14] According to Berger's group, potential causes of gaps between conclusions from RCTs and observational studies include:

- Distinct aims and endpoints in RCTs (e.g., efficacy) compared to observational studies (e.g., effectiveness).
- Differences in studied populations.
- Confounding in observational studies, especially related to differences in medication adherence, the influence of patient copays, and confounding by indication.
- Poor quality of patient-level data in observational studies.

Cautiously consider findings from an observational study that contradict prevailing pathobiologic mechanisms, particularly when confirmatory evidence from higher-quality studies (e.g., RCTs) is not available. Certain epidemiologic investigations may meet a knowledge void when it is impractical to conduct a RCT. Cross-sectional studies tend to be limited by uncertainty of the sequence of exposure and outcome, whereas well-designed, longitudinal case-control trials can inform causal inferences (if not conclusively determine causality

and its direction). A time-series study may support the relative effectiveness of an intervention in certain settings (e.g., cancer screening).[14]

Even if your manuscript relates to a single investigational or marketed product, consider constructing an "individual-treatment-agnostic" Introduction that weighs evidence concerning classes of medications, or even technologies (e.g., biological vs. smaller-molecule therapies), and their roles in consensus clinical practice guidelines (CPGs) for disease management. Including CPGs within Introductions is important to ensure not only fair balance but also the credibility of the overall essay and its relevance to practitioners. If one of your coauthors has served on CPG panels, arrange to speak with him or her to seek perspectives on issues that were "voted up or down" by the panel. Get to know the issues and even "politics," including the views of scientists who might serve as peer reviewers of your work after it has been submitted to a PRJ. (A parallel example from the world of macroeconomics is the US Federal Open Market Committee's meeting minutes, which are read avidly by investors.)

1.4.4.2 FAIR-BALANCED METHODS

Many components of a CSR, study protocol, Data Analysis Plan/Statistical Analysis Plan (DAP/SAP), or published article culminate a rational, methodical scientific process, including implicit value judgments. These judgments may inform both the fundamentals of study design and conventional statistical tests as well as the most scientifically nuanced selection of a correlational matrix structure for a generalized estimating equation (GEE) to control for intracorrelated data over time in a longitudinal observational (e.g., patient registry) study.

As detailed in Chapter 3, certain statistical issues warrant critical thinking, ideally during study design, to ensure fair balance. These include the following:

- Are observations independent? This is a common assumption of many statistical tests but may not be appropriate in certain settings. For instance, if you measure blood pressure at 3 time points in 6 different patients, you do not have 18 independent observations (they are paired or matched within patients). Similarly, data from cross-over studies are not independent because each subject serves as his or her own control; the data are paired.

- Do prespecified inferential tests match the likely character of the data? Most notably, are the data:
  - Continuous, or categorical?
  - Limited by upper or lower bounds? For example, a percentage cannot exceed 100, and a blood pressure cannot be below 0 mmHg. (These considerations may result in so-called "range restriction.")
  - Likely, or unlikely, to include outliers?
- How are the data distributed?
  - If symmetrical (normal, bell-shaped, Gaussian), parametric tests are warranted.
  - If asymmetrical (non-normal, skewed), nonparametric tests are warranted.
    - Within asymmetrical data distributions, are there certain shapes that may require novel analyses, including Poisson and geometric?
  - If the data distribution is unknown (by reviewing prior study reports):
    - Proactively specify the use of a statistical analysis (e.g., the Kolmogorov–Smirnov test[15,16]) that makes no assumptions about data distributions.
    - Graph the data or test the normality of its distribution. Relative normality or skew can be evaluated using the Shapiro–Wilk test[17] or the Microsoft Excel test of skew, as described in Chapter 3.
- What methods are proposed to adjust for any increased likelihood of spurious statistically significant associations because of multiple comparisons? One such method is that of Bonferroni.[18] If the two-tailed α is 0.050 in the prespecified analysis, and 10 tests are conducted, the adjusted α for each test is $0.050 \div 10 = 0.005$.
- What methods are used to control for potential biases and confounding (and/or residual confounding) on unmeasured variables? These may include analysis of covariance (ANCOVA), multivariate analysis, propensity score matching, sensitivity analysis, and stratification.

1.4.4.3 FAIR-BALANCED RESULTS

- Follow the "Rule of Chekhov's Gun":
  - Are all data "motivated" in the Methods section? That is, are there any new or unexpected findings that result from statistical or other analyses that were not specified in the Methods?
  - Conversely, for each analysis/endpoint specified in the Methods section, are data presented in the Results?
  - Results sections that emphasize efficacy over tolerability and safety, including economic models that do not take into account all costs to manage frequent and/or serious adverse events, are arguably not fair balanced.

1.4.4.4 FAIR-BALANCED DISCUSSION

Predicate your conclusions soundly on study data, avoiding conjecture, overinterpretation, or a "defensive," overly "argumentative," or "strenuous" tenor. Achieving fair balance often requires great finesse. Typically, we are "arguing a case," in a logical (rhetorical) sense, seeking to persuade readers of a particular conclusion or viewpoint. However, fair balance is struck only when our Discussions explicitly weigh both supportive and countervailing evidence. Such overall "reckoning" enables MWs to achieve the property of "scientific equipoise" required for acceptance of manuscripts by most PRJs.

To achieve fair balance in the Discussion section, we typically begin by offering a 1-paragraph *précis* of the findings. In general, these data should be summarized in the same order as in the Results. A typical summary sequence might run as follows: (1) primary, secondary, then tertiary or exploratory efficacy endpoints; and (2) safety and tolerability endpoints. Communicate results that are either expected or unexpected, statistically or clinically significant (or not), and compatible or incompatible with hypotheses, previously published findings, and overarching biological theory and drug mechanisms of action. How and why did the study turn out the way it did? Are there alternative explanations of the findings?

Suppose that you uncritically accept and report the finding that a short-term RCT in a small number of subjects (e.g., $N < 200$) followed up for 12 weeks failed to identify safety issues. This is akin to sending a myopic child downstairs, to poke around a large yet unfinished and cluttered basement, to see if a single Phillips-head screw is missing, and then praising him for not finding anything amiss! "Absence of evidence is not evidence of absence."

One defect frequently encountered in preliminary drafts of Discussions that erodes fair balance is the use of "judgmental" or "editorializing" modifiers. One such statement runs as follows: "*Only* 1% of our RCT's subjects experienced adverse events." That "only 1%" likely underestimates actual frequencies (and severities) of untoward effects. Patients in RCTs are often highly selected for favorable medication tolerability and adherence profiles, including few comorbidities and concomitant medications, and are monitored for shorter intervals compared to the case in clinical practice and in phase 4 pharmacovigilance monitoring. These factors seriously undermine fair balance in choosing the editorializing adverb "only."

When writing for a PRJ, avoid promotionality (Figure 1.6). Less egregious than promotional writing, and hence potentially insidious, are off-label uses—real or implied—of marketed medications. LSC sponsors employ intellectual-property attorneys to prevent such off-label reporting, but this does not free you of your obligation to maintain fair balance by being attuned to any potential (real or implied) off-label claims. When writing a "branded paper" about a marketed therapy, download the FDA US full prescribing information (USPI) or European Medicines Agency Summary of Product Characteristics (SPC), keep it handy, and cite it when necessary (including the URL and last access date). Seek FDA or other updates to labeling, which are usually available online. These may include black box warnings to avoid use of a medication in certain high-risk populations. Occasionally, a teleconference with the CA is necessary to discuss potential off-label issues.

As real-world evidence becomes increasingly influential, guidance from the FDA Modernization Act (FDAMA) §114 for health economic data specifies that observational studies should not exceed or contradict labeling. For instance, a retrospective cohort (administrative-claims database) analysis on the use of an approved medication should exclude data from patients in whom the medication is contraindicated (or has not been adequately studied) or who receive the medication in an off-label setting, including unlabeled dosages and routes of administration.

Any effects on hard, clinical endpoints should take precedence over surrogate outcome measures in data reporting. Most reports on a medication's effects on surrogate efficacy endpoints should include any off-target or countervailing pharmacodynamic data such as untoward effects or safety signals.

As discussed at greater length in Chapter 3, a major tension with which MWs need to reckon in the Discussion section is between findings from:

- Controlled studies (e.g., RCTs) with largely homogeneous patient populations selected for favorable tolerability and adherence, treated

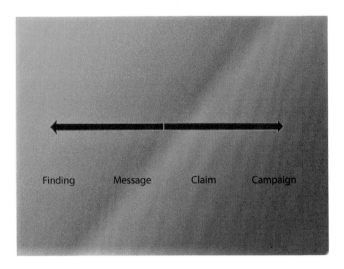

Figure 1.6 *Cave scriptor* ("Writer Beware"). Fair balance and different types of statements. Use of statements shaded in orange and red warrants greater caution than that in green. Most work by medical writers will not be included in campaigns.

for short intervals using fixed protocols, and featuring a high quality of individual-patient data and a relative freedom from bias (i.e., ascendancy of internal validity); and

- Observational studies with potentially larger and more heterogeneous patient populations, treated for longer intervals using dynamic protocols, and featuring a lower quality of individual data but arguably greater generalizability of findings to a naturalistic clinical milieu (i.e., ascendancy of external or "ecological" validity).

We typically do not need to reconcile such differences in a report of a single study but may need to do so when comparing our findings with published values or attempting to pool data from different types of trials (e.g., in meta-analyses). One study setting in my own practice that involves some potentially vexing contradictions is the RCT conducted within a (US) university hospital. On average, study subjects receive more advanced care because of the teaching-hospital setting and accumulation of wisdom. However, many US medical schools and affiliated hospitals are in urban neighborhoods and hence enroll subjects from lower socioeconomic strata. Despite receiving potentially more advanced care, these individuals may have limited resources and health literacy to adhere to their study regimens.

One might say that medications, devices, diagnostic systems, and other health-care technologies are frequently evaluated in relatively "clean," homogeneous experimental settings that optimize efficacy to meet clinical endpoints (e.g., vs. placebo + UC). In contrast, the practice of medicine is decidedly "messy" and heterogeneous. The resulting divide—often a crevasse—relates fundamentally to the aims of a study, such as earning regulatory approval of an investigational product in an RCT compared to conducting an observational study (e.g., patient registry) to discern an infrequent adverse effect.

Particular or general? Controlled or observational? Associational or causal? Prospective or retrospective? Which of the "4 P's" for study perspective (physician, patient, payer, or policymaker)? Frequentist or Bayesian? We must not only recognize but explicitly disclose, clarify, and often reconcile these tensions to achieve a fair-balanced and persuasive Discussion.

1.4.4.5 FAIR-BALANCED CONCLUSIONS

A mentor once praised my work because it did not "pablumize" the science. Ignoring, minimizing, or even neutralizing the complexity of scientific findings and concepts can reduce them to the shallow shibboleths of shills. Medical writers and editors should be "steeped in the science" and focus on drawing inferences from study findings in a statistically and logically sound manner. Drawing conclusions that are consistent with "messaging" or "claims" when composing our manuscripts puts MWs in a "cautionary zone" (Figure 1.6). Such messages may not be formulated by scientists and hence may be insufficiently precise and accurate for a PRJ. For instance, one familiar claim in direct-to-consumer advertising about novel oral anticoagulants is that they are associated with "less bleeding" than the older standard bearer for the class. One might reasonably ask, "Less what? Less frequent? Less severe? Both?" Claims cited in manuscripts for PRJs must be specifically supported by and grounded in clinical trial (typically phase 3) data and also not contradict drug labeling.

Another frequent "message" might be that a new medication is "more convenient" than its predecessors because of dosing frequency and/or administration route. Such a statement may not survive peer review. First, many RCTs do not allow subjects to express their preferences for one medication or another because doing so would compromise the study blind or require a crossover design (to compare therapies).

Second, "convenience" is a complex construct influenced by many variables, including not only dosing frequency and administration routes but the way that these factors interact with different patient characteristics. Although there are validated instruments to assess patient attitudes about medications (e.g., Treatment Satisfaction Questionnaire), I am not aware of any that evaluate "convenience" specifically. Instead, we typically need to assess convenience indirectly, through adherence, which is in turn also influenced by other factors, including tolerability and acquisition or out-of-pocket costs.

One premise that seems to be asserted as axiomatic but is not unassailable is that reducing dosing frequency necessarily results in increased "convenience" and treatment adherence. Not always!

The paper often cited (Cramer's work in *JAMA*[19]) reported that adherence declined when the dosing frequency increased from three to four times daily: 87% for once, 81% for twice, 77% for three times, and 39% for four times. Adherence may have been higher with once- through thrice-daily dosing because this frequency "synced" with meals, which are potential behavioral cues to take medication.

What about claims such as "treatment was efficacious and well tolerated." Now we are moving into a realm of extreme caution. Many journals will not allow such statements unless they derive directly from phase 3 studies and other RCTs. If you are reporting data from such a trial, make sure that any claims are within labeling for the region where the study was conducted.

If you are not reporting a pivotal RCT, qualify such statements in a specific, granular manner that is consistent with the dimensions and circumstances (e.g., design, sample population) of your study. It might seem less "verbally economical" to begin a sentence with a clause such as "Based on our ["TYPE OF STUDY"] findings, subjects receiving treatment A had more favorable responses than those receiving treatment B," rather than stating simply that "Treatment A was more efficacious than treatment B." The former sentence appropriately limits the dimensions of the claim and confers appropriate specificity to match the limited scope of a given sample population, methods, and observations.

1.5 OTHER PILLARS OF QUALITY IN MEDICAL WRITING

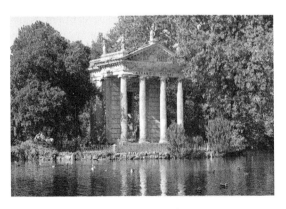

1.5.1 Brevity

Bauhaus architect Ludwig Mies van der Rohe remarked that "Less is more." A question and its answer confirm this aphorism in medical writing and editing.

Q: How many pages was Watson and Crick's report of DNA's double-helical biochemical structure?

A: < 2

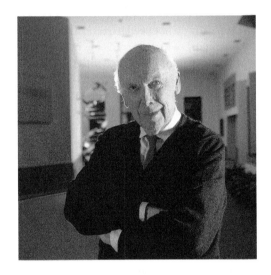

James Watson

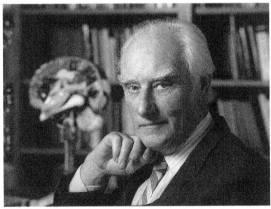

Francis Crick

Read Watson and Crick's original 1.5-page letter to *Nature* sometime. It is elegant, building to the rationale and unique (incremental) value of the research in a solid rhetorical triad. In fact, the arc of the argument is a model for our most effective

Introductions, including a problem addressed by the study and its overall objectives and rationale.

What is known ("Current foundation"): "A structure of nucleic acid has already been proposed..."
Problem/issue ("However"): "In our opinion, the structure is unsatisfactory for two reasons..."
Rationale and unique/incremental value of study/ paper ("Hence"): "We wish to put forward a radically different structure for the salt of [deoxyribonucleic] acid."[20]

Many of us are familiar with the so-called "elevator pitch," which challenges us to summarize an argument or set of ideas before reaching the fifth floor. A pedagogical exercise now making the rounds of New York City private schools is the "Six-Word Challenge." Summarize, say, your favorite vacation, or even your life, in just six words. My best vacation was in Sintra, Portugal. Six words? "Soughing cypress, tavern tawny, winsome wife." My life? "Virtuosic creativity supersedes immobilizing anxiety!" There, I did it in five! Take the Six-Word Challenge sometime and see if it culminates in more succinct written expression.

Against such pithy examples we often encounter rising verbal inflation in our daily lives. Such verbosity evidently slakes certain writers' need for "profundity" (really pseudoprofundity). But more complex is not necessarily "deeper" and certainly not clearer. For example, my photocopier/printer intermittently advises me that "Media for the held job is [sic] unavailable" [seven words]. Whatever happened to "Add paper" [two words]? Colloquial English is so saddled with "verbal inflation." With a nod to political correctness, I still often wonder why every school must be a "learning center"; and every church, temple, mosque, or synagogue a "place of worship."

It is counterproductive to choose the word "utilize" instead of "use"; "prior to" (two words) or "in advance of" (three) instead of "before" (one); "following" instead of "after" (unless something is truly following); or "in spite of the fact that" (six words) or "despite the fact that" (four words) instead of "although" (one word) or "even though" (two words). After completing a first draft manuscript, run a search function for the word "the"; many of these articles can be removed with no loss of meaning.

Be mindful of the person on the other end of your pen, including her level of fluency with English in general and certain terminology in particular. (E.M. Forster: "Only connect" with your reader.) Don't expect the reader to find the fragrant flower of key intertreatment comparisons only after wading through a thicket of thorny subordinate clauses. Don't task her to switch her eyes back and forth from a "respectively" construction located toward the end of a sentence to find its antecedent at the beginning.

1.5.1.1 LEAD WITH THE NEWS!

New York tabloids never beat around the bush (lowercase "b"!). The supersuccinct headline "Ford to City: Drop Dead" did not help Gerald R. Ford's 1976 presidential aspirations. When the "Big Apple" verged on bankruptcy, Ford decided not to allow the federal government to bail it out. John Updike's amazing seven-word *precís* for the often-elusive pleasures of golf—"perfection lying just over the next rise"—left a lasting memory that accompanies me to the first tee about 20 years after it was published.[21]

As a former arts critic for a Brooklyn, NY, newspaper, I advocate two familiar journalistic axioms: (1) "lead with the news" and (2) "don't bury the lead" (or the journalist's "lede")" (Table 1.1). Busy readers should be able to apprehend the key meaning of a sentence or paragraph—the "payoff"—up front, not at the end of a sentence (or paragraph) that leads with subordinate (e.g., methodologic) details. [The "lead-burying" counterpart of the above sentence might read "Busy readers should be able to apprehend the key meaning of a sentence or paragraph—the "payoff"—not at the end of a sentence (or paragraph) that leads with subordinate (e.g., methodological) details, but up front.]

Your "verbal crutches" may be your reader's "verbal speed bumps," driving him to set aside your paper. When was the last time you said to a friend or colleague, "Further, moreover, consequently, thus, therefore, or hence?" Consider striking them from your writing. If one sentence follows organically from its predecessor—and it should!—such "connectors" are usually unnecessary and counterproductive.

Limit pronouns and relative pronouns and liberally use "-ing" forms of verbs. Seek to consolidate words around coordinating conjunctions, which have the mnemonic "FANBOYS": "For,"

Table 1.1 Principles and examples of brevity

- "Lead with the news (outcomes and other data)." Don't "bury the lead"[a] (the journalistic term, not the metal!). Wherever you can, limit sentences to about 20 to 25 words.
  - "Flip the script." Provide "the payoff" up front. Lead with key data such as intertreatment comparisons and p values ("the news"), rather than lengthy descriptions of Methods and study design ("news analysis"; "deep background"), as I have done in this bullet point!
- Avoid wordy expressions enclosed by parentheses or em (1/M) dashes. Segregate them into a separate, second sentence.
- Do use parentheses to include key numerical data, especially comparisons, p values, and 95% confidence intervals (try to report both).
- Use indented bullets and tables/figures to limit words. However, make sure to connect graphics to text, especially if numerical values are otherwise provided only in the Abstract (e.g., numbers in figures that are not otherwise conveyed by the graphic or "narrative text" of the Results).
- Use symbols in text (if allowed by the journal's Author Guidelines) to save words; after all, many of our readers spend a sizeable proportion of their days reviewing lab and other charts!
- Avoid "connectors" (e.g., "additionally"—is it the antonym of "subtractionally?") Dispatch these "verbal apologies" if one sentence flows organically from the last (and it should!). Your "verbal crutch" might be a reader's "verbal speed bump."
- "On the other hand," use expressions such as this one to warn the reader of an imminent break in logic.

[a] To some of you, particularly dyed-in-the-wool journalists, this recommendation may be "old hat." Yet I challenge you to revisit your sentences to discover how many (if not most) do not "lead with the news" but rather "give the payoff" at the end, of either a sentence or even paragraph or manuscript section! Rather than begin five consecutive paragraphs with stultifying sentences emphasizing study design, e.g., "In one RCT... In another RCT..." use the heading "**RCTs**" above all five, and "get to the good stuff" up front: endpoints, p values, 95% CIs, and attendant study conclusions.

"And," "Nor," "But," "Or," "Yet," and "So." I favor an almost telegraphic, data-laden prose. Enclose numerical findings, such as means, standard deviations (SDs), p values, confidence intervals (CIs), and statistical test names within parentheses. The following sentence consolidates around the "FANBOYS" conjunction "but":

The patient, but not his sexual partner, should be involved in planning treatments for Peyronie's disease. [16 words]
Not:
The patient should be involved in planning treatments for Peyronie's disease, but his sexual partner should not. [17 words]

1.5.1.2 CHECK YOUR GUNNING FOG INDEX

Too frequently, MWs in search of profundity, sophistication, or even "gravitas" compose prolix, convoluted, even turgid prose. Yet it is not profound and is in fact less effective to write:

The presence of renal failure in a patient has the capacity to warrant downward drug dosage adjustments" [A 17-word "slog"]; *instead of*
Drug doses may need to be reduced in patients with renal failure. [A 12-word "breeze"].

In general, write in short (generally ≤25-word), direct, declarative, but not necessarily "simple," sentences with no variety. "Leading with the news" should include an emphasis on study data, especially p values and 95% confidence intervals for treatment comparisons, as well as the statistical test that generated each. Try not to gloss over or "neutralize" nuances and otherwise compromise needed scientific sophistication. I am often leery of MWs who promise that they "excel in reducing complex scientific concepts into simple, easy-to-understand prose." The science and practice of medicine are complex and not necessarily amenable to "reduction" to anything. Unless readers are patients or other lay audiences, your prose should clarify, but not necessarily simplify, complex concepts.

To those who are receptive to quantitative approaches, I recommend the Gunning Fog Index (http://gunning-fog-index.com). For a paragraph or passage of 100 words, it is calculated as follows:

$$0.4 \times \left(\frac{\# \, words}{sentence} \right) + 100 \left(\frac{\# \, complex \, words}{\# \, words} \right)$$

Complex words have three or more syllables (apart from proper nouns, compound words, and common suffixes). A Fog Index score ≤5 is considered elementary very easy to read; 6–14, sixth grade to college sophomore; and ≥17, graduate/very difficult.

Apart from a few statistics that can be cited readily in the Abstract, do not repeat (within Results text) numerical data presented in tables and figures. Aside from these graphics (and their titles and legends), which are self-contained units of meaning and hence need to expand key abbreviations and statistical tests used to generate p values, narrative Results text should not repeat tabulated data. However, a figure such as a scatter plot without a trendline often cannot communicate exact numerical data. When this is the case, the Results text is an appropriate place to convey summary data such as $y = mx + b$ expressions, as well as Pearson r and other correlation coefficients associating one variable to another.

A few caveats about brevity. Sometimes it vies with, and needs to be subordinated to, other principles of quality, including clarity and integrity (e.g., transparent and ethical disclosure; see below). For instance, I prefer to save words in a Results narrative by parenthetically calling out graphics, e.g., "Sociodemographic and clinical characteristics were well balanced at baseline (Table 1)." However, non–native-English-speaking researchers and others may prefer the wordier but arguably more direct "Table 1 shows that sociodemographic and clinical characteristics were well balanced at baseline." To decide which way to present findings, consult recent online content for the targeted PRJ.

1.5.2 Clarity

Clear thinking begets clear writing. To achieve clarity, we need to ensure that each segment of a manuscript "motivates" and justifies the next. The Introduction should explain the rationale, research questions, and unique (incremental) value of the study in meeting readers' educational needs.

The Introduction also helps to establish and justify key endpoints presented in the next section: Methods. Prose about endpoints and statistical analyses delineated in the Methods then "motivate" and help to organize presentation of data in the Results. Key statistically and clinically significant (and nonsignificant) findings in the Results then drive organization and overall presentation of the Discussion.

The Discussion builds to the crowning "manuscript reconciliation" in the Conclusions. As MWs, we use the Conclusions to "reckon." Were the study objectives of the research and communication met? If not, why not? Are there alternative explanations of the findings? What unique findings were reported, and what future research might assist in corroborating or extending them?

Consistent with the "IMRAD" (Introduction, Methods, Results, And Discussion) modular format of contemporary medical publications, different readers apprehend information from segments of our manuscripts in discrete ways. Many browse, pick and choose, and rarely read from the first word to the last. Some have time only to review the Abstract and Discussion. Others peruse only the Abstract, tables, and figures.

Because of these distinct cognitive styles and practices, manuscript segments should be self-contained units of meaning to optimize clarity. To "stand alone" if necessary, table titles and footnotes (and figure legends) need to be highly descriptive but not wordy. Text associated with many graphics needs to spell out the following (as examples):

- abbreviations, even if expanded in the narrative text;
- descriptive statistics of the sample population, including mean and SD for symmetrical (Gaussian, bell-shaped) data and median and range (or interquartile range) for skewed (asymmetrical) data;
- different populations analyzed, including intent-to-treat and per-protocol, and any

methods to control or adjust for patient attrition and multiple comparisons;

- p values and statistical tests that generated them;
- analysis of covariance (ANCOVA) models (and prespecified covariates) associated with any least-squares mean values; and
- which group or condition is the referent (risk ratio = 1.0) in a series of relative-risk comparisons.

1.5.2.1 METHODS SECTIONS AS THE "ROSETTA STONE" OF MANUSCRIPT CLARITY

Central to the overall organization, logic, and clarity of a manuscript is a precisely delineated Methods section. In theory, it enables other scientists to repeat your study and confirm or reject its findings (Table 1.2).

Inexplicably, Methods and hence Results sections of many papers published in PRJs are unclear because they fail to offer any "legend" or "key" for major signifiers: in the pre-GPS era, we would say "road map." Of course, it is not necessary for Methods to state that "reductions in blood pressure indicate improvements." With PROs and many other assessments, readers need to know whether an increase, decrease, or positive or negative value represents an improvement or worsening in function. Are there any normative data? What are the psychometric properties of assessment instruments? Have they been validated, and, if so, in which populations? Are there any benchmarks of clinically significant changes? Does a patient survey instrument have an MCID, especially as related to PROs and HRQOL? (See this textbook's Appendix 1 for a summary of key MCIDs.) In many cases, the MCID score represents 10% of the instrument's overall score range.

1.5.3 Cogency

1.5.3.1 THESIS STATEMENT AND TOPIC SENTENCES

The aims of both cogency and clarity are subserved by including thesis statements and topic sentences.* The thesis statement should culminate the Introduction, narrowly focusing on the study's rationale, research questions, and objectives. Effective thesis statements pinpoint the one or two vital clinical or other gaps in knowledge, as well as problems or issues met by the study being reported. Unlike the case with more generic or "secular" thesis statements (often termed simply "theses"), scientific papers do not typically set out an overarching argument, such as "Our thesis is that spastex reduces hiccupping," which cannot necessarily be refuted or corroborated by scientific evidence. Rather, the scientific paper may include a similarly worded null hypothesis, "Our null hypothesis is that [the made-up drug name] spastex does not reduce the frequency of hiccupping as measured using the HURP post-meal instrument for 21 meals before and after treatment," which can be refuted or corroborated by such data.

To help organize a cogent argument, I recommend the website from Purdue University known as the Online Writing Lab (Owl) (https://owl.english.purdue.edu/owl). It presents the Toulmin Method of logic and composition. Although not tailored to medical writing per se, it parallels the rhetorical structure of many of our papers.

First is the claim, which is the thesis being argued and is typically introduced within the first few paragraphs. Next are data—the evidence marshaled in support of the claim. From the data (Methods and Results), our papers proceed to the warrant, or bridge (in the Discussion).

Here we explain connections between our data and the claim, including biological and pharmacologic mechanisms of action and other assumptions. The bridge is strengthened by backing or foundation. In a scientific manuscript, the foundation further buttresses the warrant by comparing findings of similar studies and reports to our own.

Finally, we embrace the totality of the debate on a topic as a context for our study findings by considering counterclaims, which may also derive from the peer-reviewed literature. In the Limitations section of the Discussion, we admit counterclaims but ultimately build a rebuttal. Doing so enables us to consider and, if possible, "defeat" any objections that a reviewer (e.g., targeted PRJ or reader) might raise: the proverbial "straw man," augmenting the credibility and fair balance of our essay.

---

* This sentence did not open with "Thesis statements and topic sentences subserve the aims …" because doing so would have repeated the heading immediately above. More on this in the "Variety" section below.

Table 1.2 Methods section as the "Rosetta Stone" of manuscript clarity: Questions to answer

1. What were the study objectives and/or hypotheses (or null hypotheses [NHs])?
2. What were the study design and duration? (Consider including a study timeline or schema as Figure 1 in the Methods.)
3. How were participants screened, enrolled, randomized, treated, and monitored? In the Results, consider including a Figure 2 (Consolidated Standards of Reporting Trials [CONSORT]) patient-disposition flow diagram to account for these numbers.
4. What were the study's ethical considerations? Were randomized controlled trials (RCTs) conducted in a manner compatible with Good Clinical Practices and ethical tenets originating in the Declaration of Helsinki? Did study participants provide informed consent (or verbal assent for minors), and were the informed-consent document and protocol approved by an ethical or institutional review board? Were observational studies conducted in a manner compatible with guidance from the International Society for Pharmacoepidemiology (ISPE) and patient protections espoused in the Health Insurance Portability and Accountability Act (HIPAA) of 1996; Ethical, Legal and Social Implications (ELSI) Research Program; or the Genetic Information Nondiscrimination Act (GINA) of 2008?
5. In RCTs, what strategies and tactics were applied to effect allocation concealment, blinding, and randomization?
6. In observational studies, what strategies and tactics were employed to minimize, control, or account for confounding or bias (e.g., analysis of covariance [ANCOVA], matching, sensitivity analysis, stratification)?
7. What was the study setting? If the study was registered, what was its identifier (e.g., www.clinicaltrials.gov NCT #)?
8. What prespecified criteria were applied to include or exclude patients (or their data)?
9. For systematic reviews, what search terms were used, what reference databases (e.g., PubMed/MEDLINE/Excerpta Medica (EMBASE)/Cochrane Database of Systematic Reviews) were searched (over what interval), and what criteria were applied to include or exclude studies?
10. What methods were employed to promote data quality, including survey and other rater training; use of central laboratories; and independent data review and entry? What were tests' reliability (e.g., Cronbach's α coefficient)?
11. In retrospective cohort studies, how were the index date, as well as baseline and observational (i.e., follow-up) periods, defined? How many mutually exclusive cohorts (or subcohorts) were there?
12. If any "responder" or other qualitative modifiers are used in the Results section (e.g., "acceptable" clinical response), how were these defined quantitatively, and were imprecision boundaries included? Are they biologically sound, otherwise anchored (e.g., in terms of assessment norms or minimum clinically important differences [MCIDs]), or arbitrary?
13. In RCTs, how was the patient population size determined? Typically, one needs to know the effect size and variance in a similar study.
14. What were the key efficacy, safety, tolerability, patient-reported outcome, economic, and other assessments and their schedules? Which endpoints were prespecified as primary, secondary, tertiary, or exploratory? Which were *post hoc*? Did Methods evolve because of changes in circumstances (e.g., protocol amendments, protocol violations)?
15. How should the reader interpret Results based on changes in assessment scores? Does an increased or decreased score on an instrument indicate that function improved or worsened? What is the MCID? Are there any population norms? Were responses standardized or otherwise normalized or adjusted?

(Continued)

Table 1.2 (Continued) Methods section as the "Rosetta Stone" of manuscript clarity:
Questions to answer

16. How were patient surveys fielded? Was the survey instrument validated and/or translated into other languages (with back-translation into English)? What was the survey response rate? Did nonresponders differ from responders?

17. What were the major assumptions of any statistical models (e.g., covariates in an ANCOVA)? Linear regression analyses assume a continuous dependent variable (DV), whereas logistic regression analyses assume a categorical DV. Were analyses based on multivariable or multivariate regression models? (See Chapter 3 for further details.) In cost-effectiveness and other forecasting or modeling analyses, what were model inputs, outputs, and assumptions (e.g., discount rate)? Were these varied in any prespecified sensitivity analysis, and, if so, how?

18. What populations comprised different analysis datasets? In RCTs, these include intent-to-treat (ITT), per-protocol (PP), and safety populations. How were missing data handled (i.e., by which imputation method)?

19. For comparative relative-risk data such as odds ratios (ORs), what group was prospectively designated as the referent (i.e., had OR = 1.0)? (If a 95% confidence interval for OR overlaps 1.0, the comparison is not significant.)

20. For predictive models, what were the sensitivity, specificity, and negative and positive predictive values? What was the area-under-curve (AUC) for the receiver-operating-characteristic (ROC) curve (which plots sensitivity on the ordinate vs. 1 − specificity on the abscissa)? The AUC of the ROC curve is also known as the C-statistic and measures the model's performance (ability to discriminate diff erent variables, e.g., presence vs. absence of disease). How were models validated and tested for goodness of fit (e.g., by Hosmer–Lemeshow test for logistic regression models).

21. What were safety and tolerability endpoints? Safety endpoints include serum chemistries and hematology, vital signs (body temperature, blood pressure, pulse rate, respirations) and 12-lead electrocardiograms (ECGs), as well as any serious adverse events (SAEs). SAEs are events that cause death or hospital admission, or prolong hospital stay. Narrative text should explain whether SAEs were causally attributed to treatment (often a "judgment call" for the investigator partly according to temporal association between medication administration and occurrence of the SAE). What actions were taken, and what were the outcomes of these interventions?

22. Tolerability endpoints include treatment-emergent adverse events (TEAEs), which either first appear or worsen on treatment. Which dictionary (e.g., Medical Dictionary for Regulatory Activities [MedDRA] 17.1) was used to categorize AEs? By what system: e.g., system organ class (SOC), or preferred term (PT)?

23. Other basic statistical issues (see also Chapter 3):
    a. What were key measures of central tendency and dispersion?
    b. How were categorical and continuous data handled? Categorical analyses include the χ^2 test, whereas continuous analyses include Student's t-test.
    c. Were data normally, or non-normally, distributed? Normally distributed data warrant use of mean, SD, and parametric statistics, whereas non-normally distributed data warrant use of medians, ranges (e.g., interquartile range), and nonparametric statistics.
    d. What were the population sociodemographic and clinical characteristics? Intergroup differences in these (categorical) traits are sometimes analyzed using Fisher's Exact Test.
    e. In correlational analyses, were Spearman ρ, Kendall τ, Pearson r, or other coefficients used? Squaring the Pearson r value (i.e., r^2) determines the percent of variance in one variable explained by another.

(Continued)

Table 1.2 (Continued) Methods section as the "Rosetta Stone" of manuscript clarity: Questions to answer

f. Were Cox proportional hazards regression or Kaplan–Meier survival analyses conducted (and plots drawn)? If so, was the risk difference (or absolute-risk reduction) used to compute numbers of patients needed to be treated to benefit or harm one patient (NNT_B or NNT_H; the inverse of the absolute-risk reduction)?

g. What was the standard of statistical significance: typically, this is a two-tailed (or two-sided) α = 0.05 with a power of 80% or 90% to detect a particular treatment effect between groups. There are very few exceptions in which one-tailed testing should be contemplated (e.g., if a variable can only increase or decrease).

h. What methods were used to control or adjust for multiple comparisons? In the Bonferroni formulation, if 10 tests are conducted, and the *a priori* p value is 0.050, each test must be significant at p = 0.050 ÷ 10 = 0.005.

1.5.3.1.1 A Caveat

It is possible to overdo thesis statements. One defect frequently encountered, even in published articles, is a thesis or other introductory statement that foretells or "gives away" the study findings. Such a statement can disincentivize the reader to press on. Suppose that, in a paper, you encounter the following introductory sentence: "This article demonstrates that a new therapy significantly improved both surrogate and PRO endpoints." Would you be less inclined to read the paper? (I would!)

1.5.3.2 TOPIC SENTENCES

Strive to begin each paragraph with a summary topic sentence. Writing in this manner allows the busy practitioner to trace the arc of your argument by reading the first sentence of each paragraph in sequence. Topic sentences hence support an argument's "horizontal logic." You may choose to structure your essays and topic sentences using the Gutkin 4 × 4 Cogent Manuscript Structure Outline. (See Chapter 2.)

1.5.3.3 OVERALL GUIDANCE ON COGENCY

In addition to using topic sentences, try to repeat your manuscript's key words to assist in linking your paragraphs, organizing the material, and preventing rhetorical tangents. Undertake your writing in the same methodical manner employed when planning and conducting the study. Building a detailed, referenced outline, using abstracts from

PubMed/MEDLINE/EMBASE helps to get you started and seek input from your coauthors or other peers.

Thoughtfully select the studies to cite in order to bolster arguments. Refer to the chemist's axiom of "like dissolves like," citing studies with designs like your own (and systematic literature reviews and meta-analyses of them). To ensure compatibility between your paper and those published in the target PRJ, download a similar study report from the journal's website.

> Appraise, then apprise. Aggregate, then advocate.

Instead of mindlessly "regurgitating" published study data, assess them critically. We appraise published findings, then apprise our readers of their meaning and relevance. In the more argumentative segments of our manuscripts (Introduction and Discussion), we aggregate data pertinent to our study, including results from similar published study reports. We then advocate a certain position: in the Introduction, why our study uniquely (or incrementally) addresses a clinical problem and its report meets an educational need or fills a knowledge gap; and, in the Discussion, why the findings are consequential to practicing clinicians and other key stakeholders ("The 4 P's").

Prioritize the sequence of published results (see Figure 1.3, evidence pyramid, above) and rank the facts and concepts you report. Be a "source snob," basing your selection of cited studies largely on

Cogent essay

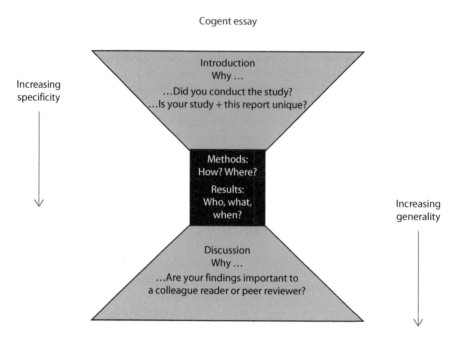

Increasing specificity

Increasing generality

Introduction
Why …
…Did you conduct the study?
…Is your study + this report unique?

Methods:
How? Where?
Results:
Who, what,
when?

Discussion
Why …
…Are your findings important to
a colleague reader or peer reviewer?

Figure 1.7 The cogent essay. "Y," inverted "Y," and "why."

journals' overall prestige, including impact factor, circulation, years in print, society affiliations, and editorial-board diversity. Yet do not be so selective as to exclude a highly relevant investigation published in a lower-tier journal, especially if the study's population and methods mirror your own or the lower-tier journal happens to be the one to which you plan to submit your manuscript!

Figure 1.7 depicts stable foundations for cogent manuscripts. The "Y" signifies decreasing generality, or increasing specificity, from the beginning of the Introduction to the statement of the unique value of the study and study objectives at the end. The "inverted Y" refers to increasing generality (decreasing specificity) from the beginning of the Discussion, which summarizes the key study findings and concludes by projecting the potential clinical implications of the findings and needed future research to extend or challenge them. The "Why" of the Introduction relates to the rationale for the study and its unique (or incremental) value in addressing a clinically important problem. In what ways are the findings meaningful to peer reviewers, readers, and other reviewers, including basic scientists, physicians, patients, payers, and policymakers?

The final check of cogency involves a retrospective "reckoning" process. We review the manuscript and "do the math" to ensure that all components and details "hang together." For instance, did the study meet all study objectives set forth in the Introduction? If not, why not? Are there any endpoints stated in the Methods that were not reported in the Results (or vice versa)? Are there any alternative explanations of the findings?

In an RCT, were sociodemographic and clinical characteristics in the different treatment or other groups well balanced? If not, why not? Is your study sample similar to the larger (general) population who might receive the treatment evaluated in your trial? Similarly, in an observational investigation with propensity score matching, how effective was the match? Were the different groups well balanced after matching? If not, why not? Does the Discussion include any speculative conclusions? Can each table and figure stand alone, adequately defining key terms such as abbreviations, p values, CIs, and statistical tests? Are most of the paragraphs strongly linked to each other and to the key words listed after the Abstract? Are there any other potential "loose ends" or tangents?

1.5.4 Variety

Write clearly and concisely but not monotonously. In general, use direct, declarative sentences that "lead with data" and subordinate less important details. Also warranting our attention is the variety of words and sentence structures, which help to propel readers through the essay. After all, pivotal findings are not discussed (and conclusions drawn) until nearly the end of the manuscript. How will you get them there? Not with dull writing!* An example follows:

Before:
Amilosantronol blocks both the RAA axis and β-adrenoceptors. Amilosantranol is the first once-daily medication for secondary prevention of major adverse cardiovascular events in its class. Amilosantranol also improves HRQOL in patients of all ages.
After:
Amilosantronol blocks both the RAA axis and β-adrenoceptors. The first once-daily medication for secondary prevention of major adverse cardiovascular events in its class, amilosantranol also improves HRQOL in patients of all ages.

In the above example, a participle ("The first once-daily...") was substituted in the second sentence to avoid repetition of the same subject. Try not to repeat nouns or modifiers within the same sentence or in two closely apposed or arrayed sentences.

Strive to avoid interminable series of sentences constructed as "Subject predicate, subject predicate." An example might be "Prostate cancer is this. Prostate cancer is that," *ad infinitum, ad nauseam.* If several paragraphs begin with the name of a disease or medication, use that word or phrase as a heading to reduce such duplication. In many cases, such as review articles, exposition is organized by study design: Instead of writing "In one RCT...In another RCT," use the heading "RCTs." If not, you may choose to subordinate the methodologic details. For example:

Treatment with an investigational farnesoid X receptor agonist reduced serum

levels of liver injury markers, according to findings from a phase 2 randomized controlled trial.

Such a sentence "leads with the news" (a principle of brevity) and appropriately places the main clause before the subordinate clause.

Although most scientific prose is, by convention, composed in the passive voice, there is nothing so bracing as a well-constructed sentence written in the active voice. I began a preliminary draft of a recent paper in the following manner, using an adroit serial construction:

Schizophrenia is a chronic, incurable, frequently disabling mental disorder characterized by severe cognitive and behavioral disturbances. These signs and symptoms can undermine patients' capacity to learn, tax their energy to work, and compromise their social interactions.

Variety may relate to:

1. Openings
2. Subjects
3. Lengths/rhythms
4. Forms of the verb "to be"

The following before-after example illustrates Points 1 and 2 above.

Before (repetitious subjects and sentence structures, and also wordy):
The diagnostic test had a low rate of false negatives (i.e., a high sensitivity). The test found 99.99%—19,249 out of 19,250 true cases—of disease.
After (varied):
The new diagnostic test had a low rate of false negatives (i.e., a high sensitivity). Of 19,250 cases of disease, 19,249 (99.99%) were correctly identified.

I have often encountered the next one in manuscripts and even published articles.

---

* Variety check: The above paragraph includes sentences of different lengths, a backward-running sentence (which uses the adverb "also" in the only correct way at the front of a sentence), an interrogative, and an exclamation.

Before (repetitious to the point of "double-talk"):

Inclusion criteria included [**??**] serum creatinine < 2.0 mg/dL, < 2-fold elevations in alkaline phosphatase and aminotransferases, and normal creatine kinase. Other inclusion criteria included [**??**] SBP < 150 mmHg and DBP < 100 mmHg.

After (varied):

Patients with serum creatinine < 2.0 mg/dL, <2-fold elevations in alkaline phosphatase and aminotransferases, and normal creatine kinase were eligible. Also included were individuals with SBP < 150 mmHg and DBP < 100 mmHg.

The "varied" example also demonstrates the only grammatically correct use of the adverb "also" to introduce a sentence.

When writing directly about complex subject matter, one may unwittingly divide paragraphs into short, choppy sentences or other monotonous rhythms. You can enhance verbal interest and more effectively engage your reader by mixing combinations of dependent markers (subordination), prepositions, transitions, and relative pronouns.

Before (choppy; a bit boring but not bad; 101 words; 10 words per sentence):

Allen's Rule helps to explain certain anthropometric data. It postulates that populations in equatorial and other tropical climates develop long limbs. This may be a result of natural selection and environmental pressures. People with long limbs are best able to exchange heat. In these populations, natural selection may also result in sickled erythrocytes. Sickle-cell anemia afflicts many persons of African race in these same climates. This disease is characterized by sickled erythrocytes. It also results from selection pressures and is inherited. It is inherited in an autosomal recessive pattern. Sickled cells protect hosts from Plasmodium infection. Plasmodium infection causes malaria.

After (a more varied and engaging prose style; 74 words; 18 words per sentence):

Allen's Rule helps to explain certain anthropometric data. Under natural-selection and environmental pressures to promote heat exchange, populations in equatorial and other tropical climates tend to develop long limbs. Sickle-cell anemia, which afflicts many persons of African race in these same climates, also develops because of selection pressures. Inherited in an autosomal recessive pattern, sickle-cell anemia is characterized by sickled erythrocytes, which protect hosts from the Plasmodium infection that causes malaria.

The second paragraph's prose is leaner and also more varied and active. To achieve greater verbal interest, it uses a prepositional phrase ("under"), two relative pronouns ("which"), linkage via subordination ("because"), and a participle ("Inherited in an autosomal pattern") to limit repetition of the verb "to be" (e.g., "...is inherited...It is inherited.")

A memorable example occurred during a boxing match between two of Muhammad Ali's greatest pugilistic foes: George Foreman and Joe Frazier. ABC Sports commentator Howard Cosell exclaimed "Down goes Frazier! Down goes Frazier!" To me, this account is so enduring because of its brevity and variety: it is a three-word, "backward-running" sentence. A preposition is followed by a verb and then the subject. Cosell's locution is also unforgettable because it "leads with the news": "Down!" Had the former attorney less thoughtfully uttered simply "Frazier goes down," I promise you that I would not be writing about it 45 years later. The drama of the moment elevated Cosell's speech, and, for that reason, I will never forget it.

1.5.5 Integrity

How do we understand integrity in our daily lives? One poignant example derives from the US sporting telecast network ESPN's "30 for 30" documentary entitled "Unguarded." The film chronicles the struggles with substance abuse and addiction of former US professional basketball player Chris Herren. Several weeks after Herren had remained "clean and sober," his wife asked him why he was no longer shaving in the shower. "Because," he replied, "I can finally look at myself in the mirror."

Powerful influences are often arrayed across the field of medical communications. To conduct ourselves with professional integrity, we must be aware of these forces and not only balance but "own" them, just as we do the study data. To avoid "clinical demagoguery," we should thoughtfully plan our studies and report data—both positive and negative, expected and unexpected—in an impartial, evidence-based manner that withstands review: first by the MW in the aforementioned "reckoning" process; then by the internal group of coauthors, especially the CA; and, finally, by journal editors and referees. It also behooves us to be "solid scientific citizens," attending scientific and other professional congresses and keeping abreast of CPGs and best practices for manuscript preparation and transparent and ethical disclosure. (See Chapter 4.)

In an invited commentary titled "Evidence-Based Medicine Has Been Hijacked," John P.A. Ioannidis of Stanford University wrote of "salami-sliced data-dredged [articles]" and the practice of "dictating [health] policy from spurious evidence."[22] In this vein, remember that *post hoc* subgroup analyses are by nature "hypothesis generating." The Limitations section should identify this sort of pitfall as well as any sources of imprecision, bias, confounding on unmeasured variables, and/or the inability to generalize conclusions to real-world clinical settings, which might otherwise distort your conclusions.

Keep up to date on controversies surrounding the interventions on which you are writing and the ways in which medical, patient-advocacy, and lay communities might view them. You should not only understand, but "own" these controversies, just as you own the literature that you review, saving .pdfs, highlighting and annotating them, and then neatly "zipping" and sharing them with your colleagues on the publication team, especially the CA.

It is also our role as communicators to "own" "shop-talk terminology" for each specialty on which we are writing. To earn the lasting respect and allegiance of your study sponsors, coauthors, and other colleagues, seek and read the latest paper and editorial on the subject matter of your paper. A visit to www.clinicaltrials.gov or https://www.guideline.gov almost always rewards you with key information about ongoing or planned RCTs and guidance related to a therapy. Stay ahead of the curve.

One way to promote study integrity is to prompt participants to disclose financial interests and intellectual contributions not only transparently but prospectively, using forms presented in Chapter 4 of this volume and provided by PRJs in Author Guidelines. Another approach is to prospectively register study protocols for ongoing studies and other forms of research also listed in Chapter 4. Registries such as ClinicalTrials.gov (for RCTs) and PROSPERO (for systematic literature reviews; https://www.crd.york.ac.uk/prospero/) help to avoid study duplication and reduce reporting bias.

To achieve ideological alignment and integrity, seek to cultivate a strong relationship with your colleagues, especially the CA. Learn her beliefs and positions on scientific issues or controversies by reviewing her recent publications and discussing the issues, ideally at an Investigator Meeting, KOMT, and beyond. Enter the CA's name and key words related to your project into your referencing software, then search the English language from the past 5 years. An ideal point of departure would be an editorial or CPG related to your topic that was bylined by the CA. Seek to cement a bond with the CA to tide the research team over issues with other authors, LSCs, and journal peer reviewers. CAs often "break ties" between authors when conflicts arise.

Figure 1.8 depicts the favorable ethical transition that I have witnessed in the development of industry-supported reviews. Ideally, the content of such publications should originate with the CA/KOL and other authors, in collaboration with the MW, and then be reviewed for factual accuracy and approved at the end of the process by representatives of the LSC. In my experience, most KOLs choose to work with an LSC or other funding entity that manufactures or markets a medication that has a favorable benefit: risk ratio, in the KOL's well-informed opinion. However, everyone—KOL, LSC, and MW—should know "what we have" in data about a new technology, and what we can and cannot say about them, as guided by labeling and CPGs.

Welcome progress toward greater transparency has resulted in both researchers and journal editors gaining access to study protocols, DAPs, SAPs, and even CSRs and "raw data." Many KOLs challenge the LSC at nearly every turn. "May I see a nonparametric analysis of these data? Do trends in transformed data run in the same direction as the raw data? Does a finding represent a class effect? How generalizable are these results to my colleagues' practices? Does a questionnaire have content validity as well as face validity?" I have heard

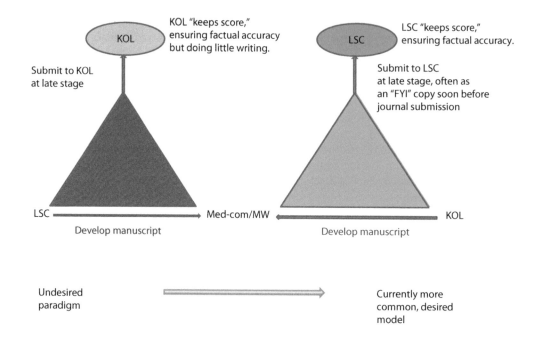

KOL "keeps score," ensuring factual accuracy but doing little writing.

LSC "keeps score," ensuring factual accuracy.

Submit to KOL at late stage

Submit to LSC at late stage, often as an "FYI" copy soon before journal submission

LSC ——→ Med-com/MW ←—— KOL

Develop manuscript   Develop manuscript

Undesired paradigm   Currently more common, desired model

Single-sponsored review articles

Figure 1.8 "Restorative evolution" of relationships among medical writers, key opinion leaders/authors, and life sciences companies over 20 years: 1990s to present. The former, undesired paradigm for writing single-sponsored review articles is depicted at left, and the more common contemporary, desired model at right. Many journals no longer accept single-sponsored reviews.
Abbreviations: FYI, for your information; KOL, key opinion leader; LSC, life sciences company; Med-Com, medical-communications company; MW, medical writer.

KOLs address these and other similar queries to LSC sponsors in order to enhance the integrity of studies and their reports.

1.5.5.1 ON THE OTHER HAND! THORNY FACTORS THAT CONTINUE TO BREACH INTEGRITY

1.5.5.1.1 Lack of meaningful author participation

One of the most prevalent deviations from ethical guidance encountered in my practice is the bylined author who merely nods approbation at each manuscript review. Sorry, but the statement "I approve," reiterated at each stage of manuscript development, does not meet authorship criteria as set forth by the International Committee of Medical Journal Editors (www.icmje.org). Of course, each author must review and approve the final manuscript, but she must also meet other criteria. These include making a substantial contribution to the conception or design of the study; acquiring and interpreting data; drafting the manuscript or offering substantive intellectual contributions (revisions, which may include only deletions); and agreeing to be accountable for, and answer any questions about, the study and its report.

Proactively distribute the ICMJE and journal disclosure forms included in Chapter 4 of this manual and in PRJ Author Guidelines to document each author's intellectual contributions. Doing this proactively, at the KOMT, notifies each potential author of the duties needed to be a bylined author.

One inauspicious sign of impending guest, gift, or "ghost" authorship is a proposed author team of >10 participants, particularly if the individuals did not serve as part of an investigative team who enrolled significant numbers of patients in an RCT. Chapter 4 presents a Committee on Publication Ethics (COPE; www.publicationethics.org) flowchart to identify and address such misconduct.

1.5.5.1.2 Potential undue influence by a study sponsor

Certain study sponsors have the privilege of reviewing both the first and final draft of a manuscript. Being "first in, last out" matters in not only the field of accounting but also matters of intellectual integrity in manuscripts. Sponsors should, and increasingly do, vet manuscripts for factual accuracy. For their part, KOLs typically wish to disclose that they were not compensated to author a single-sponsored review manuscript. Both parties often meet in a mutually agreeable middle represented by the following sort of disclosure statement on the title page of the manuscript (or in the Acknowledgments on the last page).

> The sponsor financially supported writing and editorial services by Redacteusse Inc. (Cherry Hill, NJ, USA). The sponsor reviewed and approved the final manuscript for factual accuracy and integrity, but the authors had complete autonomy over its intellectual content.

According to the GPP3 panel, the above and other relationships between sponsor, author, MW, and other supportive personnel should be delineated in formal correspondence, ideally before the KOMT.[13] The correspondence or other formal, recorded interaction between sponsor and prospective authors should also delineate the protocol for reconciling differences of opinion among members of the writing team.[13] This process should be conducted in an objective, evidence-based manner. One approach is to default the decision to the CA if participants are at loggerheads. This contingency should also be spelled out clearly at the KOMT and/or before beginning the draft.

1.5.5.1.3 The Dreaded "P Word"

Readers of this volume are unlikely to traffic in intellectual dishonesty or fraud, including fabricating data, patients, or reports. According to https://www.etymonline.com (a favorite websites!),

the term "plagiarism" is rooted in the sense of "kidnapping" content. Chapter 4 of this textbook presents COPE decision flowdiagrams to handle plagiarism and fabrication.

In the past, plagiarism was considered to be mainly a "categorical," rather than a "continuous," variable. In the words of US Supreme Court Justice Potter Stewart (referring to quite a different matter!), "I know it when I see it." Contemporary software treats plagiarism as more of a continuous variable. Software is available from https://www.crossref.org and https://www.ithenticate.com. Given this more "probabilistic" standard, MWs can quite unwittingly enter the realm of "medical transcription" via a few missteps. One ominous sign occurs when we find ourselves no longer methodically analyzing, ranking, otherwise organizing, and then reporting published findings: "appraising, then apprising" and "aggregating, then advocating." No amount of "cutting and pasting" can ever substitute for the fundamental intellectual practices of reading—and adequately contemplating, comprehending, and critically assessing—source materials in their many denotations, connotations, and nuances.

If you are in doubt about possibly "creatively borrowing" a previous text, simply quote the original text. Authors of the cited paper often convey their meaning better than you can. A "component-oriented" approach to constructing manuscripts was championed by Bruce G. Charlton. His practice entails assembling a "mosaic" of quotations excerpted directly from published papers.[23]

One "Charlton-esque" approach to summarizing study data in my own practice is to include one sentence each on:

- A problem statement and why the study was conducted and its methods chosen;
- Key study findings, including odds ratios, 95% CIs, p values, and names of statistical tests;
- A succinct quotation from the original paper's authors, typically from the last parts of the Discussion (e.g., Conclusions).

1.5.5.1.4 Other failures to disclose

Other forms of misconduct include failures of investigators or authors to: (1) communicate findings from regulatory audits of study sites; (2) seek, obtain, and disclose ethical or institutional review board approval of study protocols and/or informed-consent documents; and (3) secure written informed consent or verbal assent from study candidates (or legal guardians) before the first assessment or other procedure. No patient should be identifiable from his or her data (e.g., photographs). Methods to protect patients' rights should be disclosed not only in the Methods section of the manuscript but also in the cover correspondence accompanying manuscript submission. An example follows.

> This study was conducted in accordance with Good Clinical Practices, ethical tenets originating in the Declaration of Helsinki, and national laws (whichever conferred the greatest protection to the individual). All potential study participants and/or legal guardians provided written informed consent (or verbal assent) to participate after being informed of the potential study risks and benefits and before any study assessment or treatment. Translators and other surrogates were provided for non-native speakers and illiterate persons. Both the informed-consent document and study protocol were reviewed and approved by local institutional review boards. As per §801 of the Food and Drug Administration Amendments Act (FDAAA) of 2007, the study was registered at https://www.clinicaltrials.gov (NCT # 10µ8508λ).

Such statements are compatible with ethical disclosures concerning subject rights for an RCT report. Other types of study (e.g., observational trials) reports may state that all data were "anonymized (de-identified)," and then cite adherence to guidance from other authorities and legislation, such as the International Society for Pharmacoepidemiology (ISPE); Health Insurance Portability and Accountability Act (HIPAA) of 1996; Ethical, Legal and Social Implications (ELSI) Research Program; and the Genetic Information Nondiscrimination Act (GINA) of 2008.

1.5.6 Credibility and fidelity

These principles are mutually supportive "progeny" of Integrity: the condition of "being whole or indivisible."

With regard to Credibility, and in the words of American songwriter Don McLean, the following came as very "bad news on my doorstep" on January 15, 2009. The *New York Review of Books* (*NYROB*; in an article titled "Drug Companies & Doctors: A Story of Corruption") published these plaintive words of Dr. Marcia Angell:

> It is simply no longer possible to believe much of the clinical research that is published, or to rely on the judgment of trusted physicians or authoritative medical guidelines. I take no pleasure in this conclusion, which I reached slowly and reluctantly over my two decades as an editor of *The New England Journal of Medicine*.

Dr. Angell's contentions find support in a range of contemporary marketed medications that were discontinued or had indications retrenched (Table 1.3). In some cases of withdrawn medications or retrenched indications, "paradigmatic" (rather than strictly evidence-based) arguments were proposed.

Recent reminders of the importance of ethical conduct (e.g, transparent disclosure) include billion-dollar settlements resulting in corporate integrity agreements for some LSCs. Especially given these developments and overall climate, it behooves MWs to evaluate clinical and other data with scientific objectivity (or even initial skepticism) and to be mindful of relevant US and international law, including the Federal Food, Drug, and Cosmetic Act and False Claims Act.

Since that sad day in 2009, effective initiatives have been instituted to shore up the credibility of medical communications. Around the time of Dr. Angell's remarks, best-practices panels undertook initiatives to close the moral breach concerning industry-supported publications. In 2008, COPE was designated as a charity, named Elizabeth Wager as its secretary, and (in 2007) became a major player at the First World Conference on Research Integrity.

Other professional societies have established or updated standards for ethical conduct, including the American Medical Writers Association

Table 1.3 Selected medications that were withdrawn or had their indications retrenched

Drug (trade name)	Class	Time on US market, yr	Issues	Manufacturer/ Marketer
Accutane	Retinoid	27	Suicidal tendencies, IBD, birth defects	Hoffman La Roche
• Avandia	TZD	17	• MI, CHF	• GSK
• Rezulin		3	• Liver failure	• Parke-Davis/ Warner Lambert (now Pfizer)
Baycol	Statin	3	Rhabdomyolysis (acute renal failure secondary to myoglobinuria)	Bayer
Darvon, Darvocet	Opioid	55	Cardiotoxicity	Xanodyne
• Fen-phen	Catecholamine	• 24	• Valve disease, PH	• AHP/Wyeth (now Pfizer)
• Meridia	uptake	• 13	• CVD/CBVD	• Knoll (Meridia)
Premarin/Prempro	HRT	75	CVD, cancers	Wyeth (now Pfizer)
Raptiva	CD11a inhibitor	6	PML	Genentech
• Vioxx	COX2-I	5.3	CVD	• Merck
• Bextra		3.3	CVD, SJS	• G.D. Searle (now Pfizer)

Source: Selected data from ProCon.org (http://prescriptiondrugs.procon.org/view.resource.php?resourceID=005528).
Abbreviations: AHP, American Home Products; CBVD, cerebrovascular disease; CHF, congestive heart failure; COX, cyclo-oxygenase; CVD, cardiovascular disease; Fen-phen, fenfluramine-phentermine; GSK, GlaxoSmithKline; HRT, hormone replacement therapy; IBD, inflammatory bowel disease; MI, myocardial infarction; PH, pulmonary hypertension; PML, progressive multifocal leukoencephalopathy; SJS, Stevens–Johnson syndrome; TZD, thiazolidinedione.

(AMWA), ICMJE, and International Society for Medical Publication Professionals (ISMPP). It is my hope that adhering to the principles espoused in this chapter, particularly related to fair balance and prospective disclosure of author financial interests and intellectual contributions, will advance these efforts. Mansi articulated strategies to "close the credibility gap," most of which have been covered in this chapter. Others include publicizing all results, including negative findings and adverse events as well as efficacy data; transparently communicating statistical methods; ensuring access to study protocols (and/or DAPs/SAPs), CSRs, and other key source documents; and disclosing writing assistance from MWs in order to prevent ghostwriting or guest authorship (see Chapter 4 and https://www.publicationethics.org).[24]

"Internal fidelity" (precision) signifies consistency within a manuscript across different sections, whereas "external fidelity" (accuracy) signifies compatibility of a manuscript with published references and study data (Table 1.4). No credible manuscript contains self-evident internal inconsistencies or purported statements of fact that can be disproved with a single click on Google scholar or snopes.com!

1.6 CHAPTER SUMMARY

Millions of manuscripts are undertaken by researchers each year, often without a reliable path to publication. To improve a manuscript's likelihood of acceptance by a PRJ, this chapter encouraged you to:

- Seek and adhere to PRJ Author Guidelines and other quality standards.
- Further research the PRJ, including its Aims and Scope, and download recent online content (especially reports of studies with designs like your own).
- Reach out to PRJ editors to preview a blinded abstract, in order to gauge journal interest in receiving a full submission (and avoid *prima facie* rejection; i.e., presubmission inquiry).

Table 1.4 Fidelity in medical communications

A. Internal fidelity

1. Data should be presented consistently across segments of a manuscript; findings cited in the Abstract must match those presented in the Results narrative text, which in turn match those presented in tables or figures. (When preparing figures, use the "display numerical data labels" function in Microsoft.) Abbreviations and statistical methods used to generate p values should be defined at first mention in the text, and, separately, within figure legends and table titles or footnotes.

2. All Results should be "motivated" in the Methods. No data should be presented for the first time in the Results; conversely, no results from assessments specified in the Methods should be omitted when presenting Results. The Methods should also organize the presentation of the Results (primary, followed by secondary, tertiary, and exploratory endpoints).

3. Findings (especially numbers) not only need to be minutely correct compared to their sources but also "make sense" internally (i.e., be intuitively sound).

4. Similarly, a statement or table presenting a series of percentages should include a footnote if some percentage values do not sum to 100 because of rounding or discrepant denominators secondary to missing data for different assessments.

B. External fidelity

1. Reported data must minutely match external sources of data, including raw outputs (tables, figures, and patient listings) provided by statisticians and published references cited.

2. To help achieve such consistency, try only to reformat tables (if required) and figures from raw data. Avoid rekeystroking, which can introduce errors.

3. Any statements or claims made in the Discussion, and particularly the Conclusions, should not exceed the scope of product labeling; be vigilant for potential off-label uses—actual or implied. Discuss any such issue with the corresponding author.

- Write succinctly, clearly, and in a fair-balanced manner.
- Base your paper's conclusions on study findings, avoiding conjecture, overinterpretation, and a "defensive" or "argumentative" tenor.
- Conduct yourself ethically, transparently disclosing financial interests such as conflicts of interests (real or perceived) and intellectual contributions, and avoiding off-label promotion (and promotional writing in general).

REFERENCES

1. Björk B-C, Roos A, Lauri M. Scientific journal publishing: yearly volume and open access availability. *Information Research* 2009;14:1–14.
2. Ross JS, Tse T, Zarin DA et al. Publication of NIH funded trials registered in ClinicalTrials.gov: cross-sectional analysis. *BMJ* 2012;344:d7292.
3. Ranasinghe I, Shojaee A, Bikdeli B et al. Poorly cited articles in peer-reviewed cardiovascular journals from 1997 to 2007: analysis of 5-year citation rates. *Circulation* 2015;131:1755–62.
4. Lu S, Zhe Jin G, Uzzi B et al. The retraction penalty: evidence from the Web of Science. *Nature Sci Rep* 2013;3:3146. doi:10.1038/srep03146.
5. Steen RG, Casadevall A, Fang FC. Why has the number of scientific retractions increased? *PLoS One* 2013;8:e68397.
6. Zimmer C. A sharp rise in retractions prompts calls for reform. *The New York Times.* April 16, 2012.
7. Fang FC, Casadevall A. Retracted science and the retraction index. *Infect Immun* 2011;79:3855–9.
8. Seife C. Research misconduct identified by the US Food and Drug Administration: out of sight, out of mind, out of the peer-reviewed literature. *JAMA Intern Med* 2015;175:567–77.

9. Jacobs A. Adherence to CONSORT guidelines in papers written by professional medical writers. *J Eur Med Writers Assoc* 2010;19:196–200.

10. Woolley KL, Lew RA, Stretton S et al. Lack of involvement of medical writers and the pharmaceutical industry in publications retracted for misconduct: a systematic, controlled, retrospective study. *Curr Med Res Opin* 2011;27:1175–82.

11. Audisio RA, Stahel RA, Aapro MS et al. Successful publishing: how to get your paper accepted. *Surg Oncol* 2009;18:350–6.

12. Paulos JA. *Innumeracy: Mathematical Illiteracy and Its Consequences*. New York: Hill and Wang (Farrar, Straus and Giroux), 2001.

13. Battisti WP, Wager E, Baltzer L et al. Good publication practice for communicating company-sponsored medical research: GPP3. *Ann Intern Med* 2015;163:461–4.

14. Berger ML, Mamdani M, Atkins D et al. Good research practices for comparative effectiveness research: defining, reporting and interpreting nonrandomized studies of treatment effects using secondary data sources: the ISPOR Good Research Practices for Retrospective Database Analysis Task Force Report—Part I. *Value Health* 2009;12:1044–52.

15. Kolmogorov A. *Sulla determinazione empirica di una legge di distribuzione. G Ist Ital Attuari* 1933;4:83–91.

16. Smirnov N. Table for estimating the goodness of fit of empirical distributions. *Ann Math Stat* 1948;19:279–81.

17. Shapiro SS, Wilk MB. An analysis of variance test for normality (complete samples). *Biometrika* 1965;52:591–611.

18. Bonferroni CE. *Teoria statistica delle classi e calcolo della probabilità. Pubblicazioni del R Istituto Superiore di Scienze Economiche e Commericiali di Firenze* 1936;8:3–62.

19. Cramer JA, Mattson RH, Scheyer RD et al. How often is medication taken as prescribed? A novel assessment technique. *JAMA* 1989;261:3273–7.

20. Watson JD, Crick FHC. Molecular structure of nucleic acids; a structure for deoxyribose nucleic acid. *Nature* 1953;171:737–8.

21. Updike J, Szep P. *Golf Dreams*. New York: Alfred A. Knopf, Inc., 1996.

22. Ioannidis JPA. Evidence-based medicine has been hijacked: a report to David Sackett. *J Clin Epidemiol* 2016;73:82–6.

23. Charlton BG. How can the English-language scientific literature be made more accessible to non-native speakers? Journals should allow greater use of referenced direct quotations in 'component-oriented' scientific writing. *Med Hypotheses* 2007;69:1163–4.

24. Mansi BA, Clark J, David FS et al. Ten recommendations for closing the credibility gap in reporting industry-sponsored clinical research: a joint journal and pharmaceutical industry perspective. *Mayo Clin Proc* 2012;87:424–9.

Drafting the manuscript: Step-by-step guidelines and exercises

CHAPTER OBJECTIVES

The aims of this chapter are to:

- Consider work flow dynamics, including the all-important project kickoff meeting or teleconference (KOMT).
- Review methods of building structure and cultivating style when drafting and editing manuscripts.
- Walk through "HOW–TWA–ROA" ("How To Write A Report Of A...") exercises. How to write reports of a randomized controlled trial (RCT), observational study, health economic analysis, systematic literature review (SLR), and meta-analysis.
- Offer examples to foster writing quality (including "before/after" exercises).

2.1 WORK FLOW DYNAMICS

2.1.1 Getting started

At minimum, the following resources are strongly recommended.

- Author Guidelines (AGs), Aims & Scope, and a "template" article from the targeted peer-reviewed journal (PRJ), ideally a paper involving a topic similar to your own.
- Author disclosure forms in Word, .pdf, or other readily circulated files (Tables 2.1–2.3; selected forms available at www.icmje.org).
- Microsoft (MS) Office (or Mac-compatible version) including PowerPoint and Excel. SigmaPlot (Available at: http://sigmaplot.co.uk/products/sigmaplot/sigmaplot-details.php.

Last accessed December 31, 2017), Prism from GraphPad (Available at: https://www.graphpad.com/scientific-software/prism. Last accessed December 31, 2017), and Smartdraw (Available at: https://www.smartdraw.com. Last accessed December 31, 2017) assist in generating figures and other graphics.

- Open-source or otherwise widely available online statistical software, including R Project for Statistical Computing (Available at: https://www.r-project.org. Last accessed December 31, 2017), Vanderbilt University's P/S for power and sample size calculations (Available at: http://biostat.mc.vanderbilt.edu/wiki/Main/PowerSampleSize. Last accessed December 31, 2017), and The Cochrane Collaboration's Review Manager (RevMan) for SLRs and meta-analyses (Available at: http://community.cochrane.org/tools/review-production-tools/revman-5. Last accessed December 31, 2017).
- Off-site/cloud-based file-backup software with automatic saving of new work.
- Antivirus software.
- *American Medical Association Manual of Style,* 10th ed. (or later editions as appropriate).
- Electronic medical and generic grammar-, spell-, and consistency-checking software, including PerfectIt Pro (www.intelligentediting.com) and Grammarly® (https://www.grammarly.com/).*
- A general reference text, such as *Harrison's Internal Medicine* or *Goodman & Gilman's The Pharmacological Basis for Therapeutics.* Find prescribing information online, and cite the URLs where you accessed it (and the date accessed). Throughout the publication process, make sure that these URLs remain active and accurate.
- A textbook on biostatistics. (I recommend, and cite throughout Chapter 3, Riffenburgh's *Statistics in Medicine,* and Kirkwood and Sterne's *Essential Medical Statistics.*[1,2])
- Any other, authoritative specialty reference texts as needed to acquaint you with the disease state being discussed, including, for instance, *Braunwald's Heart Disease: A Textbook of Cardiovascular Medicine.* Use these for "deep background." Do not overuse textbooks and/or secondarily cite references in their chapter bibliographies.

- Reference search, retrieval, and management software, such as Endnote or Reference Manager (Available at: http://endnote.com. Last accessed December 31, 2017). Mendeley software (Available at: https://www.mendeley.com. Last accessed December 31, 2017), is highly useful for organizing references. Once you have obtained .pdfs of articles, you can upload them to Mendeley, which not only "reads" but organizes them into searchable content "bits." For instance, if you cannot recall which paper evaluated effects of cetirizine on frequency of sneezing (sternutation), you can type "cetirizine," "sneezing (sternutation)" or, if the database contains mainly references on cetirizine, type simply "sneezing/sternutation." Type the key term into a Mendeley window and the software will open the appropriate reference exactly at the word searched. In a word, "brilliant!"
- A subscription or other access to a high-quality nonspecialty medical journal (e.g., *Ann Intern Med, BMJ, JAMA, Lancet, N Engl J Med, The Cochrane Database of Systematic Reviews [CDSR]*) and/or "gray literature" (e.g., Medscape [https://www.medscape.com/], epocrates [http://www.epocrates.com/], UpToDate [https://www.uptodate.com/home]), preferably if they update your e-mailbox to notify you of new and noteworthy articles.
- A thirst and knack for Internet searches, especially via Google Scholar, government, regulatory, and payer websites with data on disease statistics, pharmacovigilance, ongoing clinical and observational trials (e.g., ClinicalTrials.gov and other registries), and approvals and other activities related to investigational and marketed products, and costs.
- Industriousness, self-reliance, attention to detail, a "can-do" attitude, and an abiding respect for your colleagues and their contributions.

2.1.1.2 MANAGING THE FLOW OF WORK

The term "medical writer" is often somewhat of a misnomer; we are expected not only to draft the manuscript but also "drive" the overall project, from preparing for and running the all-important KOMT to addressing final peer review (Figure 2.1). At the KOMT, distribute forms (Tables 2.1–2.3),

---

* There are too many spell checkers to endorse a single one. They include Dorland's (https://www.dorlandsonline.com/dorland/home); Medispell (http://medispell.com/); and Spellex (http://www.spellex.com/).

Table 2.1 Author disclosure form to facilitate submission of manuscript to journal

Dear Prospective Author/Contributor: Kindly complete and return the form below before the kickoff meeting or teleconference (KOMT).

Your name:	**Academic affiliation**	**Hospital affiliation (or indicate "private practice")**	**Other info. to facilitate submission**
	University:	Hospital/Medical Center/Clinic/VAMC	
Your academic degrees:	Your title:	Your title:	Log-in information for Journal Author Center:
"Honorifics" (e.g., FACP, FACS)	Department(s):	Department(s):	User ID:
	Postal address:	Postal address:	P/W:
Office assistant's information			Recommended peer reviewers (include name, institution, and E-mail address):
E-mail:	Street:	Street:	1:
Tel:	City:	City:	2:
Fax:	State/Province:	State/Province:	3:
Your office #:	Postal code:	Postal code:	
Your cell #:	Country:	Country:	
Best time(s) of day to reach you			
AM; PM			
If possible, insert jpeg of your signature in one of the following columns:			

Abbreviations: ID, identification; P/W, password; VAMC Veterans Affairs Medical Center.

Table 2.2 Form: Author intellectual contributions (based on ICMJE)

Dear Prospective Author/Contributor: To qualify for authorship, you need to check a box in each category. You must make some definitive intellectual contribution to the paper. It is not sufficient to merely approve each draft; reviewing and approving the manuscript is a necessary but not sufficient criterion of authorship. Please complete this form only after the manuscript has been completed (but before it has been submitted to the journal). If you have made contributions to the project that meet criteria in two or fewer categories, or in other categories (e.g., performed statistical analyses, conducted laboratory/pathology or other technical testing, generated figures and other graphical support, provided managerial oversight, obtained funding), be prepared to consent to have your name included in Acknowledgments at the end of the paper.

Category	Your contribution	Page #
Category I.		
Conceived/designed study	☐ **Date(s):**	N/A
Generated/acquired data	☐ **Date(s):**	N/A
Analyzed and interpreted data	☐ **Date(s):**	N/A
Category II.		
Drafted the manuscript	☐ **Date(s):**	Page(s):
Revised the manuscript for intellectual content	☐ **Date(s):**	Page(s):
Category III.		
Reviewed and approved the final manuscript	☐ **Date(s):**	N/A
Category IV.		
Agree to be accountable for the accuracy or integrity of the study report and address any questions about it.	☐ **Date(s):**	N/A

Source: Tables 2.2 and 2.3 are derived from documents authored by the International Committee of Medical Journal Editors (ICMJE) and are available at www.icmje.org.
Abbreviation: N/A, not applicable.

Table 2.3 Form: Author financial disclosures (conflicts of interests)

Your name:	Relationship with study/ms sponsor	Relationship with relevant competing or associated entity[a] (name)	USG or other government support (include grant #)	IP (Patents with USPTO numbers)
Employee of sponsor				
Otherwise compensated by study sponsor to coauthor paper				
Other compensation for coauthoring manuscript				
Equity (major ≥$10,000 or minor) holder in sponsor				
Options (major ≥$10,000 or minor) holder in sponsor				
Principal investigator				
Personal monies[b]				
Grant support (include only entities that could be affected financially by the published work, not public-funding sources)				
Academic support (last 36 mo.)				
Royalties (e.g., from patent)				
Expert testimony				

Source: Tables 2.2 and 2.3 are derived from documents authored by the International Committee of Medical Journal Editors (ICMJE) and are available at www.icmje.org. An electronic financial disclosure form that can be filled out by each author is available at: http://www.icmje.org/conflicts-of-interest. Last accessed October 28, 2017.

Abbreviations: IP, intellectual property; ms, manuscript; USG, United States government; USPTO, US Patents and Trade Office.

[a] Any commercial or other organization researching/pursuing diagnostic or treatment modalities for the overall therapeutic category (not just the narrow topic) researched by you/your study.

[b] Personal monies include fees for services rendered, generally honoraria, royalties, or fees for consulting, lectures, speakers' bureaus, expert testimony, employment, or other affiliations.

Editorial Production Calendar: 30- to 36-week cycle

May 2017

Sunday	Monday	Tuesday	Wednesday	Thursday	Friday	Saturday
	1 MW begins research for KOMT.	**2** Lancet/NEJM/ textbook: Disease state. All online searches for KOMT prep = 5 years. extend to 10 years (later) if necessary.	**3** EMBASE/ MEDLINE: Disease state x key terms (epi, nat. hx, etiology, risk factors, patho-physiology, diagnosis, treatment, HRU, costs).	**4** EMBASE/MEDLINE: Cochrane Collaboration and other systematic literature reviews/meta-analyses.	**5** Google Scholar: CPGs for disease management (US: guidelines.gov). CDC, NIH, NICE, WHO epidemiology stats.	**6**
7	**8** Online search: USPI (for branded paper); Clinicaltrials.gov (RCTs) or other websites for other types of papers (e.g., PROSPERO for SLRs)	**9** Research corresponding author (CA) point of view. Name x disease state x last 5 yr. include reviews/ editorials.	**10** Publication plan: Gap analysis on issues addressed by study report and potential peer-reviewed journals (PRJs) with interest.	**11** Publication plan: Target PRJ (pubshub.com). Any upcoming special/theme issues?	**12** Publication plan: Suitability of manuscript for upcoming congresses (abstract/poster)? Any prior presentations?	**13**
14	**15** KOMT. Decide on target journal and CA. Present "publications grid" prepa-red in prior week (Table 2.4 in this chapter).	**16** KOMT (continued) Distribute Au disclosure and other forms (Tables 2.1–2.3 in this chapter), including this calendar.	**17** KOMT (continued) Align on review/other dates/processes.Align on roles and responsibilities.	**18**	**19** Avoid *prima facie* rejection: Presubmission inquiry: MW sends blinded abstract to PRJ managing editor.	**20** MW/ME/ Administrator: retain COI and other Au disclosures on file for later PRJ submission.
21	**22** MW drafts referenced outline based on initial reference search (see Gutkin 4 × 4 outline in this chapter).	**23** MW circulates outline to publication team.	**24** MW 1:1 teleconference (t/c) with CA. Discuss outline and key issues addressed by research and report.	**25**	**26**	**27**
28	**29** MW receives outline and incorporates feedback from publication team.	**30** MW begins drafting manuscript (assumption 2,000-word study report).	**31**			

(Continued)

Figure 2.1 (a)

June 2017

Sunday	Monday	Tuesday	Wednesday	Thursday	Friday	Saturday
				1	**2** PRJ expresses interest in receiving full submission.	**3**
4	**5**	**6**	**7**	**8**	**9**	**10**
11	**12** PM: 1st draft due from MW next week. Arrange additional adequate editorial support.	**13**	**14**	**15**	**16**	**17**
18	**19**	**20** MW completes 1st draft and circulates to medical editors (MEs).	**21** MEs fact-check and copy-edit 1st draft.	**22**	**23**	**24**
25	**26**	**27**	**28**	**29** MW addresses ME queries/ comments. Discuss any issues with CA if necessary. MW/ME finalize document.	**30** MW/PM circulates 1st draft to Aus/reviewers/ team. Allow ≥ 2 weekends for review.†	†"Editorial symmetry/etiquette": If you have spent 2–3 weeks drafting the manuscript, allow others an approx. equal time frame to review!

(Continued)

Figure 2.1 (a)

July 2017

Sunday	Monday	Tuesday	Wednesday	Thursday	Friday	Saturday
						1
2	**3** PM: Comments from Aus/reviewers/team due next week. Arrange adequate editorial support.	**4**	**5**	**6**	**7**	**8**
9	**10**	**11**	**12**	**13**	**14** MW/MEs receive input from Aus/reviewers/team.	**15**
16	**17** MW/ME incorporate all input from team. CA "breaks ties."	**18**	**19**	**20**	**21**	**22**
23	**24** MW/PM submit 2nd draft for internal grantor review (medico-legal/regulatory/IP).	**25**	**26**	**27**	**28**	**29**
30	**31** MW/PM receive internal grantor review (medico-legal/regulatory/IP) comments.					

(Continued)

Figure 2.1 (a)

August 2017

Sunday	Monday	Tuesday	Wednesday	Thursday	Friday	Saturday
		1 PM: Comments from Aus/reviewers/team due next week. Arrange adequate editorial support.	**2**	**3**	**4** MW/ME incorporates internal input and circulates provisionally final document to all authors.	**5**
6	**7** MW drafts cover letter to journal editors from CA.	**8** Cover letter emphasizes originality and gaps filled. (See template in Chapter 4.)	**9** MW/ME incorporate CA input on draft cover letter to journal and request CA's login info. for PRJ Au Center.	**10** PM: Submission to PRJ next week. Arrange adequate administrative assistance (AA).	**11** MW/ME incorporate all final author input and share final document with all for files.	**12**
13	**14**	**15**	**16**	**17**	**18** PM/MW/ME/AA: SUBMIT/UPLOAD MS, COVER LETTER, AND DISCLOSURES TO PRJ (WITH SCREENSHOT CONFIRMATION).	**19** Cycle 1: 16 weeks.
20	**21** CA confirms PRJ receipt of submission to coauthors/MW/PM.	**22**	**23**	**24**	**25**	**26**
27	**28**	**29**	**30**	**31**		

(Continued)

Figure 2.1 (a)

September 2017

Sunday	Monday	Tuesday	Wednesday	Thursday	Friday	Saturday
					1	**2**
3	**4**	**5**	**6**	**7**	**8**	**9**
10	**11** PRJ accepts with referee comments. (May take from 3 to 12 weeks)	**12** PRJ rejects with referee comments. PM schedules a t/c with team to discuss options.	**13** ME/MW work with CA to address input and draft cover letter detailing responses per. reviewer and items.	**14**	**15** Hold t/c to discuss PRJ options. Seek journal with high acceptance rate and expedited-publication option.	**16** Take a conservative approach to addressing peer review. No new stat. analyses unless required (sensitivity analysis).
17	**18** CA/Aus/reviewers decide on alternative PRJ option.	**19** *Avoid prima facie* rejection. Revisit Presubmission inquiry	**20** CA/MW/ME address selected (major) peer-reviewer comments	**21**	**22**	**23** To decline new stat. analyses, it is appropriate to state that these were not prespecified in study protocol/exceed scope.
24	**25** ME/MW/PM complete tracked and clean ms + letter addressing input per reviewer and items. Circulate to Aus/team.	**26**	**27**	**28**	**29**	**30**

(Continued)

Figure 2.1 (a)

October 2017

Sunday	Monday	Tuesday	Wednesday	Thursday	Friday	Saturday
1	**2** PM: Comments from Aus/reviewer/team due next week. Arrange adequate editorial support.	**3**	**4**	**5**	**6**	**7**
8	**9** MW/MEs receive input from Aus/reviewers/team.	**10** MW/ME incorporate all input from team. CA "breaks ties."	**11**	**12**	**13**	**14**
15	**16** MW/PM submit revised manuscript for internal grantor review/medico-legal/regulatory/IP).	**17**	**18**	**19**	**20**	**21**
22	**23** MW/PM receive internal grantor review (medico-legal/regulatory/IP) comments.	**24** MW/ME incorporate internal input and circulate provisionally final document to all authors.	**25**	**26**	**27**	**28**
29	**30** MW drafts cover letter to journal editors from CA.	**31** Cover letter emphasizes unique or incremental value of study and report, including gaps filled. (See Chapter 4.)				

(Continued)

Figure 2.1 (a)

November 2017

Sunday	Monday	Tuesday	Wednesday	Thursday	Friday	Saturday
			1 MW incorporates CA input on draft cover letter to journal.	**2** PM: Submission to PRJ next week. Arrange adequate administrative assistance.	**3** MW/ME incorporate all final author input and share final document with all for files.	**4**
5	**6**	**7**	**8**	**9**	**10** PM/MW/ME/AA: SUBMIT/UPLOAD MS, COVER LETTER, AND DISCLOSURES TO PRJ (WITH SCREENSHOT CONFIRMATION).	**11**
12	**13**	**14**	**15**	**16**	**17**	**18**
19	**20**	**21**	**22**	**23**	**24** PRJ 1 accepts revised manuscript and cover letter incorporating/ addressing referee comments.	**25** Cycle 2: 14 weeks Total cycle: 30 weeks (or up to 36 weeks if journal takes longer to review manuscript).
26	**27**	**28**	**29**	**30** PRJ 2 accepts manuscript with referee comments.		See above.

AA, administrative assistant (or assistance); Au, author; CA, corresponding author; CDC, Centers for Disease Control and Prevention; COI, conflict of interests; CPG, (consensus) clinical practice guidelines; epi, epidemiology; HRU, health resource utilization; IP, intellectual property; KOMT, kickoff meeting or teleconference; ME, medical editor; MW, medical writer; nat. hx, natural history; NEJM, New England Journal of Medicine; NICE, National Institute for Health and Care Excellence; NIH, National Institutes of Health; pathophys, pathophysiology; PM, project manager; PRJ, peer-reviewed journal; PROSPERO, International Prospective Register of Systematic Reviews (UK); RCT, randomized controlled trial; SLR, systematic literature review; stat, statistical; USPI, US full prescribing information (package insert); WHO, World Health Organization.

(a)

Figure 2.1 (a) Organizing, planning, and delivering a publication for a peer-reviewed journal (PRJ). Circulate a version of this editorial calendar at the kickoff meeting or teleconference (KOMT) to align all participants' expectations, adjust timelines as necessary, and secure proactive "buy-in" as to key roles, responsibilities, and review dates. One aspect of editorial etiquette ("edi-quette"!): whenever possible, allow colleagues about the same amount of time to review a manuscript as you took to draft or polish it.
(Continued)

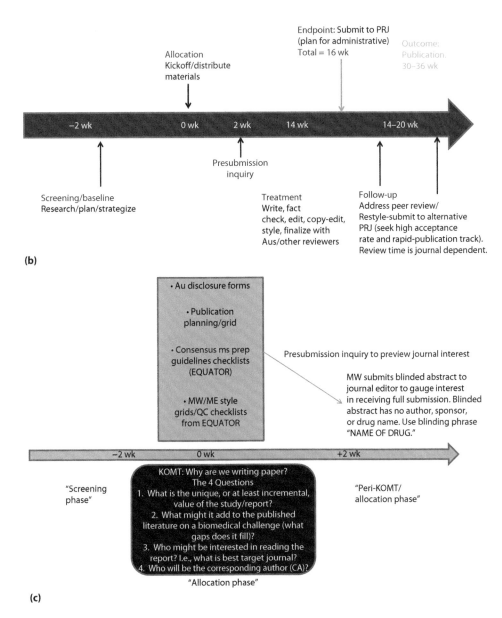

(b)

(c)

Figure 2.1 (Continued) Organizing, planning, and delivering a publication for a peer-reviewed journal (PRJ). **(b, c)** The KOMT is a pivotal event that allows the authors (Aus), overall research/publication team, medical writer (MW), project manager (PM), and medical editor (ME) to determine the all-important issues of (1) who will serve as the corresponding author (CA)? and (2) which peer-reviewed journal would be the best fit for the research and report (based on publication planning and gap analysis; See Table 2.4). The KOMT answers the broad questions "Why?" (Are we here? Did we conduct the study? Are we reporting the findings?) and "How?" (Will we organize and divide labors to submit the manuscript to a suitable PRJ?) Circulate disclosure forms (Tables 2.1–2.3) to facilitate PRJ manuscript submission, which can be a labor-intensive process. Note that the disclosure form is distributed prospectively but can be completed only retrospectively to ensure that all four International Committee of Medical Journal Editors' criteria for authorship have been met. To become most conversant with key issues addressed by the research and report—and how to engage the PRJ's readers—schedule 1:1 time with the CA.
Abbreviations: EQUATOR, Enhancing the Quality and Transparency of Health Research; QC, quality control.

including Gantt charts, to remind participants of their roles and facilitate submission of the final manuscript to the PRJ. Commercial web portals (e.g., www.pubshub.com) offer details about key parameters of thousands of journals (e.g., impact factor, time from submission to publication). Another, admittedly "old-school," approach that I often adopt is to target the "statistical mode." In other words, examine the bibliography of your outline or manuscript. Which journal is cited most frequently? Consider submitting your paper there.

2.2 STRUCTURE AND STYLE

2.2.1 Finding your voice: From Charles Darwin to Chris Matthews

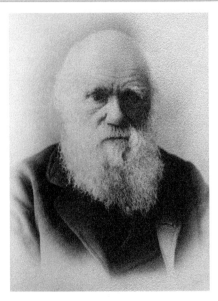

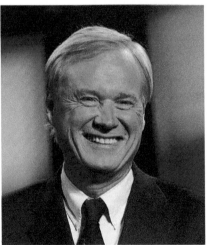

Statements in your Introduction, Results, Discussion, and Conclusions should not only report data but culminate a thoughtful, fair-balanced consideration of the findings that enables your essay to draw meaningful inferences to either improve, or otherwise inform, readers' practices. (As stated in Chapter 1, "Appraise, then apprise; aggregate, then advocate.")

To capture the essence of writing that is not only evidence based but also engaging and memorable, I refer to two solid minds separated by more than a century: naturalist Charles Darwin, who was an intellectual titan but not eminently accessible to us in modern times, and political pundit Chris Matthews who is more so. To represent the evidence-based aspect, we have the introduction to the *Sterling Signature* (2008, 2011) edition of *On the Origin of Species*. David Quammen states:

> Seldom in English prose has such a dangerous, disruptive, consequential book been so modest and affable in tone. That's because its author was himself a modest and affable man—shy in demeanor though confident of his ideas—who meant to persuade, not to declaim or intimidate. [His prose] might sound like a gentle uncle, clearing his throat, politely, about to share a few curious observations and musings over tea.

As researchers and communicators, we are almost always seeking to persuade readers of a particular point of view. However, we should do so in a Darwinian modest, calibrated, and evidence-based, if not "affable," way. Slightly rewording a famous quotation of US industrialist Henry J. Kaiser (founder of Kaiser-Permanente), "When your data speak for themselves, don't interrupt." For instance, if a therapy reduces hospital LOS from 10 to 7 days, it is better to report the 3-day (rather than a 30%) reduction in LOS. The 3-day reduction is more likely to have subject-matter "hooks" in terms of direct health-care costs.

While striving for an ideal of tempered, evidence-based expression, we also need to engage our readers by being original and, if possible, memorable. The reach and salience of our work are driven largely by its likelihood of being cited by others. To convey the original, engaging, and enduring qualities of desirable medical writing, we turn to Chris Matthews. This former

Table 2.4 Example of a publication/journal options grid ("long list"): Brief report manuscript on adherence to an oral antidiabetic drug

Journal	Impact factor	Circulation	Acceptance %	$T_{Sub \to Pub}$* wk	Brief reports? (data provided if yes)?
Acta Diabetologica.	3.34	1,000 (print) 118,247 (downloads)	25	5–12	Max words text = 1,000 No abstract Max. refs = 5 Max. tables/figures = 2
Clinical Endocrinology.	3.327	191 (print)	43	14	No brief reports.
Diabetes.	8.684	1,600 (print)	18	12–26	Max. words text = 2,000 Max. refs = 25 Max. tables/figures = 4
Diabetes and Vascular Disease Research.	3.417	923 (print)	25	7–10	Max. words text = 1,500 Max. refs = 10–12 Max. tables/figures = 1
Diabetes Care.	11.857	6,600 (print)	13	9–24	No brief communications.
Diabetes Research and Clinical Practice.	3.639	23 (print)	39	7–17	Max. words text = 1,000 (w/summary ≤50 words)
Diabetic Medicine.	3.054	854 (print) 16,047 (monthly downloads)	67	18	Max. words text = 1,500 (w/ structured abstract) Max. refs = 20 Max. tables/figures = 2
Diabetes, Obesity and Metabolism.	6.715	11,000 (print)	20	4–13	Max. words = 1,200 (w/180-word unstructured abstract) Max. refs = 12 Max. tables/figures = 2
Endocrine Practice.	2.347	4,400 (print)	35	13–16	Commentaries. Max. words text = 1,500 Max. refs = 15 Max. tables/figures = 1
Endocrine Reviews.	15.745	763 (print)	30	12–24	Commentaries Max. words text = 1,000 Max. refs = 8 0 tables/figures
Endocrinology.	4.286	1,398 (print)	30	24–28	Max. words text = 2,400

(Continued)

Table 2.4 (Continued) Example of a publication/journal options grid ("long list"): Brief report manuscript on adherence to an oral antidiabetic drug

Journal	Impact factor	Circulation	Acceptance %	$T_{Sub \to Pub}$,* wk	Brief reports (data provided if yes)?
European Journal of Endocrinology.	4.101	800 (print)	25	16–18	No brief reports.
International Journal of Endocrinology.	2.510	N/A	25	15	No brief reports.
Journal of Clinical Endocrinology and Metabolism.	5.455	6,925 (print)	25	20	Commentaries Max. words text = 1,000 Max. refs = 8 0 tables/figures
Journal of Diabetes and its Complications.	2.056	9,199 (average monthly visits)	40	4–18	Max. words text = 1,000 (w/summary ≤50 words). Max. refs = 20.
Journal of Endocrinology.	4.706	850 (print)	20	13	No brief reports.
Metabolism.	5.777	38 (print) 17,225 (average monthly visits)	39	5–16	Max. words text = 1,500 (w/structured abstract). Max. refs = 20. Max. tables/figures = 2.
Pancreas.	2.967	12,815 (average monthly visits)	50	9–25	Yes, but no posted max. words (except summary of ≤50 words).
Primary Care Diabetes.	1.381	2,757 (average monthly visits) 850 (print) 40,000 (average monthly users worldwide)	43	11–41	Max. words text = 1,000 Max. refs = 20

Source: Data available from PubsHub, An ICON plc Company. Available by subscription at: https://journalsand congresses.pubshub.com. Last accessed February 9, 2018.

Note: "Author Team: Journal aims/scope, free recent on-line content, and editorial contact information are provided under separate cover."

Abbreviation: NA, not available.

*$T_{Sub \to Pub}$, time from manuscript submission to publication or posting ahead of print, including under assumptions of expedited publication.

speechwriter for President Jimmy Carter and chief of staff to Speaker of the House Thomas "Tip" O'Neill closes his MSNBC telecast "Hardball" with a segment that challenges his guests to "Tell Me Something I Don't [Already] Know."

Similarly, by evaluating data and arriving at your own unique and original synthesis—in short, by telling your readers "something they don't know"—you not only engage their interest but also enliven and increase the intellectual currency of your work.

Review literature critically, fashion your own creative synthesis, and then target it appropriately to your likely readers. I find "raw" statistics—millions of patients with a condition; billions of dollars spent on its management—eminently forgettable compared to relationships, trends, and rankings.

2.2.2 Examples of both evidence-based and memorable prose

Take the following statement summarizing clinical data:

Diaphragmatic bleeding frequency was 6% in the spastex, compared to 12% in the treatment-as-usual (TAU) arm (p = 0.047) of patients with involuntary noisome hiccup syndrome (INHS).*

Is this the most impactful statement for a clinician (e.g., gastroenterologist) caring for many patients with INHS? It would be completely acceptable in the Results section of a study report but perhaps not as consequential in a summary of a prior study presented in an Introduction or Discussion. From these data, we can compute the *risk difference* or *absolute risk reduction* and then easily calculate the number of patients that a clinician would need to treat to benefit one by preventing a single bleeding episode (NNT_B). NNT_B is calculated as the inverse of the difference in absolute risk between the two treatment arms, in this case:

$$NNT_B = \frac{1}{0.12 - 0.06} = \mathbf{16.7}$$

A clinician would need to treat 17 patients with spastex (vs. TAU) to prevent a single episode of diaphragmatic bleeding.

What about incidence rate and prevalence? It is often sufficiently illuminating to report each—as numbers of new cases per 100,000 person-years for the former and as a percentage (not a number of patients) for the latter—in your Introduction. By combining them, you can reach an original creative synthesis:

Influenza virus has a high incidence and low prevalence, which are consistent with an acute but curable and overall effectively managed condition. Such disorders are not compatible with a crossover or other multiphase study, because many patients will no longer harbor the virus after the first phase. Type 2 diabetes mellitus has a lower incidence and higher prevalence, which are consistent with a chronic, incurable, and suboptimally managed condition. Such disorders are compatible with a crossover or other multiphase study because subjects will continue to have diabetes for a prolonged period (*ad vitam*).

Calculating the attributable proportion of a risk factor in exposed (vs. unexposed) individuals is another way to offer a more meaningfully descriptive and memorable "snapshot" of a cohort or other population. For instance, let us say that we know the following data, under the assumption that highly spiced meals can cause INHS:

The incidence of INHS was 7/100,000 among patients in the INHS-IV-COHORT study who consumed highly spiced foods at least once weekly, compared to 3/100,000 in those who consumed spicy diets less frequently.

$$\text{Attributable Proportion} = \frac{\text{Incidence}_{exposed} - \text{Incidence}_{unexposed}}{\text{Incidence}_{exposed}}$$

$$\text{Attributable Proportion} = 100 \times \frac{7 - 3}{7} = \mathbf{57.1\%}$$

---

* Also termed "Smelly Hicupping Disorder," this clinical syndrome has been completely fabricated by me for teaching purposes (and a little levity).

This value can also be computed from the rate ratio (RR; rate in exposed vs. unexposed) as:

$$\text{Attributable Proportion} = \frac{RR - 1}{RR}$$

In the entire INHS-IV-COHORT, approximately 57% of all incident episodes of INHS would be attributable to consuming highly spiced foods (i.e., attributable risk). Approximately 43% of individuals in this cohort would experience episodes of INHS without consuming such foods (i.e., inherent risk). Attributable proportion can also be computed if the incidence and risk or rate ratio are known. Like other methods, this form of analysis has certain limitations.

Consider the following statistics about suicide in the United States. Which do you find more impactful (and why)?

- Each year, 21,334 Americans commit suicide using firearms.
- Suicide is the leading cause of firearm deaths in the United States; each year more than 60% of Americans who die by gunshots are committing suicide.

For most readers, the second sentence has a far more affecting, tangible (almost "moral") dimension, whereas the first is eminently forgettable. (However, some public policy scientists may be more interested in the first sentence; make sure to research your likely readers, as described below.) Another example follows.

- Each year, 44,193 Americans commit suicide.
- Suicide is the 10th-ranked cause of death in Americans (n = 44,193)

Your choice of words (especially active, memorable verbs) and original synthesis of data can make the difference between memorable and forgettable facts. I recently wrote:

Patients with schizophrenia shoulder a disproportionate burden of suicide. The US prevalence of schizophrenia is only about 1.0% compared to 6.7% for major depressive disorder and more than 10% for anxiety disorders. Yet about 33% of Americans with schizophrenia attempt suicide and 10% ultimately take their own lives. (Centers for Disease Control and Prevention: Available at: https://www.cdc.gov/mentalhealth/basics/burden.htm. Last accessed December 31, 2017.)

Describing the cellular and molecular microenvironment of non–small-cell lung cancer, I recently referred to the fact that the carcinoma recruits fibroblasts to "cement a nearly impervious bulwark that protects against surveillance by host tumor-infiltrating immune cells."

When seeking to introduce memorable facts to engage your readers, be mindful of their clinical and other points of view and likely interests. Though largely "intuitive," this guidance is often ignored. For example, the following epidemiologic data might be of interest to a family physician, who treats patients from infancy through advanced age:

- Suicide is the 3rd-ranked cause of death among persons aged 10 to 14 years, 2nd in those aged 15 to 34, 4th in those aged 35 to 44, 5th in those aged 45 to 54, 8th in those aged 55 to 64, and 17th in those aged ≥65 years.
- In the past decade, the incidence of suicide among Americans aged 35 to 64 increased by nearly one-third. The sharpest increases were observed in men in their 50s and women in their early 60s.

A pediatrician might be especially interested to learn the following:

Not only is suicide the 2nd- to 3rd-ranked cause of death in US adolescents and young adults (behind only accidents and homicides), but some studies estimate that one-third to one-half of community-dwelling young people also inflict wounds on themselves without suicidal intent.

Psychiatrists may be most interested in knowing that:

- More than 90% of suicide decedents had a diagnosable psychiatric condition (especially major depressive disorder or treatment-resistant depression) at death.
- Veterans of military combat may be more likely than age-matched civilians to commit suicide, because veterans meet criteria of Joiner's Interpersonal Theory, including a perceived low sense of "belongingness" and burdensomeness to others, as well as an ability to endure the discomfort that might be required in killing oneself.

Almost all readers would be interested in learning that:

- Because of medical surveillance bias, suicide is a problem of largely untold dimensions. Many patients, especially members of certain ethnoracial minority groups and veterans of military combat, experience stigma about mental illness and hence do not report or seek medical attention for suicidality.

Readers of a health economics and outcomes research (HEOR) journal might be more inclined to read the following, from former US National Institute of Mental Health (NIMH) director Thomas Insell (Available at: https://www.nimh.nih.gov/about/direc tors/thomas-insel/blog/2011/the-global-cost-of-men tal-illness.shtml. Last accessed December 31, 2017).

The Agency for Healthcare Research and Quality cites a cost of $57.5 billion (2006) for mental health care in the (United States), equivalent to the cost of cancer care. But unlike cancer, much of the economic burden of mental illness is not the cost of care, but the loss of income [because of] unemployment, expenses for social supports, and a range of indirect costs due to a chronic disability that begins early in life.

Some HEOR readers are payers and chiefly interested in direct health-care costs. Research your targeted PRJ's websites and online publication-planning sites (e.g., www.pubshub.com) to understand the PRJ's circulation and numbers of different types of readers, including physicians (providers), patients, payers, and policymakers. (The "4 Ps" of reader perspectives.)

As a digression related to memorable introductory statistics, I remember once driving with my father along one of the many highways and byways of New Jersey. We observed that roadside sound barriers were being erected, and my dad stated that the project was costing New Jersey taxpayers "$1 million per mile."

Such "neat and tidy" relationships in Introductions (and Discussions) are so memorable that they linger with readers long after being read. Examples in medicine that I have read over the years include the facts that:

- On a population (not necessarily per-patient) basis, there is a 20% reduction in the annual incidence of ischemic cardiovascular disease for every 1-mmol/L decline in low-density lipoprotein cholesterol (LDL-C) on treatment with HMG-CoA reductase inhibitors (i.e., statins).
- Risks of percutaneous ("needle-stick") viral transmission are 30% for hepatitis B, 3% for hepatitis C, and 0.3% for HIV. [These relationships were true when I read the statement but have now been updated.]
- For every 30-day gap in antipsychotic medication adherence, there is a 10-fold increase in the incidence of relapse in patients with newly diagnosed schizophrenia.

Typically, try to exclude from manuscripts statistics such as "every 30 seconds an American experiences a myocardial infarction." Such statements often originate from patient-advocacy groups and shed more heat (emotion) than light (intellect) on a problem. They can, however, confer "gravitas" and command attention. During a recent presentation to a life sciences company (LSC), including several representatives of Medical Affairs, the room grew quieter and the participants more attentive after I announced that, "During my 1-hour talk, 5 Americans will die by suicide [1 every 13 minutes; CDC data]."

2.3 STRUCTURING THE OUTLINE

2.3.1 "Scaffolding": The Gutkin 4 × 4 cogent manuscript structure outline

Using references identified by PubMed/MEDLINE/EMBASE/CDSR and other literature searches, develop a detailed and referenced outline. The "4 × 4" structure refers to four headings (Introduction, Methods, Results, Discussion) with four subheadings each (Table 2.5). If a congress abstract is available, it should be introduced as the Abstract segment of the outline. If figures or tables from an existing congress poster are available, introduce them in the outline (after ensuring with the statistician that they are final and "clean").

Table 2.6 summarizes key considerations when preparing the report of a randomized controlled trial (RCT).

2.3.1.1 INTRODUCTION

The chief aim of the Introduction is to develop the scientific rationale for the study, its objectives, and, in some cases, hypotheses and outcome measures. The Introduction builds to a thesis statement, which sets forth issues or problems that the study and its report uniquely (or incrementally, compared to prior published literature) address.

One formulation or idea flow for the Introduction runs along the lines of typical review articles in the *New England Journal of Medicine*, which cover, in sequence (and often using one paragraph each):

- Disease state definitions and clinical or humanistic dimensions.
- Public health dimensions (incidence, mortality, prevalence, and costs).
- Normal physiology, homeostasis, pathophysiology, and natural history.
- Etiology, risk factors (and protective factors, if applicable), and genetics.

- Consensus diagnostic and treatment embodied in clinical practice guidelines (CPGs).

Readers of specialty journals are well acquainted with such introductory facts. For these readers, craft an introduction that quickly builds to the rationale and objectives of the study and its report.

Aims* of Introductions should be to delineate the dimensions of a disease state; its contemporary consensus diagnosis and management; and any potential ongoing issues or clinical challenges. The Introduction should culminate in clear objectives that guide the rest of the manuscript.

In my practice, I have received draft Introductions that were:

- Vague, "diffuse," and unfocused: did not build to a study rationale and objectives.
- Tangential: did not use key words and themes to link paragraphs and organize the essay.
- Overly argumentative (not gently persuasive in the Darwinian spirit): foretold the findings or a controversy reviewed in the Discussion, in a "defensive" or "strenuous" manner that included value judgments, superlatives, or other non–evidence-based statements.
- Innocuous: not necessarily bad but bombastic and inconsequential, never "hooking" potential readers with ongoing challenges related to their practices in an RCT or failing to characterize the "situation on the ground" in a regional pharmacoepidemiology (real-world evidence [RWE]) paper.

Table 2.7 defines key epidemiologic terms frequently cited in Introductions, including incidence proportion, attack rate, secondary attack rate, incidence rate, point prevalence, and period prevalence.[3] Prevalences should be reported as proportions (%) of a population, not as numbers of people with a disease, as is so often encountered even in published articles. Clarify whether you mean point or lifetime prevalence.

---

* In medical writing, the word "aim" is a noun, not a verb. The "aim" of the study corresponds to its objectives, but researchers do not "aim" to determine one thing or another.

Table 2.5 Gutkin 4 × 4 (4 major headings × 4 subheadings in each) cogent manuscript structure outline[a]

Each Roman numeral below becomes a heading (H), and each capital letter becomes one paragraph (¶) or more. Each topic sentence (**TS**) provides "horizontal logic." The reader of your outline or essay should be able to progress from one topic sentence to the next and appreciate the arc of your argument.

I. **Introduction (250–500 words) H**
   A. Disease state, definitions, and basic epidemiology **1–2¶**, each with a **TS**
   B. Pathophysiology/etiology/natural history/genetics **1–3¶**, each with a **TS**
   C. Consensus diagnostic and management guidelines **1¶** with a **TS**
   D. **Thesis statement**: clinical problem/educational need and unique or incremental value in addressing it study rationale and objectives **1¶/TS**

II. **Methods (250–750 words) H**
   A. Study design/setting/participants/ethics **1–3¶**, each with a **TS**
   B. Interventions **1¶** with a **TS**
   C. Assessments/outcome measures **1–3¶**, each with a **TS**
   D. Statistical methods **1–4¶**, each with a **TS**

III. **Results (250–750 words) H**
   A. Patient disposition **1¶** with a **TS**
   B. Baseline characteristics **1¶** with a **TS**
   C. Efficacy outcome measures **1–2¶**, each with a **TS**
   D. Tolerability/Safety **1¶–2¶**, each with a **TS**

IV. **Discussion (500–1,000 words) H**
   A. Key findings: $p < 0.05$ and >0.05; expected and unexpected; meeting or not meeting endpoints/MCIDs (and why) **1–3¶**, each with a **TS**
   B. Relationship to published literature (narrowly construed, as it relates to study design and findings), as well as potential clinical implications, and alternative explanations, of the data, **1–3¶**, each with a **TS**
   C. Potential study strengths and limitations **1–2¶**, each with a **TS**
   D. Conclusions: clinical implications and needs for future research **1¶**, with a **TS**

Abbreviation: MCID, minimum clinically important difference.

[a] Consult journal author guidelines and online content. Refer to checklists in Chapter 4 to adapt this basic structure to other forms of study reports (e.g., Consolidated Standards of Reporting Trials [CONSORT] for randomized controlled trials and Strengthening the Reporting of Observational Studies in Epidemiology [STROBE] for observational studies). Collaborate with the corresponding author to formulate the outline. Circulate it to all potential authors, request their feedback, and record/date the input (including deletions). Outlines should be referenced and include newly generated figures and tables or "table shells."

In your Introduction, strive to include (and cite) CPGs, which help to orient readers concerning diagnosis and management of the disease. When doing so, find something specific and not uniformly applicable, trivial, or innocuous. An example of the former is "phosphodiesterase type 5 inhibitors constitute first-line therapies for erectile dysfunction, irrespective of its etiology or concomitant chronic conditions." This statement is consequential to clinical decision making. Conversely an innocuous introductory sentence might include a banality ("throwaway") such as "Objectives of therapy for erectile dysfunction are to enhance quality of life while minimizing adverse effects." This is true of virtually any disease's management!

Leave readers with concepts that they did not learn in medical school or early training. For example, a statement such as "Risperidone is an atypical antipsychotic that functions as a central serotonin ($5\text{-}HT_{2A}$) antagonist at lower doses and dopamine (D_2) receptor antagonist at higher doses" is more valuable to most practitioners than one such as "Schizophrenia results from excess brain dopamine."

Table 2.6 Considerations when drafting a randomized controlled trial report

Disclosures	Introduction	Methods	Statistical issues and methods	Results	Strengths	Limitations
Registration. Clinicaltrials.gov (NCT ID #).	**Historical perspective:** the "saga" of the disease; management advances over the years; and limitations/ongoing challenges of current modalities.	**Study setting** (e.g., number and locations of centers). **Eligibility criteria. Ethics (IRB/ICD). Study schema/timeline** (Figure 2.5).	Attrition (MAR MCAR) and imputation method (e.g., LOCF).	**Baseline characteristics** (Table 2.8). Segregate categorical and continuous variables. Define ITT, PP, other populations.	Random allocation, blinding, and placebo control largely preclude bias or confounding.	Ecological validity/generalizability to real-world treatment settings.
Previous presentation (all manuscripts).	If nonspecialty journal: Allocate 2–4 paragraphs for disease state, then build to problem/objectives (250–750 words).	**Efficacy endpoints** (primary, secondary, tertiary, exploratory). **Prespecified subgroup analyses. Safety/tolerability endpoints.**	Type 1 or 2 Error Multiple comparisons (Bonferroni).	**Efficacy endpoints:** reported in same sequence as "motivated" in Methods: primary, secondary, tertiary, exploratory. **Text: report p values, 95% CIs, and test that generated each p value.**	High quality of patient-level data.	Highly selected patient population (tolerability, adherence, and overall treatment response may be overestimated).
Funding statement and author financial disclosures/conflicts of interests (all manuscripts).	If specialty journal: Build swiftly to problem/objectives (100–200 words), e.g., 1 sentence on disease state; 1–3 development; last 1–2 on problem/issues and objectives.	**Assessments** (can use summary table for assessment schedule by visit) and their biometric/psychometric properties and implications (e.g., MCID for PROs).	Parametric or nonparametric analyses: plot data, test for skew (Microsoft Excel, see Chapter 4); use Shapiro–Wilk test to determine if distribution is normal or non-normal.	Efficacy graphics: tables, figures (e.g., pie, bar, linear regression, forest, Kaplan–Meier, box-whisker).	Guidance on endpoints (FDA).	Protocol-based (inflexible) treatment regimens.
Author contributions (ICMJE; all manuscripts).	• **What is known?** • **What is the issue/problem/gap?** • **How does this study/report address the issue/fill the gap? What does it add to existing knowledge?**	**Populations** (total, intent-to-treat, per-protocol, safety).	ANCOVA often does not control for disease severity or age.	**Safety/tolerability endpoints:** See Table 2.9 for terminology. **Safety:** narrative text and shift tables. **Tolerability:** frequency table (MedDRA PT/SOC; Table 2.10).		RCTs are typically not powered to determine intertreatment differences in infrequent adverse events and of insufficient duration to determine differences in safety parameters.

Abbreviations: ANCOVA, analysis of covariance; FDA, Food and Drug Administration; ICD, informed consent document; ICMJE, International Committee of Medical Journal Editors; IRB, institutional review board; ITT, intent-to-treat; LOCF, last observation carried forward; MAR, missing at random; MCAR, missing completely at random; MCID, minimum clinically important difference; MedDRA, Medical Dictionary of Regulatory Activities (www.meddra.org); PP, per-protocol; PRO, patient-reported outcome; PT, preferred term; SOC, system organ class.

Table 2.7 Measures of morbidity that are often used—and misused—in introductions

Measure	Numerator	Denominator
Incidence proportion (or attack rate or risk).	Number of new cases of disease during specified time interval.	Number in population at start of interval.
Secondary attack rate.	Number of new cases among contacts.	Total number of contacts.
Incidence rate (or person-time rate).	Number of new cases of disease during a specified time interval.	Summed person-years of observation or average population during time interval.
Point prevalence.	Number of current cases (new and pre-existing) at a specified point in time.	Number in population at the same specified point in time.
Period prevalence.	Number of current cases (new and pre-existing) over a specified period of time.	Number in the average or mid-interval population.

Source: Centers for Disease Control and Prevention. In: *Principles of Epidemiology in Public Health Practice: An Introduction to Applied Epidemiology and Biostatistics*. 3rd ed. Atlanta, GA: CDC, 2016. Available at: http://cdc.gov/ophss/csels/dsepd/ss1978/lesson3/section2.html. Last accessed December 31, 2017.[3]

2.3.1.2 METHODS

As mentioned in Chapter 1, the Methods section is the linchpin of "internal fidelity" and represents the "Rosetta Stone of Clarity" for the entire manuscript. The purpose of the Methods section is to enable the reader to understand (and, ideally, replicate) your investigation, with reference to the justifications for, and meanings of, the pivotal efficacy, safety, tolerability, patient-reported outcome (PRO), and/or pharmacoeconomic endpoints. The Methods section delineates the overall logic of the paper and helps the reader or other reviewer (e.g., PRJ referee) to follow it.

In the pre–GPS era, Methods sections were identified as "road maps," in that they elucidated study assessments and outcomes in sufficient detail for the reader to understand if: (1) an increase or decrease signifies an improvement or worsening in function; (2) there are normative values associated with no disease or other impairment; and (3) there are any threshold values that represent minimum clinically important differences (MCIDs).

2.3.1.2.1 Internal fidelity: "Rule of Chekhov's Gun"

If you say in the first chapter that there is a rifle hanging on the wall, in the second or third chapter it absolutely must go off. If it's not going to be fired, it shouldn't be hanging there.

Anton Chekhov

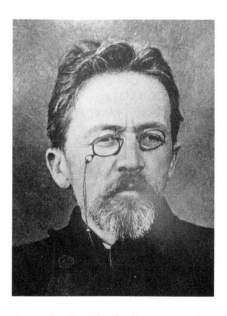

Reporting of scientific findings must be internally consistent (i.e., have "internal fidelity"). If the Methods section mentions a study objective or endpoint, the Results section must include a value for that outcome variable irrespective of whether it is statistically or clinically significant. Conversely, the Results section should not present any value that was not mentioned or "motivated" in the Methods. A cogent Methods section also determines the sequence in which data are presented in the Results.

Statistical methods are considered in detail within Chapter 3 of this textbook. In my practice, I have found that the names of many statistical tests are "buried" in footnotes or other obscure sections of a CSR or raw statistical output. Only after reviewing these data might you learn the key covariates in an analysis of covariance (ANCOVA) or that, say, Fisher's Exact Test, Student's t-test, or Mann–Whitney's U test was performed. Include such data not only in the Methods text but also in footnotes to tables or legends to figures.

2.3.1.3 RESULTS

Report the findings concisely, and in the same sequence as presented ("motivated") within the Methods section (Rule of Chekhov's Gun). One sequence of data flow for RCTs runs as follows: (1) patient disposition (including a Consolidated Standards for Reporting Trials (CONSORT) patient-disposition flow diagram if possible), (2) baseline characteristics (example in Table 2.8), (3) efficacy, (4) tolerability (Tables 2.9 and 2.10), and (5) safety.

Because of the modular organization of contemporary scientific papers (and divergent styles of readers in apprehending information) tables and figures must be self-contained units of meaning (stand-alones). Some readers access information from papers largely by jumping from one table or figure to the next. For these readers, abbreviations and statistical methods used to generate p values (and other statistical details such as covariates in an ANCOVA model) need to be defined within figure legends and table titles or footnotes, as well as in the Methods text. For each endpoint identified in the Methods, a p value should be presented in narrative text, table, or figure, regardless of whether the test result is statistically significant ($p < 0.05$).

Tolerability and safety are often confused but are not synonymous. Tolerability typically includes adverse events (AEs) or treatment-emergent adverse events (TEAEs), which first appear, or are present at baseline and worsen, after treatment initiation. Adverse events should be elicited via open-ended questioning by the investigator or other appropriately trained trial personnel at each study visit. Definitions of different tolerability terms are presented in Table 2.9.[4]

Avoid "judgmental," non–evidence-based modifiers that might make the modest and affable Darwin blush. For instance, the Food and Drug Administration (FDA) has no standard for the term "well tolerated"; it is what I term an "unanchored judgmental" adverb. Rather than use such

a loose modifier, convey incidences (usually in descending order of frequency) of the most salient AEs, often in a table.

Safety includes serious adverse events (SAEs). Chapter 4 provides tables to guide you in reporting harms in RCTs.[5] An SAE report in a manuscript should detail how the SAE presented, actions taken, outcomes of these interventions, and whether investigators judged the SAE to be related to treatment. This last inference is based largely on temporal patterns of the patient's taking the medication and then experiencing the SAE, or discontinuing the regimen and then not experiencing it.

Other key safety parameters include mean changes from baseline to end of treatment or study in laboratory parameters (e.g., chemistries, hematology) as well as any outliers, such as numbers (%) of patients with values ≥5 times the upper limit of normal (≥5 × ULN). Individual or group changes (often in so-called "shift tables") in 12-lead electrocardiography (ECG) and vital signs (pulse rate, blood pressure, respiration rate, body temperature) are also subsumed under the rubric of safety.

2.3.1.4 DISCUSSION

A thoughtful, fair-balanced, and well-organized Discussion helps the reader to understand the findings and their ramifications. Such a Discussion should meet the following objectives.

- Recap key findings and probe their implications and relationships to the hypotheses and endpoints [**1–3 paragraphs**]. What is the single statement that will convey the most lasting meaning? Were study objectives or outcome measures met? If not, why not? How do the findings address a scientific problem or controversy and advance the field or readers' practices? Do they confirm or violate hypotheses (e.g., reject the null hypothesis or accept the alternative hypothesis)? Are findings clinically as well as statistically significant? (Do associated effects meet or exceed MCIDs?) If prespecified subgroup analyses were conducted, did any patient segments derive special benefits, or experience more adverse consequences, from treatment?
- Compare the data to results from similarly designed and other recent (past 1–5 years) and pivotal studies using the same agent (or related agents from the same pharmacologic class)

Table 2.8 Example of a baseline characteristics table for a randomized controlled trial. Baseline characteristics of subjects with involuntary noisome hiccup syndrome (INHS) in the NO-MO-BURP-PLS! Trial[a]

Characteristic	Spastex + placebo group (n = 848)	TAU[b] + placebo group (n = 459)	Total (N = 1,307)
Mean (SD) age, yr	55.3 (11.2)	57.2 (9.3)	56.0 (10.6)
Mean (SD) body mass index, kg/m²	28.0 (4.3)	29.4 (4.7)	28.5 (4.5)
Mean (SD) daily hiccup frequency	8.6 (0.6)	7.6 (1.6)	8.1 (1.4)
Mean (SD) INHS severity score[c]	14.9 (6.3)	13.1 (6.4)	14.3 (6.3)
With gastric pH, n (%)			
<7.0	820 (98.7)	186 (41.1)	1,006 (78.3)
7.0–10.0	9 (1.1)	209 (46.1)	218 (17.0)
>10.0	2 (0.2)	58 (12.8)	60 (4.7)
Age (yr), n (%)[b,d]			
<50	274 (32.3)	91 (19.8)	365 (27.9)
50–64	402 (47.5)	274 (59.7)	676 (51.7)
65–74	146 (17.2)	86 (18.7)	232 (17.8)
≥75	26 (3.1)	8 (1.7)	34 (2.6)
Daily treatments, n (%)			
Placebo	250 (29.5)	146 (31.8)	396 (30.3)
Spastex 2.5 mg	79 (9.3)	117 (25.5)	196 (15.0)
Spastex 5 mg	519 (61.2)	196 (42.7)	715 (54.7)
Ethnoracial identity, n (%)[b,d]			
Caucasian	728 (85.8)	367 (80.0)	1,095 (83.8)
African	21 (2.5)	11 (2.4)	32 (2.4)
Hispanic	80 (9.4)	68 (14.8)	148 (11.3)
Native American/other	19 (2.2)	13 (2.8)	32 (2.4)
INHS severity, n (%)[d]			
Mild	313 (36.9)	141 (30.7)	454 (34.7)
Moderate	235 (27.7)	126 (27.5)	361 (27.6)
Severe	293 (34.6)	191 (41.6)	484 (37.0)
Unknown	7 (0.8)	1 (0.2)	8 (0.6)
INHS duration, n (%)[d]			
3–5 mo.	29 (3.4)	9 (2.0)	38 (2.9)
6–11 mo.	70 (8.3)	36 (7.8)	106 (8.1)
≥1 yr	749 (88.3)	414 (90.2)	1,163 (89.0)
INHS etiology, n (%)			
Organic	346 (40.8)	330 (71.9)	676 (51.7)
Psychogenic	127 (15.0)	5 (1.1)	132 (10.1)
Mixed	316 (37.3)	118 (25.7)	434 (33.2)
Unknown	59 (7.0)	6 (1.3)	65 (5.0)
Comorbidity/history, n (%)			
GERD	254 (30.0)	265 (57.7)	—
Hiatal hernia	14 (1.7)	13 (2.8)	—

Note: GERD, gastroesophageal reflux disorder. For Consolidated Standards of Reporting [Clinical] Trials (CONSORT) patient flow diagram related to these data, see Figure 2.6.

[a] Intent-to-treat population; denominators vary across characteristics and reflect numbers of subjects with available data for each.

[b] The treatment-as-usual (TAU) group comprises patients receiving placebo + proton pump inhibitors, histamine₂ (H₂) blockers, and/or over-the-counter antacids for INHS.

[c] Lower scores denote more serious disease with worse effects on diaphragmatic function.

[d] Some percentages do not add to 100 because of rounding.

Table 2.9 Common terms in tolerability and safety defined according to the International Conference on (now Council for) Harmonisation (ICH)

Term	Definition
ADR	Preapproval: "All noxious and unintended responses to a medicinal product related to any dose." Postapproval: "A response to a drug which is noxious on and unintended and which occurs at doses normally used in man for prophylaxis, diagnosis, or therapy of disease or for modification of physiological function."
AE	"Any untoward medical occurrence in a patient or clinical investigation subject administered a pharmaceutical product and which does not necessarily have to have a causal relationship with this treatment."
AESI	"An adverse event of special interest (serious or nonserious) is one of scientific and medical concern specific to the sponsor's product or program, for which ongoing monitoring and rapid communication by the investigator to the sponsor can be appropriate. Such an event might warrant further investigation in order to characterize and understand it. Depending on the nature of the event, rapid communication by the trial sponsor to other parties (e.g., regulators) might also be warranted. (This definition is covered by ICH E2F guidance.[b])"
SAE[a]	"A serious adverse event (experience) or reaction is any untoward medical occurrence that, at any dose: results in death; is life threatening; requires [hospitalization] or prolongation of existing [hospitalization]; results in persistent or significant disability/incapacity; or is a congenital anomaly/birth defect."
UAE	"An adverse reaction, the nature or severity of which is not consistent with information in the relevant source documents."

Source: International Conference on Harmonisation. *ICH Harmonised Tripartite Guideline: Clinical Safety Data Management: Definitions and Standards for Expedited Reporting E2A.* Available at: https://www.ich.org/fileadmin/Public_Web_Site/ICH_Products/Guidelines/Efficacy/E2A/Step4/E2A_Guideline.pdf. Last accessed December 31, 2017.[4]

Abbreviations: ADR, adverse drug event; AE, adverse event; AESI, AE of special interest; SAE, serious AE; UAE, unexpected AE.

[a] The terms "serious" and "severe" are not synonymous. "Severe" signifies a step up in intensity from mild and moderate. "Serious" is based on an outcome or event in a patient that is associated with threats to her survival and/or function.

[b] In characterizing overall adverse reaction experience, nonspecific terms that lack a commonly understood or precise meaning are discouraged, because use of such terms can be misleading. For example, the phrase [well tolerated] is a vague and subjective judgment about a drug's adverse reaction profile for which there are no commonly understood parameters. Specific frequency ranges (e.g., adverse reactions occurring in <1/500) provide more precise information about incidence." (From ICH E2F.)

[1–3 paragraphs]. Which findings are consistent with, or divergent from, published data? Do results in general confirm or violate expectations based on the literature? In what ways do the present analysis and its findings improve on prior methodologies and results?

- Probe the potential clinical implications of the findings and how they might fit into contemporary patient care, referring to recent CPGs if appropriate [1–2 paragraphs].
- Appraise potential strengths and limitations related to study design, statistical methods, baseline patient populations and other factors, which render the study more or less generalizable to populations related to readers' practices [1–2 paragraphs]. What questions could the study address or not address? Do error, bias, confounding, or other factors undermine confidence in the findings? What types of future studies are warranted to confirm, reject, or extend them? (See Chapter 3 for more on issues in study design.) Are there any other potential mechanisms or lines of evidence that could provide an alternative explanation of the findings?

- **Conclude the argument,** crystallizing the key information, including pivotal findings, potential limitations, and plausible future research avenues [1 paragraph].

Table 2.10 Example of a tolerability table. Frequencies of treatment-emergent adverse events (TEAEs) in the NO-MO-BURP-PLS! Trial (12-week data)

TEAE[a]	No. (%)		
	Spastex + placebo (n = 846)	TAU[b] + placebo (n = 458)	Total (N = 1,304)[c]
≥1 TEAE	324 (38.3)	166 (36.2)	490 (37.6)
Headache	47 (5.6)	19 (4.1)	66 (5.1)
GERD	44 (5.2)	18 (3.9)	62 (4.8)
Dyspepsia	42 (5.0)	16 (3.5)	58 (4.4)
Nasal congestion	34 (4.0)	14 (3.1)	48 (3.7)
Nasopharyngitis	18 (2.1)	9 (2.0)	27 (2.1)
Influenza	12 (1.4)	6 (1.3)	18 (1.4)
URI	12 (1.4)	6 (1.3)	18 (1.4)
Dizziness	9 (1.1)	0	9 (0.7)
Bronchitis	9 (1.1)	0	9 (0.7)

Note: GERD, gastroesophageal reflux disorder; URI, upper-respiratory-tract infection.

[a] Treatment-emergent adverse events (TEAEs; Medical Dictionary for Regulatory Activities (MedDRA) 14.0 preferred terms), occurring in ≥2% patients in any treatment group (or with higher frequency in the active-treatment group), presented in descending order of frequency, in the safety population.

[b] The treatment-as-usual (TAU) group comprised patients receiving placebo + proton pump inhibitors (PPIs), histamine$_2$ (H$_2$) blockers, and/or over-the-counter antacids for involuntary noisome hiccup syndrome (INHS). Some patients had more than one TEAE.

[c] The total N value is smaller than that for efficacy (Table 2.8) because the safety population comprised all subjects who were randomized and received at least one dose of study treatment (safety population) rather than those randomized to one group or another (intent-to-treat population).

Chapter 3 delves into potential study limitations, error, bias, and confounding factors, and considers ways in which to account, control, or otherwise adjust for them. In a *New England Journal of Medicine* article, Avorn referred to RCTs and observational studies as the "yin and yang of drug research" (Figure 2.2).[6]

Randomized controlled trials are ideal for establishing a medication's efficacy but are typically conducted in a highly "selected" population that chooses and enrolls patients who tolerate and adhere to medication regimens optimally. Investigators painstakingly maximize the quality of individual patient data. Such studies are also typically not powered or of sufficient duration to discern intertreatment disparities in TEAEs and safety signals, particularly infrequent ones. In addition to a perhaps somewhat exaggerated homogeneous population of study participants, treatment is typically inflexible and protocol driven, rather than dynamic, as in most readers' "real-world" practices. Although ideal to demonstrate treatment efficacy, RCTs have limited ecological validity, or generalizability to typical care settings.

In contrast to RCTs, observational studies are conducted in a more familiar and typical (naturalistic) clinical milieu, enabling enrollment of more subjects who can be monitored for longer intervals. However, such studies may be "associational" in nature, unable to conclusively determine causality and also susceptible to biases, confounding factors, and other statistical issues.

Unlike RCTs, retrospective cohort (observational) studies involving administrative (pharmacy) claims databases typically lack high-quality individual patient-level data. Because of their retrospective nature and failure to randomize patients, such studies may also be subject to various forms of bias and confounding on unmeasured variables. Propensity score matching (PSM) is one statistical approach to limit such biases and adjust for potential imbalances resulting from the failure to randomly allocate patients to treatments.

Methodological heterogeneity may occur when pooling data from studies with fundamentally disparate methods and populations. Measured by the I^2 statistic (among other methods), heterogeneity can undermine the strength of conclusions drawn

Strengths
- Highly selected patient populations (high chance of showing p<0.05 effect vs. placebo)
- "Criterion standard" for assessing efficacy
- Can be registered to avoid selective reporting

Limitations
- Generalizability of findings (external/ecological validity)? Certain patients under-represented; protocol dissimilar to clinical practice (placebo/randomization)
- Short duration; limited number of patients (may be difficult to identify AEs in <1/100 to <1/1,000) Surrogate endpoints

(a)

Strengths
- Can involve large numbers of typical patients in routine-care setting (high external/ecological validity/generalizability of findings)
- Can monitor patients over prolonged intervals
- Hence, can identify AEs in <1/100 to <1/1,000
- Can focus on specific vulnerable populations

Limitations
- Susceptible to bias and confounding
  - Underlying differences among patients treated with different drugs
  - Patient selection/differences in adherence
- Lower quality of individual patient data
- Typically cannot determine causality

(b)

Figure 2.2 Randomized controlled trials **(a)** and observational (also known as "real-world evidence [RWE]) studies **(b)** as the "yin and yang of drug research."[6]

by meta-analyses and other pooled-data analyses. Finally, SLRs may be influenced by publication bias, whereby smaller studies need to report greater treatment effect sizes in order to be published; some journals are less likely to publish study reports of negative (null) findings. Publication bias can be assessed using funnel plots, in which the average treatment effect size in each study is plotted on the abscissa (x-axis) and precision (the standard error or number of subjects) on the ordinate (y-axis). Asymmetrical funnel plots suggest publication bias.

Most progress in pharmaceutical research is incremental. Hence, even the advent of a new class of medications or an innovative new agent or technology that promises to be "best in class" should not prompt overly zealous or, worse yet, promotional writing. Hew closely to the most up-to-date product labeling. Most medications are members of families (pharma-cological classes); writing that "derogates" one

member may tarnish the entire family, including the medication being considered in your paper. Discussions that unduly emphasize benefits over risks (e.g., adverse events), are speculative, or bear the merest whiff of promotionality will likely not survive journal peer review.

2.3.1.4.1 Before-after exercises in discussions (and results)

Before (promotional)-after (balanced) exercises follow:

Promotional: The dose of spastex does not need to be reduced in patients aged ≥65 years, whereas other agents in the anticholinergic class must be adjusted in older patients.

Neutral: The dose of spastex does not need to be reduced in patients aged ≥65 years.

Neutral: Agent X has a terminal elimination half-life of 16 hours.

Promotional: Agent X is the only member of its pharmacologic class whose terminal elimination half-life exceeds 10 hours.

Or (worse, speculative and misleading): Agent X may offer longer-term benefits on patient-reported outcomes and be associated with enhanced convenience and higher adherence because of less frequent dosing.

Not necessarily. On a pharmacodynamic basis, Agent X may confer not only more durable benefits on efficacy endpoints but also longer-lived adverse events, potentially *compromising* patient-reported outcomes in some individuals. Regarding the "enhanced convenience" of "less frequent dosing," I am aware of no well-validated instrument that measures patient convenience. The original publication on adherence and dosing frequency, by Cramer and co-workers,[7] found that adherence fell off substantially when dosing frequency increased from three to four times daily.

Avoid "unanchored superlatives." For example:

According to the American Society of Hematology, the International Normalized Ratio is the criterion standard (or reference standard or method of choice) to measure coagulation.

Not:

The International Normalized Ratio is the gold standard to measure coagulation.

In our study, treatment with Agent X was associated with a reduced incidence of outcome D compared to therapy with Agent Y.

Not:

Treatment with Agent X was superior to Agent Y in reducing outcome D.

Be careful about inaccurate "causal implications" of verbs. Observational studies typically cannot prove causation or its direction.

In our observational study, treatment with Agent X was associated with a lower 5-year disease event rate compared to therapy with Agent Y.

Not:

In our observational study, treatment Agent X reduced the 5-year disease event rate compared to therapy with Agent Y.

Biased writing can also result from narrowly discussing the efficacy profile of a medication (e.g., the one manufactured and/or marketed by the study grantor) without considering its potential adverse effects or other costs (humanistic or economic). However, it is reasonable and appropriate to use study findings to help identify certain patient subgroups who might derive special treatment benefits based on disease-centered, PRO, or other key endpoints.

2.3.1.5 CONCLUSIONS

"Clinch" your essay as concisely and precisely as you began it. As a lesson, I refer to the "Lads from Liverpool" for one of the most elegant "clinchers" ever penned, in music or any other creative endeavor:

And in the end; The love you take,
Is equal to the love…You make.

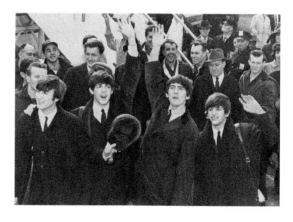

Paul turned what could have been an afterthought or pastiche into an unforgettable axiom. The last recorded Beatles' album (*Abbey Road*) was arguably the most creative and collaborative, with everyone working "frightfully well" together (according to producer George Martin). To "clinch" the work, Paul penned the above (at least nearly) heroic couplet, drawing deeply from the roots of English literature, reaching back as far as Chaucer. The phrasing is almost mathematically elegant. You can almost put a "QED" (*quod erat demonstrandum*) at the end of the verse.

One takeaway from this example, apart from the reminder that "brevity is the soul of wit?" Creative work, including medical writing, is enriched by collaboration. Especially when challenged by a problem in a study or its report, reach out to your colleagues early and often, including, most importantly, the corresponding author (CA). In many instances, only a fresh pair of eyes from a peer is needed. In short, "No man [or woman] is an island!"

Avoid conclusions that exceed the scope and aims of the predefined (*a priori*) protocol, including off-label (or beyond-label) claims, conjecture, and failure to distinguish between surrogate measures and hard outcomes such as morbidity and mortality. Undertake the previously mentioned "reckoning" process. How well do the Results answer the study's questions and meet its prespecified objectives (from the Introduction)? Which findings were expected or unexpected and statistically (and/or clinically) significant? Are there alternative explanations for the findings? What future research could help to further evaluate and challenge or extend the findings?

2.4 HOW TO WRITE A REPORT OF A … ("HOW–TWA–ROA") STUDY

2.4.1 Overview

This section focuses on building high-quality study report manuscripts. Like Chapter 4, which provides quality-control checklists for preparing different manuscripts, the next section summarizes my own guidance to prepare diverse types of study reports, organized below in descending order of evidence quality (Chapter 1 evidence pyramid). Types of papers are summarized below in descending order of evidence quality according to the medical evidence pyramid presented in Chapter 1.

2.4.2 HOW–TWA–ROA … Systematic literature review (SLR) or meta-analysis

See Chapter 4, Tables 4.15 and 4.19.[8–10]

2.4.2.1 CONSIDERATIONS WHEN CONDUCTING A SYSTEMATIC LITERATURE REVIEW OR META-ANALYSIS AND INTERPRETING THE FINDINGS

The chief advantage of conducting an SLR or meta-analysis is that it enables the researcher to pool data from multiple trials in order to increase statistical power and hence more readily test hypotheses. Two potential pitfalls are heterogeneity and publication bias. The former occurs if study designs, populations, and other factors are so disparate across the included studies that they are not necessarily all measuring the same treatment effect or other variable being reported. Heterogeneity can also occur if data from patient subgroups differ meaningfully from findings in the overall (general) population.

To evaluate heterogeneity in meta-analyses, Cochran's Q is calculated by summing the squared deviation of each investigation's estimate within the overall meta-analysis and weighting each trial's contribution in an identical manner to the method in the overall analysis. The Cochran Q statistic is then compared with the χ^2 distribution in k number of studies with $k-1$ degrees of freedom to generate p values.[11]

Of a more recent vintage, and increasingly more frequently employed in meta-analyses to evaluate heterogeneity, is the I^2. One advantage of using this statistic is that it can be directly compared between meta-analyses with distinct types of outcomes and disparate numbers of patients.[11] I^2 ranges from 0 to 1.0 (or 0 to 100%). A score of 0 indicates no observed heterogeneity, whereas higher numbers indicate rising heterogeneity.

In practice, I^2 values exceeding 0.75 (75%) are typically considered to be consistent with an unacceptable degree of heterogeneity. Although I have previously stated that you should avoid such "unanchored" modifiers (e.g., "acceptable, unacceptable"), another similar example is a frequent rule of thumb in the literature on prognostic models: a c-statistic (area under the receiver operating characteristics curve [AUC ROC]) exceeding 0.70 is consistent with acceptable model performance in discriminating one predicted outcome from another.

Publication bias may occur because smaller studies must report a greater effect size (vs. larger studies) to be published by a PRJ. In the absence of such bias, the precision in projecting a treatment effect should increase with rising sample sizes of the contributing studies. In this setting, a plot of precision (e.g., standard error; number of study participants) on the y-axis against effect size on the x-axis should show that the smallest studies (i.e., with the lowest N values) loosely scatter at the bottom, whereas the largest ones cluster narrowly at the top. When a plot has this inverted-funnel shape and is symmetrical, publication bias is unlikely.[12,13] In addition to publication bias, potential contributors to asymmetrical funnel plots include[12]:

- Artifacts related to choice of treatment effect measure
- Citation bias
- Data irregularities, including poor study design, insufficient analyses, and fraud
- Disparate intensities of interventions across trials
- Difference in sample populations' underlying risk
- Location bias
- Multiple-publication bias
- Random probability

When conducting an SLR or a meta-analysis, you may choose to visit the UK National Institute of Health Research's International Prospective Register of Systematic Reviews (PROSPERO) website to register your study or determine if similar ones have been or are being performed (Available at: https://www.crd.york.ac.uk/PROSPERO. Last accessed December 31, 2017). Before conducting your literature search using EMBASE/PubMed/ MEDLINE and other, more specifically subject-related databases, electronically scan the CDSR and other published reviews to confirm that a review like your own has not been conducted. If it has, define your objectives to build on (or further evaluate) the prior findings and conclusions.

Of course, it is a fool's errand for you and your colleagues to consider all papers on a particular disease state or therapy. Published papers need to be reduced, consolidated, organized, and prioritized.

A proven way over potentially immobilizing anxiety about covering all relevant papers is to "divide and conquer." This maxim has a twofold meaning concerning SLRs and meta-analyses,

from broadest to most specific in nature. First, don't go it alone. Find a few committed researchers who are willing to share the load with you. Second, work with your colleagues to focus your research team on a discrete scope for the review. This scope should in turn be translated into a manageable number of SLR objectives. Limits must be imposed, including English-language articles in PRJs from the previous 5 to 10 years that are related to a limited number of key search words or terms and publication types.

An example of a PRISMA (Available at: http:// www.prisma-statement.org. Last accessed December 31, 2017) flow diagram is provided in Figure 2.3. When conducting your literature searches with EndNote or Reference Manager software, use the "tab delimited" function to export the search results into a Microsoft Excel file, then share it with your colleagues to review. It is often wise to include three independent reviewers to determine different articles' relevance and suitability for inclusion in the SLR or meta-analyses, including one to "break ties" (as mentioned above, this can be the CA).

Software from the Cochrane Community (Review Manager [RevMan] 5) is available to generate pivotal data for a meta-analysis (Available at: http://community.cochrane.org/tools/review-production-tools/revman-5/revman-5-download. Last accessed December 31, 2017). As shown in Figure 2.4, data on each study of a meta-analysis on our hypothetical disease INHS can be entered, after which the software generates odds ratios and 95% confidence interval (CI) values, a forest plot, a funnel plot, and I^2 values. The I^2 value in the example (71%) is consistent with substantial heterogeneity in effects of spastex (vs. treatment as usual) on patients with (vs. without) congenital disease. The funnel plot is somewhat asymmetrical, suggesting publication bias.

2.4.3 HOW–TWA–ROA … Randomized controlled trial (RCT)

See Chapter 4, Tables 4.21–4.25.[14–16]

2.4.3.1 INTRODUCTION

Download recent online content from the target PRJ so that you understand its readers and their likely educational needs and become acquainted with the current issues and approaches to them (Table 2.6). These activities are supported by

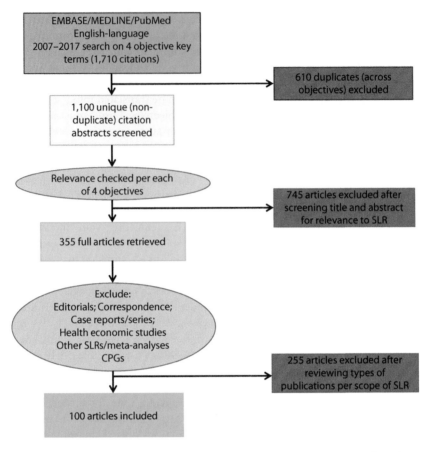

Figure 2.3 PRISMA flow diagram for a systematic literature review. PRISMA, Preferred Reporting Items for Systematic Reviews and Meta-Analyses.
Source: Available at: http://www.prisma-statement.org. Last accessed December 31, 2017.

reviewing the published literature and presented data, and discussing these with the CA.

Typically (for a clinical study), your aim in the Introduction is to (very concisely) summarize a disease and its contemporary management, identify gaps and other limitations in such management, and hence "motivate" the need for (and aims of) the current research and its report. ("This…but that…therefore this study….") Build to a clinical problem and/or deficiency in knowledge and how your study and report are unique or of incremental value in addressing them.

Most PRJs allot approximately 100 to 500 words for the Introduction, especially in the setting of a maximum 2,000-word manuscript. Citing a Cochrane review or other recent SLR or meta-analysis can help to set the stage for your report by providing an overview of previously published data, with an emphasis on the highest-quality studies.

If consensus CPGs are available and applicable—particularly if issued by the professional society that also sponsors the targeted PRJ or authored by members of the research/publication teams—try to cite them in an incisive, clinically consequential way.

Even if your introduction focuses on clinical development of a particular medication, including phase 1 to 3 study data related to the grantor LSC's investigational product, strive to render the introduction otherwise "individual-treatment–agnostic." For instance, CPGs often feature stepped-care treatment algorithms comprising classes of medications without emphasizing individual agents. Citing a landmark study that compares multiple therapies for a condition may offer a widely applicable frame of reference for the broadest swath of readers and practitioners. In the field of schizophrenia, for example, the Clinical Antipsychotic Trials of Intervention Effectiveness (CATIE) study—which compared

Ferrous 2015

Methods	Observational study (electronic medical records [EMR] review)
Participants	1,188
Interventions	Spastex versus TAU
Outcomes	Hiccup frequency (%)
Notes	

Plumbous 2009

Methods	Patient registry
Participants	4,444
Interventions	Spastex versus TAU
Outcomes	Hiccup frequency (%)
Notes	

Stannous 2013

Methods	Open-label extension study
Participants	88
Interventions	Spastex versus TAU
Outcomes	Hiccup frequency (%)
Notes	

(a)

	Spastex			TAU	
Study or subgroup	Mean [percent]	SD [percent]	Total	Mean [percent]	SD [percent]
Ferrous 2015	22.2	10.1	0	72.2	36.1
Plumbous 2009	14.1	4.2	0	71.3	8.1
Cupric 2016	17.3	14	0	65.7	60.1
Chromic 2017	28.8	30	0	78.4	54.8
Stannous 2013	19.4	22.4	0	62.3	68.7

(b)

Characteristics of studies

Characteristics of included studies

Chromic 2017

Methods	Randomized controlled trial
Participants	150
Interventions	Spastex versus TAU
Outcomes	Hiccup frequency (%)
Notes	

Cupric 2016

Methods	Observational study (administrative claims database analysis)
Participants	425
Interventions	Spastex versus TAU
Outcomes	Hiccup frequency (%)
Notes	

(c)

Figure 2.4 Data inputs and outputs for a meta-analysis using RevMan 5 software. **(a–c)** Study inputs. *Source:* Images of figures from Cochrane Review Manager 5 (RevMan) [Computer program]. Reprinted with permission from The Cochrane Collaboration (www.cochrane.org).

(Continued)

clinical outcomes using a range of first- and second-generation oral antipsychotics in patients with chronic schizophrenia—has been cited more than 5,000 times since its publication in 2005.[17]

You may be provided with a clinical study report (CSR) by the trial grantor, typically an LSC. Although typically useful in outlining the subject matter addressed by the study, the Introduction from a CSR represents the LSC's point of view. To appropriately orient the Introduction and align it with the viewpoint of the PRJ, review recent online content of the PRJ and, if possible (beginning before, during, or soon after the KOMT), discuss the study with the CA and/or other key researchers. Review the Statistical Methods of the CSR, study protocol, or data/statistical analysis plan (DAP/SAP) to understand why certain statistical approaches and tests were chosen. At the KOMT, you may be able

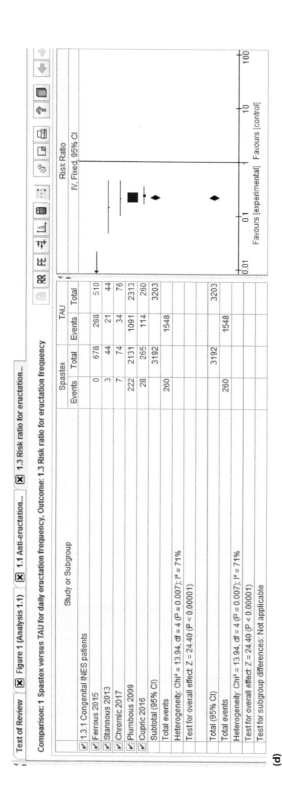

(d)

Figure 2.4 (Continued) Data inputs and outputs for a meta-analysis using RevMan 5 software. **(d)** Event frequencies in patients with congenital INHS, including forest plot. The statistically significant I^2 value of 0.71 (I^2 ranges from 0 to 1.0 or 0 to 100%) indicates substantial heterogeneity between patients with acquired versus congenital INHS.

Source: Images of figures from Cochrane Review Manager 5 (RevMan) [Computer program]. Reprinted with permission from The Cochrane Collaboration (www.cochrane.org).

(Continued)

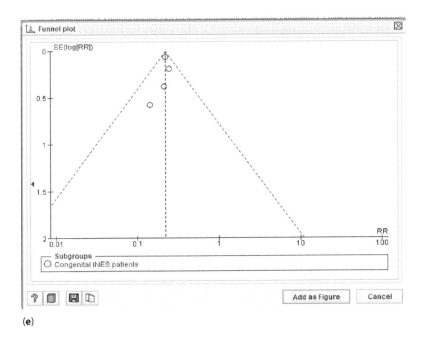

(e)

Figure 2.4 (Continued) Data inputs and outputs for a meta-analysis using RevMan 5 software. **(e)** The funnel plot is asymmetrical, suggesting publication bias.
Source: Images of figures from Cochrane Review Manager 5 (RevMan) [Computer program]. Reprinted with permission from The Cochrane Collaboration (www.cochrane.org). RevMan 5 software is available at: http://www.community.cochrane.org/tools/review-productiontools/revman-5. Last accessed December 31, 2017.

to ask the biostatistician about such issues. Perhaps the most important objective of the KOMT is to target a PRJ to publish the findings, because this decision informs manuscript development, formatting. and other key editorial activities.

2.4.3.2 METHODS

If study objectives could not be specified in the Introduction, delineate them at the outset of the Methods section.

Briefly characterize the study setting, including numbers and locations of study sites and study dates, such as dates of first subject enrolled or randomized and last subject followed up. If data on numbers of subjects at each site are available, include them in the Results, not the Methods. Detailing the study setting is especially important for international trials because responses to assessments may vary by culture and certain demographic traits. Detail patient eligibility criteria and ensure that these are consistent with any product labeling in the countries where study sites are located. Graphing a "schema" and timeline may help to summarize study design, especially if it is complex and not the

typical parallel-group, randomized, double-blind, placebo-controlled trial (Figure 2.5).

The Study Setting section may include statements about ethics and protection of patient rights and safety. Review the CSR or protocol to identify these. Increasingly, PRJs are requesting that the actual informed-consent document (ICD) be included along with the submitted manuscript. A typical ethics statement runs along the following lines:

The study was conducted in a manner consistent with ethical tenets originating in the Declaration of Helsinki (DOH; seventh revision, 2013). Each potential subject provided written informed consent after receiving an explanation of the potential risks and benefits of participating in the study but before undergoing any study procedure (assessment or intervention). The informed-consent document (ICD) and study protocol were reviewed and approved by local institutional review boards (IRBs) before study onset.

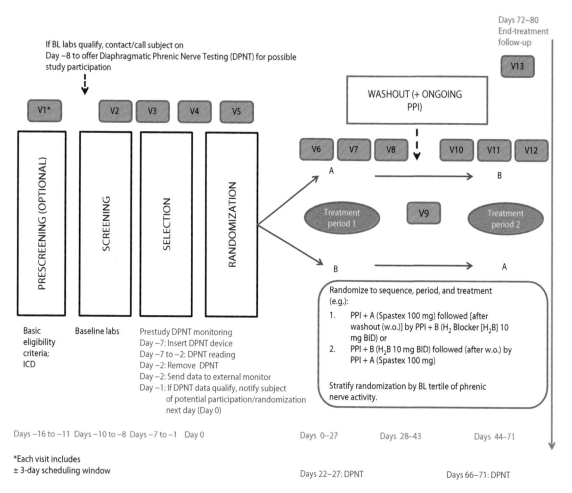

Figure 2.5 Example study schema and timeline for an actively controlled crossover clinical trial involving assessments of diaphragmatic phrenic nerve activity in patients with involuntary noisome hiccup syndrome (INHS). In general, crossover trial designs have greater statistical power (i.e., smaller needed sample sizes) compared to parallel-group studies because each subject serves as his or her own control. Paired statistical tests are warranted because each observation in the same subject receiving two different treatments (e.g., active treatment vs. placebo or usual-care) is not independent of others in the same individual.

Abbreviations: BL, baseline; H_2, histamine type 2; H_2B, histamine type 2 blocker; ICD, informed-consent document; PPI, proton pump inhibitor; V, visit.

The DOH transcends local and national law, falling within the domain of the World Medical Association.

Devote most of the Methods section to assessment measures, including their schedule and attributes. Begin by defining the intent-to-treat (ITT), per-protocol (PP), and safety populations. The ITT population includes all patients who are randomly allocated to one study treatment or another, irrespective of whether treatment is received. Using this population may help to avoid artifacts associated with crossover and attrition due to non-missing-at-random (non–MAR) dropouts. The PP population encompasses individuals who completed the study according to protocol, typically with perfect adherence, and is often used to assess efficacy. The safety population encompasses all subjects who were randomized and received one dose or more of study treatment.

Organize outcome measures by efficacy (primary, followed by secondary, tertiary, and exploratory) and then safety/tolerability. If you are reporting subgroup analyses, disclose if these were prespecified in the study protocol and/or included statistical adjustment for multiple comparisons (e.g., Bonferroni correction) or were *post hoc*; subgroup analyses are intrinsically hypothesis generating. If pressed for words, include a table detailing the efficacy/safety/tolerability assessment schedule in a supplementary online appendix.

Safety assessments are typically conducted at baseline (e.g., prescreening, screening) and end of treatment or soon afterward. They include a medical history (with concurrent conditions and medications), physical examination, vital signs, laboratory panels (serum chemistries, hematology, urinalysis), and 12-lead ECG. Blood pressure and pulse rate are typically measured at each study visit. Any adverse events (AEs) can be elicited by open-ended questioning, at each visit after randomization.

Are efficacy outcome measures hard clinical endpoints (e.g., all-cause and disease-specific mortality), or surrogate variables? If the former, Kaplan–Meier survival or other (e.g., Cox) analyses may be warranted. For certain PROs and other, more subjective endpoints provide a verbal "legend" or "road map": does an increase or decrease in scores on an instrument indicate improvement, or worsening? Are any changes associated with normal—or otherwise reliably improved—functional status or health-related quality of life (HRQOL) on PROs? These include thresholds for MCIDs.

For an RCT, it is often appropriate to include one or more null hypothesis (NH; often expressed as H_0) as well as an alternative hypothesis [AH; often expressed as H_1 (H_N)] for each. Be careful about using categorical, "responder [or target achievement] analyses" as the major NH. Unless the target or responder criterion is widely recognized as biologically relevant, defining the endpoint as a "percentage of patients with [*choose measure*] greater [or less] than [*choose threshold*]" is not necessarily statistically valid because it categorizes an intrinsically continuous variable. If this sort of analysis is formulated, include (and report) precision limits (e.g., 95% CI) around the threshold for response in the report.

Graphing data and asking a few basic questions may help to inform your discussions with biostatisticians and other scientists at the KOMT and afterward:

- How was sample size calculated? The main data needed (typically derived from similar previous trials) are treatment effect size, variance, α level, power $(1 - \beta)$, and nature of data (paired or independent). See Chapter 3 to learn about using P/S software to determine sample sizes.

- How were statistical methods selected? Typically, Fisher's exact test is used for baseline categorical characteristics (descriptive analyses in relatively small numbers of subjects), Student's (Gosset's) *t*-test for continuous variables, and χ^2 for categorical variables. These tests and analysis of variance (ANOVA) can be run using Microsoft Excel, as shown in Chapter 3. However, choice of tests (especially parametric vs. nonparametric) is also dependent on the relative normality or skew of the data, which can be assessed by plotting the data, using Microsoft Excel, or conducting the Shapiro–Wilk test.

- Which methods were used to impute missing data? In the past, the last observation carried forward (LOCF) convention was relied on, but, increasingly, multiple imputation and other approaches are advocated. (See Chapter 3.)

- What methods were used to control for potential covariates? Typically, an ANCOVA with treatment and study site as potential covariates is conducted; however, ANCOVAs often do not include other, potentially influential baseline variables, such as baseline patient age, number of comorbidities, and duration or severity of disease.

2.4.3.3 RESULTS

To ensure "external fidelity (consistency/accuracy)," request original data tables (in Word- or other software-compatible format) from the statistician. Avoid rekeystroking data, which can introduce errors. After "setting" your tables, review with an editor and be alert to any duplication of rows or columns of data, which often indicate human transcription errors.

Include a Consolidated Standards of Reporting Trials (CONSORT) patient flow diagram (Available at: http://www.consort-statement.org. Last accessed December 31, 2017; Figure 2.6); a baseline characteristics table (Table 2.8); efficacy tables or figures that address every endpoint "motivated" in the Methods (and in the same sequence), including numerical data in text for figures that do not include numbers; and a tolerability (AE frequency) table (Table 2.10).

Safety can be covered either in shift tables showing changes in mean values for study populations

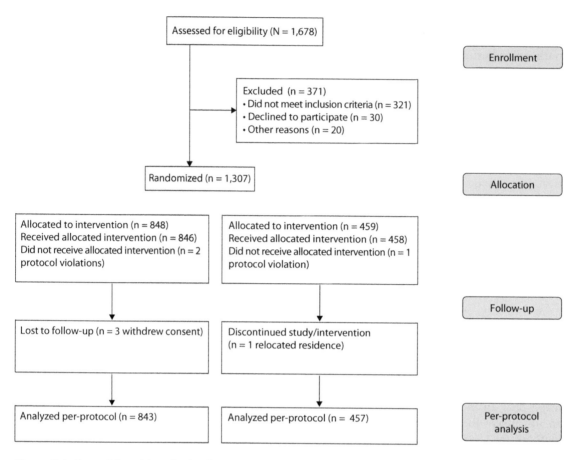

Figure 2.6 Consolidated Standards of Reporting [Clinical] Trials (CONSORT) patient disposition flow diagram for a randomized controlled trial involving spastex for involuntary noisome hiccup syndrome (INHS).

by treatment group and/or in narrative text. Safety parameters include vital signs, 12-lead ECGs, laboratory panels, as well as serious adverse events (SAEs) and how they resolved? Investigators typically decide if SAEs were related to treatment according to their temporal pattern regarding drug administration, dosing, and/or discontinuation.

As appropriate for normally distributed data, report the mean, standard deviation (SD), 95% confidence interval (CI), p value, and the statistical test used to generate it. For non-normal (skewed) distributions, report the median and interquartile range (IQR), or other measure of variability. Physicians may be particularly interested in SD or IQR as indices of treatment variability across different patient subgroups or even within individual patients over time. Make sure that the comparison giving rise to a p value is clear. In many cases you will have pairwise Student t-tests between two treatment groups for

continuous data and χ^2 for categorical data. In other instances, you are testing effects of a treatment across three or more groups such as different-dose recipients, in which case an ANOVA is typically more appropriate. When effects of treatment are compared in an ANCOVA that controls for baseline covariates, we typically compare least-square means of changes from baseline to visit or study termination.

2.4.3.4 DISCUSSION

Ask yourself the following pivotal questions.

- How well balanced were the groups at baseline? How effective was randomization?
- How representative of, and consistent with, readers' practices (and other larger populations) was the population? Compare baseline characteristics to epidemiologic statistics and/or baseline characteristics of other related studies.

- Which NHs were rejected, which AHs accepted, and which subgroup analyses generated new hypotheses?
- Which study objectives were (or were not) met? If not, why not?
- Were the findings expected, or unexpected? Why?
- What future studies are warranted to evaluate, corroborate, and/or extend (or refute) the findings?
- Are there alternative explanations for the findings?

2.4.4 HOW–TWA–ROA … Observational study

See Chapter 4, Table 4.26.[18]

2.4.4.1 OVERVIEW

Table 2.11 summarizes key considerations when drafting an observational study report.

The main guideline for preparing observational study reports, including retrospective cohort analyses of administrative claims and electronic medical records (EMR), case series, and patient registries, is Strengthening the Reporting of Observational Studies in Epidemiology (STROBE).[18] These have been specifically adapted to certain types of studies, including genetic association investigations (STROBE–STREGA).

As mentioned earlier in this chapter, Avorn referred to observational studies and RCTs, as "the yin and yang of drug research."[6] Figure 2.2 illustrates the complementarity of these forms of research. Randomized controlled trials optimize the quality of individual-patient data, often to maximize efficacy in registration trials; however, the findings may not be generalizable to naturalistic treatment settings, including more heterogeneous patient populations treated with dynamic (vs. protocol-based, fixed) regimens. Conversely, observational studies may have lower patient-level data quality but view the patient "in situ," optimizing ecological validity: generalizability to naturalistic care settings of PRJ readers.

By the same token, observational studies may also be subject to certain forms of bias or confounding or residual confounding on unmeasured variables, which the RCT design typically excludes. One frequent finding is confounding by severity, which may result because treatment allocation is not randomized and patient groups differ in systematic,

but not necessarily immediately evident, ways. An example might be an observational study's finding that patients with more severe, and/or recurrent, coronary heart disease (CHD) have superior clinical outcomes compared to those with less severe disease who have yet to experience a clinical event (i.e., secondary vs. primary prevention). Patients with more severe CHD may be more likely to receive specialty or other more advanced forms of care that optimize outcomes compared to their less ill counterparts.

With the passage of the 21st Century Cures Act (US HR 34; especially §3022), real-world evidence (RWE) is likely to occupy a more central role in future US biomedical research and even regulatory approval.[19,20] RWE includes retrospective cohort studies such as administrative claims database and EMR database analyses, case series, and patient registries. Like other observational studies, patient registries enable larger numbers of patients to be followed over longer periods of time (vs. RCTs) and hence may be well suited to evaluate infrequent safety signals in pharmacovigilance audits or other studies.

2.4.4.2 INTRODUCTION

As with other Introductions, build to a problem, issue, or gap that your study addresses and follow with the study's (and report's) aims. Whether to draft a longer (clinically comprehensive), or shorter (problem-focused) Introduction depends largely on the subject matter and journal AGs (and online PRJ content). Frequently a published observational study has identifiable objections that a novel study design can overcome.

For instance, I was involved in research comparing two intravenous antibiotics for community-acquired pneumonia. By conducting a de novo PSM procedure, we found that formerly reported differences between antibiotics in terms of health resource utilization (HRU) were biased away from the null by methodological issues in the previous study.[21] I have also contributed to research on rheumatoid arthritis (RA) in a "real-world" cohort (patient registry study) that included many individuals with long durations of illness and otherwise greater heterogeneity of demographic and clinical characteristics compared to recent-onset RA populations in most other clinical trials; many study subjects with recent-onset RA were followed for shorter intervals in RCTs compared to our observational (registry) study.[22]

Table 2.11 Considerations when drafting an observational study report

Disclosures	Introduction	Methods	Statistical issues and methods	Results	Strengths	Limitations
	• What is known? • What is the issue/problem/gap? • How does this study/report address the issue/fill gap? • "Situation on the ground": local epidemiologic, clinical, and other data and guidelines.	Devote most of the Methods to describe the setting (e.g., which health plan/electronic health claims database/EMR setting/registry) patient profiles (eligibility criteria).	Biases are possible given lack of randomization/control/blinding. Propensity score matching (PSM) is one statistical approach to adjust/control. Disclose methods of PSM (e.g., greedy match).	Adherence (e.g., MPR, PDC and % with MPR/PDC > 0.80/80%).	"Real-world evidence": high ecological validity and generalizability of findings to actual clinical practice: Less "selected" patient populations. Dynamic treatment (vs. rigid, protocol-based in RCTs).	Associational data: cannot necessarily infer causality or its direction.
Registration. WHO Registry Network (Available at: http://www.who.int/ictrp/network/en. Last accessed December 31, 2017). US AHRQ Registry of Registries (Available at: https://patientregistry.ahrq.gov. Last accessed December 31, 2017). Previous presentation (all manuscripts).		Explicitly and clearly identify: 1. the cohort(s) and/or subcohort(s) 2. the baseline or "look-back" period 3. the all-important index date (see Figure 2.7) 4. the follow-up observational period	Attrition Use of mixed models may conserve patient data (do not lose a patient from analysis if missing a single datum or small number of observations.	Health-care utilization • Hospitalization/LOS • Relapse • DME use • Office visits • Medications prescribed	Potential statistical power: can observe many patients "in situ." Because there is no study blind, patients can also be surveyed concerning e.g., treatment preferences.	Potential biases (see Chapter 3 of this manual): • Channeling • Treatment by indication • Selection • Immortal time Possible confounding on unmeasured variables
Conflicts of interests (all manuscripts).			Intracorrelated longitudinal data in registries require special statistical models (e.g., GEE). Disclose the correlational matrix structure.	Other clinical and subjective outcome measures (importance of MCIDs for PROs; see Appendix 1 of this textbook).	Potential value in pharmacovigilance: can not only observe more patients (vs. typical RCT) but monitor them for longer intervals.	• Lower quality (or limited) patient-level data (e.g., in claims analyses) • Prescription claims ≠ medications taken • ICD-9-CM, ICD-10, and Read (UK) codes are intended for reimbursement, not case ascertainment, purposes (coding errors are possible).
Author contributions (ICMJE; all manuscripts).					Registries particularly useful to study <1/100 to <1/1,000 disease events or safety signals.	Cross-sectional studies: may not be suited to assess frequently waxing and waning disorders.

Abbreviations: AHRQ, Agency for Healthcare Research and Quality; DME, durable medical equipment; EMR, electronic medical records; GEE, generalized estimating equation; ICD, International Classification of Diseases; ICMJE, International Committee of Medical Journal Editors; LOS, length of stay; MCID, minimum clinically important difference; MPR, medication possession ratio; PDC, proportion of days covered; PRO, patient reported outcome; WHO, World Health Organization.

One caveat to practitioners: unlike RCTs, RWE studies often do not have neat and tidy CSRs to summarize methods and results. As early as possible, by the KOMT or shortly thereafter, request a protocol, DAP/SAP, and/or "table shells" from the researchers, including the biostatistician.

2.4.4.3 METHODS

The null and alternative hypotheses of RCTs typically give way to assumptions and other premises in observational, and especially health economic (HE), trials. In retrospective cohort studies, it is most important to clearly define the cohorts (and/or subcohorts) being compared as well as the baseline, index, and follow-up periods. Figure 2.7 is an example of a schema and timeline for a hypothetical observational study on INHS. In this example, the index date is the first day on which an electronically linked health claim for INHS—a prescription for spastex—was recorded.

In parallel to the CONSORT patient flow diagram in an RCT (Figure 2.6), observational study reports may include a flow diagram that is based largely on eligibility criteria informed by reimbursement codes (e.g., *International Classification of Diseases, 10th ed* [ICD-10] in the United States and Read codes in the United Kingdom; Figure 2.8). However, eligibility criteria tend to be much less stringent in observational studies, enabling investigations of more heterogeneous, real-world sample populations.

Unlike RCTs, which typically determine medication efficacy, observational studies can provide data on effectiveness in a typical clinical setting.

Other measures relate to HRU, including medication adherence. Adherence is typically assessed via the medication possession ratio (MPR) and the proportion of days covered (PDC), which range from 0 to 100%. Acceptable adherence is often defined as an MPR > 0.80 or a PDC > 80%. The PDC may be less susceptible to overestimation of adherence and may be overall more reliable than MPR because the numerator of the PDC is the number of days covered in a given interval, whereas the numerator of the MPR is the sum of days supply for all fills in a given interval. However, prescriptions filled cannot necessarily be equated to medications taken as prescribed. Other HRU data may include hospitalization, length of stay (LOS), relapse/rehospitalization, and durable medical equipment (DME) use. Although some of these data may inform HE and outcomes research (HEOR), indirect health-care cost data are not typically available and/or included.

Observational studies typically are better suited than RCTs to assess PROs. Allowing randomized patients to express treatment preferences might require crossover studies and compromise the RCT study blind. Strive to fully characterize any patient survey instruments, scales, or subscales, including whether an increase or decrease signifies an improvement or worsening; any psychometric data; validation (including any back-translated survey instruments in international studies); normative values; sensitivity, specificity, *c*-statistic, negative predictive value, and positive predictive value; and MCIDs. These data can be omitted if the study report is destined for a journal read by specialists well acquainted with such information.

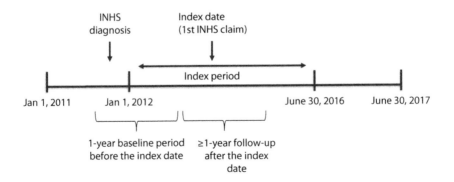

Figure 2.7 Example study schema and timeline for a retrospective cohort study on spastex for involuntary noisome hiccup syndrome (INHS). Ensure that the Methods text defines (1) the study cohorts (and/or any subcohorts), (2) the baseline ("look-back") period, and (3) perhaps most importantly, the index date/period.

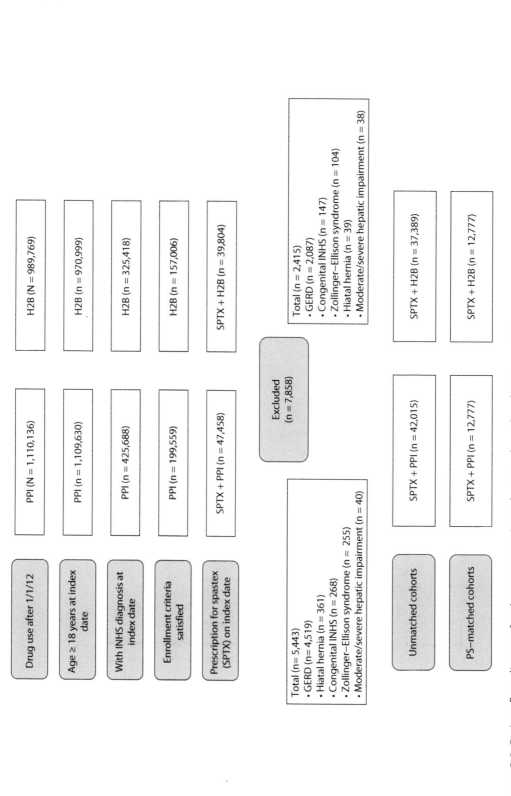

Figure 2.8 Patient flow diagram for the retrospective cohort study outlined in Figure 2.7.
Abbreviations: GERD, gastroesophageal reflux disease; H2B, histamine type 2 blocker; INHS, involuntary noisome hiccup syndrome; PPI, proton pump inhibitor; PS, propensity-score; SPTX, spastex.

To determine this, download recent online content from the targeted PRJ and discuss the matter at the KOMT.

According to the FDA Modernization Act (FDAMA), observational or RWE studies involving marketed products should not violate product labeling, in letter or spirit. For instance, eligibility criteria for patients studied in a claims database analysis should not include individuals for whom medications are contraindicated or in populations in whom the therapy has not been adequately studied; or off-label indications, dosages, or administration routes.

2.4.4.4 RESULTS

Regression analyses are frequently conducted when analyzing observational data. However, correlations between independent and dependent variables (IVs/DVs) do not necessarily imply causation and are most conservatively reported as "associations between," rather than "effects of," IVs on DVs.

2.4.4.5 DISCUSSION

One potential limitation of observational studies can be identified from their study design, schema, or timeline (Figure 2.7). In many cases, the baseline period is relatively short: on the order of 1 to 2 years. Such a relatively brief "look-back" interval may not capture data from patients treated many years before the index date. In our example, patients included during the short baseline period who received spastex on the index date may have overall more severe disease than those whose disease was effectively managed (or even cured) earlier, by older medications such as proton pump inhibitors and H_2-blockers. Channeling (allocation) bias may result when patients with more advanced disease are more likely to receive a new medication (in our case, spastex), hence spuriously associating its use with a previously unknown comorbidity.[23]

Another, perhaps more subtle, and less frequently cited, limitation of certain observational studies relates to adherence. Most health claims database analyses require that a patient be enrolled for at least 1 year before and after the index date. Because continuity of care may be associated with higher adherence, MPR and PDC values may be inflated in some such database analyses.[24–26]

2.4.5 HOW–TWA–ROA … Health economic and outcomes research (HEOR) study

See Chapter 4, Table 4.34.[27,28]

2.4.5.1 INTRODUCTION

The economic value of a health intervention—which is generally understood as a health outcome achieved per unit of currency allocated—may inform decisions at the individual patient, prescriber, health plan, policymaking, or even societal perspective.

Findings from HEOR analyses involving economic modelling often relate to discrete transition states and transition probabilities (TPs), which are in turn informed by published clinical trials—particularly findings from Kaplan–Meier survival analyses. Different forms of modelling may also use stochastic mathematics and other approaches to deal with random probability and project future health outcomes according to different treatment alternatives.

Apart from the model structure (e.g., discrete-time or continuous-time Markov chain [DTMC, CTMC]), model inputs, and model outputs, arguably the most important facet of an HEOR study and its report is the perspective taken. If the analysis is conducted from the societal perspective, both direct and indirect costs are important. Indirect costs include productivity losses due to disability and/or premature mortality. Direct health-care costs include HRU (hospitalization, LOS), prescriptions, DME use, and outpatient care.

Certain prescribers, payers, and policymakers are more interested in direct health-care costs, including incremental cost-effectiveness and cost-utility ratios (ICERs, ICURs) for one treatment compared to another. Health plan administrators are often concerned about the budget impact of introducing a new health technology in the future compared to the current situation in which the new technology has not been introduced. Many of these outcomes fall within the domains of cost-effectiveness analysis (CEA), cost-utility analysis (CUA), and budget impact analysis or model (BIA/BIM).

Transitions between different health states are informed by TPs, which in turn derive from clinical-trial data, including numbers of subjects available: alive and not censored at several time points within a Kaplan–Meier plot. TPs are described by a transition matrix.

Health economic models typically include a base-case scenario and a sensitivity analysis (SA) in which assumptions are systematically varied and effects on projected outcomes evaluated. One example is the discount rate. Because health benefits of certain therapies may not be realized for several years in the future, costs of these interventions are typically discounted (often at 3%). An SA might vary the discount rate to 1% or 5% and reassess HE outcomes.

2.4.5.2 METHODS

Methods should detail the

- Model structure, perspective, and time horizon;
- Model ratification and/or validation by payers or policymakers;
- Model inputs;
- Model outputs;
- Effects of varying key assumptions (e.g. discount rate) in an SA, including the discount rate;
- Type of SA (e.g., deterministic, probabilistic).

Cost-effectiveness analyses typically compare the incremental ratios of the costs of a clinical benefit divided by the benefit itself, for two or more interventions. When expressing CEA data as ICERs, the numerator is the computed allocation (in US dollars or other currencies) to achieve a clinical benefit, and the denominator is that benefit, including years of life saved (YOLS).

Health is a function of both the quality and quantity of life. If patients rate their HRQOL as better when receiving one health intervention compared to another, we may have the basis for a CEA. The numerator is again the calculated allocation to achieve an HRQOL or other benefit, and the denominator is the number of quality-adjusted life years (QALYs). QALYs are expressed on a scale from 0 (death) or even negative numbers ("worse than dead") to 1.0 (perfect health) and are weighted by time trade-offs. If a patient would prefer to live 5 years while receiving a new medication associated with a health

utility value of 0.8 (4.0 QALYs) at an annual cost of $10,000, compared to 6 years on a previous therapy with a utility value of 0.6 (3.6 QALYs) at an annual cost of $800, the ICUR value would be:

$$\text{Incremental cost-utility ratio} = $$
$$\frac{\$10,000 - \$800}{4.0 - 3.6\,\text{QALY}} = \$23,000/\text{QALY}$$

Different societies around the world hold different perspectives on the cost-effectiveness or cost-utility of one intervention compared to another. Willingness-to-pay (WTP) thresholds are operative when there is a discrete, positive ICER or ICUR value for the comparison between two treatments. For the example above, the ICER value of $23,000/QALY might not exceed most countries' WTP thresholds. If, on the other hand, one therapy is less expensive than the other *and* is associated with greater clinical benefits in terms of either YOLS or QALYs, that therapy is said to "dominate" the other, and WTP cut points do not come into play. In the "Cavalier argot" of US NBA star LeBron James, we have the proverbial "slam dunk."

A BIM assesses the impact of introducing a new health intervention on the (frequently 5-year) budget of a health plan or other well-defined population, compared to a referent scenario in which the technology is not introduced (Figure 2.9).[28]

One variable that may arise in BIMs that is not typically encountered in a CEA or CUA is that the epidemiologic profile of the disorder in the population can change because of the new technology being introduced to a large number of health plan members. Such a shift may include a reduced incidence of an infectious or other disease after introducing a vaccine, or a decreased prevalence of a chronic disease after introducing a more effective medication. A cohort- or patient-level, condition-specific model can account for patients entering and leaving the eligible population (i.e., changing size of population), as well as changes in case mixes, disease severity, and resultant costs of managing a disorder.

Key elements of a BIM include[28]

- Any restricted access to therapies
- Costs of all therapies and any projected changes
- Time horizon

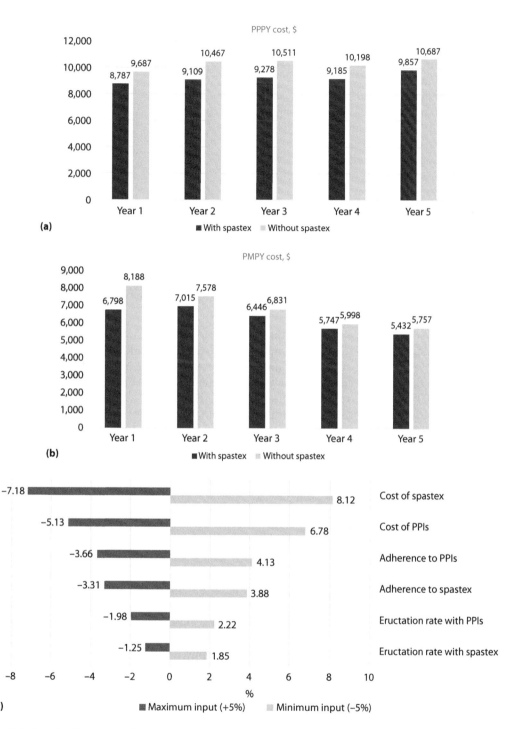

Figure 2.9 Results from hypothetical budget impact model: effects on prices to a health plan of introducing a new treatment (spastex) compared to the situation before or without doing so (referent or treatment as usual, including proton pump inhibitors and H₂ blockers). **(a)**: Price per patient (with involuntary noisome hiccup syndrome [INHS]) per year (PPPY) after versus before introducing spastex. **(b)**: Price per member (with or without INHS) per year (PMPY) after versus before introducing spastex. **(c)**: Tornado plot showing the effects, on budget impact, of varying key assumptions by 5% in sensitivity analyses.

- Health plan features, including the size of the eligible population and the current and projected case mix after introducing the new intervention:
  - Model inputs;
  - Model outputs;
  - Model ratification/validation, including face validity with decision makers and verification of all calculations;
  - Projected uptake/penetration of the new intervention and any changes in use of already available therapies;
  - Sensitivity analysis (SA): effects of varying key assumptions such as discount rate in an overall analysis that projects alternative scenarios selected using the budget holder's perspective;
  - Type of SA, including deterministic versus probabilistic.

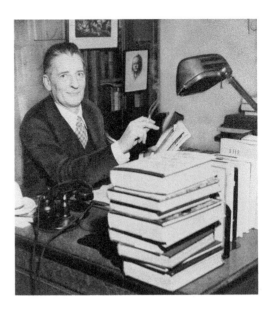

Figure 2.9c shows a "tornado plot" of hypothetical SA data in a BIM. BIMs need to be user friendly. Not only should they present outcomes in familiar ways that are relevant to budget holders and other decision makers, but certain assumptions should be subject to changes by the user; typically, the flexibility is indicated by "drop-down" menu options in a Microsoft Excel spreadsheet. The user can hence examine the effects of changing different combinations of assumptions on model outputs. After constructing a BIM, quality-test it using alternative software platforms or iterations rather than only the one used to develop the model. Users can and will use numerous software applications.

2.5 RHETORICAL EXERCISES AND "BEFORE-AFTER" EXAMPLES TO ENHANCE PROSE STYLE

2.5.1 Motivation

[Anyone] who wishes to become a good writer should endeavour, before he allows himself to be tempted by the more showy qualities, to be direct, simple, brief, vigorous, and lucid.

Henry Watson Fowler

After surveying work by bloggers, I was dismayed to "learn" that there is "grammar you don't have to pay attention to" or "phony grammar." As a dyed-in-the-Harris-tweed (and nearly lifelong) grammarian, I had to take an antiemetic and lie down.

I awoke refreshed to the singularly symmetrical beauty of medical writing: the rigor and conventions of both the "medical," including empiricism and sound scientific logic; and the "writing," including cogent organization and rhetorical elegance.

Both aspects—the medical and the writing—attracted me to the profession before it really was one. I have read and absorbed messages from manuals by not only the American Medical Association and Council for Biology Editors (edited by Edward Huth) but also by great English prose stylists who were not scientists: William Strunk and E.B. White in *Elements of Style*; H.W. Fowler in *Modern English Usage*; and Wilson Follett in *Modern American Usage*, which was completed posthumously by his colleagues (writers, editors, and prose stylists) Jacques Barzun, Carlos Baker, Frederick W. Dupee, Dudley Fitts, James D. Hart, Phyllis McGinley, and Lionel Trilling.

Do the lessons of these great books go to the graves with their authors? Perhaps. There are many niceties on which Follett insisted that are now all but obsolete. I freely concede that medical writing is typically tempered and straightforward. Shorter is usually sweeter. As a co-worker once said to me, "C'mon, Gutkin, this isn't Proust." Point taken. However, MWs benefit from connecting to the larger tradition of their rhetorical forebears and striving for noble ideals in prose.

Given the advent of newfangled communications, including tweets and texts, some might assert that we are masters of the English language. Perhaps when communicating via PDAs. Medical journals, however, are governed by what is termed "standard written English." In this context, MWs are stewards—not masters—of the language. As with most other distinctions, it is a matter of context. Writing for peer-reviewed journals is compatible with a learned, if not always formal, tenor. The day you find "LOL" or "IMHO" in *The Lancet*, we can talk about "phony grammar."

To optimize your written work, seek an editor who shares your passion for not only accurate and precise, but also elegant and memorable, expression. Consider contacting the Editorial Freelancers Association (Available at: http://www.the-efa.org/. Last accessed December 31, 2017.), American Medical Writers Association (http://www.amwa.org. Last accessed December 31, 2017), and International Society for Medical Publication Professionals (Available at: http://www.ismpp.org. Last accessed December 31, 2017.). Carefully review the editor's comments for any patterns of errors in your work, including verbosity, "crutch" phrases, lapses into jargon, and other infelicities.

2.5.1.1 OVERVIEW

The next section will reinforce principles of quality discussed in Chapter 1 by presenting before-after examples and exercises "ripped" from my own practice of nearly 30 years.

2.5.2 Brevity

Our first rhetorical example includes drafts of President Abraham Lincoln's Inaugural Address. Secretary of State William Seward (of "Seward's Folly" fame) seems to have had some difficulty "coming to the point" in his first draft! As usual, Honest Abe both pared down verbiage while elevating the emotional appeal of the rhetoric[29]:

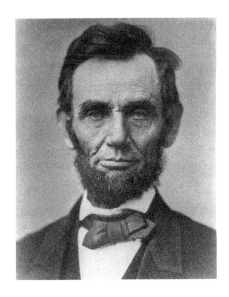

- Draft of Lincoln's Inaugural Address by Secretary of State William Seward: "We are not, <u>we must not be</u>, aliens or enemies, but fellow-countrymen and brethren. Although passion has strained our bonds of affection too hardly, <u>they must not, I am sure they will not be</u>, broken. The mystic chords which, <u>proceeding from so many battle-fields and so many patriot graves</u>, pass through all the hearts and all the hearths in this broad continent of ours, will yet harmonize in their ancient music when breathed upon by the guardian angels of the nation." [82 words; underlined clauses distract!]
- Lincoln's Inaugural Address: "We are not enemies but friends. We must not be enemies. Though passion may have strained it must not break our bonds of affection. The mystic chords of memory, <u>stretching from every battlefield and patriot grave to every living heart and hearthstone all over this broad land</u>, will yet swell the chorus of the Union, when again touched, as surely they will be, by the better angels of our nature." [70 words; underlined clauses build!]

Next is an example from a medical journal article. It strikes me as masterly in its simplicity:

Telephone ownership introduces a bias irreconcilable by recourse to sociodemographic and health status measures.

In the foregoing example, there are no nonessential pronouns or relative clauses. It reads almost like Henry David Thoreau (from the Conclusion of *Walden*):

If one advances confidently in the direction of his dreams, and endeavors to live the life which he has imagined, he will meet with success unexpected in common hours.[30]

The frequent version of the sentence about telephone ownership, which I have encountered all too often in first drafts?

Telephone ownership introduces a bias <u>that does not have the ability to be</u> reconciled by <u>reverting back</u> to sociodemographic and health status measures.

The first example is simple, elegant, and memorable, manifesting thoughtful organization and expression. The second is a wordy, convoluted, "pseudoprofound" mess. The first example is the pith of sophisticated thought and analysis, whereas the second is quasierudite and a dim assortment of wind-blown chaff.

Write most prose in short, simple declarative sentences, but also try to introduce sentence variety to engage and maintain the interest of readers. Try to mix in some sentences with structures other than "subject-predicate, subject-predicate" *ad infinitum, ad nauseam*. If the journal targeted permits, mix in some "lambent flashes" of active voice among the "dense wood" of the passive. However, when mixing in active voice, be cautious about subject-predicate agreement. For instance:

On further examination, we determined that cortisol levels were consistent with hypothalamic-pituitary-adrenal (HPA) axis disturbance.

Not:

On further examination, cortisol levels [*this is a borderline dangling participle*] were determined to be [*They were? What was the mark of their determination?*] consistent with hypothalamic-pituitary-adrenal (HPA) axis disturbance.

Erythema and erosions can complicate visualization of Barrett's esophagus. [*OK: concise but somewhat passive*]
Or:
When assessing Barrett's esophagus, the clinician may find that erythema and erosions complicate visualization. [*OK: active but somewhat wordy*]
Or:
Visualization of Barrett's esophagus is complicated, at times, by the presence of erythema and erosions. [*OK but wordy and passive*]
But not:
When attempting to visualize Barrett's esophagus, erythema and erosions can complicate matters. [!] [*Dangling modifier!*]
Undesired (verbose):
The rates of recanalization with adjunctive regimens that combined IAT with IVT have been substantially higher than those <u>that</u> have been reported <u>for those patients who underwent</u> IVT monotherapy. [*29 words and cites no numerical data*]
Desired (consolidated):
Recanalization rates with IAT-IVT (79% TIMI 3–4) exceeded those previously reported with IVT alone (<20% TIMI 3–4). [*17 words and cites key numerical data*]
Undesired (verbose):
PROACT II was the first randomized trial <u>in which IAT was shown to have benefit</u> in patients <u>who have had</u> an ischemic stroke caused by occlusion of the MCA, <u>as well as in patients whose treatment has been initiated more than three</u> hours after the onset of symptoms. [*48 words*]
Desired (consolidated):
PROACT II was the first randomized trial <u>showing</u> benefits of IAT in patients with:

(1) ischemic stroke secondary to MCA occlusion and (2) treatment initiation > 3 hours after symptom onset. [*30 words*]

Bulleted lists also foster readers' access to (apprehension of) data and help to rid verbiage. Take, for example, the following drug manufacturers' labels, before and after the advent of the plain-language movement in government communications.

Undesired (old warning label, verbose):
Do not take this product unless directed by a physician, if you have a kidney problem such as acute interstitial nephritis, or if you have Cogan's syndrome or increased frequency of urination due to enlargement of the prostate gland.

Desired (new warning label, consolidated):
Ask a doctor before use if you have:

- Cogan's syndrome;
- a kidney problem such as acute interstitial nephritis; or
- increased frequency of urination because of an enlarged prostate gland.

In Introductions, make sure that statements are adequately and accurately referenced:

Alleles of single-nucleotide polymorphisms were associated with high plasma levels of Lp(a).[38,119] (Hypothetical references)

Not (unless the number of references is at a critical minimum):
Alleles of single-nucleotide polymorphisms have been shown to be associated with high plasma levels of Lp(a). *[Stating "have been shown to be" without including references raises questions with readers or peer reviewers.]*

In most cases, I advocate dispensing with pronouns and using "ing" verb forms to avoid wordy pronoun constructions.

For instance:

The group randomized to placebo also received usual care.

Not:
Those subjects who were randomized to placebo also received usual care.

Eliminate terms that have been stated or strongly suggested by context, in order to consolidate. For example:

A total of 100 patients received intensive and 75, intermediate, therapy. [OK]

Individuals with marked hypo- or hypertension were excluded from study. [OK]

But not:
The subject's vital signs were monitored and her chart updated.

The foregoing example of an attempt to consolidate words is prohibited because the subject of the compound sentence changes from plural ("vital signs were") to an implied singular ("her chart was" updated).

Not:
Eligible subjects were randomized to treatment with an ACE inhibitor, angiotensin$_{II}$ receptor blocker, or placebo.

The problem here is that subjects are not "treated with" placebo. Rephrase as follows:

Eligible subjects were randomized to receive an ACE inhibitor, angiotensin$_{II}$ blocker, or placebo.

Or:
Eligible subjects were randomized to the ACE inhibitor, angiotensin$_{II}$ blocker, or placebo arm.

Consider the following expendable (vs. succinct) phrases; many of these are identified in the *American Medical Association (AMA) Manual of Style*, 10th edition.[31]

Expendable phrases

In other words
It goes without saying that
Needless to say
To be sure
First and foremost

Redundant or incomparable/insuperable terms

Adequate enough
Advanced planning
Aggregate (combine, fuse) together
Brief in duration
Completely full (empty)
Consensus of opinion
Distinguish the difference

Redundant or incomparable/insuperable terms

Each individual person
Eliminate altogether
Empty out
Enter into
Equally as well as (should be just
    "equally"
Estimated at about (approximately)
Evolve over time
Fairly/very/most unique
Fellow colleagues
Fewer in number (quantity)
Filled to capacity
First initiated
Future plan
General rule
Green in color (tint/hue)
Improved [increased] the quality of
Indurated (tender) on palpation
    (hard/tender)
Interval of time (interval; period)
Large (small, bulky) in size
Lift (raise) up
Near to
Oval (square, round, lenticular) in
    shape
Own personal view
Perfect circle
Period of time, time period
Personal friend
Plan of action
Precede in time
Predict (project) in advance
Raise up
Reassessed again
Revert back
Rough (smooth) in texture
Skin rash
Soft (firm) in consistency
Sour (sweet, bitter) tasting
Still continues (remains)
Sum total
True fact
Very (quite, most) unique
Uniformly consistent

Be aware of sentences beginning with variants of "It" + forms of the verb "to be." Most are dispensable and "lead burying."

Prolix:

It has been demonstrated that
It is important (interesting) to note that
It may be stated (said, concluded) that
It stands to reason that
It was found (shown, demonstrated) that
The result was noteworthy (remarkable)
    because...

Prolix versus succinct

As a consequence (result) of	Because/Consequently
As long as	If
At this point in time	Now, while
Brought to fruition	Caused (elicited; but not "produced"; save the "produce" for the market; studies do not "produce" results!!)
Carry out	Conduct (perform)
Commented to the effect that	Said (stated, commented)
Despite (or in spite of) the fact that	Although, even though, though
Draws to a close	Ends (terminates)
Fall off	Decrease (decline, but not "diminish," which has an emotional/moral connotation)
File a lawsuit against	Sue
Following/subsequent to	After (unless "following" is actually meant, and it usually isn't!!)
Have an effect on	Affect (but not "effect," the verb form of which means "to cause")
In advance of	Before
In cases in which	When
In close proximity to (vicinity of)	Near
In order to; in an effort to	To (however, you can use "in order to" if you have already used "to" in a sentence "in order to" avoid repetition...)
In (with) regard to	About (regarding, concerning)

(Continued)

Prolix versus succinct (Continued)	
In those areas where	Where
Look at (in Methods or Introductions)	Assess, evaluate, examine, investigate, study
Most well	Best
Not remotely close to	Far from
Prior to	Before
Produce an inhibitory effect on	Inhibit
The majority of	Most

2.5.2.1 CONCISE *"MA NON TROPPO"*

Efforts to communicate tersely should not result in oversimplification or a failure to communicate the intrinsic complexities of a phenomenon—a practice referred to as "pablumizing." Strive for elegance and clarity without oversimplifying descriptions of key scientific details.

Also in the context of oversimplifying, one often encounters a form of "ellipsis" (a sort of short-handed deletion) in medical communications that runs approximately as follows:

> Study findings support that [*what?*] anti–CRP antibody titers are predictors of rapid radiographic progression in RA.

This, I am afraid, is so terse as to lose sense and should be reworded as

> Study findings support the conclusion that anti–CRP antibody titers are predictors of rapid radiographic progression in RA.

2.5.3 Variety

The best medical writing is varied and engaging while also being direct and forceful. To engage the reader and sustain his interest, seek to mix in different words, sentence structures, and active voice where appropriate.

For instance, be aware of the following sort of defect in a series of paragraphs:

> Par. 1: ED is a source of distress to many men, leading them to withdraw from otherwise fulfilling relationships…

> Par. 2: ED often causes rancor with one's partner, compromising interpersonal relationships and quality of life….

> Par. 3: ED is commonly caused by endothelial dysfunction in penile vascular beds…

One way around this quadruple repetition?

Heading: Erectile dysfunction (ED)

> Par. 1: A source of distress to many men, ED often leads them to withdraw from otherwise fulfilling relationships…

> Par. 2: ED often causes rancor with one's partner, compromising interpersonal relationships and quality of life…

> Par. 3: Endothelial dysfunction in penile and other vascular beds is a common cause of ED.

Backward-running sentences (e.g., with predicate preceding subject) can also increase variety and verbal interest. For example:

> This study enrolled patients with a history of myocardial infarction or unstable angina. Also eligible were (*predicate first*) individuals with ST-segment depression. [*Subject second*]

2.5.4 General prose style

In journalistic terms, "Lead with the news" (outcomes); don't "bury the lead (or the journalist's "lede")." While also remembering to vary sentence structure, try to give the reader the "pay-off" (i.e., outcomes) up front, not after a long-winded description of methods via subordinate clauses, unless the journal's AGs, online content, and/or the overall structure and style of the essay dictate otherwise.

> Treatment with dalteparin for 6 days significantly reduced the incidence of pulmonary embolism (vs. placebo) in subjects with deep-vein thrombosis who were enrolled in this randomized double-blind controlled trial. [*OK: Payoff for reader is up front.*]

Not (the lead-burying):

Subjects who were enrolled in this randomized double-blind controlled study in subjects with deep-vein thrombosis showed that treatment with dalteparin for 6 days significantly reduced the incidence of pulmonary embolism (vs. placebo). [*A tough slog*]

Spastex significantly reduced mean BURP scores (by 25%; p = 0.03 vs. placebo) in a multicenter, randomized double-blind, controlled study. [*OK: Payoff for reader is up front.*]

Not (the lead-burying):

In a multicenter, randomized double-blind, controlled study, spastex significantly reduced mean BURP scores (by 25%; p = 0.03 vs. placebo).

In many cases, an intervening clause is nonrestrictive; it adds nonessential information and does not redefine the subject as plural. For instance:

The patient, together with his loved ones, makes the final decision about end-of-life care. [*Correct*]

Comparisons in medical writing can also lead to imprecise agreement, with potential distortions of meaning. Examples follow.

Like other nephrologists, George Bakris is concerned about prerenal azotemia. [*OK*]

Not:

Like nephrologists, George Bakris is concerned about prerenal azotemia. [*Implies that Bakris is not a nephrologist!*]

Or:

Like all nephrologists, George Bakris is concerned about prerenal azotemia. [*Compares Bakris to himself!*]

As a pediatrician, Robert Pantell recognizes his role of educating youngsters.

Not:

As a pediatrician, it is Robert Pantell's recognized role to educate youngsters.

Strive to avoid dehumanizing and jargon-laden prose, even if doing so requires that you add words. Patients are not defined by their diseases.

Most HMG-CoA reductase inhibitor (statins) have not been investigated in children or adolescents (or "youngsters"). [*OK*]

Not:

Most HMG-CoA reductase inhibitors have not been investigated in pediatric patients.

But:

Clinicians should try to educate patients with diabetes (or hypertension).

Not:

Clinicians should try to educate diabetes (or hypertension) patients.

Or (even worse):

Clinicians should try to educate diabetics (or hypertensives).

Another way to enhance prose style is to connect clauses in parallel-structured series. We often miss opportunities to do so. For instance:

Schizophrenia can make it more difficult for patients to reason, learn, interact, and take care of themselves. [*Direct and well constructed*]

Not:

Schizophrenia has the ability to [*wordy construction*] compromise patients' capacity for reason, to attain degrees, and also limits their [*unclear antecedent; whose?*] interpersonal interactions and self-care.

Be mindful of agreement between singular and plural:

Study participants experienced significantly greater health-related quality of life after being randomized to daily treatment with either spastex 2.5 or 5 mg.

Not (implies treatment with both dosages):

Study participants experienced significantly greater health-related quality of life after being randomized to daily treatment with spastex 2.5 and 5 mg.

Sentences differing only in punctuation (commas) may convey vastly different meanings:

LDL-C increased by a mean of 8.3 mg/dL, and TG decreased by a mean of 1.7 mg/dL, from baseline to week 52.
Not:

LDL-C increased by a mean of 8.3 mg/dL, and TG decreased by a mean of 1.7 mg/dL from baseline to week 52. [*By distinct proximities of the phrases, this sentence implies that only TG was measured from baseline to week 52. Commas or parentheses signifying nonrestrictive clauses, as shown in the former example above, are necessary.*]

Predicates often do not match antecedents, and we commit "plural effusions."

Subject-verb agreement is often lacking in first drafts. On some level, this defect is endemic to medical writing, with its fluid shifts between considerations of individuals and groups.

A total of 1,112 women and their husband participated in this placebo-controlled trial. [!]

[*Apologies for my indelicacy here, but he must be very busy!*]

I find that the following plural-singular usage is objectionable:

Each physician inserted a catheter into his patient's pulmonary artery. [*OK*]
Or:

Physicians inserted catheters into their patients' pulmonary arteries. [*OK*]
Not:

Physicians inserted a catheter into their patients' pulmonary artery. [*Hmn? Do the patients share a single, "communal" pulmonary artery?*]

Predicates frequently do not agree with subjects because an intervening clause distracts us. Attention must be paid! For instance:

Treatment with oral antihypertensives, such as calcium channel blockers and β-blockers, were recommended.

Be careful: the subject/antecedent is "Treatment," which is singular. The above sort of disagreement occurs frequently in published papers.

OK:

Treatment with an ARB was at least as effective as, if not more effective than, therapy with an ACE inhibitor.
Or:

Treatment with an ARB was at least as effective as with an ACE inhibitor, if not more so.
Not:

Treatment with an ARB was at least if not more effective than therapy with an ACE inhibitor.

Less than 10% of patients experienced treatment-emergent adverse events.
Should be reworded as:

Fewer than 10% of patients experienced treatment-emergent adverse events.

Although "10%" can be considered as a singular quantity, the fact that "patients" are individuals who can be counted favors the use of "fewer than." However,

Less than 10% of body surface area was affected by plaque psoriasis after treatment.

is also correct because body surface area is indivisible and cannot be counted.

A cohort of 128 patients with RA were followed up for a cohort mean of 10 years.
Should be reworded as:

A cohort of 128 patients with RA was followed up for a cohort mean of 10 years.

because the overall cohort (not the individual participants) is being referenced.

The next example was excerpted from a published paper:

A significant increase in serum total testosterone, prostate-specific antigen, hematocrit, hemoglobin, and total bilirubin were seen in the treatment arm.

Should have been reworded as:

Significant increases in serum total testosterone, prostate-specific antigen, hematocrit, hemoglobin, and total bilirubin were seen in the treatment arm.

unless the intended meaning was that there was a (singular) significant increase in all components combined, in which case the verb form should have been "was."

The tolerability of both patches was also evaluated in this study.
Should have been reworded as:

The tolerability profiles of both patches were also evaluated in this study.

The singular "tolerability" in the first sentence suggests that both patches were worn at once. The plural "tolerability profiles" suggests that more than one patch was evaluated and/or compared.

However, added, nonrestrictive clauses offset by commas do not imply a plural antecedent:

The patient, together with his physician, family, and other caregivers [*nonrestrictive clause*], chooses the treatment course.

is correct, but so is the following (restrictive clause):

The patient, his physician, family, and other caregivers [restrictive clause] choose the treatment course.

However:

The presence of anti-citrullinated protein antibodies are powerful predictive factors for development and progression of RA.
Should be reworded as:

The presence of anti-citrullinated protein antibodies is a powerful predictive factor for development and progression of RA.
Or:

Anti-citrullinated protein antibodies are powerful predictive factors for development and progression of RA.

By convention, certain fundamentally plural medical terms warrant use of the singular:

In the case of ectopic pregnancy, D & C is indicated.
H & E is used to stain granulomas.
The H & P is warranted to discern histories of comorbidities.

However,

Hemoglobin and testosterone levels were determined, and QOL [*omission of form of the verb "to be" implies continued use of "were" even though "QOL" is singular*] surveyed, at regular intervals for 24 months.
Should be reworded as:

Hemoglobin and testosterone levels were determined, and QOL was surveyed, at regular intervals for 24 months.

In each of the preceding sentences, commas are placed before "at regular intervals" to signify nonrestrictive clauses. Absent these commas, the sentence would imply that only QOL was surveyed at regular intervals.

Dangling and "Warring" Clauses: "You Had Me at Hello; You Lost Me at Although."

Be leery of long introductory clauses, including those beginning with "Although."

From a published paper, we have the following:

Although the prognosis of patients with CHF is poor even with optimal management, suboptimal diagnosis, investigation, and treatment of heart failure and comorbidities (e.g., coronary artery disease) in community-dwelling patients contribute to poor survival.
[*The reader gets lost after "optimal management."*]
Should have been reworded as:

Suboptimal diagnosis, investigation, and treatment of heart failure and comorbidities (e.g., coronary artery disease) contribute to poor survival in community-dwelling patients, even though the prognosis of patients with CHF is poor even with optimal management.

Or recast as two sentences:

Suboptimal diagnosis, investigation, and treatment of heart failure and comorbidities (e.g., coronary artery disease) contribute to poor survival in community-dwelling patients. On the other hand, the prognosis of patients with heart failure is poor even with optimal management.

More egregious (and often risible) are long introductory clauses that dangle:

After scrubbing in for the surgery, our eyes noticed that there were no size 7 latex gloves. [!]

2.5.5 Before-after examples on general prose style from my practice

I consulted with an author of a review and offered the following revisions (among others). Notice how my edits to "lead with the news" (and not "bury the lead") not only reduce verbose sentences but also help to organize paragraphs, by moving otherwise buried concluding sentences to the fronts of paragraphs (as topic sentences).

Before: "Buries the Lead"

In one of the largest, the long term prospective Malmo study (19), baseline serum creatinine, incidence of smoking and low BMI, plasma glucose, pulse pressure, and frequency of antihypertensive therapy were all higher in the subpopulation of 40- to 55-year-old men who had orthostatic hypotension at the onset.

After: "Flips the Script," Uses Last Sentence in the "Before" as the Leading (Topic) Sentence in the "After"

The Malmo study (19) showed that the following factors were elevated in a subpopulation of men with OH at study onset:

- baseline serum creatinine
- incidence of smoking and low body mass index (BMI)

- plasma glucose
- pulse pressure
- frequency of antihypertensive therapy.

The Malmo trial was among the largest long-term prospective trials of men aged 40–55 years with OH.

Before:

Since hypertension is associated with orthostatic hypotension, and the target organ damage associated with hypertension (left-ventricular hypertrophy with impaired diastolic filling, central vascular rigidity, stroke and other cerebrovascular changes, and congestive heart failure) may all contribute, in a causative fashion, to OH, even the directionality of the association is uncertain.

After:

Even the directionality of the association between OH and target organ damage (TOD) is uncertain.

Hypertension is directly associated with OH. Findings of TOD associated with hypertension may also contribute in a causal manner to OH. These manifestations include left-ventricular hypertrophy (LVH) with impaired diastolic filling; central vascular rigidity; stroke and other cerebrovascular changes; and congestive heart failure.

2.6 BEFORE-AFTER EXERCISES, BY MANUSCRIPT SEGMENT

2.6.1 Article title

This section illustrates principles of high-quality writing and editing, using "before" (raw; red font and hypothetical author queries to address errors) and "after" (refined; green font) exercises and examples. When drafting titles avoid declarative sentences that convey the study's results because they can reduce the reader's motivation to read the paper. Do include the study design if possible.

Not:

Treatment with spastex improves diaphragmatic function without causing off-target anticholinergic effects in patients with involuntary noisome hiccup syndrome: a randomized controlled trial

But:

Can treatment with spastex improve diaphragmatic function without causing off-target anticholinergic effects in patients with involuntary noisome hiccup syndrome? A randomized controlled trial.

Or (most simple and preferred):

Effects of treatment with spastex on diaphragmatic function in patients with involuntary noisome hiccup syndrome: a randomized controlled trial.

2.6.2 Abstract

2.6.2.1 "HELP READERS TO FIND YOUR ARTICLE"

Major considerations are summarized in Box 2.1. Structured abstracts are typically 250 to 300 words, represent a microcosm of the overall essay, and may include (1) Introduction/Background; (2) Objectives; (3) Methods; (4) Results; (5) Discussion; (6) Study Limitations; and (7) Conclusions. The chief requirement is to include your key words and other terms that search engines will locate. I always try to include at least one comparison and/or p value.

2.6.3 Acknowledgments: Before and after editing

Before: Raw

Acknowledgment

We are indebted to Ms. Smyrna Smulewicz for preparing the manuscript and to Dr. Hamish Heimstich for reviewing and commenting on it.

This is all very nice on the surface but woefully deficient overall.

After: Refined

Acknowledgments
Financial disclosures

This study and the present report were supported financially by Apex Pharmaceuticals, Inc. (Weston-Upon-Super Mare, UK), which provided study medications and had a role in study design; data acquisition and analysis; and the decision to report the findings. Apex Pharmaceuticals Inc. reviewed the manuscript for accuracy, but the authors had final autonomy over decisions related to its content.

C.R. has served as a paid consultant to, and a recipient of honoraria, lecture payments (service on speakers' bureaus), and travel support from Apex Pharmaceuticals. She has received lecture payments from, and served on speakers' bureaus for, Astragal Pharma (Cleveland, UK) and T-farma Technologies (Hoddesdon, Hertfordshire, UK). She is also a board member for Kittrec Kickyzer (Marske-by-the-Sea, UK). W.G. is the recipient of a grant from the US National Institutes of Health (NIH; Grant # 24-88482). He has also served as an expert witness for Kittrec Kickyzer. R.D. and T.M.I. are employees of, and stock or shareholders (minor) in, Apex Pharmaceuticals. Z.Q. has received fees from Apex Pharmaceuticals for participating in review activities such as data safety monitoring boards, statistical analysis, and endpoint committees. A.M. has served as an expert witness for T-farma. J.K. has no financial interests to disclose.

Assistance in manuscript preparation was provided by Ms. Smyrna Smulewicz, Bristol University (UK), with support from Apex Pharmaceuticals, Inc. Hamish Heimstich, MD, PhD (Bristol University, UK) reviewed and commented on the manuscript.

Author contributions

Category 1

All authors made substantial contributions to the conception and design of the work, as well as acquisition, analysis, and interpretation of data.

Category 2

(a) Drafting the article: W.G. with assistance from Ms. Smulewicz.

(b) Revising it for intellectual content: All authors and Dr. Heimstich.

BOX 2.1: Before-after exercise to enhance search engine (and hence reader) access to your article via its abstract

THE IMPORTANCE OF SEARCH ENGINES

Google and Google Scholar are the principal search engines by which people find your article online. The search engine is now the first "port of call" for researchers, and it is of paramount importance that your article can be found easily in search engine results. Taking some simple steps to optimize your article abstract for search engines can help your work to be discovered, read, used, and cited in others' work. This, in turn, helps with the ISI Impact Factor of the journal in which your article is published, further raising the visibility of your article.

There are more than 100 factors that a search engine will look at before deciding how to rank your article in their search results, but the starting point is the content that you write.

WHAT DO SEARCH ENGINES SEEK?

Today's search engines use complex, proprietary mathematical algorithms that change every month to keep their search results as accurate as possible. They take into account more than 100 different factors and do not disclose the weighting or importance of each. Below are a few of the elements considered today by search engines:

- the volume of incoming links from related websites
- page titles
- quality of content
- relevance
- page descriptions
- quantity of content
- technical precision of source code
- functional vs. broken hyperlinks
- volume and consistency of searches time within website
- page views
- revisits
- click-throughs
- technical user features
- uniqueness
- key words
- spelling

WHAT CAN YOU DO TO HELP?

Repeat key phrases in the abstract while writing naturally

Search engines look at the abstract page of your article, which is free for everyone to review online. Your abstract is not only the "sales pitch" that tempts researchers to read your article, it is also the information that gives a search engine all the data it needs to be able to find your article and rank it in the search results page. Try to repeat the key descriptive phrases. Try to imagine the phrases a researcher might search for if your paper would be of interest to him or her. Focus on three or four key phrases in your abstract.

Get the title right (see also above)

Ensure that the key phrase for your topic is contained in your article title. Make sure that your title is descriptive, unambiguous, accurate, and reads well. Remember that people search on key phrases, not just single words, e.g., "women's health," not "health."

Choose your key words carefully

Include your three or four key phrases and add at least three or four more. Where more than one phrase (or abbreviation) is often used to describe the same thing, include both/all variants, e.g., drug names (proprietary and generic).

Summary

- What key phrases would you give a search engine if you were searching for your own article?
- Write for your audience, but be mindful of how search engines work also.
- Write a clear title with your main key phrase in it.
- Write an abstract and choose key words reiterating three or four key phrases.
- Keep it natural. Google will un-index your article if you go overboard in repeating terms.

The better you write your abstract, the better chance you give your article to appear high up in the search results rankings. This is vitally important, because researchers will rarely investigate beyond the first 20 results from Google.

BEFORE: EXAMPLE OF AN ABSTRACT NOT OPTIMIZED FOR SEARCH ENGINES

The following abstract's article could not be found in Google Scholar after searching on a variety of phrases around the subject of the article: the representation of youth anti-war protests. The words highlighted below are the only terms repeated, and these were unlikely to help someone researching this subject to find this article via Google.

Peace Children

Debate over the role that young people should play in politics reflects different conceptions of childhood and adult concerns about loss of authority and political hegemony. Coverage of demonstrations against the Second Iraq War by the British national press echoes adult discourse on the nature of childhood and exposes the limits set on political activity. Analysis of news-text and images reveals concerns about the political competence of youth, their susceptibility to manipulation and the requirement for social control. Approval of youth's right to protest was often conditional on the cause espoused.

Key Words: childhood • Second Iraq War

Key points:

- The title is meaningless outside the context of the printed journal issue. It might appeal to certain readers but not to online search engines.
- The title does not include key terms or phrases such as "youth anti-war protests."
- The Abstract does not repeat key phrases used within the title or article and presents Google with no patterns to search.
- Key words play a reduced role in SEO [search engine optimization] but still have influence. In the above Abstract, only two key words were provided, and the article's key phrases were not listed.
- Many other factors influence ranking, but the content above was written in a way that offered the article a very poor chance of being found online through search engines.

AFTER: EXAMPLE OF AN ABSTRACT OPTIMIZED FOR SEARCH ENGINES

The following abstract's article emerged at the top of Google Scholar's search of "depression X folic acid." These are words that researchers are likely to search on. The search terms are highlighted below so that you can discern the patterns of repeated phrases that Google searches.

Treatment of depression: Time to consider folic acid and vitamin B_{12}

We review the findings in major **depression**: of a low plasma and particularly red cell folate, but also of low vitamin B_{12} status. Both low folate and low vitamin B_{12} status have been found in studies of **depression**, and an association between **depression** and low levels of the two vitamins is found in studies of the general population. Low plasma or serum folate has also been found in patients with recurrent mood disorders treated by lithium. A link between **depression**: and low folate has similarly been found in patients with alcoholism. Hong Kong and Taiwanese populations with traditional Chinese diets (rich in folate), including patients with major **depression**, have high serum folate concentrations. However, patients in these countries have very low lifetime rates of major **depression**. Low folate levels are furthermore linked to a poor response to antidepressants, whereas treatment with **folic acid** is shown to improve such responses. A recent study also suggests that high vitamin B_{12} status may be associated with better treatment outcome. Folate and vitamin B_{12} are major determinants of one-carbon metabolism, in which S-adenosylmethionine (SAM) is formed. SAM donates methyl groups that are crucial for neurological function. Increased plasma homocysteine is a functional marker of both folate and vitamin B_{12} deficiency. Increased homocysteine levels are found in patients with **depression**. In a large population study from Norway increased plasma homocysteine was associated with increased risk of **depression**: but not anxiety. There is now substantial evidence of a common decrease in serum/erythrocyte folate, serum vitamin B_{12} and an increase in plasma homocysteine in **depression**. Further, the *MTHFR C677T* polymorphism that impairs homocysteine metabolism is over-represented among depressive patients, which strengthens the association. On the basis of current data, we suggest that oral doses of both folic acid (800 µg daily) and vitamin B_{12} (1 mg daily) should be tried to improve treatment outcomes in **depression**.

Key Words: cobalamin • **depression**: • diet • folate • **folic acid** • homocysteine • one carbon-metabolism • S-adenosylmethionine • vitamin B_{12}

Key points:

- Clear and descriptive title includes main key terms or phrases.
- Abstract repeats key phrases in a contextually natural way.
- Key terms or phrases are repeated in the Key Words field.
- Many other factors influence ranking, but the foregoing content was written in a way that gives it the best chance of being found online through search engines.

Source: Help Readers Find Your Article. Retrieved from https://us.sagepub.com/en-us/nam/help-readers-find-your-article. Reprinted by permission of SAGE Publications, Inc., 2455 Teller Road, Thousand Oaks, CA 91320-2234. Last accessed April 16, 2017.

Following are major ICMJE categories for author-ship or contributorship. Categories 1, 2, 6, and 8 must be met to qualify for authorship. It is not sufficient to approve each draft; some substantive intellectual contribution must be made (e.g., addition, deletion, or other revision of text).

(1) Conception and design of the study and/or acquisition of data; Analysis and interpretation of data; (2) Drafting the manuscript or critical revision for important intellectual content; (3) Obtaining of funding; (4) Provision of study materials or patients; (5) Administrative, technical, or logistic support; (6) Final approval of the article; (7) Statistical expertise; (8) Agreement to be accountable for all aspects of the work, in ensuring that questions related to the accuracy or integrity of any part of the work are appropriately investigated and resolved.[32]

2.6.4 References

Before: Raw (with author queries)

1. Lieberman JA, Stroup TS, McEvoy JP et al. Effectiveness of antipsychotic drugs in patients with chronic schizophrenia. *N Engl J Med* 2005;353:1209–1223.
2. Wessels T, Grunler D, Bunk C et al. Changes in the treatment of acute psychosis in a German public hospital from 1998 to 2004. *Psychiatr Q* 2007;78:91.
3. World Health Report 2001 on mental health.
4. Lieberman JA, Stroup TS, McEvoy JP et al. Effectiveness of antipsychotic drugs in patients with chronic schizophrenia. *N Engl J Med* 2005;353:1209–1223.
5. Weiden PJ. Discontinuing and switching antipsychotic medications: understanding the CATIE schizophrenia trial. *J Clin Psychiatry* 2007;68:S12–S19.
6. Kane J, Canas F, Kramer M et al. Treatment of schizophrenia with paliperidone extended-release tablets: A 6-week placebo-controlled trial. *Schizophr Res* 2007;90:161–147.
7. Hamish Heimstich, personal communication, May 4, 2013.
8. DOF, Astragal Pharma.

After: Refined

1. Lieberman JA, Stroup TS, McEvoy JP et al. Effectiveness of antipsychotic drugs in patients with chronic schizophrenia. *N Engl J Med* 2005;353:1209–23. [Note: 1/N dash, not hyphens, for page ranges.]
2. Wessels T, Grunler D, Bunk C et al. Changes in the treatment of acute psychosis in a German public hospital from 1998 to 2004. *Psychiatr Q* 2007;78:91–9.
3. World Health Organization. The World Health Report 2001. Mental health: new understanding, new hope. Available at: http://www.who.int/whr/2001/en/whr01_en.pdf?ua=1. Accessed January 29, 2014.
4. Weiden PJ. Discontinuing and switching antipsychotic medications: understanding the CATIE schizophrenia trial. *J Clin Psychiatry* 2007;68(Suppl 1):S12–S19.
5. Kane J, Canas F, Kramer M et al. Treatment of schizophrenia with paliperidone extended-release tablets: A 6-week placebo-controlled trial. *Schizophr Res* 2007;90:147–61.

2.6.5 Tables: Before and after editing

Before: Raw

Table X Baseline characteristics of patients with involuntary noisome hiccup syndrome

Characteristic	Placebo (n = 69)	Spastex 5 mg (n = 146)
Age	51.9 ± 10.4	52.2 ± 10.9
BMI	27.7 ± 3.4	27. 9 ± 4.7
Race, n (%)		
Caucasian	69 (100.0)	144 (98.6)
Black		
Hispanic		
Asian	0.000 (0.000)	2 (1.4)
Disease etiology, no. (%)		
Psychogenic	9 (13.0)	22 (15.1)
Organic	23 (33.3)	40 (27.4)
Mixed	27 (39.1)	61 (41.8)
Unknown	10 (14.5)	23 (15.8)
Disease duration (time since diagnosis), n (%)		
3–6 months	6 (8.7)	10 (6.8)
6–12 months	14 (20.3)	33 (22.6)
>12 months	49 (71.0)	103 (70.5)
Mean ± SD INHS severity domain score	15.9 ± 6.2	15.5 ± 6.0
Categorical severity (categories of severity domain scores), n (%)		
Mild (17–30)	31 (44.9)	64 (43.8)
Moderate (11–17)	22 (31.9)	47 (32.2)
Severe (1–11)	16 (23.2)	35 (24.0)
Comorbidities, no. (%)		
Gastroduodenal ulcer	20 (29.0)	46 (31.5)
Gastroesophageal reflex	6 (8.7)	17 (11.6)
Zollinger–Ellison syndrome	6 (8.7)	19 (13.0)
Barrett's esophagus	1 (1.4)	1 (0.7)
Mean ± SD phrenic nerve parameters		
DPNT > 1.0; no. (%) with values (AU)		
≤1.67	26 (38.8)	63 (43.8)
1.67–2.07	18 (26.9)	50 (34.7)
≥2.07	23 (34.3)	31 (21.5)

Note: Margin and queries and highlights indicate author-remediable defects that should be flagged and/or addressed.

Many questionable items need to be footnoted in the above table to explain internal inconsistencies. See the footnote in the "after" example below.

After: Refined

Table X Baseline characteristics of patients with involuntary noisome hiccup syndrome (INHS)[a]

Characteristic	Spastex 5 mg (n = 146)	Placebo (n = 69)
Mean ± SD age, yr	52.2 ± 10.9	51.9 ± 10.4
Mean ± SD body mass index, kg/m^2	27. 9 ± 4.7	27.7 ± 3.4
Mean ± SD INHS severity score	15.5 ± 6.0	15.9 ± 6.2
Race, no. (%)		
Caucasian	144 (98.6)	69 (100.0)
Asian	2 (1.4)	0
Etiology, no. (%)[b]		
Psychogenic	22 (15.1)	9 (13.0)
Organic	40 (27.4)	23 (33.3)
Mixed	61 (41.8)	27 (39.1)
Unknown	23 (15.8)	10 (14.5)
Disease duration (time since diagnosis), no. (%) with[b]:		
3–5 mo.	10 (6.8)	6 (8.7)
6–11 mo.	33 (22.6)	14 (20.3)
≥12 mo.	103 (70.5)	49 (71.0)
Severity (categories of severity domain scores), no. (%) with:		
Mild (17–30)	64 (43.8)	31 (44.9)
Moderate (11–16)	47 (32.2)	22 (31.9)
Severe (1–10)	35 (24.0)	16 (23.2)
Comorbidities, no. (%)		
Gastroduodenal ulcer	46 (31.5)[c]	20 (29.0)
Gastroesophageal reflex	17 (11.6)[c]	6 (8.7)
Zollinger–Ellison syndrome	19 (13.0)[c]	6 (8.7)
Barrett's esophagus	1 (0.7)	1 (1.4)
Mean ± SD phrenic nerve parameters		
DPNT > 1.0; no. (%) with values (AU)		
<1.67	65 (44.5)	28 (40.6)
1.67–2.07	50 (34.2)	18 (26.1)
>2.07	31 (21.2)	23 (33.3)

Abbreviations: AU, arbitrary units; DPNT, direct phrenic-nerve test.

[a] Intent-to-treat (ITT) population (N = 215): placebo (n = 69), spastex (n = 146); 2 subjects without follow-up data were excluded from all outcome analyses except for adverse events.

[b] Some percentages do not sum to 100 because of rounding.

[c] $p < 0.05$ by Fisher's exact test.

2.7 PUTTING IT ALL TOGETHER: A REPRESENTATIVE (FICTITIOUS) STUDY REPORT FOR A MULTISPECIALTY JOURNAL*

Effects of the anticholinergic agent spastex in patients with involuntary noisome hiccup syndrome: A randomized controlled trial in a naturalistic setting

INTRODUCTION

[1 DISEASE DEFINITIONS/EPIDEMIOLOGY:]

Involuntary noisome hiccup syndrome (INHS) is a neuromuscular disorder of the thoracic diaphragm. Also termed smelly hiccupping disorder (SHD), INHS represents the second-ranked cause of reduced quality of life among diners in Eastern European restaurants.[1–3] Noisy, fetid, and often frankly offensive hiccupping (often with purulent sialorrhea) is virtually pathognomonic for INHS.

[2 NORMAL PHYSIOLOGY:]

The diaphragm receives blood supply from branches of the internal thoracic, superior phrenic, lower internal intercostal, and inferior phrenic arteries. It is innervated mainly by the (cervical) phrenic nerve (C3, C4, C5).[4]

[3 DISEASE STATE: ETIOLOGY/NATURAL HISTORY/GENETICS:]

Smelly hiccupping disorder has a complex etiology. Potential causes result in slowed digestion and can be divided by their propensities to occur postprandially. Non–meal-related causes include gastroparesis, pyloric obstruction, and pregnancy, whereas meal-related causes include acid reflux, hiatal hernia, and hypochlorhydria potentially secondary to *Helicobacter pylori* infection.[5] Meal-related belching is especially frequent after patients consume heavily spiced Hungarian Gulyás (goulash) and more often becomes chronic. The disorder has an autosomal recessive inheritance pattern, with a carrier allele frequency of 0.04%.[6]

[4 IDENTIFY "GAPS" IN RESEARCH AND BUILD TO PROBLEM/THESIS STATEMENT/STUDY RATIONALE AND THE UNIQUE/INCREMENTAL VALUE OF THE STUDY AND ITS REPORT:]

Largely because of halitosis and embarrassment, most patients with INHS do not seek health care. It has been difficult to recruit them for clinical studies, and there are as yet no consensus practice guidelines to manage INHS. A *Cochrane Collaboration* review[7] found only three high-quality studies[8–10] supporting the clinical utility of anticholinergic medications in general[8,9] (and spastex hydrochloride [HCl] in particular[10]) in reducing the frequency and severity of INHS. Another study,[11] with a small and atypical sample population, found no significant difference between treatment with spastex and placebo (+ usual care [UC]). However, the overall unadjusted odds ratio (OR) was 0.78 (p = 0.04; 95% CI = 0.74–0.82) for the likelihood of audible diaphragmatic spasms across these four studies, which involved 288 patients receiving anticholinergic agents compared to placebo and/or UC (referent; OR = 1.0).

[5 THESIS STATEMENT AND OBJECTIVES:]

Because of the challenges in motivating individuals with INHS to seek medical attention, the present study uniquely assessed large numbers of subjects by examining them "in situ": within a Budapest restaurant serving heavily spiced Hungarian goulash to Eastern European families. The chief aim of this study was to determine if once-daily treatment with spastex could reduce the frequency and severity of hiccupping in an Eastern European population.

(Continued)

---

* This text of a hypothetical study report cites references and calls out graphics that would likely be part of an actual manuscript but are not included here, to keep the exercise brief.

(Continued)

METHODS

Study design and setting

This randomized double-blind placebo-controlled trial (RCT) was conducted in a reserved and temperature-controlled private room of the Budapest restaurant Éshpítészpince from April 1, to June 30, 2018.

Participants

Study candidates were recruited from five large Hungarian gastroenterologic practices but were not specifically compensated for participation (apart from free suppers at Éshpítészpince). Previously untreated patients with ≥2-year histories of noisy, loathsomely smelling hiccupping, before or after meals, with or without purulent sialorrhea, were eligible. Consistent with draft labeling for spastex, exclusion criteria comprised: patients who were ages 18–25 or >65; had ulcerative colitis, Crohn's disease, inflammatory bowel disease, or porphyria; or had renal or hepatic disorders. Also ineligible were pregnant women. Also excluded were patients with congenital INHS, Barrett's esophagus, certain neuromuscular disorders (e.g., myositis), and a history of hospitalization for disabling hiccups.

Ethics

The trial was conducted in accordance with Good Clinical Practices and ethical tenets originating in the Declaration of Helsinki. All study participants were explicitly apprised of the study's potential benefits and risks, then provided written informed consent before any study assessment or treatment. Both the informed-consent document and study protocol were reviewed and approved by local institutional review boards.

Interventions

Subjects were randomized 1:1 (by computerized block randomization) to receive spastex 1.0 mg or placebo (+ UC) once daily for 12 weeks.

Assessments and outcome measures

The primary efficacy outcome measure was change in the frequency of audible hiccups (by trained assessors posing as wait-staff) by each patient, assessed as number of audible hiccups within 3 hours after a standardized test meal, from baseline to week 12. The severity of belching was determined by assessor ratings of noise (secondary efficacy endpoint) and smell (tertiary efficacy endpoint), as graded on a scale from 0 (no noise or smell) to 10 (unbearable noise or smell). Decreases in these measures are compatible with reduced hiccup severity. According to prior field work in Eastern European populations,[12] the minimum clinically important difference (MCID) threshold for decreases in hourly hiccupping frequency associated with increased health-related quality of life (on the SF-36) is 25%. As an exploratory endpoint, we conducted a responder analysis to compare changes from baseline to week 12 in proportions of subjects experiencing a ≥25% (95% CI = 20%–30%) decrease in hiccupping frequency. Treatment adherence was assessed by pill count at week 12.

Safety and tolerability

Laboratory panels (chemistries, hematology), vital signs (pulse rate, blood pressure, body temperature, respiration rate), and 12-lead electrocardiograms (ECGs) were assessed at baseline and week 12.

(Continued)

(*Continued*)

Any adverse events (AEs) were elicited at each study visit using open-ended questioning and categorized by preferred terms using the Medical Dictionary for Regulatory Activities (MedDRA 17.1). The study design and timeline are depicted in Figure 1 (study schema).

Statistical methods

Baseline characteristics were designated as continuous (mean ± standard deviation [SD]) or categorical (number, %) variables. Intergroup differences in baseline characteristics were assessed using Fisher's Exact Test.

For inferential statistics concerning efficacy endpoints, we put forth three null hypotheses (NHs): H_{0a}: There is no significant difference in changes in hiccupping frequency (H_{0a}), subjective ratings of noise (H_{0b}), or subjective ratings of smell (H_{0c}) from baseline to week 12 in patients randomized to once-daily spastex or placebo for 12 weeks. Alternative hypotheses were that there were significant changes on active treatment compared to placebo.

Previous studies[13–15] documented that frequencies of hiccupping are normally distributed. Mean (± SD) changes in hourly hiccup counts from baseline to week 12 in the actively treated and control groups (primary endpoint) were compared using Student's t-tests.

Hiccupping severity data are asymmetrically distributed because many patients who have INHS with predominant purulent sialorrhea have less noisy and smelly belches; median severity is greater than the mean. Hence, intergroup comparisons for changes in assessors' ratings of noise (secondary endpoint) and smell (tertiary endpoint) from baseline to week 12 were conducted using Mann–Whitney's U Test. The exploratory efficacy endpoint was evaluated using a χ^2 test.

No RCT of pharmacotherapies in untreated patients has been conducted, largely precluding sample size calculations in the present trial. Efficacy analyses were conducted in both the intent-to-treat (ITT) population (subjects randomized to either treatment) and per-protocol population (subjects who completed the protocol without violations). Safety analyses were conducted in subjects who received at least one dose of active treatment or placebo. All statistical tests were two-tailed at $\alpha = 0.05$. Statistical analyses were conducted using SAS version 9.1 (SAS Institute, Cary, NC, USA).

RESULTS

Patient disposition

A total of 108 study candidates were screened, 100 (92.6%) randomized, and 90 (90%) completed the protocol (45 in each group; Figure 2). [CONSORT patient flow diagram.[33]]

Baseline characteristics

Sociodemographic and clinical characteristics were well balanced in the two treatment groups at baseline (Table 1).

Efficacy

Treatment with spastex significantly reduced 3-hour hiccup counts from baseline to week 12. The mean (SD) change was −11.2 ± 1.1 in the spastex group compared to +0.8 ± 0.2 in the control group (p = 0.024 by Student's t-test; Table 2). However, reductions in hiccupping severity (ratings of noise and smell) did not differ significantly between groups (Table 2).

(*Continued*)

(Continued)

Significantly higher proportions of subjects in the spastex (vs. control) group experienced ≥25% reductions in hiccupping frequency (Figure 3). For all endpoints, findings in the per-protocol population were similar to those in the ITT population. Treatment adherence was similar in the actively treated (79%) and placebo (82%) groups.

Tolerability and safety

The most frequent AE was dyspepsia, but no single AE occurred in ≥5% of subjects in either group (Table 3).

There were no clinically significant differences between groups in mean frequencies of abnormal laboratory results, vital signs, or ECGs. A single subject (in the placebo + UC group) experienced a serious adverse event at the baseline assessment, after consuming his meal: emesis and diarrhea requiring hospitalization. A fecal culture returned *Clostridium perfringens*, but triplicate immunologic fecal occult blood tests were negative. After rehydration and rest, the patient recovered within 36 hours and completed the study protocol. The investigator considered the event to be unrelated to study treatment.

DISCUSSION

For the first time to our knowledge, we conducted a trial in a controlled yet naturalistic setting to determine whether daily treatment with the investigational oral anticholinergic agent spastex significantly reduces the frequency of hiccupping (vs. placebo + UC) in previously untreated patients with INHS. Significantly higher proportions of actively treated (vs. control) subjects achieved ≥25% decreases from baseline in hiccupping frequency, an emerging MCID threshold.

The severity of hiccupping, by subjective assessment of noise and smell, was not significantly decreased by spastex (vs. placebo + UC) from baseline to week 12. One potential reason for this somewhat unexpected finding is that measures of noise and smell on the 11-point rating scale varied widely in all subjects both at baseline (SD for noise = 4.3; SD for smell = 3.6) and 12 weeks (SD for noise = 5.2; SD for smell = 4.1). In fact, even in the relatively controlled setting of a private room, Éshpítészpince is a busy and noisy eatery redolent of spices. Baseline values of Cronbach's α (0.34 for noise and 0.18 for smell) and the more recently developed ω coefficient[16,34] (corresponding values of 0.36 and 0.20) for reliability of ratings were low. We hope that the overall favorable experience reported by our subjects in this study will enable other investigators to examine hiccupping severity under more controlled settings better suited to discriminate noise and smell, ideally by more objective methods.

During the 12 weeks of this study, no safety or tolerability issues were identified. The leading AE (dyspepsia) was likely attributable to off-target (extradiaphragmatic) effects. However, certain patients with higher susceptibility to anticholinergic effects were excluded; many of these individuals had congenital INHS and/or received treatment with atropine, phenothiazines, or antispasmodics. Our study was also underpowered to discern infrequent (<1/100 to <1/1,000) adverse events, such as lower-limb paralysis, which has been observed in some Eastern European patients with INHS dining frequently in Budapest eateries. This phenomenon was observed mainly in the 1990s and was ascribed to the unscrupulous practice of restaurateurs who spiked their paprika with lead oxide to enhance the spice's color.

Many patients with INHS are embarrassed and halitotic, and hence do not seek medical attention, let alone volunteer for clinical trials. Only four high-quality trials have been conducted in patients with INHS; findings from three were broadly consistent with our results,[8–10] whereas data

(Continued)

(Continued)

from the fourth did not include hypothesis testing.[11] This last study's population included an arguably more difficult-to-treat population, with a higher mean age, median number of comorbidities and concomitant medications, and mean frequency of congenital INHS.

POTENTIAL STUDY STRENGTHS AND LIMITATIONS

A unique strength of our trial was its RCT design, which largely excludes biases. At the same time, our study was pragmatically executed in a naturalistic setting, which promotes ecological validity and generalizability of the findings to actual social settings in which patients are often troubled by their signs and symptoms. The fact that we were able to randomize 100/108 (93%) study candidates—of whom 90 (90%) completed protocol—attests to the acceptability of the experimental paradigm to the subjects.

A high degree of error in subjective ratings of the noise and smell associated with study participants' hiccups may have limited the precision of severity assessments. Our study did not assess effects of INHS on those most adversely affected, apart from patients: their loved ones. We have fielded a new subjective rating scale (NO–MO–BURPS–PLS) to evaluate such effects.[17] These individuals may be better able to discriminate changes in levels of noise and smell associated with their loved ones' hiccups compared to highly educated and trained study personnel who were unacquainted with subjects. Our eligibility criteria were also somewhat stringent, resulting in a relatively homogeneous sample population. Finally, the duration of the present study was only 12 weeks, arguably too short an observation window to discern intertreatment differences in adverse events and safety signals occurring in <1/100 to <1/1,000 subjects. The long-term safety and tolerability profiles of spastex are being evaluated in a 52-week extension study (NCT # 108Σ984; available at www.clinicaltrials.gov).

CONCLUSIONS

For the first time in both a controlled and naturalistic experimental setting, this study demonstrated that once-daily treatment with the investigational oral anticholinergic agent spastex significantly reduced the frequency of hiccupping compared to placebo (+UC) from baseline to 12 weeks. Future studies, in larger and more heterogeneous sample populations, are needed to reject, corroborate, or extend our findings. An ongoing 52-week extension study, which is being conducted by our group (NCT # 108Σ984), should provide complementary long-term safety and tolerability findings.

REFERENCES

1. Riffenburgh RH. *Statistics in Medicine.* 3rd ed. Academic Press, 2012.
2. Kirkwood BR, Sterne JAC. *Essential Medical Statistics.* 2nd ed. Malden, MA: Blackwell Science, 2007.
3. Centers for Disease Control and Prevention. In: *Principles of Epidemiology in Public Health Practice: An Introduction to Applied Epidemiology and Biostatistics.* 3rd ed. Atlanta, GA: CDC, 2016: Available at: http://www.cdc.gov/ophss/csels/dsepd/ss1978/lesson3/section2.html. Last accessed April 16, 2017.
4. International Conference on Harmonisation. ICH Harmonised Tripartite Guideline: Clinical Safety Data Management: Definitions and Standards for Expedited Reporting 2A. Available at: https://www.ich.org/fileadmin/Public_Web_Site/ICH_Products/Guidelines/Efficacy/E2A/Step4/E2A_Guideline.pdf. Last accessed October 23, 2017.

5. Kelly WN, Arellano FM, Barnes J et al. Guidelines for submitting adverse event report for publication. *Drug Saf* 2007;30:367–73.

6. Avorn J. In defense of pharmaco-epidemiology—Embracing the yin and yang of drug research. *N Engl J Med* 2007;357:2219–21.

7. Cramer JA, Mattson RH, Prevey ML et al. How often is medication taken as prescribed? A novel assessment technique. *JAMA* 1989;261:3273–7.

8. Moher D, Liberati A, Tetzlaff J et al. Preferred reporting items for systematic reviews and meta-analyses: The PRISMA statement. *PLoS Med* 2009;6:e1000097.

9. Stroup DF, Berlin JA, Morton SC et al. Meta-analysis of observational studies in epidemiology: A proposal for reporting. Meta-analysis of Observational Studies in Epidemiology (MOOSE) group. *JAMA* 2000;283:2008–12.

10. Moher D, Cook DJ, Eastwood S et al. Improving the quality of reports of meta-analyses of randomised controlled trials: The QUOROM statement. Quality of Reporting of Meta-analyses. *Lancet* 1999;354:1896–900.

11. Higgins JP, Thompson SG, Deeks JJ et al. Measuring inconsistency in meta-analyses. *BMJ* 2003;327:557–60.

12. Egger M, Smith GD, Schneider M et al. Bias in meta-analysis detected by a simple, graphical test. *BMJ* 1997;315:629–34.

13. Egger M, Smith GD. Meta-analysis: Potential and promise. *BMJ* 1997;315:1371–4.

14. Moher D, Schulz KF, Altman DG. The CONSORT statement: Revised recommendations for improving the quality of reports of parallel-group randomised trials. *Lancet* 2001;357:1191–4.

15. Moher D, Hopewell S, Schulz KF et al. CONSORT 2010 explanation and elaboration: Updated guidelines for reporting parallel group randomised trials. *BMJ* 2010;340:c869.

16. Schulz KF, Altman DG, Moher D. CONSORT 2010 statement: Updated guidelines for reporting parallel group randomized trials. *Ann Intern Med* 2010;152:726-32.

17. Lieberman JA, Stroup TS, McEvoy JP et al for the Clinical Antipsychotic Intervention Effectiveness (CATIE) Investigators. Effectiveness of antipsychotic drugs in patients with chronic schizophrenia. *N Engl J Med* 2005;353:1209–23.

18. Vandenbroucke JP, von EE, Altman DG et al. Strengthening the Reporting of Observational Studies in Epidemiology (STROBE): Explanation and elaboration. *PLoS Med* 2007;4:e297.

19. Hudson KL, Collins FS. The 21st Century Cures Act—A view from the NIH. *N Engl J Med* 2016;372:1–3.

20. Avorn J, Kesselheim AS. The 21st Century Cures Act—Will it take us back in time? *N Eng J Med* 2016;372:2473–5.

21. Friedman H, Xong S, Crespi S et al. Comparative analysis of length of stay, total costs, and treatment success between intravenous moxifloxacin 400 mg and levofloxacin 750 mg among hospitalized patients with community-acquired pneumonia. *Value Health* 2009;12:1135–43.

22. Alemao E, Joo S, Kawabata H et al. Effects of achieving target measures in RA on functional status, quality of life and resource utilization: Analysis of clinical practice data. *Arthritis Care Res (Hoboken)* 2016;68;308–17.

23. Petri H, Urquhart J. Channeling bias in the interpretation of drug effects. *Stat Med* 1991;10:577–81.

24. Chen CC, Cheng SH. Continuity of care and changes in medication adherence among patients with newly diagnosed diabetes. *Am J Manag Care* 2016;22:136–42.

25. Warren JR, Falster MO, Tran B et al. Association of continuity of primary care and statin adherence. *PLoS One* 2015;10:e0140008.

26. Hansen RA, Voils CI, Farley JF et al. Prescriber continuity and medication adherence for complex patients. *Ann Pharmacother* 2015;49:293–302.

27. Husereau D, Drummond M, Petrou S et al. Consolidated Health Economic Evaluation Reporting Standards (CHEERS) statement. *Value Health* 2013;14:367–72.

28. Sullivan SD, Mauskopf JA, Augustovski F et al. Budget impact analysis—Principles of Good Practice: Report of the ISPOR 2012 Budget Impact Good Practice II Task Force. *Value Health* 2014;17:5–14.

29. Lepore J. The speech: Have inaugural addresses been getting worse? *The New Yorker*, January 12, 2009;49-53. Available at: http://www.newyorker.com/magazine/2009/01/12/the-speech. Last accessed April 16, 2017.

30. Thoreau HD. *Walden, Civil Disobedience, and Other Writings.* New York: W.W. Norton, 2008.

31. *American Medical Association Manual of Style*. 10th ed. Chicago, IL: American Medical Association, 2007.

32. Ivanis A, Hren D, Sambunjak D et al. Quantification of authors' contributions and eligibility for authorship: Randomized study in a general medical journal. *J Gen Intern Med* 2008;23:1303–10.

33. Moher D, Schulz KF, Altman D. The CONSORT statement: Revised recommendations for improving the quality of reports of parallel-group randomized trials. *JAMA* 2001;285:1987–91.

34. Dunn TJ, Baguley T, Brunsden V. From alpha to omega: A practical solution to the pervasive problem of internal consistency estimation. *Br J Psychol.* 2014;105:399–412.

APPENDIX: "DICTION-ERR-Y"— A GUIDE TO BETTER USAGE

"Diction-Err-Y": Of "plural effusions" and other peculiarities of medical writing's "singular" syntax and semantics

IUVIF: Infrequently used verbs that I favor (often to introduce greater rhetorical variety).

FUVIA: Frequently used verbs that I abhor (when overused).

Abate: IUVIF. What transient effects do with time or continued treatment.

Accident: This term may be imprecise or misleading. What is usually meant? Injury, trauma, shooting, or collision.

Do not use "cerebrovascular accident" to mean stroke. Stroke is preventable and not an accident. Prefer cerebrovascular incident (CVI).

Acquaint: IUVIF, e.g.,

This review will acquaint the reader with emerging diagnostic methods.

Acronyms vs. abbreviations: Acronyms are abbreviations that spell words (or easily spoken "quasi-words"). AIDS, CONSORT, NASA, RANKL, and SARS are examples. All others (e.g., MI, NIDDM) are just abbreviations. All acronyms are abbreviations, but not vice versa; being an abbreviation is a necessary but not sufficient condition of being an acronym. If permitted by the targeted journal, include a list of abbreviations and acronyms at the front of your manuscript. Try not to exceed a 0.5% abbreviation: text ratio (e.g., ≤10 abbreviations in a 2,000-word paper). Define/expand all abbreviations in tables and figures, even if they have been defined in the text. Tables and figures need to function as discrete/self-contained units of meaning for readers who apprehend most or all information from graphics.

Active voice; Use, misuse: Most journals encourage you to use passive voice, which has a solid foundation in medical writing. To encourage sentence variety and reader interest, however, I advocate that you introduce active voice when you can. Do it carefully, however, maintaining parallel structure and subject-predicate agreement.

Not:

After controlling for covariates, women were more likely than men of all ages to respond to β-blockers.

But:

After controlling for covariates, we found that women were more likely than men of all ages to respond to β-blockers.

Acute, chronic: These terms describe diseases or conditions, not treatments. Treatment may be longterm but not chronic; urgent but not acute. In at least two major disorders, the term "acute" has a specific physiologic definition not completely encompassed by its meaning of "short-term": "acute abdomen" refers to severe abdominal pain within 24 hours that has an unclear etiology, with a differential diagnosis that includes abdominal aortic aneurysm, appendicitis, pyelonephritis, pancreatitis, cholecystitis, diverticulitis, ovarian torsion, ectopic pregnancy, and ischemia. A more precise term in some cases is acute peritonitis, which results from infection of the peritoneal lining of the abdominal cavity. "Acute coronary syndromes" refer to cardiovascular conditions associated with acute myocardial ischemia, including 12-lead electrocardiographic ST-segment-elevation myocardial infarction (STEMI).

Additionally: PLEASE AVOID. PLEASE?! For example, "Additionally, we reviewed study report data." Additionally? As opposed to "Subtractionally?" Ditto "Hopefully, I will write a sound paper" (unless you are filled with hope). "Historically, elders have received suboptimal care," and others.

In general, be leery of connecting introductory modifiers such as "Moreover" and "Further." If one sentence or paragraph flows organically from the last, these "verbal crutches" are not only unnecessary but potentially distracting. "On the other hand," use an expression such as this one (or "However") to mark a departure in logic from the previous sentence or paragraph.

Ad libitum: (or *Ad lib*) At liberty, freely, at one's pleasure, as much as desired.

Laboratory animals drank water *ad libitum.*

Adverbs vs. conjoined adjectives:

Don't hyphenate adverbs (which modify the verb "to be"):

Thank you, waiter; this steak is well done. [*correct, no hyphen*]

Conjoined adjectives (two words modifying a noun) do require a hyphen:

Waiter, please bring me a well-done steak.

Never hyphenate an adverbial ("-ly") construction. Hyphenate only conjoined adjectives.

This is a smoothly flowing sentence.

Not:

Smoothly flowing sentences drive any argument.

But:

Enjoy your hard-earned paycheck [*conjoined adjective requires hyphen*].

Having perused many of my reviews, my readers are well informed [*adverb does not require hyphen*].

Not:

Having perused many of Gutkin's reviews, our readers are well-informed.

But:

Gutkin's reviews have built a well-informed readership.

Involuntary noisome hiccupping syndrome has an adverse effect on well-being.

[*Stet the hyphen because it appears this way in the dictionary.*]

Ad vitam: For life.

Attempt to optimize treatment adherence because the medications will be taken *ad vitam*.

Affect/effect: Affect (n.): the patient with major depression often has a flat affect.

> **Affect (v.):** to influence. Treatment affected disease incidence.
>
> **Effect (n.):** One adverse effect of treatment was rash.
>
> **Effect (v.):** Treatment effected a favorable outcome.

Age referents: Seniors, elders, or the elderly are ≥65 years of age.

Adults (men, women) are ≥18.

Adolescents are 12 to 17 years of age.

Children (not "pediatric patients") are below the age of 18 or 21 (depending on location/society) years, infants 5

weeks to 1 year; and neonates (newborns) birth to 4 to 5 weeks. Toddlers are 1 to 3 years of age and preschoolers 3 to 5.

Agreement: Subject-predicate disagreement often occurs in medical writing because of the high frequency of intervening phrases and shifts in voice from plural to individual (and back!); only in our field could I coin the term "plural effusion" to characterize these defects.

Not:

The rising incidence of stroke, congestive heart failure, and end-stage renal disease has signalled a need to increase awareness and treatment of hypertension. [*Unless you mean that the incidence of the combined outcome of stroke, CHF, and ESRD, in which case the sentence should specify "incidence of the combined outcome of..."*]

But:

The rising incidences of stroke, congestive heart failure, and end-stage renal disease have signalled a need to increase awareness and treatment of hypertension.

Introduction of nonrestrictive clauses, which add information but do not define or limit their antecedents, does not change the number of the subject, e.g.,

The patient, together with his partner, is capable of making a decision about ED therapy.

And:

The patient and his partner are capable of making a decision about ED therapy.

Difficulty with gender issues often can be resolved by switching from a singular to plural subject.

Physicians must make up their own minds.

Or:

A physician must make up her own mind.

Not:

A physician must make up his or her own mind. [*grammatically correct but unwieldy*].

However, indiscriminately rendering plural subjects that would be better handled as singular can also create distracting connotations (even if strictly correct).

Each patient with ED and his wife gave informed consent.

Not:

Patients with ED and their wife gave informed consent.

Aim (n., not v.): Typically use as a noun but not a verb.

Our aim was to evaluate anti-inflammatory effects.

Not:

We aimed to evaluate anti-inflammatory effects.

All: ≠ each.

Compared to patients treated by FPs, those receiving care from specialists had significantly lower frequencies of emergency-department visits (22% vs. 87%), hospital admissions (10% vs. 38%), and durable-equipment use (p < 0.05 for <u>each</u>).

[p < 0.05 for "all" would imply that endpoints were combined or that the test was for the overall trend.]

Alleviate vs. ameliorate: The verb "alleviate" means to lessen or relieve.

"Ameliorate" signifies improvement.

Treatment with spastex alleviated symptoms of involuntary noisome hiccup syndrome (INHS).

Not:

Treatment with spastex ameliorated symptoms of INHS.

But:

Treatment with spastex ameliorated diaphragmatic function in patients with INHS.

Also: Also frowned upon is the use of "Also, (with a comma)" as an adverbial at the head of a sentence. The use of "Also" (without a comma) in the prior sentence is the only permissible exception.

Although: Use at the head of a sentence to introduce a subordinate clause.

Not:

I have never received a speeding ticket, although I typically drive my Ferrari at 154 mph.

But:

Although I typically drive my Ferrari at 154 mph, I have never received a speeding ticket.

Amenable: For example, "amenable to treatment" is an antonym of "refractory to treatment." Both are IUVIFs!

Among: For comparisons involving more than two entities (between is suitable only for two entities).

Among patients with impaired glucose tolerance, losing weight is frequently recommended.

Amongst: Archaic (avoid). Others include "proven" (in the sense of "this study has proven" but not in the sense of "this medication has proven benefits in elderly patients") and "towards."

Ampersand: Prefer "and" to &. Exceptions include company names and certain medical terms, such as D&C, H&P, and H&E.

Anatomic terms, implied: Be sensitive to possibly distracting medical connotations of otherwise commonplace modifiers.

Not:

Undergoing <u>knee</u> replacement should be a <u>joint</u> decision of the surgeon and patient.

[The word "joint" is distracting in this context.]

Patients with <u>rotator-cuff</u> injury in the active treatment <u>arm</u> received the new device.

[The word "arm" is distracting in this context.]

and/or: Think carefully about whether you mean "and," "or," or "and/or." Frequently, "or" will suffice.

About 10% of patients randomized to spastex 5 mg or phragoph 50 mg experienced treatment-emergent dizziness.

or

Use of nitrates or nitric oxide donors contraindicates spastex treatment.

Spastex treatment may improve quality of life for the patient and/or his caregiver.

Appraise: IUVIF.

Apt/liable: In most cases, prefer "likely" as a more neutral descriptor.

As (≠ because): "As" has a time connotation. (So does "since," which should not be substituted for "because," and "while," which should not be substituted for "whereas.")

Not:

Please confirm the veracity of this statement <u>as</u> the backup patient listing differs. *[This may take some fortunate "timing!"]*

But:

Please confirm the veracity of this statement <u>because</u> the backup patient listing differs. *[This usage is time neutral.]*

As (vs. so): "As" is used for positive comparisons, "so" for negative ones.

Warfarin is as effective as LMWHs in preventing DVT in elderly ACS patients.

Or:

Esteemed Professor Eliot Bookbinder was not so patient as to indulge questions from uninformed students.

Ascribe: IUVIF for "attribute."

Assent: Adults give informed consent; children/minors, verbal assent.

Assure: ≠ ensure. "Ensure" is a neutral term meaning "to make certain." "Assure" carries a psychological connotation ("the physician assured his patient that the injection would not hurt"). Insure is restricted to the meaning of indemnifying against loss.

As though: See "like."

Attend, attended: ≠ "seen." A patient is attended by a physician. This involves much more than "being eyeballed." ("Seen" is also jargony.)

Back formations: Avoid.

Because of hypervolemia, diuresis was instituted. Patients who received surgery fared better.

Not:

The patient was diuresed due to *[this is also wrong usage of "due to," which needs to follow the verb "to be"]* **to hypervolemia.**

The operated group fared better.

Based on: Avoid at the head of sentence. Substitute "On the basis of" in most instances.

On the basis of these findings, the MIRACLE investigators concluded that biventricular pacing enhances survival in heart failure patients with low ejection fractions.

Not:

<u>Based on these findings, the MIRACLE investigators</u> concluded that biventricular pacing enhances survival in heart failure patients with low ejection fractions. *[How can the "MIRACLE investigators" be "based on" anything?]*

Because: Not synonymous with "since," which has a time connotation.

Because of: Substitute this for "due to" or "since" when causal attribution is intended.

Before: One word versus "prior to" (two words) or "in advance of" (three)!

"Borderline-significant": Avoid. A p value is either below its prespecified critical value (usually < 0.05) or it is not. This type of phrase amounts to a "statistical apology." Instead, simply report p values and confidence intervals, and allow the reader to judge.

Breastfeed: ≠ the verb "nurse" (i.e., connotation of RN, NP).

Bullet points: Useful to augment reader apprehension of data, especially when clauses are "buried" in longer sentences.

Burning: Unless we actually imply a scalding, we typically mean "a burning sensation."

Can: Preferred over the wordy "has the potential to," "has the capacity to," or "has the ability to."

Cause: IUVIFs:

Elicit

Induce

Precipitate

Prompt

Spawn

Trigger

FUVIA: "Produce"

Center around: Sorry, no. Something "centers on" or "revolves around" but does not "center around."

Claudicant: A patient with intermittent claudication.

Clinician: Person who works in clinics, not just a physician (e.g., RN, NP, PA).

Comparable: ≠ "similar." In its strict sense, comparable means "able to be compared." Virtually any two entities are "comparable." Vexed by "apples-to-oranges" comparisons? Why? Both are fruits. Both are nutritious and promote digestive health. Both grow on trees.

Ergo, totally comparable, though not entirely similar!

Compared with: "Compared with" or "compared to" is acceptable. If a sentence is short (<15 words), use "than"; if longer, use "compared to" or "as/when compared to."

It is often preferable to use "compared to" in order to avoid repetition of the word "with" in the same sentence.

On average, men <u>with</u> below-normal dihydrotestosterone levels grew significantly more new hair on the vertex compared <u>to</u> their counterparts <u>with</u> elevated DHT. *[Writing "to" here avoids triplicate use of "with" in same sentence.]*

Comprise/compose: Groups either *comprise* their elements or are *composed of* them; they are not "comprised of" them.

Concur: One concurs *in* an opinion or *with* another person (not *vice versa*).

Conduct: IUVIF. Studies, electrocardiography, and laboratory analyses are "conducted" (also "performed," or "carried out").

Confer [to/on]: IUVIF.

Confidence interval/CI: Because CIs may contain negative values, and both the "minus" sign and range symbol can be 1/N dashes, there are different styles for CIs.

For intervals with positive values: The odds ratio was 4.9 (95% CI, 3.8–6.1).

For intervals with negative values: The treatment effect was 0.2% (95% CI, –0.1%, 0.3% or –0.1% to 0.3%).

Comparisons: If one of the items being compared already has the word "with," use "compared to" or "as against" (British). It often works out nicely to start a sentence with "Compared to."

Examples:

> **Patients with metabolic syndrome are, on average, at higher risk of adverse cardiovascular events compared to their age-matched counterparts.**

Consolidate words using short parentheses to set off data in the correct location within sentences:

> **Compared to placebo (12%), drug Y enabled a significantly higher proportion of patients to achieve goal (48%; p<0.001).**

Comport (with): IUVIF.

The data do not comport with the prevailing biological theory.

Others: The data are not "compatible" or "concordant" with prevailing biological theory. Commensurate has a slightly different meaning:

Salary for either gender should be commensurate with experience.

Conjoined adjectives: Adjectives comprising more than one word often need to be hyphenated, e.g.,

The late Charles Janeway was well informed [*not "well-informed"*] about immune effector cell mechanisms. It was difficult to find someone better informed.

Or:

To learn more about immune effector cells in the aftermath of Janeway's passing, we will now need to consult other well-informed scientists.

and

drug-induced effects

not

drug induced effects (*which has a vastly different meaning!*)

The medication was well tolerated; it was a well-tolerated medication.

Controlled: Diseases, not patients, are "controlled" or "managed" ("cases" are also managed). Avoid such dehumanizing language.

Currently: ≠ "presently" (which means "soon"). "At present" is also OK.

Dashes:

em (1/M) dash: Don't overuse. Strive to keep clauses within these dashes (and parentheses) short (<10 words). Sentences with unwieldy clauses enclosed in (1/M) dashes often need to be recast as two (or more) sentences.

en (1/N) dash: Use with unequally weighted three-term conjoined adjectives. Non–insulin-dependent diabetes.

But:

very low density lipoprotein cholesterol

Negative symbols and ranges (in parentheses) are expressed using en dashes, not hyphens.

Data: Data *are* **plural;** *datum* **is singular. Alt.:** findings.

These data need to be confirmed in a RCT.

Not:

This data needs to be confirmed in a RCT.

Decrease: IUVIFs:

Attenuate

Downregulate

Lessen

Lower

Note: "diminish" ≠ "decrease."

Diminish has a non-numeric/subjective connotation:

Stroke survivors report diminished self-esteem.

or

The death of any patient diminishes morale on the entire ward.

not

Treatment with losartan diminishes blood pressure in patients with hypertension.

Dehumanizing: Patients should not be defined by their diseases, ages, or other clinical data. Diseases and cases are managed, not patients.

Children and adolescents (or "youngsters") provided verbal assent rather than written informed consent.

Not:

Pediatric patients provided verbal assent rather than written informed consent.

Patients with diabetes and hypertension were randomized to intensive therapy.

Not:

Diabetes and hypertension patients were randomized to intensive therapy.

Or (even worse!):

Diabetics and hypertensives were randomized to intensive therapy.

Patients also do not "fail to achieve" or attain certain potentially disease-reducing cut points. After all, is the failure all theirs, or does the health-care system not deserve to shoulder some of the "failure?"

Not:

Despite intensive therapy with medications from three pharmacological classes, the patient failed to achieve JNC-V target blood pressure.

But:

Despite intensive therapy with medications from three pharmacological classes, the patient's blood pressure remained above the JNC-V target.

I also object to the term "treatment-naïve" or, worse, just "naïve." Patients either have or have not been treated.

In most instances, you can substitute "untreated" (or unexposed) for "naïve."

Demonstrated/demonstrable/documented (*argumentative*): Clinical trials test hypotheses and address research questions. They are not designed *a priori* to "demonstrate" or "document" anything. However, if these terms must be used, please observe the following.

Clinical trials of medications, not the medications themselves, demonstrate effects. Hence:

Clinical trials have demonstrated the efficacy of antisense agents.

not

Antisense agents have demonstrated efficacy in clinical trials.

However, an agent may have "demonstrable" efficacy or effectiveness on the basis of clinical trials or experience.

Denote: IUVIF. Also: "signify." Strict definition, as opposed to "connote."

Depressor: Adjective. Blood pressure–lowering. Antonym is "pressor."

Despite (or, worse, in spite of) the fact that: Use "even though" or "although." "Despite the fact that" is wordy (four words vs. one or two).

Determined: Sometimes this verb is combined with forms of the verb "to be," in a passive construction that is not only wordy but also distracting:

Not:

> The mean systolic pressor effect of aerobic exercise in the placebo group <u>was determined to be</u> +5.8 mmHg.
>
> *[There is no stopping that pressor effect when it is "determined to be" +5.8 mmHg!]*

But:

> The mean systolic pressor effect of aerobic exercise in the placebo group was +5.8 mmHg.

df: Degrees of freedom; no need to expand this abbreviation, SD, or SE (and certain other oft-used abbreviations, e.g., DNA, RNA).

Diabetes: I prefer type 2 (with "mellitus" at first mention only; DM2) over non–insulin-dependent (NIDDM), which defines the condition by what it isn't.

"Diabetic" (n.) and other objectionable (dehumanizing) labels: Use "patient with diabetes" rather than "diabetic" per American Diabetes Association. Ditto "asthmatic," "epileptic," and "hypertensive." People are not defined by their health problems. They also should not be referred to as "cases" unless you intend the limited statistical sense (e.g., number of "incident cases"). Diseases, not patients with these diseases, are managed. Other dehumanizers include "patients on a drug" rather than "patients using [or taking] a drug."

Diagnose: Diagnose a condition, not a patient; the patient is evaluated or examined.

Disclose: IUVIF.

Discrete vs. discreet: "Discrete" means "independent" or "separate." "Discreet" signifies a sense of care or caution.

Different: One effect may be "different from" another but is not "different than" it. UK usage permits both similar and different "to."

Disinterested: A disinterested party is impartial. Someone without interest is uninterested. If you're quite uninterested in this, you may not be disinterested.

Document: Never use this verb (or "well documented") without citing references! As a noun, this is an imprecise term for which article, study report, case series, or other names of communications should be substituted.

Argumentative. As mentioned above, I have encountered published articles referring to a study's aim being to "document" effects of a medication. Remember, the prospective aim of a study is typically to test hypotheses or address research questions, not to "document" anything. Testing hypotheses is in the appropriate, fair-balanced province of "clinical equipoise," whereas documenting findings or conclusions reaches into the dangerous realm of deductive argument. In hindsight, however, we can say that a study "documented" effects.

Double verbs (*"pseudoprofoundly passive" clutter*):

Not:

> Sound <u>interpretation</u> of data <u>can be achieved</u> when all observations are independent. *[12 words]*

But:

> Data <u>can be interpreted</u> soundly when all observations are independent. *[10 words]*

Due to: Can be used as an adverb, typically after the verb "to be." However, it should not be used in other instances because it implies a false modification. In most cases, substitute "because of" or "owing to."

> Cough is largely due to the effects of ACE inhibitors on kinin levels.

Not:

> Due to patient attrition, the ITT population was larger than the evaluable population. *[Was the ITT population "due to" patient attrition?" No.]*

But:

> Because of patient attrition, the ITT population was larger than the evaluable population.

and:

> Coughs due to cold can be managed using OTC medications.

"Due to" is often used in the same lazy manner as "which" (see below):

Not:

Epidemiologic data such as the point prevalence of dyspepsia are difficult to interpret <u>due to</u> heterogeneity between studies and, particularly, differences in disease definitions. *[The phrase "due to" "floats" without an immediately identifiable antecedent.]*

But:

Epidemiologic data such as the point prevalence of dyspepsia are difficult to interpret <u>because of</u> heterogeneity between studies and, particularly, differences in disease definitions.

The other permissible use of "due to" is outside of the realm of "to be" verbs. In a sentence such as "Coughs due to cold are manageable": "due to" is acceptable because it is functioning as an adverb modifying the verb "to be": Coughs that are due to cold….

Echo: IUVIF. To signify agreement of data or opinions.

Echoing data from previous trials, the present study demonstrated that C-reactive protein is a reliable risk marker for inflammatory disease.

Editorializing: Do not "spin" data.

Rhabdomyolysis occurred in 0.1% of patients.

Not:

Rhabdomyolysis occurred in <u>only</u> 0.1% of patients.

Effects (title): Be careful when using this term to summarize study results. If a study is observational, the results are typically of an associational, not causal, nature; in this setting, the term "effects" may be inappropriate and warrant replacement with more "associational" language.

e.g., i.e., etc.: *exempli gratia, id est, et cetera*

Each should be enclosed in parentheses and separated by a comma (not the word "and"). Never use "etc." if the remaining/implied conditions are not clearly understood. Use "e.g.," "i.e.," and "etc." only in short parentheticals. Never combine "e.g.," and "etc.," in the same parenthesis.

Examples follow.

We treated patients with upper-airway inflammatory diseases (e.g., PAR).

Or:

The results were consistent across sexes (i.e., male, female).

Not:

We evaluated reproductive-tract inflammatory conditions (e.g., PID, etc.).

Not:

We treated patients who had chronic illnesses (e.g., major depressive disorder consistent with the definition established by the Diagnostic and Statistical Manual [DSM IV] and not by the American Psychiatric Association [APA], which is subject to industry bias). *[This parenthesis is much too long and needs to be recast as a separate sentence.]*

Ellipses: Omitting a verb (often of the infinitive "to be") where it is understood in a series is fine if the subject of the verb does not change.

The diagnosis was established and intervention [was] instituted.

And:

Tests were performed and the results [were] noted in the chart.

Not:

Tests were performed and the report updated. (*The word "report" is singular; hence it requires the singular verb "was."*)

Endpoint: Used chiefly to signify an outcome measure. If you are using this term to signify the date of completion of a study, it is preferable to state:

The present study was conducted from August 11, 2010 (first patient enrolled) to August 10, 2011 (last patient follow-up visit).

Not

The endpoint of the present study was August 10, 2011. *[Distracting by connotation of "endpoint" to "outcome measure."]*

Epidemic: A condition that affects many persons in a defined area and is temporary or time limited is an epidemic. A pandemic spans more than one geographic region (e.g., continent).

Be careful not to overuse. For example, some journal peer reviewers object to statements such as "Because of the growing diabetes epidemic [or pandemic]…." These are not true epidemics/pandemics. In most settings of evidence-based study reports, restrict the use of these words to their intended, infectious-disease contexts.

Eponyms: Use the singular together with a brief parenthetical descriptor, such as:

Turner syndrome (gonadal dysgenesis)

Oppenheim disease (amyotonia congenita)

Follow contemporary standard usage (journal or other style guides) for use of possessive.

The patient developed Parkinson's disease at the age of 61.

Or:

The patient developed parkinsonian signs and symptoms at the age of 61.

Not

The patient developed Parkinsonian signs and symptoms at the age of 61.

Eskimo: Unacceptable racial designation (by analogy to American Indian, which should be replaced with Native American). Substitute "Alaska Native," "Aleut," or "Inuit" (as appropriate).

Etiology: ≠ "cause." Etiology is the study or overall perspective on causes.

Sternutation (sneezing) has a complex etiology.

Not

The etiology of sternutation is antigen-induced irritation of the mucous membranes lining the nose and throat.

Ex ante: Literally "before the event": based on or referring to predictions rather than actual data.

Exculpate: IUVIF. Antonyms = impugn, inculpate.

Follow: Patients are observed or monitored, not "followed." Cases and clinical courses are followed. Avoid patient and reader paranoia.

Following: If you mean "after," use "after." And you usually do mean "after" unless something is truly being followed, in a spatial rather than temporal sense. See also "prior to" (before).

For: Often sets up wordy or passive expressions. As an example, see the text below, from a major consensus guideline concerning manuscript preparation:

Not:

Describe any methods <u>for inferring</u> genotypes or haplotypes.

But:

Describe any methods <u>to infer</u> genotypes and haplotypes.

Fore (overused): Even nongolfers understand that the expression "fore" alerts those ahead of a player that an errant ball is on its way.

"Fore" as a prefix relates to events in the future, e.g., "forewarned is forearmed."

However, the correct spellings of other similar words that have the sense of "doing without" rather than a future event do not include the "e." Examples include "forbear" (verb), "forfeit," "forgo," "forsake," and "forswear."

Forme fruste: An attenuated or atypical disease manifestation.

Antonym is *forme pleine*.

Foster: IUVIF. Others: facilitate, promote.

Gave (provided) the ability to: Allowed or enabled.

Gender: Don't overuse the terms *male* and *female*. Substitute the age-appropriate terms for "male patient" and "female patient," i.e., men and women (≥18 years old) or girls and boys (or youngsters) if ages <18.

Gerund/participle: Use "ing" expressions to economize words. Be careful, because these may set up run-on sentences:

Write the journal requesting an investigation into ethical issues related to a submitted or published manuscript.

[Who is doing the requesting, the person being directed by this sentence, or the journal?]

Greek symbols: Generally, use Greek symbols for generic scientific concepts but not in proper nouns (e.g., drug names). Examples follow.

There is no convincing evidence to support first-line use of β-adrenoceptor blockers [*at first mention;* "β-blockers" *thereafter*] to manage uncomplicated hypertension.

Statistical significance was computed at a two-sided $\alpha = 0.05$.

But not:

Patients with hepatitis C were randomized to placebo or interferon-2-α *[Should be "alfa" as a proper noun (drug name).]*

Or:

Some patients with respiratory diseases are eligible for treatment with β-methasone. *[Should be "betamethasone."]*

Has been shown [demonstrated] to: Redundant at worst, wordy at best; delete if you are citing references and use only if you are not or cannot (e.g., in an abstract).

Bivalirudin is an effective and well-tolerated treatment for acute coronary syndromes.[1–4] (Hypothetical references, here and below.)

Or:

Studies have shown that bivalirudin is an effective and well-tolerated treatment for acute coronary syndromes. *[In the abstract, where references cannot be cited.]*

Not:

Bivalirudin has been shown to be an effective and well-tolerated treatment for acute coronary syndromes.[1–4]

Has the ability to; has the capacity to: Can.

Healthily vs. healthfully: Only a patient is healthy. His or her diet or other regimen may be healthful, in the sense of promoting health, but not healthy.

Heart/kidney/liver failure: A patient is encountered "in" (not "with") heart (cardiac), kidney (renal), or liver (hepatic) failure.

Homogeneous: Don't forget that second "e." People often write or say "homogenous" (*does it have something to do with milk?*).

Hyphen vs. dash: Most prefixes, including "non," "de," "co," "post," "anti," "ultra," "under," and "over" should not be hyphenated unless the same letter follows.

A hyphen is not the same as a "minus" sign. The minus sign is a (1/N) dash (–), which you access from the "symbols" tool in MS Word.

Never hyphenate an adverbial: a "highly publicized study," never a "highly publicized study." See also conjoined adjectives. Use (1/N) dashes to express ranges or to "weight" a conjoined adjective (e.g., "non–drug-dependent," "obsessive-compulsive–like symptoms").

Hyphenate if failing to do so leads to an unintended meaning:

> **Our management approach given these symptoms was to re-treat.** *[Not "retreat"]*

Given the major salary increase and many fringe benefits in the new contract, I decided to re-sign. *[Not "resign"]*

A lesion may form and "re-form." *[Not "reform"]*

Remember also that you can be "detail oriented" (not "detail-oriented") in the adverbial sense, or a "detail-oriented person" in the conjoined adjectival sense.

Avoid lengthy clauses enclosed by (1/M) dashes (or parentheses).

Use a 1/N dash if more than word is modifying another (even when abbreviated):

Nitric oxide–mediated vasodilation reduces total peripheral resistance.

NO–mediated vasodilation reduces total peripheral resistance.

(See also "Dashes," page 105.)

Impart: IUVIF (also: confer [to]).

Imperatives: Avoid expressions such as "the physician should [can]." These read as "preachy" or condescending. Rephrase in passive voice if possible.

Imply/infer: The writer or speaker implies. The audience or reader infers.

Impugn: IUVIF. Synonym = inculpate; antonym = exculpate.

The close temporal association with serious adverse events impugned [inculpated] active treatment as a cause.

Improve (ameliorate) the quality of: Redundant/wordy. Improve or ameliorate means to increase the quality. One can "increase the quality" but not "improve the quality."

Indeed: "A friend in need is a friend indeed." I object to beginning many sentences with "Indeed." Doing so may represent a verbal crutch and a facile attempt to confer "gravitas." Avoid.

Including: Use a comma before if introducing a list.

Increase: IUVIF (depending on context):

Augment

Elevate

Heighten

Potentiate

Raise

Upregulate

Inculpate: IUVIF. Antonym: "exculpate." Synonym "impugn."

Infinitives, split: Strive to avoid them and not to promote their use.

Inflate (or exaggerate): IUVIF to reduce words compared to, e.g., "bias may have spuriously elevated our estimates."

In order to: Use just "to" in most cases. Use "in order to" if "to" is used earlier in the sentence and there is no way to avoid having a second "to" in the sentence.

Institute: IUVIF. Treatment, therapy, or care is instituted. For example,

In the event of rhabdomyolysis, institute mannitol diuresis.

Insuperable attributes: Each of the following uses is incorrect because the adjectives are categorical rather than continuous in nature (present or absent but not different degrees):

We sat in a perfect circle.

This trial had a very [most] unique design.

Intended: Be careful. Use of this modifier may imply that an objective was established but not met.

Interrogate: IUVIF. One may interrogate a clinical database to seek answers to problems.

Irrespective: Or "regardless," but not "irregardless."

It (starting sentence): In a letter to me, the late rhetorician William Safire stated, "Sentences beginning with 'It is' are boring." Try to avoid and/or recast.

Pomposity, not zeal for clear communication, prompts writers to be verbose.

Not:

It is pomposity and not zeal for clear communication that prompts writers to be verbose.

Niacin causes untoward cutaneous effects.[1-5] (Hypothetical references)

Not:

It has been demonstrated that [or "It is important to note that; It should be observed that; It is undeniable that; It has been shown that; It has been found that"] niacin causes untoward cutaneous effects.

When composing a style manual, <u>it is the tendency of</u> some authors to excessively rely on the guidance of Luddites.

[This sentence has two defects. Can you detect them? Take a moment, then examine the sentence below.]

But:

When composing a style manual, some <u>authors</u> *[in the above, the phrase "it is the tendency" was not only wordy but also did not agree with its antecedent ("authors")* <u>tend to rely excessively</u> *[split infinitive in the above]* on the guidance of Luddites.

Italic vs. Roman: Do not italicize expressions that have been well assimilated into English (e.g., in vivo, in vitro, vice versa). Italicize panel letters in more exotic Latin or foreign phrases (e.g., *ex ante, forme fruste*).

Lead/led: I hate to do this but have to!

Get the "Lead" Out!: The past tense of the verb "to lead" is "led."

You might be surprised to learn how many times we encounter this as "lead," e.g., "Our study lead to the following conclusions." Oh, really? Elemental lead (Pb), or alloyed with something else?

Please come down from the "ferrous wheel" and spell the word correctly!

"Leading": There is only one leader. Avoid examples such as "obesity is the third-leading cause of cardiovascular disease." How can this be so? Substitute the verb "ranked" for "leading."

Leading zero: I include this in all decimals, including p values. However, defer to the prevailing style of the journal targeted.

In a table, avoid using, e.g., 0.0, 0.00 even if these are consistent with the number of significant figures elsewhere in the table. Doing so strikes me as the height (or nadir?) of pedantry. Zero is just that: 0!

Like: In the 1970s, grammarians had a field day with an advertising campaign purporting that a tobacco product "tastes good, like a cigarette should." Use "as" in most such cases.

Not:

Like I said, the data are inadequate to draw a conclusion.

But:

As I said, the data are inadequate to draw a conclusion.

Look at, looking at: In my world (standard written, not colloquial, English), reviews and studies don't "look at" anything. They evaluate, assess, evaluate, investigate, test, examine, probe, ascertain, or appraise.

MACE: A terrific medical acronym.

Major adverse cardiac events—typically CAD death, nonfatal MI, and/or revascularization. Expand at first mention.

MACE rates declined in actively treated subjects.

Manage (dehumanizing): Diseases, disorders, conditions, syndromes, or cases are managed. Patients receive treatment, therapy, or care, but are not "managed."

Matching placebo: Redundant. If it doesn't match, it's not a placebo.

Mathematical operators, numbers: Use whenever you can (next to units of measure) to reduce numbers of words...See journal style.

Unless expressly prohibited by journal style, use Arabic numerals to express quantities of 10 or higher (≥10) or with units (of time or other measure), the 1/N dash for ranges, and mathematical operators (>, <) in parentheses. Avoid these practices when the entity is unitless or the context dictates Roman numerals.

Treatment with more than two [not >2] agents in this class is not recommended.

The normal range for LDL cholesterol is 0–130 mg/dL.

Not:

Normal values for LDL cholesterol range from 0–130 mg/dL.

Not:

Platelet counts in the range of 100,000/mm³ are considered normal. [*One value does not constitute a range.*]

Spell a number when in opposition to another digit, even if the first number is zero to nine:

On the third day of Christmas, my purchasing manager gave to me: three 25-mL syringes, two 5-L bags of O negative, and a partridge in a pear tree.

Me vs. my: American users of gerunds/participles tend to use the possessive "my," whereas British users tend to use "me." Adapt according to journal style:

US: I hope you don't mind my taking your patient's pulse.

UK: I hope you don't mind me taking your patient's pulse.

Medical misspellings: Some misspellings "fly under the radar" of electronic spellcheckers because they are also valid words:

Complaint (compliant), compliant (complaint), creatine (creatinine; *and vice versa, check meaning*), dairy (diary), infraction (infarction), inoccuous or inocuous (*should be "innocuous"*), innoculate (*should be "inoculate"*), relive (relieve), and trail (trial).

Menopause: Menopause, or the climacteric (cessation of menses), is a time of life and not a medical condition. Are there signs and symptoms associated with the virtual cessation of estrogen output? Of course. Is there possibly even a manageable "postmenopausal syndrome," including acute hot flushes and vaginal atrophy? Arguably. But "menopause" or "post-menopause" as a medical condition? I am not persuaded. Ditto "partial androgen deficiency of the aging male." Each of these expressions is, on its face, potentially judgmental, refers to populations (rather than individual patients), and may spuriously suggest a "need to replenish" "deficient" levels of the reproductive hormone.

Mild-to-moderate: ≠ "mild or moderate." Use only to imply a continuum.

Minimum effective dose: Like "coronary heart disease," this term is so misleading that one almost needs to rethink it to fathom the users' true intent. Substitute "minimum dose effective."

Minuscule: This is the preferred (first-listed) spelling, not "miniscule."

Mitigate: ≠ "militate against." The former has a favorable resonance (e.g., to lessen or "commute" something noxious), whereas the latter suggests an undermining or countervailing force.

Modifiers: dangling, misplaced, wayward:

Walking down the ward, our pagers went off simultaneously.

Driving through Boston, our eyes saw Brigham and Women's.

But:

Driving through Boston, we got carsick and went to Brigham and Women's.

Not:

As a nurse practitioner, it is my obligation (no antecedent) to write correct prescriptions.

But:

As a nurse practitioner, I have an obligation to write correct prescriptions.

And:

Trials using statins to lower LDL cholesterol have reported 25% to 35% reductions in CHD events, including death, nonfatal MI, revascularization, and unstable angina, after 5 years of treatment ….

Not:

Trials using statins to lower LDL cholesterol have reported 25% to 35% reductions in <u>CHD events</u> after 5 years of treatment, <u>including</u> death, nonfatal MI, revascularization, and unstable angina….

Braunwald reported at the American College of Cardiology congress that 12 placebo controls with atrial fibrillation in the WARSS trial experienced strokes.

Not:

Braunwald reported that 12 patients with atrial fibrillation in the WARSS trial experienced strokes at the American College of Cardiology congress. (?!)

Monitor: Patients are not monitored or "followed"; adverse events and clinical conditions are monitored, whereas patients receive follow-up. The use of "elevated index of clinical suspicion" is permitted if there is no "monitoring" of "suspicious" patients.

Mortality/mortality rate: Sorry to be grim, but mortality is 100%; death is inevitable. (However, watch this space for future developments!)

No medication or other intervention can reduce mortality, though it may reduce "premature mortality" or mortality over a certain time span (i.e., "mortality rate"). Therefore, only a mortality rate (or mortality over some time interval or age-standardized mortality rate) should be reported.

The 2-year crude mortality rate was 75% lower in the actively treated compared with the control study arm.

Not:

Mortality was 75% lower in the treated group compared with controls.

Conversely, "longevity" and "survival" are not categorical variables (dead, or not dead?) but continuous ones (how many years lived?). Hence, it is permissible and even desirable to state that a medication increased longevity (expressed as mean [SD] or median [IQR] years of life). Longevity has an unfixed, variable upper (right) limit, unlike mortality, which is fixed. Hence, a medication can increase longevity but cannot reduce mortality (only premature mortality, death over a specified interval, or the mortality rate).

Most well: = Best.

The Lowry method is the best-known protein assay.

Not:

The Lowry method is the most-well-known protein assay.

Nadir: Useful antonym to "peak."

Nauseous vs. nauseated: A person can be nauseated or experience nausea. However, the term "nauseous" refers to something causing disgust or nausea, not the state of being nauseated.

Neither, nor: "Neither, nor" constructions often warrant singular verb forms (unless each entity is plural). Do not use "nor" without "neither." Nor should you start a sentence with "nor" (unless it's "Nor-… epinephrine!")

Number at front of sentence: Avoid spelling out, particularly if you then must also spell the unit of measure. Rephrase to introduce the Arabic numeral.

A total of 66 (22%) of 300 patients had fever.

In all, 66 (22%) of 300 patients had fever.

Or:

Of 300 patients, 66 (22%) had fever.

Not:

Sixty-six (22%) of 300 patients had fever.

Object (n.): A topic is the "object" (not "subject") of consideration, because it is the entity that is being considered or debated.

Of the: Wordy and usually can be deleted. Yet, it is amazing how frequently one finds this in writing, even in highly authoritative consensus guidelines. It adds nothing but verbal clutter!

Not:

All <u>of the</u> items in the CONSORT guidelines should be followed.

But:

All items in the CONSORT guidelines should be followed.

Or (more active and concise)

Follow all items in the CONSORT guidelines.

Optimalization [*sic*]: I have seen it published. Should be "optimization."

Or (restrictive): To signify nonrestrictive clauses, each of the following sentences should have a comma before the word "or":

Are the data paired or unpaired? *[Yes, they must be!]*

But:

Are the data paired, or unpaired?

"Mr. Gutkin, would you like the lobster bisque or the coquille St. Jacques?" *[Yes, please!]*

Pancreata: Plural of pancreas.

Parallel structure: I cherish elegant serial expressions, which reflect thoughtful analysis with adroit synthesis by the writer. In a serial expression, use the same forms of verbs throughout:

Exercising at or near VO_{2max} augments collateral circulation, lowers heart rate, and builds lean muscle mass. *[Lovely!]*

Not (what one usually encounters:)

Exercising at or near VO_{2max} **augments collateral circulation, heart rate is lower, and lean muscle mass is increased.**

Patient vs. subject: Individuals become patients after developing illnesses. Once enrolled in clinical trials, they become study participants or subjects. The generic "individual" covers all contexts, although it represents an adaption of an adjective as a noun and may hence be objectionable to some.

"Patient" vs. "data": In observational studies, it is sometimes tempting to write "patients were eligible if...." or "patients were censored if..." In fact, such intransitive verbs often relate only to patients' data. To state that "patients were eligible if" may connote a prospective study design rather than an actual retrospective design, misleading readers.

Regimens [*not patients*] **are switched.**

I also too frequently see patients dehumanized in the following type of usage:

We treated only patients that [*should be "who"*] **were eligible.**

Pediatric patients (dehumanizing and imprecise): Avoid. Substitute age-appropriate terms (e.g., infant, adolescent; see **"Age referents"**on page 101)..

Pauci-: This prefix signifies a small number, by analogy to "paucity." (E.g., "Late Lyme disease often presents with pauciarticular arthritis.")

Phagocytose: Not "phagocytize." (I have encountered the latter in published papers.)

Place on (*dehumanizing and jargony*): Do not use when referring to administering or instituting treatment.

Not:

For pain management, the patient was placed on a PCA pump.

[In the words of former US talk-show host David Letterman, "and you know how painful that can be!"]

But:

For pain management, the patient received a PCA pump.

Potentiate: IUVIF. Approximate antonym of "attenuate."

Practicable: An action that can be practiced is "practicable."

Presently: Means "soon." "Currently" means now.

I will visit the metabolic ward presently.

At present, I am evaluating a patient for diabetic ketoacidosis in the metabolic ward.

Pressor: Adjective. Blood-pressure–raising effect. Antonym is depressor.

Presume vs. assume: Presumption has a lower level of certainty compared to assumption. An American has the "presumption (not "assumption") of innocence until proven guilty."

Prevalence: Should be expressed as a percentage or ratio, not a number.

Need to specify point versus period versus lifetime (see Table 2.7).

The point prevalence of whooping cough is 0.1% of the immunized, and 1% of the nonimmunized, US population.

Or:

Approximately 1 million Americans will experience whooping cough at some time in their lives.

Not:

The prevalence of whooping cough in the United States is 750,000.

Primum non nocere: Latin for "First do no harm." This phrase is not found anywhere in the Hippocratic Oath.

Prior to, in advance of: Substitute "before." Also "after" instead of "following" or "subsequent to."

Principal vs. principle: The "principal" is your "pal." Principle is a belief or property.

Probability (observed): I once committed the following to a manuscript and was scolded (and "scalded!") by an über-statistician:

> "The observed probability differed widely from the projected probability."

The problem? Only frequencies (not probabilities) are observed.

I reworded to:

The observed frequency differed widely from the projected probability.

Proclivity/propensity: The evidence-based and more neutral (non anthropomorphic) term is "imbalance." For instance

The study population had a slight imbalance [*not "proclivity" or "propensity"*] of women (female: male ratio = 1.18).

On the other hand,

Veterans of foreign military conflicts may have a lower propensity of reporting major depressive disorder because they experience stigma.

[Or:]

Veterans are less apt to report major depressive disorder because they experience stigma.

Produce (v.): FUVIA. If you want to be a "producer," go to Hollywood (or Bollywood!). This is a grossly overused verb in medical communications. Avoid "these studies produced the following results…" or, worse, "this drug has produced favorable efficacy and tolerability data."

Proper nouns/names: Avoid capitalizing nouns that are not names.

The Framingham Heart Study was highly influential.

But:

As shown by the Framingham study, low HDL cholesterol is associated with increased cardiovascular risk.

Dr. Morton Pram is chief of pediatrics [*not "Chief of Pediatrics"*] at Immaculate Conception Hospital.

But:

Dr. Morton Pram is the Donna Shalala Distinguished Chair of Pediatrics at Immaculate Conception Hospital. [*Given the pediatric discipline, this may be a "High Chair" if not a "high-chair!"*]

Proven: Archaic as the past form of the verb "to prove."

However, the use of "proven" in the adjectival form is permissible.

This study has proved that positive inotropes are indicated in emergent care of low-output syndrome.

Or:

Positive inotropes have proven benefits in emergent care of low-output syndrome.

But not:

This study has proven that positive inotropes are indicated in emergent care of low-output syndrome.

Providing that: Should be "provided that" if used in this limited logical/rhetorical sense.

Punctuation: Use the serial comma before "and." [Don't be a "serial killer."] Place both commas and periods inside quotation marks and reference numbers, semicolons, and colons outside (unless otherwise stipulated by PRJ AGs). Use a semicolon to separate two very closely related sentences or to help punctuate longer or complex series, especially those with components including "and" or "or." Use a colon to introduce a series.

Symptoms of seasonal allergic rhinitis include:

- **congestion**
- **runny nose and**
- **itchy eyes.**

Or:

Symptoms of seasonal allergic rhinitis include

- **congestion, which is believed to be secondary to histamine-induced vasodilation with increased perfusion;**

- **runny nose, which may be related to leukotriene- and histamine-induced rises in secretory activity; and**

- **itchy eyes.**

p value: Unless otherwise advised, use roman lower case "p" because it is the most efficient way (even after factoring in the time to program a "macro"). Use p = 0.04 with the leading 0 and space on either side of the operator. Many journals require that p values be preceded by the test used (e.g., ANOVA, Student's *t*-test) and degrees of freedom, which is indicated as a subscript, e.g., $\chi_3^2 = 15.5$; p = 0.02. Report both the p value and the 95% CI or other prespecified confidence interval.

Always try to report the actual p value rather than a category, e.g., p = 0.039; not p < 0.05

p = 0.067; not p > 0.05 or p = NS.

Prefer two-tailed/sided over one-tailed/sided p values; there is usually no statistical benefit of using one-tailed/sided tests.

Race/ethnicity: Racial characteristics are genetic; ethnicities, cultural.

What makes a group an ethnicity is that they are not in the majority of a population.

Persons of African descent include African Americans and Afro-Caribbeans.

Persons of African descent, of course, are not necessarily African *Americans* (e.g., in a European population!).

"Asian" encompasses East Asian (Islander) and Southeast Asian (Islander).

"Eurasian" includes persons from India and Pakistan.

"Alaska Natives" include Aleuts and Inuits.

"Latino" or "Hispanic" is a term of ethnicity, not race.

Conversely "non-Hispanic white (or black)" is a racial term.

Ranked: See "leading."

Rash (redundant): "Skin rash" or "cutaneous rash" is redundant.

Rather than, Instead of: Maintain parallel construction before and after.

Rather than escalate the dose of either drug, introduce an adjunctive treatment with a complementary MOA.

Not:

Rather than **escalating** the dose of either drug, **introduce** an adjunctive treatment with a complementary MOA.

Redundant, wordy

Advanced planning
Brief in time (or duration)
Consensus of opinion (or general consensus)
Draws to a close [*concludes*]; brings to fruition [*completes*]
Due to the fact that [*because*]
During the time that [*during, while*]
Each individual person
Fellow colleagues
Fewer in number
Fill to capacity
General rule (or general consensus)
Green in color (or hue, tint)
Had (or exerted) an effect on [*affected, influenced*]
Heralds the onset of [*predicts*]
In close proximity to [*near*]
In terms of, in regard to [*about or concerning*]
Major breakthrough
Majority of [most]
Matching placebo
Mild or moderate in severity
Out of: 4 (10%) of 40, not 4 (10%) out of 40
Precede in time
Produce an inhibitory effect on [*inhibit*]
Skin (or cutaneous) rash
Small in size (or extent)
Smooth in texture
Soft in consistency
Sour tasting
Sum total
Tender to palpation (or to the touch)
Uniformly consistent

Refractory (dehumanizing): A condition, not a patient, may be refractory to treatment.

Regimen: Fine alternative for a pharmacotherapy. It should include both the drug and dosage (with administration route and frequency). Do not confuse with "regime," which does not always carry a health connotation. Regimens ("not patients") are switched (or altered).

Registrant: A participant in a patient registry.

Regurgitate (figurative): Don't. If numerical data are reported in Results tables, there is no need to repeat them in the Results text. Instead, point out the key relationships (e.g., trends, directions, p values) and refer readers to the table. If, on the other hand, the only data are contained within a figure that does not disclose numbers, but you have numerical data used to generate the figure, try to include them.

Relative to: Unless someone is truly related (e.g., a kindred to a proband), do not substitute "relative to" for "compared to/with."

Repeat (adj.): ≠ "repeated." If a test is repeated, state the number of repetitions.

A second MRI suggested a meningeal lesion.

Not:

Repeat MRI suggested a meningeal lesion.

Repeated words, prolix: *Not:*

Results **from** this study and **from** published reports support the same conclusion.

But:

Results from this study and published reports support the same conclusion.

From an online policy:

Not:

"We protect **your** privacy, **your** data, and put you in control."

[Nonparallel construction and needless repetition of "your!"]

But:

"We protect your privacy and data, and put you in control."

However, in the "Amidah" of the Jewish prayer book is the phrase "G-d of Abraham, G-d of Isaac, and G-d of Jacob." Why? The repetition signifies that each prophet had his own, individual relationship with the deity.

Respectively: Avoid such constructions. Forces the reader to go back in sentence to find the antecedents.

Restrictive clauses: A restrictive-clause riddle:

Q: How would you survive in the desert with no food?

A: On the "sand which is" there!

Be careful when using restrictive clauses. They can undermine meaning and set up infelicitous expression (e.g., run-on sentences).

Not:

The patient was referred to the operating room (OR) where he underwent open reduction and internal fixation for a fractured right femur. *[Implies that the patient visited more than one OR.]*

An errant US bomb exploded in a Kunduz, Afghanistan hospital killing 100 patients. *[Implies that the hospital was killing patients!]*

Robust: Prefer to use mainly in the strict biostatistical sense of not being affected by changes in assumptions. Do not overuse as a way of exaggerating the importance of findings.

Run-on sentence (ROS): Often set into motion by repetition of "ing" forms of verbs and relative pronouns.

Two witches make a curse, whereas two "whiches" often make a ROS.

Salt: ≠ "sodium." Typically, we mention the salts with which drugs are formulated only at first mention unless a complex formulation might otherwise be confused.

Define at first mention, then use chemical name afterward. For example, "Sildenafil citrate has been available to men with erectile dysfunction for nearly 20 years. A contingent agonist of the male sexual response, sildenafil was the first US–approved PDE5 inhibitor for this indication."

Salubrious: Healthful.

Salutary: Favorable, especially to patients' health. Antonym: deleterious

Saw, seen: ≠ attended or treated. A patient is attended or treated by a physician, which constitutes much more than "being seen" (which is also jargony).

Sign (vs. symptom): Symptoms (or complaints) are experienced by patients, whereas signs are observed by clinicians and/or via tests.

Marked rises in CK are signs of statin-induced myopathy.

And:

Myalgia that cannot be attributed to physical exertion may be a symptom of evolving statin-induced rhabdomyolysis.

Not:

Ipsilateral pupil dilation is a symptom of elevated intracranial pressure and/or cerebral edema after stroke.

Not:

Myalgia is a sign of incipient rhabdomyolysis.

Set (singular/plural): Because of a strong connotation of singularity, each of the following is correct:

> A battery of tests <u>was</u> administered.
>
> The H&P <u>did</u> not raise suspicion of tropical infection.
>
> D&C <u>is</u> indicated to assess a potential ectopic pregnancy.

Since: ≠ "because"; use the latter to signify causality. "Since" has a time connotation. See also "whereas"/while."

SI Units: Use Standard International Units (e.g., mmol/l) for most, non–US or non–UK publications. Consult peer-reviewed journal Author Guidelines (PRJ AGs).

If the PRJ AG permits, provide SI–English unit conversion factors, especially in table footnotes.

Subject: Individuals or patients enrolled in a study are subjects or study participants. Also useful as a verb.

The study design was subject to bias.

Writers drawing conclusions from biased findings may be subjected to a scolding by the journal referees!

A topic being debated is the "object," not "subject," of consideration. (It is the thing being considered, and hence an object, not subject.)

Such as: Use a comma before if introducing a list in the nonrestrictive (adding, nonessential) sense (first example below) and no comma if introducing a particular quality or attribute in the restrictive (naming or defining) sense (second example).

Symptoms of asthma, such as wheezing and cough, are amenable to inhaled corticosteroid treatment.

But:

Lower-airway symptoms such as bronchiectasis are often refractory to antihistamines.

Technique (vs. method): Technique is the level of one's prowess, not a method.

The methods relied on enrollment of surgeons with acceptable technique.

Tense: What bad writing makes me! Be as consistent as you can but not so rigid as to preclude rational shifts. For instance, you may use the past tense when discussing data in a study and the present tense when describing or reporting a stable or persistent quality or attribute.

A CDC registry showed that indiscriminate use of broad-spectrum antibiotics increased the likelihood of vancomycin-resistant staphylococci.

But:

Indiscriminate use of broad-spectrum antibiotics increases the likelihood of vancomycin-resistant staphylococci, according to a CDC registry.

The Scandinavian Simvastatin Survival Study demonstrated that statin therapy significantly reduced the probability of recurrent MI (vs. placebo and usual care) and was well tolerated.

But:

Statin therapy significantly reduces the probability of recurrent MI (vs. placebo and usual care) and is well tolerated, according to findings from the Scandinavian Simvastatin Survival Study.

That: Often can be deleted in the interest of verbal economy (as can the pronoun "who").

Aspirin was both effective and well tolerated in a double-blind trial of 38 patients <u>discontinuing</u> therapy because of adverse events.

The: In general, I object to the practice of capitalizing "The" ("The Johns Hopkins Hospital") unless this is the actual institutional identity. In many instances, "the" can be omitted. The article in "The Netherlands" is "The" national identity and hence should not be omitted.

The (*wordy*): The (hospital, clinic). American users tend to state, "The patient was admitted to <u>the</u> hospital (or was hospitalized)" or "The patient was seen in <u>the</u> clinic." UK users tend to leave out what Americans (wrongly, in my view) believe is a necessary article ("the"). I prefer the UK version because it is more concise and equally clear:

The patient was seen in clinic, then admitted to hospital.

Patients were randomly allocated to receive spastex or placebo.

Not:

The patients were randomly allocated to receive spastex or placebo. *[What purpose does "the" serve?]*

Not

Aspirin was both effective and well tolerated in a double-blind trial that involved 38 patients who had discontinued prior therapy because of adverse events.

Also

Thomson Reuters warrants that, if used properly, the *Physicians' Desk Reference* should help to prevent prescribing errors. *[The comma "that" is needed.]*

It is often possible to remove relative pronouns:

Medication-adherent patients *(not "Patients who adhered to medication regimens")* had superior outcomes.

Those which (who; *wordy*): Avoid. Use the word "those" freely to economize:

Patients receiving PUVA exhibited lower PASI scores than those receiving topical coal tar.

Or (much better because more consolidated):

Patients receiving PUVA (vs. topical coal tar) exhibited lower PASI.

Not:

Those patients who received PUVA exhibited lower PASI scores compared with those patients who received PUVA alone.

To (caveat): Positioned at the head of a sentence, this preposition often sets up a dangling modifier:

Not:

To evaluate the effects of spastex on belching frequency, patients were randomized (2:1) to active treatment or placebo.

But:

To evaluate the effects of spastex on belching frequency, we randomized patients (2:1) to active treatment or placebo.

Toward: Favor over the archaic "towards."

Toxic/dehumanizing: Toxicity is a condition. As with "case," "diabetic," or "hypertensive," a patient is not reducible to his or her "toxicity."

The patient's acitretin toxicity manifested as cheilitis.

Not:

She was toxic from her retinoid, so we lowered her acitretin dose. *[This is also jargon.]*

Trade (proprietary) names: Avoid unless journal style calls for these, in which case include in parentheses only at the first mention of the generic/chemical name, along with the manufacturer. However, do not use a trade name in an article title unless expressly permitted or required by the journal.

Treatment/treated: Only the active-treatment group is "treated." The control group "receives placebo (or usual care)."

Utilize/employ: FUVIA. These have specific connotations. If you mean "use," use "use." (!)

Vasodilation: Preferred over "vasodilatation." Adjectival is "vasodilator," not "vasodilatory."

Versus/vs.: Use abbreviation "vs." only in parentheses or tables. Avoid using "vs." or "versus" in text, especially display type (e.g., manuscript titles). Substitute "compared with," "compared to," "as compared with" (in longer sentences), or "as against" (UK). In short comparisons, it is permissible to use "than." See "Comparisons" above.

Which: The antecedent of "which" must be clear. Typically, it is inferred to be the immediately preceding clause. "Which" is often used in a rhetorically lazy manner:

Not:

Cholestyramine is nonsystemic, which suggests that it will be better tolerated by many patients. *[Huh? There is no antecedent.]*

But:

Ezetimibe has a favorable tolerability profile, which may be consistent with superior patient acceptance compared to bile acid sequestrants.

[The antecedent is clearly "profile," which is correctly placed immediately before "which."]

While: Has a time connotation. (See also above "since/because.") Substitute "whereas" or "although" if these are the intended meanings.

Who have (wordy) Patients with diabetes (*not the dehumanizing "Diabetics"*) may experience fatigue.

Not:

Patients (*or, worse "Those patients"*) who have diabetes may experience fatigue.

Years' experience: I have 30 years of experience as a medical writer. Hence, I also have the "experience of 30 years" or 30 years' experience (possessive). Check your CV!

3

Biostatistics: Issues in study design, analysis, and reporting

CHAPTER OBJECTIVES

The aims of this chapter are to:

- Introduce methodologies of biostatistics, including both the potential strengths and limitations of different study designs.
- Discuss the implications, on the selection of statistical tests, of different types of data, including continuous versus categorical and paired versus unpaired, and their distributions, such as normal versus skewed.
- Explain the nature of hypothesis testing and answer the question, "What does a p value signify?"
- Work through exercises that highlight the underlying principles and logic of statistical tests via "old-school" (paper-and-pencil) means, and do-it-yourself guidance to perform selected statistical tests and projections using Microsoft Excel's functions and other widely available programs.

Statistics is the grammar of science.

Karl Pearson

3.1 STATISTICS: *STURM UND DRANG*

Biostatistics (henceforth "statistics") is rife with terminology and concepts that can confuse even the most experienced scientists and communicators.

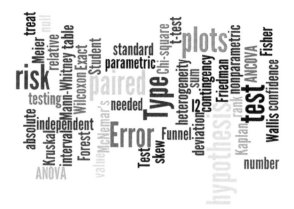

This chapter systematically and methodically walks you through the basics of scientific logic and statistical testing, but first, to get you started, a brief digression into a common and easy form of "small talk."

When folks complain about the weather, I am often reminded of statistics. For many, the issue is being "left in the dark" (or cold) about imminent ambient conditions. With few exceptions, no topic "leads" the evening news like impending storms or cleaning up in their aftermath: the wrath (or other acts) of G-d. Why do you suppose that is? Ruined outdoor plans? Frostbitten houseplants? "External locus of control?" Difficulty "avoiding a draft?"

The connection to statistics? Weather forecasts are based on statistical models to project the likelihood of future events based on limited data. A major challenge to meteorologists, and, more importantly to us, medical writers (MWs) and other researchers and communicators, is to not only comprehend but clearly disclose the statistical methods used to estimate outcomes.

In science, we rarely reason deductively based on sure logical principles but rather inductively and empirically, based on an often-challenging limit of evidence. Readers of our work need to understand these parameters. E.T. Jaynes has written that scientists must accept the ascendancy of a less certain, probabilistic, form of "plausible reasoning" (*epagoge*) over Aristotle's brand of deductive reasoning (*apodeixis*).[1] The latter includes rock-solid syllogisms such as:

> "If *A* is true, then *B* is true
> <u>*A* is true</u>
> Ergo, B is true;
> *and*:
> If *A* is true, then *B* is true
> <u>*B* is false</u>
> Ergo, *A* is false."[1]

In the above context, weather forecasts are based on predictive statistical models whose logic and inner workings are often played closely to the TV meteorologist's vest (which, for a very long time, could never be green!). These include parameters of accuracy, reliability, and precision. We sometimes focus on preponderant probabilities (e.g., "a 90% chance of rain") and brush off the "other 10%."

Compared to these "prognostic peccadilloes," the more enduring anomalies are the big "hits and misses": failures to disclose the structures, parameters, and assumptions of statistical models and their outputs.

In 2015, a storm of epic proportions was predicted in my corner of the world. The purported "Historic Weather Event of 2015?" Never happened! In the parlance of statistics, the prediction of this "non-event" is termed a "false positive." Tests and models with high specificity tend to filter these out and rather detect true negatives. In the realm of population screening, highly specific tests accurately identify individuals without disease, helping to ensure that healthy people do not receive a treatment that could potentially harm them. For instance, in cervical cancer screening, a false-positive human papillomavirus screening result could lead to colposcopy, which may cause a woman not only anxiety about the procedure but also potential, though infrequent, complications at a later date.

On the other hand, my recollection is that Hurricane Sandy, which actually did blight my region of the northeastern United States, reached much greater dimensions than predicted. Along with our neighbors, my family and I heated our home from the hearth for the better part of 2 weeks. Statisticians term such underestimates "false negatives." Tests and models with high sensitivity tend to filter these out and rather detect true positives. In the same screening example, highly sensitive tests accurately identify patients with a disease, helping to ensure that they are appropriately treated.

The idea of "plausible reasoning" was developed by Hungarian mathematician George Pólya (Pólya György; December 13, 1887–September 7, 1985).[2] In plausible reasoning, within our scientific investigations, we often encounter a premise such as the following[1]:

"If A is true, then B is true
B is true
Ergo, A becomes more plausible."[1]

Consistent with our meteorological example, Jaynes offers the following[1]:

A = "It will start to rain by 8 AM at the latest."
B = "The sky will become cloudy before 8 AM."[1]

What happens if we observe clouds at 7:45 AM? Although we're not certain of imminent rain, we may change our behaviors, such as digging out our "brolly" ("bumbershoot"), "Mac," and "wellies," under the strong suspicion of its arrival. (I use British slang when thinking about rainy weather!) As Jaynes points out, when the human brain intuitively projects from limited data it may assess the degree of plausibility by factoring in other variables from previous experiences. These experiences might include the darkness of the clouds, a damp smell in the air, or even pain in an arthritic joint. Whereas these considerations relate largely to human intuition, other factors could be built into a

statistical model of the likelihood of rain between 7:45 and 8 AM, including changes in barometric pressure during this interval.

Other weak syllogisms that we often accept in science as forms of plausible reasoning run as follows[1]:

"If A is true, then B is true
A is false
Ergo, B becomes less plausible;
or (the even weaker):
If A is true, then B becomes more plausible
B is true
Ergo, A becomes more plausible."[1]

The lesson for researchers in biological sciences: participants in (and reporters of) statistical analyses? It is not sufficient to employ statistics. To be completely transparent and accountable, we must also disclose the requirements, assumptions, and other parameters of our tests, models, and resulting data. Failing this, we risk eliciting *"sturm and drang"* in our readers, including journal referees, key opinion leaders (KOLs), other clinicians, patients and patient advocacy groups, regulatory authorities, third-party payers, and health policymakers. In many cases, a certain statistical assessment or model is chosen from among many other, perfectly suitable alternatives; these choices are not free of value judgments. It was only during the run-up to Hurricane Sandy that I learned of the presence of competing forecasting models: US and European.

3.1.1 Micro … Starting small

The word "statistics" has three "t"s and two "i"s: Cross and dot them!

In Biblical terms, the most important chapter to MWs and medical editors (MEs) is not Genesis, Exodus, Leviticus, or Deuteronomy but "Numbers!" Numbers of patients or observations in studies and their reported data often vary considerably across different populations and analyses (e.g., safety, intent-to-treat [ITT], per-protocol [PP] populations). Information concerning certain variables is inevitably missing or incomplete, leading us to a plurality of denominators for percentages and other calculations. (These disparities often need to be footnoted in tables.)

Of most medical communications submitted for peer review, my "back-of-napkin" estimate is that 75% of journalistic "column inches" comprise words; the rest are numbers, tables, graphs, and other non-verbal signifiers. Yet many MWs and even scientific researchers experience anxiety (or even dread) about statistics and thus profess or feign ignorance. They do so at their own peril, because, in many ways, statisticians often hold the "keys to the kingdom" of research—and hence dictate the way we report it.

This chapter helps you to understand the logic and "mechanics" of statistical analyses, including implications, for choosing statistical tests, of different types (e.g., continuous vs. categorical) and distributions (e.g., symmetrical vs. asymmetrical) of data; as well as different forms of statistical error, bias, and confounding, and ways to adjust for or control them. In the terminology introduced in Chapter 1 ("Literacy" vs. "Numeracy"), the previous chapters were intended largely to increase the "literacy of the numerate," whereas this one seeks to augment the "numeracy of the literate." [Just as Chapter 4 of the "Gutkin Manual" conveys consensus guidelines to prepare different types of study reports, guidance for many statistical procedures can be found in the Statistical Analyses and Methods in the Published Literature (SAMPL) guidelines. (Available at: www.equator-network. org/reporting-guidelines/sampl/. Last accessed March 10, 2018.)

Nothing scuttles the enterprise of a writing project so readily as evident, and usually avoidable, errors in conducting, and reporting data from, statistical analyses (Table 3.1).[3] These mishaps include defects in study design, inadequate understanding and documentation of methods, as well as reporting of data that are either imprecise (i.e., "internally inconsistent") or inaccurate (i.e., "externally inconsistent").

In his excellent textbook *Statistics in Medicine* (which I strongly recommend), Dr. Robert H. Riffenburgh cites four desirable properties of statistics.[4] (I have added the fifth and sixth below.)

- Unbiased: After computing the statistic for a parameter from all samples of differing numbers (n) from a population, we would find that the mean equals the parameter.
- Sufficient: The statistic provided is the most informative possible for a study sample population.
- Efficient: Minimum error results from estimates of the parameter using the statistic.
- Consistent: As the sample size (of the study population) approaches the overall (real-world, general) population, the estimate converges on the parameter.
- Consequential: Statistical significance should not be equated with (or claimed as) clinical significance; the latter should be based on quantitative and validated thresholds (e.g., minimum clinically important differences [MCIDs]; see Appendix 1 of the "Gutkin Manual.")
- Defensible: The selection of a test or overall analysis should be sound and unassailable from statistical, biological, and clinical perspectives. One example of indefensible analyses is to categorize an inherently continuous outcome measure without providing boundaries for precision and statistical confidence. Such categorizations of continuous measures should also comport with prevailing biological theory. For instance, serum uric acid (sUA) levels represent a continuous variable. Suppose that investigators evaluating a new medication for gout target, in an efficacy "responder analysis," a mean sUA level after treatment of < 8 mg/dL. The problem? Evidence suggests that sUA levels < 6 mg/dL are associated with freedom from acute attacks of gout and reduction of proinflammatory monosodium urate (MSU) crystals in joints and soft tissues, including tophi.[5] In this case, the researchers established an overly conservative efficacy threshold (< 8 mg/dL). Had they established a cut-point of sUA < 6 mg/dL (ideally with accompanying confidence or other precision limits), their analysis strategy would have been defensible.

"Measure twice; cut once."
Familiar carpenter's watchwords.

On the rare occasions when I have a "2 × 4" and nails in my hands, a blood transfusion is usually in the offing! That said, planning a statistical analysis is arguably more consequential than drafting a manuscript. Although both processes are often iterative, the consequences of a poor Statistical Analysis Plan or Data Analysis Plan (SAP/DAP), once codified as a study protocol, may be irrevocable. After your initially planned statistical test returns a statistically nonsignificant (p > 0.05) result, you might be tempted to repeat the test,

Table 3.1 Common avoidable statistical errors in reports of medical research

Defect	Example
Study design.	Did not clearly state study aims and primary outcome measures.
	Failed to report number of participants or observations (sample size; did not report numbers of withdrawals or subjects with missing/unavailable data).
	Did not perform/report an *a priori* sample size calculation/effect-size estimation (power calculation).
	Did not state *a priori* the null hypothesis (for studies in which inferential statistics are performed).
	Failed to use and report randomization (method of randomization not clearly stated).
	Failed to use and report blinding.
	Failed to report initial equality of baseline characteristics and comparability of study groups.
	Used inappropriate control group.
	Inappropriately tested for equality of baseline characteristics.
Data analysis.	Used wrong statistical tests: tests were incompatible with the type of data examined; unpaired tests were employed for paired data (or vice versa); inappropriately used parametric methods for skewed data (or nonparametric methods for normally distributed data); used inappropriate test for the hypothesis evaluated.
	Inflation of Type 1 Error: failed to correct for multiple comparisons; inappropriately conducted *post hoc* subgroup analyses.
	Typical errors with Student's *t*-test: failed to prove test assumptions; used unequal sample sizes for paired *t*-tests; improperly conducted multiple pair-wise comparisons of more than two groups; used an unpaired *t*-test for paired data (or vice versa).
	Typical errors with χ^2 test: no Yates-continuity correction reported in presence of small numbers; used χ^2 test when numbers in a cell were n < 5; did not explicitly state the null hypothesis tested; did not use multivariate techniques to adjust for confounding factors.
Methods Documentation.	Did not clearly and correctly specify/define all statistical tests; failed to state number of tails (i.e., one-tailed or two-tailed *t*-tests); failed to state if test was paired or unpaired.
	Specified an unusual or obscure method without explaining or citing a reference.
	Did not specify which test was applied to a given set of data if more than one test was performed.
Data presentation.	Inadequately described basic data in graphics/figures, tables, and numerical text: measure of central tendency without measure of dispersion (e.g., mean without SD; median without range or IQR); used mean (SD) to describe skewed (non-normally distributed) data; failed to define "±" notation for variability; did not include error bars (or did not label them).
	Inappropriately/poorly reported results: presented p values without confidence intervals (CIs); CIs presented for each group rather than intergroup contrasts; presented p values as p = NS, p < 0.05 or p > 0.5 without providing actual/exact p values (where exact p values are available); provided numerical information to an unrealistic level of precision or significant figures.

(Continued)

Table 3.1 (Continued) Common avoidable statistical errors in reports of medical research

Defect	Example
Data interpretation.	Results interpreted wrongly: statistically "nonsignificant" result interpreted as "no effect" or "no difference"; statistically significant result interpreted as clinically significant; drew conclusions not supported by the study methods and data; claimed statistical significance without mentioning the statistical test or conducting the needed analysis.
	Results interpreted poorly: reported statistically nonsignificant results without mentioning possible Type 2 Error; did not discuss potential issue of multiple comparisons and other factors that require statistical adjustment or control; did not disclose or discuss potential sources of bias and effects of confounding on unmeasured variables; did not explore the potential effects of study limitations (bias toward or away from the null) and how they might be neutralized or addressed in future studies.

Source: Reproduced with permission from Strasak AM, Zaman Q, Pfeiffer KP et al. Statistical errors in medical research: a review of common pitfalls. *Swiss Med Wkly* 2007;137:44–9.[3] Permission granted by EMH Swiss Medical Publishers Ltd. on the basis of the Creative Commons Attribution-NonCommercial-NoDerivatives 4.0 International License.
Abbreviations: IQR, interquartile range; SD, standard deviation; SE, standard error; SEM, standard error of the mean.

while modifying various parameters, until you observe a p value < 0.05. By the same token, however, you should be prepared to do the same if your first analysis returns a comparison that is p < 0.05 (and then watch as your initially statistically significant p value fades into obscurity).

Paralleling writing, statistical analyses should not only reflect—but culminate—planning and thoughtful analysis, establishing and adhering to prespecified parameters and other widely recognized conventions. According to the "Rule of Chekhov's Gun" (Chapters 1 and 2), all planned analyses (and endpoints) stated in the Methods must be reported in the Results; and, conversely, any outcome data presented in the Results must be "motivated" in the Methods, including elements of the SAP/DAP.

Just as each sentence, paragraph, and overall essay should be logically organized and thoughtfully planned, an internal logic should inform the SAP/DAP and protocol. In a typically *a priori* way, we specify our outcome measures (endpoints) and MCIDs between treatments or exposures that we seek to evaluate or demonstrate based on published literature. We then set forth the statistical level of confidence that we wish to have in our findings (typically, 95%) and project the number of patients needed to compare groups with a certain level of statistical power (typically, 80%) and at a two-tailed $\alpha = 0.05$. Each of these limits is consistent with standard practice but also largely arbitrary and modifiable.

As with our overall prose, we must be mindful of internal and external "fidelity" concerning data (see also Chapter 1). The published medical literature is not immune from violations of these fundamental requirements of data integrity. A brisk survey of even prestigious peer-reviewed journals will return examples of the following:

- "Internal infidelities":
  - Abstract data deviate from those in text (Results narrative)
  - Abstract data deviate from those in tables and figures
  - Data in narrative text deviate from those in tables and figures
  - Data in references are internally inconsistent; citation numbers in text or the bibliography are duplicated or out of sequence.
- "External infidelities":
  - Cited numbers in text deviate from data in published references
  - Data in tables and figures deviate from patient listings, including within clinical study reports and other, less burnished (the term in pharma is "cleaned") outputs
  - Citations (publication data, e.g., page ranges, website addresses of Food and Drug Administration [FDA] full prescribing information (or package inserts [USPIs]) and European Medicines

Agency's Summaries of Product Characteristics [EMA's SPCs], congress, and other information for presentations/posters) deviate from actual published references, websites, and other sources.

In some cases, infidelities result because values from tables or figures that are cited in the Abstract or narrative Results text of a manuscript are later consigned to Appendices, which readers may or may not review. Of course, an entire editorial industry, aided by supportive software packages, is devoted to aligning these various aspects. However, MWs should give our editorial colleagues a head start by being mindful of these potential defects. One hallmark of inconsistency is duplicated text or numbers, especially a string of identical values in adjoining columns or rows of a table. Because human beings are not immune from such errors, request that statisticians share their data tables and figures with you in editable files that you can gently modify and format but not rekeystroke (unless a SAS or other statistical output is simply too "raw"). Rekeystroking increases the margin of error.

Anyone who doubts the importance of forethought, planning, and "fidelity" in scientific endeavors should revisit the debacle of a 1999 $125 million mission to Mars, which seriously missed its mark. Different engineering teams (the California mission navigation team vs. the Colorado Mars Climate Orbiter team at Lockheed Martin) used English versus Standard International (metric) units when computing a pivotal operation of the spacecraft. The lack of "internal fidelity" between these approaches doomed the mission. Internal fidelity results from a kind of borderline-obsessive level of concern, which in turn motivates compulsive checks and rechecks (within reason and timelines!). As I like to say, we researchers and communicators need to "vet, sweat, and occasionally fret" our data to ensure such fidelity; we "number all references and reference all numbers." Of the errant NASA launch, Edward Weiler, Associate Administrator for Space Science, remarked

> People sometimes make errors ... The problem here was not the error, it was the failure of NASA's systems engineering, and the *checks and balances in our processes to detect the error*. That's why we lost the spacecraft [emphases mine].

3.2 THE NATURE AND DISTRIBUTIONS OF DATA AND THEIR IMPLICATIONS FOR STATISTICAL ANALYSES

Much of inferential statistics (hypothesis testing) involves evaluations of whether two groups are drawn from the same population. Such testing follows pre-specified conventions and rules concerning the probabilities with which a null hypothesis (NH)—that two or more experimental groups are not different from each other—is rejected. We assume the NH with a sense of "clinical equipoise." Statistical tests do not confirm a hypothesis but rather reject or fail to reject a prespecified NH, which is usually expressed as a statement or premise introduced by the symbol H_0. If the NH is rejected, we typically accept an alternative hypothesis (AH; H_1), that the two sample populations are significantly different.

The selection of an appropriate statistical test is dependent on the character and distribution of the data (Figure 3.1 and Table 3.2).[6]

Questions to ask when selecting a statistical test include the following:

- **Q: Are data continuous, or categorical?**
  A simple example is provided by the elevator. Your choices on the outside are categorical (dichotomous or binary): up or down. On the inside, they are continuous: floors 1 through 21. Some variables can be expressed either continuously or categorically. An observer can identify a color as blue (i.e., categorical variable), but the approximate wavelength of this color ranges from 415 to 495 nm (i.e., continuous variable).
- **Q: Are data paired, or unpaired?** If a study examines the effects of a medication on blood pressure (BP) compared to usual care in a crossover or "before-after" study design of 10 patients, the individual patient data are paired. Each BP reading from the same subject is clearly not independent of others from him or her at different times; they are also much more likely to approximate other intraindividual values rather than data from other patients. Studies that randomly allocate two unrelated groups of subjects to two different treatments result in unpaired (independent) data.
- **Q: Are data nominal, ordinal, interval, or ratio?** For nominal data, variables are mutually exclusive and often non-numeric, with

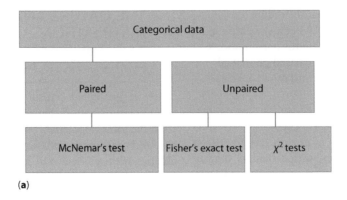

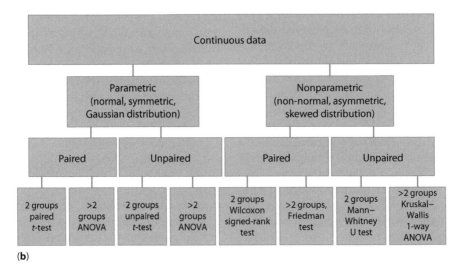

Figure 3.1 Statistical tests of categorical **(a)** and continuous **(b)** data. ANOVA, analysis of variance. *Source:* Reproduced with permission from du Prel JB et al.[6] Reprinted from *Dtsch Arztebl Int.*, 107, du Prel JB et al., Choosing statistical tests: part 12 of a series on evaluation of scientific publications, pp 343–8. Copyright © 2010 with permission from the German Medical Association.

no strict order to groupings. Examples include eye color, gender, and geographic region of residence. Tests of nominal data include:

- χ^2 (chi-squared) or Fisher's exact test for two independent (unpaired) treatment groups
- McNemar's test for paired study settings in which subjects serve as their own controls (e.g., before-after, crossover)
- Cochran Q for more than one treatment in the same subject (i.e., paired setting)
- Contingency coefficients to associate variables with more than two levels.

The term "ordinal" expresses the "order" (or rank) between variables but not necessarily any relationship between them. Examples of ordinal data include a (Likert-type) customer survey that asks a subject to grade satisfaction on a scale from 1 (very dissatisfied) to 10 (very satisfied). Although a score of 7 implies greater satisfaction than 5, and 5 implies greater satisfaction than 3, the 2-unit difference between 7 and 5 cannot be equated to that between 5 and 3. Tests of ordinal data include:

- Mann–Whitney U test for two treatment groups
- Kruskal–Wallis test
- Wilcoxon signed-rank test for study settings such as when subjects serve as their own controls (e.g., before-after, crossover).

Table 3.2 Statistical tests of association

No. of dependent variables	Nature of independent variables (IVs)	Nature of dependent variables (DVs)	Statistical test
1	0 IVs (1 population)	Interval and normal	One-sample t-test
		Ordinal or interval	One-sample median
		Categorical (two categories)	Binomial test
		Categorical	χ^2 goodness-of-fit
1	1 IV with 2 levels (independent groups)	Interval and normal	2-independent sample t-test
		Ordinal or interval	Wilcoxon–Mann–Whitney test
		Categorical	χ^2 test
			Fisher's exact test
1	1 IV with 2+ levels (independent groups)	Interval and normal	One-way ANOVA
		Ordinal or interval	Kruskal–Wallis test
		Categorical	χ^2 test
1	1 IV with 2 levels (dependent/ matched groups)	Interval and normal	Paired t-test
		Ordinal or interval	Wilcoxon signed-rank test
		Categorical	McNemar test
1	1 IV with 2+ levels (dependent/matched groups)	Interval and normal	One-way repeated-measures ANOVA
		Ordinal or interval	Friedman test
		Categorical	Repeated-measures logistic regression
1	2+ IVs (independent groups)	Interval and normal	Factorial ANOVA
		Ordinal or interval	Ordered logistic regression
		Categorical	Factorial logistic regression
1	1 interval IV	Interval and normal	Correlation
		Interval and normal	Simple linear regression
		Ordinal or interval	Nonparametric correlation
		Categorical	Simple logistic regression
1	1+ interval IVs and 1+ categorical IVs	Interval and normal	Multiple regression
			ANCOVA
		Categorical	Multiple logistic regression
			Discriminant analysis
2+	1 IV with 2+ levels (independent groups)	Interval and normal	One-way MANOVA
		Interval and normal	Multivariate multiple linear regression

(Continued)

Table 3.2 (Continued) Statistical tests of association

No. of dependent variables	Nature of independent variables (IVs)	Nature of dependent variables (DVs)	Statistical test
2 sets of 2+	0	Interval and normal	Factor analysis
	0	Interval and normal	Canonical correlation

Source: Adapted with permission from UCLA Institute for Digital Research and Education (IDRE). Choosing the correct statistical test in SAS, STATA, SPSS, and R. "What statistical test should I use?" Available at: https://stats. idre.ucla.edu/. Last accessed November 1, 2017.
Abbreviations: ANCOVA, analysis of covariance; ANOVA, analysis of variance; MANOVA, multivariate ANOVA.

- Friedman's test statistic for paired data
- Spearman rank correlation to associate two variables.

Interval data do reflect meaningful differences between variables. The difference between 30 and 20 grams of fat is equivalent to the difference between 20 and 10. Tests of interval data include:

- Unpaired Student's t-test for two treatment groups
- Analysis of variance (ANOVA) for three or more treatment groups
- Paired Student's t-test for study settings in which subjects serve as their own controls (e.g., before-after, crossover)
- Repeated-measures ANOVA for more than one treatment in the same subject
- Linear regression or Pearson product moment correlation to associate two variables.

Finally, ratio variables retain features of interval data but also have a clear definition of 0; when the variable equals 0, none of the variable exists. The anthropometric variable of body weight is a ratio variable. Relationships between such data can be determined by dividing one variable by another. A body weight of 100 kg is twice that of 50 kg. Other questions to ask about data to help select a statistical test follow.

- Q: Is the data distribution symmetrical (i.e., normal, Gaussian or bell-curved) or asymmetrical (e.g., non-normal, skewed)? The former typically warrants parametric statistical tests,

whereas the latter typically warrants nonparametric tests.
- Q: What is the likelihood of observing extreme results (i.e., "outliers")? Statistical tests of extremely infrequent events (e.g., rare diseases) and other less frequent data distributions may be related to Poisson or hypergeometric rather than normal distributions. Are there upper or lower limits on the data (potential range restriction via ceiling or floor effects)?
- Q: For tests of association (a) How many dependent variables (DVs; 1, 2, or 2+) are there? (b) How many levels of independent variables (IVs) are there? (c) What are the nature and distribution of dependent variables (e.g., categorical, interval, ordinal, normally distributed)? See Table 3.2 for further details.

3.3 SIGNAL VERSUS NOISE*; CONFIDENCE VERSUS DOUBT

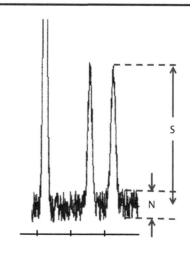

---

* The Signal and the Noise: Why So Many Predictions Fail—But Some Don't (New York: Penguin Books; 2015) is also the title of a work by statistician and über-prognosticator Nate Silver.

When evaluating scientific findings, including distributions of data, we need to segregate true, systematic effects of treatments or exposures (i.e., "the signal") from normal biological variability and random probability (i.e., "the noise"). One of the most influential forms of statistical testing is analysis of variance (ANOVA). It partitions effects due to treatment ("signal") from those due to random probability or biological variation ("noise"). In more precise statistical terms, ANOVA comprises the ratio of variance (i.e., how widely data are spread or dispersed) due to a treatment or exposure (mean square variance between groups), in the numerator, divided by the variance due to random probability or biological variation, in the denominator (mean square variance within groups).

A major challenge of biostatistics is to determine our level of confidence that findings from one study can be generalized to more heterogeneous populations of patients with a similar disease or condition. Such extrapolation from the specific to the general is the hallmark of inductive inferences, which are foundations for scientific advances. To meet this challenge, we test the likelihood that a mean value in our study population (e.g., a treatment effect of active therapy vs. placebo and/or usual care [UC]) would fall within a range of values in the overall (general) population exposed to the same conditions. This is the basis for "confidence," and we typically (but arbitrarily) define it at a 95% level (i.e., 95% confidence interval [CI]).

The challenge of discriminating signal from noise brings to mind concepts in Christian theology. In the New Testament, Christ revisits "Doubting Thomas" to convince him that He had been resurrected as a deity. In the process of canonization, the so-called "Devil's Advocate" needed to be convinced of a given candidate's saintliness.

As scientists and communicators, we often invest too much faith, if not raw emotion, in our own data; we fail to view our findings with appropriate empiricism and skepticism. Doctrine or even dogma may replace or outrace evidence. When designing or reporting a study, practitioners should consider, "How might a disinterested (that word means 'impartial,' not 'uninterested') peer reviewer, or even a scientist who 'plays for the other side' view the study findings (Table 3.3)?" "The other side" might include a proponent of an opposing school of thought concerning the science or even the manufacturer or marketer of a different medication or class of medications to manage a disease.

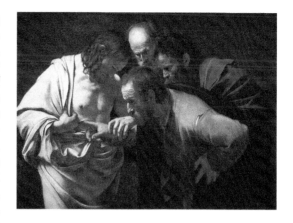

3.3.1 Statisticians are frequentists (unless they are Bayesian!)

Statistics deals not in "platonic verities" but rather probabilities, which are projected or estimated but never observed, as well as frequencies of categorical data and means of continuous data, which are observed. We conventionally (but arbitrarily) consider a result to be statistically significant if the likelihood of its occurring by random probability (chance) or biological variability alone is <5%.

Once we have rejected the NH, we can say that "confidence" in our findings has supplanted doubt. In the true statistical denotation, if we conduct a study 20 times, the population mean would be within the confidence limits of the sample population 19 times. Wider CIs signify a greater variance, dispersion, or spread to the data and hence less precision or statistical confidence. In statistical terms, the sample mean is denoted by m or $\bar{x}$ and the true overall population mean by μ.

If the 95% threshold CI for a difference between two means (e.g., data from two treatment arms) overlaps 0, or a relative risk (e.g., risk ratio [RR]) overlaps 1.0, the finding is not statistically significant at $p < 0.05$. When the 95% CIs for two means do not overlap, there is a statistically significant difference between them. The wider the CI, the less confidence we place in the effects of one treatment or exposure compared to another. If the CIs are very wide, it may prompt the researcher to consider reassessing the data using other (e.g., nonparametric) methods or retesting other key parameters.

Table 3.3 "Curb your enthusiasm" and other potential objections from journal referees

Study design	Your conclusion	Potential objection
Randomized controlled trial (RCT).	Medication was "robustly" efficacious. Study demonstrated "good" (or "acceptable") efficacy.	Avoid "judgmental" and qualitative ("good") modifiers. Seek to "anchor" any such descriptors in normative or other clinical data (e.g., term results "clinically important" if PRO endpoints meet literature definitions/thresholds for [MCIDs]).
	Medication was safe and well tolerated.	Unless vital signs (pulse rate, BP, body temperature, respiration rate), 12-lead ECG, laboratory panels, and severe adverse events were assessed, and there were no clinically meaningful differences between groups, one cannot necessarily assert safety. Clinical trials are often not powered or of sufficient duration to discern intergroup differences in infrequent adverse events that can jeopardize health on long-term medication use.
	Medication's effect was highly statistically significant.	Attach no modifiers/judgments to p values; just report them.
	Medication's effect was not significant (p = NS) or was "borderline significant" (p = 0.059).	If possible, provide actual p value (e.g., $p = 0.068$), not $p > 0.05$ or $p = NS$. Avoid phrases such as "borderline significant" and "approached significance." If $p < 0.05$, the finding is significant; if $p \geq 0.05$, then it is not (presuming that $\alpha = 0.05$). Other modifiers imply apologies or "retrospective rationalizations."
	Medication was effective.	"Effectiveness" is typically assessed in naturalistic, "real-world" ("pragmatic") studies.
Post hoc subgroup analyses of RCTs.	Statistically significant findings confirmed our hypotheses.	Post hoc subgroup analyses generate but do not reject or confirm hypotheses. In addition, hypothesis testing should seek to reject or fail to reject a null hypothesis, not confirm it.
	Effects of medication were significant ($p < 0.05$ vs. placebo) in 4 out of 10 subpopulations.	In subgroup analyses, statistically significant findings may result from random probability when performing multiple tests. Bonferroni adjustment divides study α level by number of tests (e.g., $p < 0.005$ for 10 tests in this case).
Observational studies.	Trends were identified for patients with certain conditions.	Paucity of high-quality patient-level data in administrative-claims database analysis (may need EMR analysis or survey). Typically fairly short "look-back" or baseline periods (~1 year) often limit a study to incident or more recently presenting (vs. chronic or prevalent) disease.
	Trends were identified for patients with certain conditions.	ICD codes were developed for reimbursement, not case ascertainment, purposes. Chart records of certain prescriptions may also introduce bias when used to identify patients with a disease.

(Continued)

Table 3.3 (Continued) "Curb your enthusiasm" and other potential objections from journal referees

Study design	Your conclusion	Potential objection
Observational studies (continued).	Adherence was high in a retrospective cohort (administrative-claims) study.	Adherence may be overestimated by a requirement that patients remain enrolled in health plan for a minimum period, because adherence is positively associated with continuity of care.
	Adherence was high in a survey of a patient advocacy group.	Selection bias may result from surveying such an organization, which may include higher proportions of patients who are highly motivated (and have sufficient economic resources) to improve their health status. Higher adherence would be expected.
	Improvements in outcomes were greater than expected in patients with more severe disease.	Confounding by severity may result in more severely ill patients' receiving more intensive care.
Systematic reviews/ meta-analyses.	Treatment effect/trend was identified across studies.	Possible publication bias. Studies with null or negative findings less likely to be reported. Use funnel plots to assess and exclude this form of bias.
	No treatment effect/ trend was identified across studies.	Possible methodologic heterogeneity militates against pooling data from different studies. Use I^2 or other test to assess and exclude.

Abbreviations: BP, blood pressure, ECG, electrocardiography; EMR, electronic medical records; ICD, International Classification of Diseases (US; UK Read codes); MCID, minimum clinically important difference; NS, not (statistically) significant; PRO, patient-reported outcome.

3.3.2 Overview of study designs: What we can and cannot (or should not) say in fair-balanced discussion sections

Only a fair-balanced, credible manuscript has a "favorable prognosis" with journal peer reviewers (Chapter 1). Pivotal to achieving fair balance in Discussions is to comprehensively present potential study strengths and limitations.

Figure 3.2 presents prevalent, and perhaps under-recognized, strengths and limitations of common study designs. The first step in study planning (formulating an SAP/DAP or protocol) is to recognize and seek to control, adjust, account for, or otherwise minimize (if not neutralize) the overall influence of study limitations on findings, especially their generalizability to naturalistic health-care settings. A pivotal challenge often taken up by peer reviewers relates to "ecological validity." There are typically at least two sample populations in our studies—such as cases and controls, as well as actively treated subjects and placebo controls or UC recipients. How do findings in these populations relate to the overall general population?

Without unduly constraining, undermining, or abrogating a study report's conclusions, we need to acknowledge these factors and their potential effects on the findings. Do the limitations result in possible underestimation (bias toward the null) or overestimation (bias away from the null) of treatment effects? What future research is needed to address the limitations?

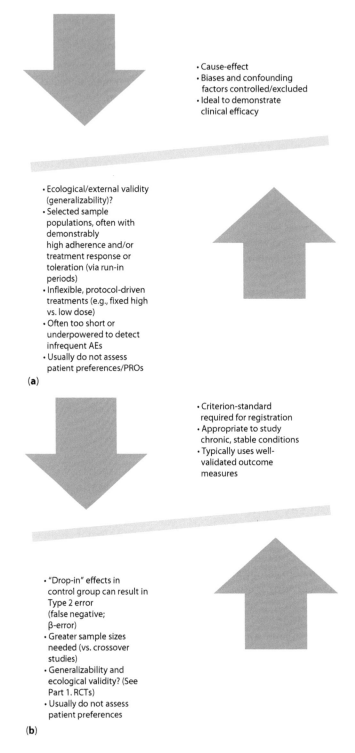

Figure 3.2 Potential strengths and limitations of common study designs. These issues should be considered in the Limitations subsection of the Discussion. The objective is to consider the strengths and limitations and, if possible, argue as to why the limitations do not abolish the overall conclusions. **(a)**: RCTs; **(b)**: parallel-group RCTs. (*Continued*)

- "Ecologically valid" data (more generalizable to "real-world" practice settings than are RCTs)
- Can accrue data from large numbers of patients, often followed for prolonged durations
- Dynamic, rather than protocol-driven (rigid) treatment protocols
- Liberal eligibility criteria
- More likely to assess patient preferences/PROs

- No cause-effect
- Advanced statistical methods (e.g., propensity score matching) often required to control for biases + unmeasured residual confounding factors that could otherwise be neutralized by randomizing

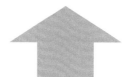

(c)

- ↓Needed sample size vs. parallel-group: each subject serves as own control
- Can neutralize any "period effects" by randomizing both treatment and sequence (cannot accomplish this using simple before-after study design)
- Minimizes between-patient variation
- Can assess patient preferences for one treatment vs. another

- May lengthen study because of washout period and the fact that each subject must undergo two treatment phases
- Ethical concerns about treatment-free "washout" (should include some form of usual care during washout)
- Not always possible to blind the crossover
- Possible carryover effects from inadequate washout (can test for and minimize this effect statistically); in most cases, 5+ X half-life washout is needed
- Not appropriate to study acute/serious conditions that can cause >20% patient attrition (e.g., mortality), or be cured before the second phase

(d)

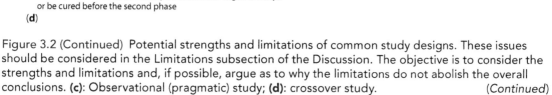

Figure 3.2 (Continued) Potential strengths and limitations of common study designs. These issues should be considered in the Limitations subsection of the Discussion. The objective is to consider the strengths and limitations and, if possible, argue as to why the limitations do not abolish the overall conclusions. **(c)**: Observational (pragmatic) study; **(d)**: crossover study.   (*Continued*)

- Can assess "real-world" treatment effectiveness
- Suitable to compare effectiveness of different interventions in pragmatic, "real-world" setting
- Enables effectiveness assessments where randomization at the individual patient level is impossible or inappropriate

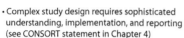

- Complex study design requires sophisticated understanding, implementation, and reporting (see CONSORT statement in Chapter 4)
- ↑ Number of subjects required (vs. randomization at individual patient level) because of intracluster correlations, necessitating nonstandard sample size calculations
- Design can compromise autonomous decision making: some subjects may not have access to certain procedures or treatments available at other study sites
- Potentially complicated ethics/informed consent
- Design should not be employed if the same conclusions can be reached via individual randomization

(e)

- Quick, simple "snapshot"
- Data collected only once
- Well suited to patient surveys and multiple-prevalence estimates
- Evaluates multiple outcomes, exposures, associations
- Well suited to descriptive analyses, hypothesis generation, and planning and allocating resources

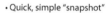

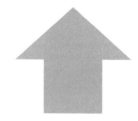

- No "natural history"; may not be well suited to assess diseases with waxing-waning (relapsing-remitting) character over time
- Potential problems of migration and low response rates can affect prevalence estimates
- Potential survival bias, misclassification because of recall bias, and adverse effects of low responses
- Unsuitable for assessing infrequent/rare or short-duration (acute) conditions
- Unsuitable for assessing disease incidence
- Associations may be difficult to interpret, e.g., did observed outcome come after the exposure, or did the outcome actually cause or contribute to the exposure?

(f)

Figure 3.2 (Continued) Potential strengths and limitations of common study designs. These issues should be considered in the Limitations subsection of the Discussion. The objective is to consider the strengths and limitations and, if possible, argue as to why the limitations do not abolish the overall conclusions. **(e)**: cluster RCT; **(f)**: cross-sectional. *(Continued)*

- Can assess treatment
  effects on disease
  trajectory over sustained
  intervals (natural history)
- Can assess disease
  incidence
- Can evaluate
  infrequent diseases
  and AEs (if sample sizes are
  adequate)

- Possible maturation and
  practice effects
- Longitudinal data from
  each subject are
  intracorrelated
  (increasing statistical
  complexity and
  necessitating special
  analyses; e.g., generalized
  estimating equations)

(g)

Figure 3.2 (Continued) Potential strengths and limitations of common study designs. These issues should be considered in the Limitations subsection of the Discussion. The objective is to consider the strengths and limitations and, if possible, argue that the limitations do not abolish the overall conclusions. **(g)**: Longitudinal study.

Source: Selected data from the University of North Carolina MCH Public Health Social Work Leadership Training Program (Available at: https://ssw.unc.edu/mch/node/221; Last accessed November 1, 2017) and Velengtas P, Mohr P, Meisner DA, eds. *Making Informed Decisions: Assessing the Strengths and Weaknesses of Study Designs and Analytic Methods for Comparative Effectiveness Research: A Briefing Document for Stakeholders: Weaknesses of Study Designs.* National Pharmaceutical Council February 2012. Available at: http://www.npcnow.org/publication/making-informed-decisions-assessing-strengths-and-weaknesses-study-designs-and-analytic. Last accessed November 1, 2017.

Abbreviations: AE, adverse event; CONSORT, Consolidated Standards of Reporting Trials; PRO, patient-reported outcome; RCT, randomized controlled trial.

3.4 THE FUNDAMENTALS: DESCRIPTIVE STATISTICS, INCLUDING DATA DISTRIBUTIONS AND MEASURES OF CENTRAL TENDENCY AND DISPERSION (ERROR)

3.4.1 Data distributions and their contours

The type of data distribution, including, most prominently, its relative symmetry, influences selection of statistical tests. A normal, symmetrical, bell-shaped data distribution is well suited to parametric testing.

German mathematician Johann Carl Friedrich Gauss was a royal surveyor and astronomer to the King of Prussia. Gauss was considered by many to have been the "greatest mathematician since antiquity." He is credited with the discovery of the normal distribution curve.

Gauss and his co-workers repeated survey measurements many times. Not only did frequencies of observations tend to cluster around a measure of central tendency, or center of a data set, but observations with increasing distances from this measure occurred with progressively decreasing frequencies and approached an asymptote (lower limit) of 0. In a normal bell-shaped, or Gaussian distribution, 68.27% of data fall within 1 standard deviation (SD) on either

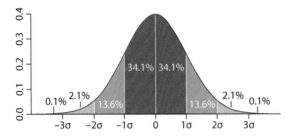

Figure 3.3 Normal, bell-shaped, symmetrical, Gaussian data distribution. In such frequency distributions, the mean is identical to the median. Approximately 68% of all values fall within ±1 standard deviation (SD) of the mean; 95%, within ±2 SDs, and 99.7% within 3 SDs.

side of the mean, 95.45% within ±2 SDs, and 99.73% within ±3 standard deviations (SDs) (Figure 3.3).

An example is a frequency distribution for male height. There are about 120 million adult men in the United States. Their mean height is 5'10," and the SD is 3 inches (3"). Because we are discussing the total male population, it is appropriate to refer to the mean as μ. The corresponding denotation for SD in the total population is σ.

At −3σ (9 inches below the US mean), we have comedic actor Danny DeVito (5'0") and, at +3σ (~9 inches above the US mean), we have basketball legend Michael Jordan (6'6"). Approximately 0.14% of adult men (168,000 each) are shorter than DeVito or taller than Jordan (total of 0.28% + 99.7% ≈ 100.0%). At 7'1", ex–NBA star Shaquille O'Neal is about +5σ (15") above the US mean. The proportion of values outside of 5σ is only 1 in 1,744,278 (× 120,000,000) = 68. Fewer than 70 American men are as tall as, or taller than, Shaquille O'Neal.

Some non-normal or asymmetrical data distributions have "tails": certain outliers skew the distributions and hence necessitate nonparametric testing. For instance, if a billionaire investor enters a lecture hall to deliver an address, he skews the frequency distribution for mean income of the audience to the right compared to the rest of us millionaires or "thousand-aires" (or "million-heirs" or "thousand-heirs!"). The outlying data point imparts a right-hand tail or positive skew. In such a distribution, the mean value increases, but the median (middle) value is less affected. When the mean exceeds the median, we have a right-skewed (positive) distribution, and vice versa for a left-skewed (negative) distribution.

The relative skew of a univariate data distribution can be computed using the following formula (Fisher–Pearson coefficient).

$$Skew = \frac{\sum (x_i - \bar{x})^3 / n}{s^3}$$

where x_i = each observation, $\bar{x}$ = mean, n = number of data points, and s = SD. The "sigma" operator tells us to sum all values. As a rough guide, values exceeding −1 (left-skewed) or +1 (right-skewed) indicate highly skewed distributions; values between −1 and −0.5 or between +0.5 and +1 indicate moderately skewed distributions; and values between −0.5 and +0.5, nonskewed (i.e., normal, symmetrical) distributions.[7] A less quantitative approach to determine the shape or symmetry of the distribution would be to plot the data. (In fact, if the number of observations is manageable, it is often a good idea to plot your data!)

Figure 3.4 shows how to compute the skew of a data distribution using Microsoft Excel.

A related concept is kurtosis, or the relative "tailedness" of a frequency distribution. (For a review, see Westfall PH.[8]) This construct was developed by major statistical progenitor ("stater-familias!") Karl Pearson. The higher the kurtosis, the more the data distribution is determined by extreme, infrequent deviations from the mean. A normal distribution has kurtosis = 3 and is termed mesokurtic (or mesokurtotic). Leptokurtic (or leptokurtotic) distributions have kurtosis > 3, with kurtosis > 3, with more data in (wider/heavier) tails. Laplace, Poisson, and exponential distributions are leptokurtic. Platykurtic distributions have kurtosis <3, with less marked ("thinner") tails (extreme deviations). (Think of a platypus.) Kurtosis can also be computed using Microsoft Excel. (See "KURT" under the "Statistical Equations" subtab.)

Because of the Central Limit Theorem, independent, random data distributions approximate a bell-shaped curve as sample sizes increase, even if the initial population distribution is not normal. Even an asymmetrical distribution—a binomial plot of outcomes that can be only one of two options (e.g., heads, or tails; disease present, or absent)—also approximates a normal distribution (asymptotically) as numbers of observations increase. This was recognized by de Moivre and Laplace as a special case of the Central Limit Theorem.

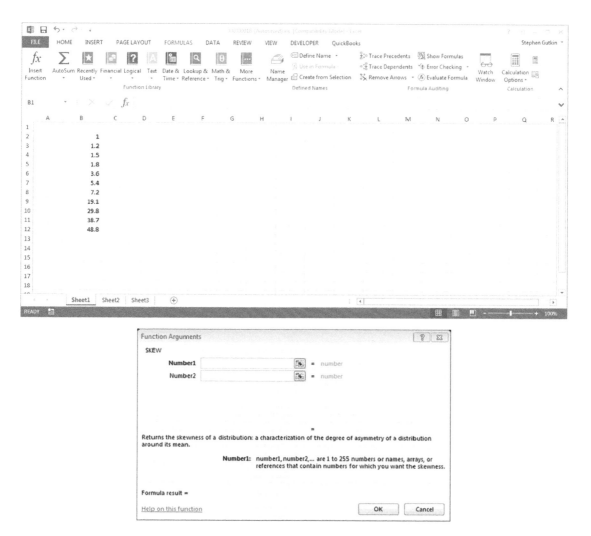

Figure 3.4 Using Microsoft Excel to compute skew (asymmetry). *(Continued)*

Suppose that we flip a coin several times in a row. We might put forth an NH as follows:

H_0: The frequency distribution of observed "heads" does not differ significantly from the population of observed "tails" at a two-sided $\alpha = 0.05$; the coin is fair.

The AH may be expressed as:

H_i: The frequency distribution of observed "heads" differs significantly from the population of observed "tails" at a two-sided $\alpha = 0.05$; the coin is not fair.

Now suppose that we flip the coin 100 times. We would expect a total of 50 ± 5 heads (i.e., SD = 5). Based on known relationships concerning normal data distributions, an observed frequency of 45 to 55 heads (i.e., 1 SD on either side of the mean) would be expected in 68% of repetitions. To evaluate our NH, we could set confidence limits of 40 to 60 heads, because these values would fall within approximately 2 SDs (exactly 1.96 SDs) of the mean and hence would be expected in approximately 95% of experiments.[9]

What if we get 80 heads? Should we begin to wonder if the coin has been adulterated? In fact, results of coin flips are not normally distributed but are described by a binomial distribution because

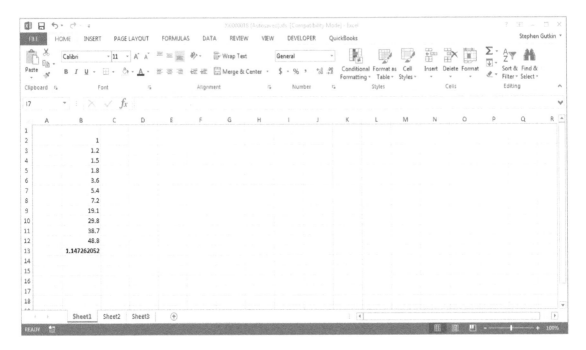

Figure 3.4 (Continued) Using Microsoft Excel to compute skew (asymmetry). The value exceeds +1, suggesting a highly (right-; positively) skewed distribution.

only two outcomes are possible for each observation: heads, or tails. In fact, if a "fair" coin is flipped N times, the probability of getting a certain number of "heads" is given by the following equation[10]:

$$Pr(x) = \frac{N!}{x!(N-x)!}\pi^x(1-\pi)^{N-x}$$

where x = the number of heads; N = the number of flips; and π = the probability of getting heads with a fair coin (0.5). The data distribution for a binomial function differs markedly from the usual bell shape.

In this case, the probability of returning 80 heads in 100 flips is far below 1%, and is computed as follows:

$$Pr(x) = \frac{N!}{x!(N-x)!}\pi^x(1-\pi)^{N-x}$$

$$Pr(x) = \frac{100!}{80!(100-80)!}0.5^{80}(1-0.5)^{100-80}$$

$$Pr(x) = 4.23 \times 10^{-10}$$

Hence, the probability of getting 80 heads in 100 coin tosses is approximately 4 in 10 million.

Eighty heads lie 6 SDs (6 × SD = 5) to the right of the expected mean of 50. The expected frequency of events falling beyond 6 SDs in a normal distribution would be 1 in approximately 507 million. We reject the NH: it is statistically significantly unlikely (p is much lower than 0.05) that the coin is fair. Note that we have not 100% proved that the coin has been "doctored" but have rather rejected the NH that it is fair with much more than 95% confidence.

Another distribution of data that deviates sharply from the normal, Gaussian plot is the Poisson distribution. It plots infrequent events observed over a fixed time interval. Originally put forth by mathematician Siméon Denis Poisson to estimate the number of nineteenth-century French citizens who were wrongfully convicted, the test found further application when Ladislaus Bortkiewicz used it to estimate numbers of Prussian cavalry injured or killed by horse kicks, an even more infrequent event. Applications of the Poisson distribution in contemporary statistics include assessments of other very infrequent events, such as pregnancies among oral-contraceptive users.

In summary, mathematical relationships and their attendant data plots or distributions affect statistical analyses, including pivotal assumptions, parameters, and inferences. The Central Limit Theorem has an equalizing or leveling effect, because, even initially asymmetrical (non-normal) distributions tend to become more symmetrical, normal, bell-shaped, or Gaussian, with increasing numbers of independent, random observations.

3.4.2 Measures of central tendency

3.4.2.1 ARITHMETIC MEAN

The mean is the most appropriate measure of a population's central tendency when independent observations are normally distributed. Parametric statistical tests for normally distributed continuous data include Student's t-test and the aforementioned ANOVA.

Watier and colleagues reported a thoughtful analysis of the mean ("What does the mean mean?"[11]) that largely exceeds the purview of this chapter but which I recommend to deepen your understanding of the mean. It included the following, thought-provoking conceptualizations: (1) Socialist, (2) Fulcrum, (3) Algebraic, (4) Geometric, and (5) Vector.

In the conventional sense, the mean is the average of all observations: their sum divided by the total number of observations:

$$\bar{X} = \frac{\sum_{i=1}^{n} x_i}{n}$$

where $\bar{x}$ is the sample population mean; x_i is each observation; Σ tells us to sum all observations; and n is the total number of observations. Figure 3.5 shows how to compute the mean of a data series using Microsoft Excel.

From Watier and colleagues, the algebraic form of the "least-squares" conceptualization of the mean is given as:

$$SS(c) = \sum_{i=1}^{n} (x_i - c)^2$$

where c is the value that minimizes the above quadratic function of differences from each observation, in order to minimize the distance of each value (x_i) from the center (c = least-squares mean) and hence also "minimize the sum of squared deviations" (see "Dispersion," below).[11]

3.4.2.2 GEOMETRIC MEAN

What if we wish to compute the central tendency of differences across very disparate scales? An example would be comparing changes in mean ratings of satisfaction among patients after receiving treatment A compared to treatment B using three very different scales in which we want to weight each score equally. One scale is the Treatment Satisfaction Questionnaire for Medication (TSQM-9),[12] which assesses patients' treatment satisfaction on a scale from 0 (not satisfied) to 100 (most satisfied). Another is a simple visual analog scale (VAS), which goes from 0 (not satisfied) to 10 (most satisfied). A third is a new scale that rates satisfaction from 0 (not satisfied) to 1.0 (satisfied).

Let us further suppose that we want to compute the mean change in all scales and that these changes are +40 on the TSQM-9, +4 on the VAS, and +0.4 on the new scale. Proportionately each of these is a 40% change. However, if we added the changes and divided by three, the influence of changes on the TSQM-9 (+40) would predominate. Calculating an unadjusted, arithmetic mean would result in a value of 14.8:

$$\frac{40 + 4 + 0.4}{3} = 14.8$$

The change in the TSQM-9 is overly weighting and, hence, in effect, skewing the mean.

To avoid this form of skew, we calculate the geometric mean as the cube root of the product of the three measures across the three different scales:

$$\textbf{Geometric mean} = \left(\prod_{i=1}^{N} \bar{x}_i \right)^{1/N}$$

where Π tells us to multiply each mean, and then take the Nth root of the number of means:

$$GM = (40 \times 4 \times 0.4)^{1/3} = 4$$

By using the geometric mean, we effectively normalize and better balance the disparate ranges being averaged, such that a change in any of the three scales does not predominate or overly weight the summary output.

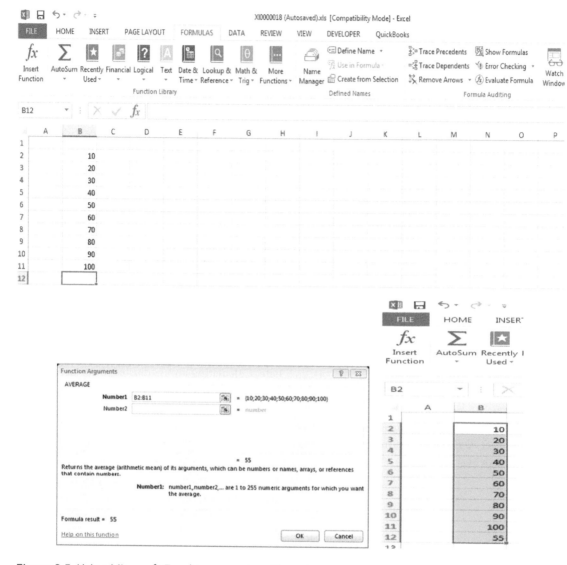

Figure 3.5 Using Microsoft Excel to compute arithmetic mean.

3.4.2.3 MODE

The value that occurs most frequently in a data distribution is termed the mode. In a symmetrical distribution, the mode, mean, and median are one and the same value.

3.4.2.4 MEDIAN

When independent observations are skewed, or non-normally distributed, the median—or middle—value most effectively conveys the population's central tendency.

The median divides a distribution into two equal aspects. If there is an odd number of observations, the median is simply the middle value. If there is

an even number of observations, the median is the average of the two middle ones.[13]

3.4.3 Measures of dispersion ("error")

3.4.3.1 STANDARD DEVIATION (SD)

Also termed "s" in the sample population (or "σ" in the overall population), SD is a measure of error, in the sense of dispersion or spread, in a distribution that is computed using the sum of the difference between each observation and the mean ($\bar{x}$ in the sample population and μ in the true or total population).

If the SD is narrow, we are confident that each data estimate is close to its population value.[4]

The SD statistic for the sample population is given as the square root of the variance:

$$s = \sqrt{\frac{\sum_{i=1}^{N}(x_i - \bar{x})^2}{n-1}}$$

where n is the number of subjects or observations; x_i is any observation in a distribution or data set; and $\bar{x}$ is the sample population's mean.

SD is expressed as a ± value associated with the mean and is expressed using the same units as the mean [e.g., mean (SD) blood glucose = 110 (1.5) mg/dL or 110 ± 1.5 mg/dL].

Figure 3.6 shows how to compute SD using Microsoft Excel.

3.4.3.2 VARIANCE

The square of the SD is another important term related to data dispersion: variance (s^2 in a sample population and σ^2 in the true population).[14] The statistic is given as

$$\text{Variance}(s^2) = \frac{\sum (x_i - \bar{x})^2}{(n-i)}$$

where x is each observation; $\bar{x}$ is the mean; n is the number of observations; and Σ tells us to sum the deviations from each observation to the mean.

3.4.3.3 STANDARD ERROR OF THE MEAN (SEM)

We are rarely if ever able to measure the mean and SD of a true population but rather measure these values in a smaller, sample (study) population. The mean of the sample population is denoted by $\bar{x}$ and the mean of the population by μ. The standard deviation of the sample population is denoted by s and the SD of the entire population by σ.[13]

SEM is computed as follows:

$$\text{SEM} = \frac{s}{\sqrt{n}}$$

Examining the equations above, we see that, unless there is a single study participant or observation, the SEM is always smaller than the SD— much smaller as sample sizes increase.

3.4.3.4 95% CONFIDENCE INTERVAL (CI)

Returning to our example above, the 95% CI can be expressed as follows. Let us say that we perform 20 independent experiments on a population and compute 95% CIs for each estimate of the mean. The 95% CI tells us that 19 (95%) of these CIs would include the population mean (μ). Another way to express this concept is that within 2 SEs (standard errors) outside of μ, 95% of the values for sample means would fall. A third explanation is that our percentage level of confidence in the fact that the CI includes the true population mean (μ) is computed as $100 \times (1 - \alpha)$. Typically, $\alpha = 0.05$.

In a normal distribution, 95% of sample means $\bar{x}$ fall within ± 1.96 SEs above and below the population mean (μ). There is a 95% likelihood that the range (CI) between

$\bar{x} - (1.96 \times \text{SE})$ and $\bar{x} + (1.96 \times \text{SE})$ includes the population mean. $\bar{x} - (1.96 \times \text{SE})$ is the lower confidence limit, and $\bar{x} + (1.96 \times \text{SE})$ is the upper confidence limit.

Figure 3.7 shows how to compute 95% CI using Microsoft Excel.

Just as we typically use $\alpha = 0.05$ and $p < 0.05$ to determine statistical significance, the 95% CI is arbitrary. To compute 90% CIs and 99% CIs, the following equations apply[13]:

$$90\% \text{ CI} = \bar{x} - (1.64 \times \text{SE}) \text{ to } \bar{x} + (1.64 \times \text{SE})$$

$$99\% \text{ CI} = \bar{x} - (2.58 \times \text{SE}) \text{ to } \bar{x} + (2.58 \times \text{SE})$$

When data distributions are sharply skewed, the scale may need to be transformed, nonparametric CIs computed, or bootstrap methods employed.[13]

3.4.3.5 CONVERTING 95% CI TO SE AND SD

From a 95% CI for a difference between groups for two distinct interventions [e.g., experimental (E) and control (C)] in a typical Student's t-test (see below)], we can compute SE and SD as follows:

$$\text{SE} = \frac{\text{Upper limit of 95\% CI} - \text{Lower limit of 95\% CI}}{3.92}$$

For 99% CIs, the denominator would be 5.15 and for 90% CIs, 3.29.

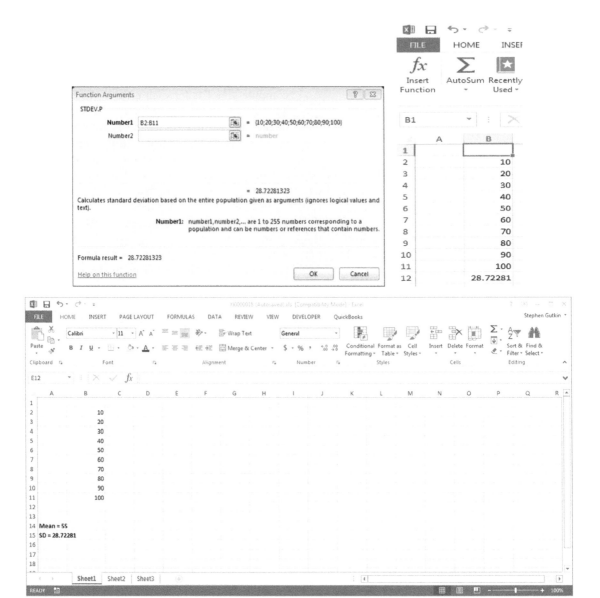

Figure 3.6 Using Microsoft Excel to compute standard deviation.

From the SE for the difference in means, we can compute the within-group SD. In the equation below, N_E signifies the number of subjects in the experimental group (or comparator 1) and N_C, the number in the control group (or comparator group 2).

$$SD = \frac{SE}{\sqrt{\dfrac{1}{N_E} + \dfrac{1}{N_C}}}$$

3.4.3.6 INTERQUARTILE RANGE (IQR)

Standard deviation is the typical measure of dispersion accompanying the mean, whereas some measure of range (e.g., IQR) typically accompanies the median. The range alone is based on only two measures (minimum and maximum) and hence conveys little information about the overall dispersion if the lower limit is very small or upper limit very large. In addition, the range increases as the number of outliers increases. The IQR denotes the dispersion of the middle 50% of the distribution—typically the

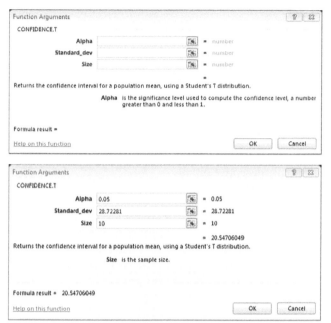

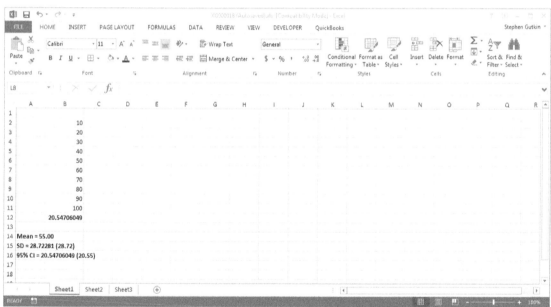

Figure 3.7 Using Microsoft Excel to compute the 95% confidence interval (CI) of a mean with a Student's *t*-distribution.

distance or spread of data from the lower (25%) to the upper (75%) quartile—and is less influenced by increased outliers.[13]

3.4.4 Degrees of freedom (*df*)

Degrees of freedom relate to the number of calculations that can be made "freely" without limiting other allocations. The sum of squared deviations in the variance calculation is divided by $n - 1$ rather than n. The denominator quantity of $n - 1$ is referred to as the number of degrees of freedom (*df*) of the variance. The number of *df* is $n - 1$, rather than n, because $n - 1$ is the number of deviations $(x - \bar{x})$ that are independent of each other.

3.5 STATISTICAL ERROR

Fortunately—and sometimes both regrettably and regretfully—our minds are adroit at finding trends and other patterns in information while often overlooking or minimizing the possibility that random probability or biological variation might explain the findings equally well. When I lecture, I say that, as a MW, "I know my [study/data] limitations" and "have two hands: 'on one hand; and on the other hand.'" What are the potentially deceptive pitfalls that we need to recognize and avoid?

3.5.1 Types 1 and 2 Errors

Type 1 Error is also termed false positive, α Error, and Error of the First Kind. Type 2 Error is also termed false negative, β Error, and Error of the Second Kind. In general, α signifies the risk of a false-positive outcome, and β signifies the risk of a false negative.

Type 1 Error occurs when we reject an NH that is not false (i.e., "false positive"), sometimes because of our choice of α significance levels.

When we fail to reject an NH that is in fact false (i.e., "false negative"), sometimes because of inadequate sample size/statistical power, we commit a Type 2 Error. To better understand Types 1 and 2 Errors in a study of normally distributed samples, suppose that we wish to determine if a new therapy improves a surrogate endpoint compared to placebo and UC in a clinical trial. The null hypothesis (NH; H_0) is that it does not, and that the actively treated and placebo samples derive from the same overall population. An alternative hypothesis (H_1) is that the new intervention does improve this endpoint (vs. placebo). By convention, we set a confidence value of $\alpha = 0.05$, which relates to the rate of false positives that we are willing to accept. In addition to α, which signifies the probability that a difference is not due to chance or biological variability, we have β, which relates to the rate of false negatives (Type 2 Errors) that we are willing to accept.

Statistical power is the likelihood that a test will reject an NH that is false. By convention the statistical power is usually designated as 80%, or $1 - \beta = 1 - 0.2$. This implies that we are willing to accept a false-negative rate of 20%.

Much less common are Type 3 Errors, in which the premise being tested is fallacious: we are asking an incorrect or inappropriate question. This circumstance exemplifies the true, philosophical sense of "question begging": we may commence an experiment from equivocal or frankly false premises or assumptions. (When people say that an idea "begs" a question, they almost always mean "prompts.")

3.5.1.1 TYPES 1 AND 2 ERRORS AND FUNDAMENTALS IN COMPUTING SAMPLE SIZE

The above considerations of Types 1 and 2 Errors connect to a larger, study design issue: computing sample sizes (Figure 3.8).[15] To do this, we typically need to know two major properties of populations from similar studies (e.g., based on published literature): effect size (differences between group means) and variance (s^2). For example, if we compare ex-smokers to a control group of never smokers effectively treated in the same pulmonology practice, we might minimize effect size because improvements in controls' lung function might be greater than expected because of the specialty-care setting and hence blunt or minimize their differences from cases in the same practice who recently quit smoking; that is, such case and control selection might attenuate the expected effect size.

Hence, we would expect the effect size—the disparity between mean spirometric changes in cases (quitters) compared to controls (never smokers)—to be higher when sampling controls from a healthy, community screening group (vs. a pulmonology practice). On the other hand, we would expect variance of the community to be smaller than that of the pulmonology practice, which includes both relatively healthy individuals and those with marked deficits in lung function.

By increasing the expected effect size and reducing the variance, we should have a greater chance of rejecting an NH (of no significant difference in spirometry between quitters and never smokers) using a smaller number of otherwise healthy, community-based never-smoker controls, compared to their counterparts drawn from the same pulmonology practice.

For a continuous outcome and samples of equal sizes in two groups, let us assume, by

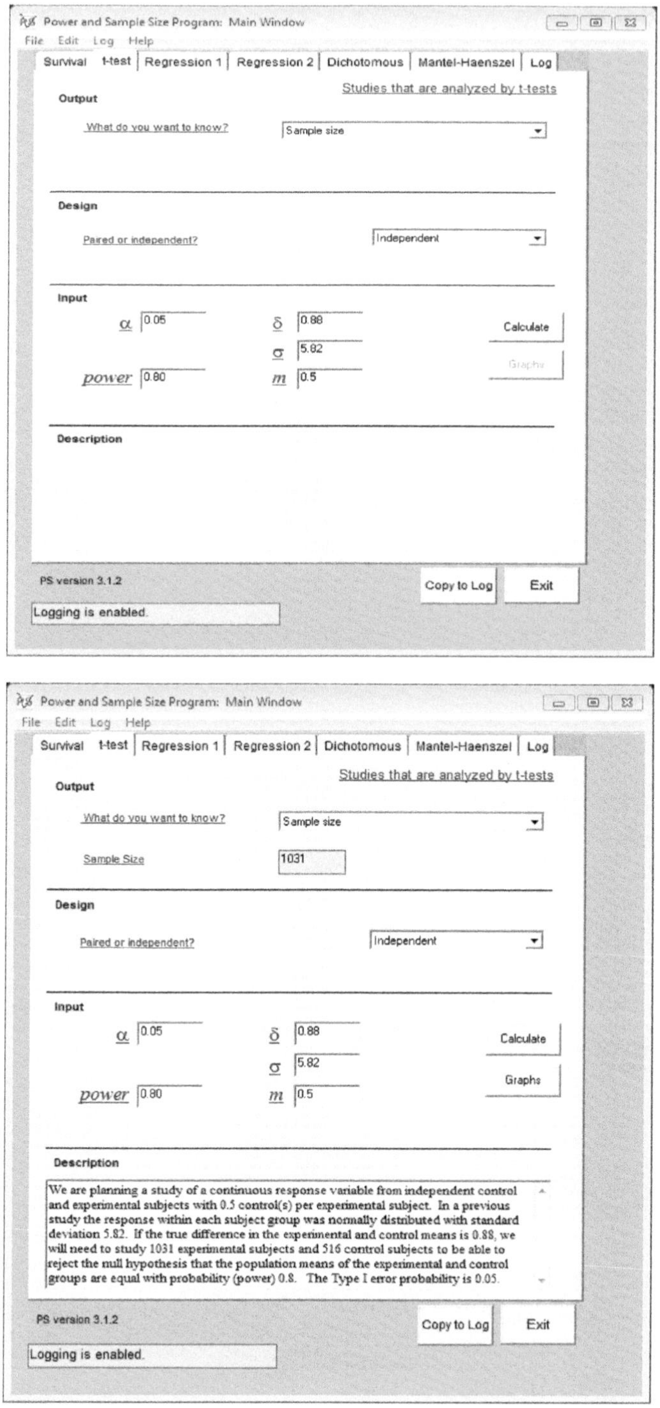

(a)

Figure 3.8 Using the software package P/S (from Vanderbilt University) to compute sample sizes for Student's *t*-test. The P/S software program is attributed to Drs. William D. Dupont and Dale Plummer's **(a)** Independent data (e.g., parallel-group study). (*Continued*)

(b)

Figure 3.8 (Continued) Using the software package P/S (from Vanderbilt University) to compute sample sizes. The P/S software program is attributed to Drs. William D. Dupont and Dale Plummer's **(b)** Paired data (crossover study). Note that, with other parameters being equal, the crossover study requires fewer study participants; it has intrinsically higher statistical power than the parallel-group study because each subject in the crossover study serves as his or her own control.

Source: From Vanderbilt University; Available at: biostat.mc.vanderbilt.edu/wiki/Main/PowerSample Size. Last accessed November 1, 2017.

convention, that we will use a two-sided $\alpha = 0.05$ and power = 0.80 (1 − β, where β is the conventionally acceptable false-negative rate = 0.20). As presented by Noordzij and colleagues,[15] we may wish to determine sample sizes to compare the effects of two antihypertensive agents. A difference in BP between population means ($\mu_2 - \mu_1$) of 15 mmHg is considered to be clinically meaningful, and we know from prior studies that BP in similar patients examined in similar ways is normally distributed and has an SD (s) of 20 mmHg [or variance (s^2) = 400 mmHg]. Sample size is computed as[15]:

$$n = \frac{2[(a+b)^2 \times s^2]}{(\mu_1 - \mu_2)^2}$$

where a is a conventional multiplier for $\alpha = 0.05$ (1.96); and b is a conventional multiplier for power (1 − β) = 0.80 (0.842 in this case)

$$n = \frac{2(1.96 + 0.842)^2 \times 20^2}{(15)^2}$$
$$n = 27.9$$

We need to enroll 28 study participants in each group.

Figure 3.8 shows how to conduct sample-size calculations using software from Vanderbilt University (P/S; Department of Biostatistics. P/S: Power and Sample Size Calculation. Dupont WD, Plummer WD Jr.).

3.5.1.2 WHAT P VALUES SIGNIFY (AND DON'T)

As mentioned, we never prove or disprove an NH. We set a limit of confidence (typically 5%) that two samples of subjects or observations derive from the same population. A p value < 0.05 tells us that it is statistically significantly unlikely that two samples of subjects or observations derive from the same overall population. Another way to express the meaning of a p value < 0.05 is that, based on random probability and biological variability alone, we would expect to find the observed results fewer than 5 times if we performed the same experiment 100 times. A p < 0.05 also signifies that there is less than a 5% chance of observing a difference as high as that observed if the NH were true: if the means of the two populations were not different.

A p < 0.05 does not signify that there is a ≥95% chance that the alternative hypothesis is true or that there is a ≥95% chance that the observed difference between sample means represents a true difference between population means. A p value > 0.05 implies only that we have failed to reject the NH, not that the NH is true.[16]

A significant p value per se is also not necessarily meaningful and is certainly not necessarily clinically meaningful. A value = 0.0001 is not necessarily "more significant" biologically or clinically than a p = 0.0100. As with other scientific observations, p values are open to interpretation. The former implies that, if we performed the same experiment 10,000 times, it would return the same results by chance or biological variability 1 time, whereas the latter implies that it would return the same results 100 times. A p value for a comparison may be < 0.05, but the difference may not be clinically meaningful. Changes in patient-reported outcomes (PROs) for frequent disabling conditions that are considered to be appreciable and relevant to the patient are designated by MCIDs. (See Appendix 1 of this textbook for a table of MCIDs.)

3.6 HUMAN ERROR: DEFECTS IN LOGIC

3.6.1 The null hypothesis as an example of "plausible reasoning"

Further work by Jaynes[1] offers the following scenario to confer an intuitive understanding of the probabilistic nature of hypothesis testing.

Suppose some dark night a policeman walks down a street, apparently deserted. Suddenly he hears a burglar alarm, looks across the street, and sees a jewelry store with a broken window. Then a gentleman wearing a black mask comes crawling out through the broken window, carrying a bag, which turns out to be full of expensive jewelry. The policeman doesn't hesitate at all in deciding that this gentleman is dishonest. But by what reasoning process does he arrive at this conclusion?[1]

The policeman cannot prove that the man emerging from the jewelry store is a criminal. We could imagine an alternative explanation. The owner of the jewelry store may have been at a costume ball, wearing a black mask as per the dress protocol. In walks German-descended Windsor Princess Michael of Kent (Marie Christine Anna Agnes Hedwig Ida von Reibnitz), completely "bereft of bling." Somehow, it seems, she was unable to open her safe at the hotel and could not access her diamond tiara. Could the jewelry store proprietor help her? Whereupon the merchant jaunts to his store but realizes that it is Saturday evening, and of course he is not carrying his shop key. So, he breaks the window, enters the premises, and fills a bag with jewelry to lend Princess Michael, leading him into the waiting cuffs of the properly skeptical constable.

The premise put forth above is analogous to the NH (H_0). Our AH (H_1) would be that this is a "garden-variety" burglary. If the police officer encountered this scenario 100 times, he could be quite confident that the explanation of the "jewelry owner breaking into his own store while wearing a mask from a costume ball (H_0)" would hold true fewer than 5 times. The NH (H_0) is rejected and the AH (H_1) accepted.

3.6.2 Problems with logic: Denying the antecedent and affirming the consequent

Other "logical fallacies" to which medical research and writing may be prone are "Denying the antecedent" (i.e., "inverse error," "fallacy of the inverse") and "Affirming the consequent," (i.e., "converse error," "fallacy of the converse," "confusion of necessity and sufficiency").

The logical defect of denying the antecedent can be represented as follows:

$$\text{If } A, \text{ then } B$$
$$\underline{\text{Not } A}$$
$$\text{Ergo, not } B$$

An example from life follows. If it is raining, my car gets wet. (If A, then B). It is not raining. (Not A.) Therefore, my car is not wet. (Not B.) Untrue: I might have taken it to the car wash. A plausible medical example follows. If a patient has tophi (MSU crystal deposits), he has gout. (If A, then B.) The patient does not have tophi (Not A). Therefore, he does not have gout (Not B). This conclusion is demonstrably false. Although tophi are pathognomonic for gout, only 25% of patients with gout have tophi.

The logical fallacy of "affirming the consequent" can be represented as follows:

$$\text{If } A, \text{ then } B$$
$$\underline{B}$$
$$\text{Ergo, } A$$

An example from life follows. If it is raining, my car gets wet. (If A, then B.) My car is wet (B); therefore, it is raining. (A.) Untrue: once again, a visit to the car wash disproves the syllogism. Premises can be true without their "logical" conclusions also being true.

A plausible medical example follows. If a patient has progressive diabetic nephropathy, she experiences acute tubular atrophy and tubulointerstitial fibrosis. (If A, then B.) The patient has tubular atrophy and tubulointerstitial fibrosis. (B.) Therefore, she has progressive diabetic nephropathy. (A.) This conclusion is patently false because there are many causes of acute tubulointerstitial nephritis other than diabetic nephropathy, including acute allergic reactions to medications (e.g., certain nonsteroidal anti-inflammatory drugs and antibiotics), certain autoimmune diseases, infections (e.g., *Legionella pneumophila*, *Streptococcus*), and collagen vascular diseases (e.g., sarcoidosis), as well as progressive diabetic nephropathy.

This textbook emphasizes the value of identifying, reviewing, and potentially citing consensus clinical guidelines for diagnosis and management of diseases. In fact, one way that the practice of medicine is shaped is by reference, by the many (practitioners) to the practices of the few: a "vanguard" of leading, widely published, clinicians (also sometimes termed "key opinion leaders"). However, it is often the "outliers" who advance science—people such as Galileo in physics and astronomy, whose advocacy of heliocentrism resulted in his condemnation for heresy and house arrest (in Arcetri, near Florence) in 1633, and, much more recently, by the late Robert Atkins, who challenged the "high-carbohydrate diet" orthodoxy. The logical fallacy of over-reliance on the opinions of experts is known as *Ipse Dixit*. (Latin: "He, himself, said it.")

3.6.3 *Post hoc ergo propter hoc* ("after this, therefore because of this")

In recent years much human capital could have been saved by recognizing the folly of an argument that ran "because low values of a surrogate physiologic measurement are associated with increased risk, raising them through treatment will reduce the risk." Two prominent examples were based on associations between both low levels of high-density lipoprotein cholesterol (HDL-C), and of estrogen after the climacteric, and increased risk of cardiovascular disease (CVD).

In the former case, low HDL-C may have been more of a disease marker than a risk factor. Paraoxonase-1, which is genetically encoded and resides within the HDL particle, hydrolyzes inflammatory phospholipids and has other antioxidant functions.[17] Enhanced levels (and function) of the HDL particle may be responsible for reducing CVD risk. The cholesterol may have been "along for the ride," in that high levels of HDL-C are consistent with a favorable "destination" of the cholesterol: through the reverse cholesterol transport pathway to hepatic excretion.

The association may also have been confounded by a biological variable related to both the exposure (low HDL-C) and the outcome/disease (increased CVD risk): insulin resistance and postprandial hypertriglyceridemia (which is in turn associated with low HDL-C via the enzymatic activity of cholesteryl ester transport protein).

3.7 INTRODUCTION TO CONFOUNDING AND BIAS

3.7.1 Confounding

The spurious effects of a third, often unmeasured or "stealth" variable (C) on an evident association between two others: the exposure (E) and the outcome (O; e.g., disease) is termed confounding. Confounding variables must not lie within the proposed path of causation between E and D but must also be associated with both E and O.

Let us consider a colorful (and hypothetical) example of confounding. Among other things, including the musky scents of perfumes, the Asian palm civet (*Paradoxurus hermaphroditus*) is known for a very expensive "dung coffee" that is derived from the animal's excrement (containing digested cherries).

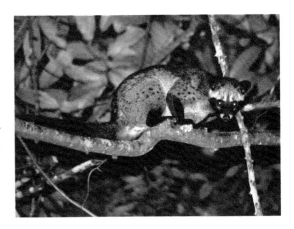

Suppose that a case-control study finds that adults who drank the exotic, Indonesian coffee kopi luwak for ≥10 years experienced a significantly reduced (relative risk reduction = 72%) 10-year mortality rate, with a hazard ratio (HR) of 0.28 (95% CI = 0.16–0.32; p = 0.003) compared to their counterparts who consumed regular coffee. Suppose that the Pearson r for the correlation between kopi luwak consumption and reduced 10-year mortality rate is 0.98, which implies that approximately 96% of the variance in excess mortality is explained by kopi luwak consumption. Have the researchers found the proverbial "Fountain of Youth?" Not so fast!

These hypothetical associational findings are likely confounded by an unmeasured variable. As mentioned above, confounding occurs when a third, unmeasured, factor (C) is shared by both the exposure and outcome (or by independent and dependent variables) and hence speciously influences their association. By definition, a confounding variable cannot lie on the causal pathway from exposure to outcome.

In this case, the unmeasured confounder is socioeconomic status (SES; Figure 3.9) as measured

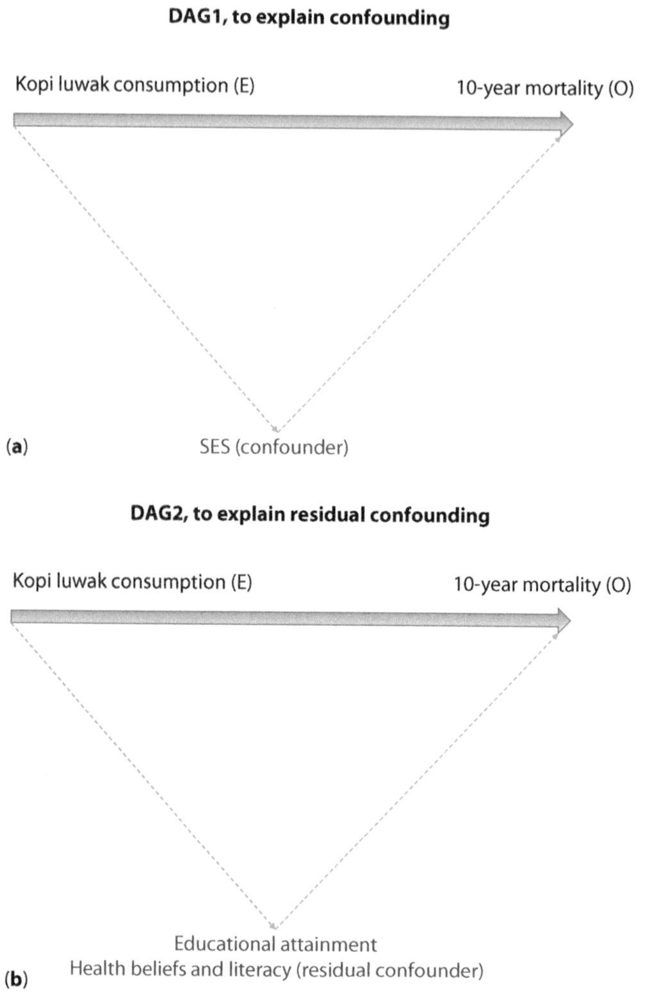

DAG1, to explain confounding

Kopi luwak consumption (E)   10-year mortality (O)

(a)   SES (confounder)

DAG2, to explain residual confounding

Kopi luwak consumption (E)   10-year mortality (O)

Educational attainment
(b)   Health beliefs and literacy (residual confounder)

Figure 3.9 Directed acyclic graphs (DAGs) to explain confounding (a) and residual confounding (b).

by annual income. Kopi luwak is sold for up to $500 per pound in the United States. Adults who can afford to "shell out so many beans" for their morning "cup of Joe" likely have more abundant economic resources to afford high-quality medical care. The confounding might be less marked in countries with government-funded health care.

Perhaps the most effective way to neutralize the potentially confounding effect (in this case, SES) on the reported association between kopi luwak consumption and reduced 10-year mortality rates would be to conduct a prospective randomized controlled trial (RCT) with stratified randomization on SES and double-blinded assignment to either kopi luwak or "garden-variety arabica." Other methods might include propensity score matching (PSM), which essentially "simulates randomization," in order to balance the kopi luwak and regular-coffee drinkers in terms of their SES. Further statistical approaches include analyses of covariance (ANCOVA) and other statistical models.

What if we continued to find a statistically significant ($p = 0.049$), albeit weakened (Pearson $r = 0.44$), association between consumption of "dung coffee" and reduced 10-year mortality rate, even after propensity score matching (PSM) or other modeling to adjust for SES? We may now be in the presence of "residual confounding." Are there any other factors associated with the primary confounding variable (SES, as measured by annual income) that might help to increase life expectancy in kopi luwak drinkers? In fact there are, including more advanced educational attainment, although many people have of course succeeded without a high-school or university degree, including Ben Franklin, Charles Dickens, Henry Ford, Walt Disney, John D. Rockefeller, and Richard Branson. Educational attainment is often associated with sound, health-promoting beliefs and behaviors, including continuing to take medications for diseases that are largely asymptomatic in the near term, to prevent potentially catastrophic events in the longer term.

A parallel example termed acquisition bias or medical surveillance bias is a possible finding of an increased incidence of diagnosed endometrial cancer in women receiving estrogen-containing regimens after the climacteric. The confounding factor is frequency of visits and pelvic examinations; clinicians prescribing hormonal therapy may schedule more frequent office visits and conduct more frequent pelvic examinations. Taken together these factors might tend to increase the probability of diagnosing endometrial cancer, biasing the association between hormone use and endometrial cancer away from the null.[18]

Confounding may include what is termed a "collider variable." An example of this form of confounding occurs when the incidence of diagnosed gastric cancer is increased among users of aspirin. The collider variable is melena; users of the antiplatelet medication are more likely to present with dark, tarry, or bloody stools, which in turn may increase the index of clinical suspicion for (and also augment efforts to detect) gastric cancer. In the aggregate, these factors could bias the association between aspirin use and the incidence of diagnosed gastric cancer away from the null, inflating diagnostic yield.[18]

Ways to minimize medical surveillance bias include (1) stratifying the analysis by disease severity or the type or frequency of health-care interventions; (2) masking exposure status before ascertaining outcomes (i.e., blinding medical surveillance); and (3) selecting cases and controls from among populations of patients undergoing similar treatments or diagnostic protocols.

Continuing in the above vein, most observational research establishes associations but not causality. A form of *post hoc ergo propter hoc* logic

informs assignment (by RCT investigators) of causality for adverse events to certain therapies based on temporal associations. Observational studies can evaluate associations but cannot conclusively ascribe causality or its direction (i.e., cause→effect or effect→cause).

As strong as correlations between two variables might be, including Pearson r or Spearman ρ coefficients approaching 1.0 or –1.0, they are not, strictly, considered to be evidence of cause and effect. When titling reports of such observational/ uncontrolled studies, I prefer to assume a conservative posture about causality, avoiding phrases such as "The effects of [e.g., treatment or exposure on a measured outcome]" in favor of phrases such as "Associations between [e.g., treatment or exposure] and a measured outcome." It may be tempting to infer causality, in part because of the terminology used in certain analyses: if one variable is found to be "dependent" on another, "independent" variable, it is not too difficult to take the next ostensibly logical step: that they are causally related. They may be, and they may not be! (This topic, and probability theory and inferential statistics in general, is examined at great length by Judea Pearl in his work *Causality: Models, Reasoning and Inference*, 2nd ed., Cambridge, UK: Cambridge University Press; 2009.)

In my practice of reporting observational (real-world-evidence [RWE]) studies, I often encounter confounding by severity.[19] Study participants with the most pronounced disease symptoms and signs, and poorest perceived prognoses, may receive the highest-quality care, including referrals to specialists and/or academic institutions (Tables 3.4 and 3.5; types of bias).[20] Despite being sicker, these patients may experience better outcomes than their counterparts with less advanced disease, who may, on average, receive less intensive or less advanced care. The confounder (C; severity) is associated with the exposure (E; intervention) and the outcome (O).

3.7.2 Simpson's Paradox and Lord's Paradox

The classic pedagogical example of Simpson's Paradox is the well-documented rise in the incidence of lung cancer, which correlated with increases in sales of automobiles, in the 1950s.

Table 3.4 Examples of bias. Part 1: Selection bias

Bias	Definition/Context	Example or effect (bias toward or away from null) and how to accommodate or neutralize
Inappropriate definition of eligible population.		
Ascertainment bias (can be caused) by:	Types of patients aggregated do not exemplify cases derived from the true general population.	Detection rate of an infrequent adverse or other event increased versus published literature because study protocol specifies more frequent MD visits/assessments. Bias away from the null.
Competing risks.	2+ outcomes are mutually exclusive in a single patient.	Causes of death. Premature death from one condition reduces mortality due to a related disorder (bias toward the null). Can be avoided by using cause-specific outcomes and removing/censoring certain causes of death (i.e. net probability of mortality).
Health-care access bias.	Hospitalized patients do not exemplify cases in community.	
Popularity bias.	Patients are admitted according to curiosity of providers in certain diseases.	
Centripetal bias.	Patients are drawn to a certain hospital or clinic because of provider reputation.	
Referral-filter bias.	Complex cases are preferentially referred to academic or tertiary-care centers.	
Diagnostic/ treatment access bias.	Patients have freer access to certain institutions because of socioeconomic, geographic, or cultural reasons.	
Neyman bias (i.e., incidence-prevalence bias, selective survival bias).	A series of survivors is selected that represents an erroneous frequency of exposure because the exposure is associated with prognostic factors or is itself a prognostic factor.	For example, the association between excessive drinking and stroke might be biased to the null if, in a case-control study, patients are interviewed about drinking habits after a stroke and heavy drinkers have a higher stroke mortality rate. The remaining (surviving) stroke cases would have a spuriously reduced frequency of drinking.

(Continued)

Table 3.4 (Continued) Examples of bias. Part 1: Selection bias

Bias	Definition/Context	Example or effect (bias toward or away from null) and how to accommodate or neutralize
Spectrum bias (diagnostic tests; purity diagnostic bias).	When assessing a diagnostic test's validity, researchers may include only unambiguous cases (test positives) and controls (negatives).	Sensitivity and specificity are spuriously elevated. An example may occur when patients with certain comorbidities are omitted, and the original cases are hence under-represented.
Inappropriate definition of eligible population.		
Survivor treatment selection bias.	In observational studies, a retrospective analysis can result in a direct association between a treatment and life expectancy if patients with longer survival have an increased likelihood of receiving that treatment.	
Healthy-worker effect.	Occupational studies may be biased because employed individuals tend to be healthier when compared to the overall population, including the unemployed.	
In case-control studies:		
Berkson's bias (also termed hospital patient bias).	Differential hospitalization rates create a distinct exposure distribution between hospitalized cases and other cases or controls. Patients with different medical conditions may also have different hospitalization rates.	May be less likely to occur in incidence-density studies, in which prevalent or previously diagnosed cases are excluded and only recently diagnosed cases are included. Can be avoided by choosing both cases and controls from the community.
Exclusion bias.	Cases with a disease and concomitant conditions are included, whereas controls without these illnesses are excluded.	Possible bias away from the null. Exclusion bias may elicit a specious association between administration of an investigational product and survival because patients with serious adverse events (often during a treatment-free run-in period) are excluded from exposure to the new medication.

(Continued)

Table 3.4 (Continued) Examples of bias. Part 1: Selection bias

Bias	Definition/Context	Example or effect (bias toward or away from null) and how to accommodate or neutralize
Inclusion bias.	In case-control studies of inpatients, controls may have conditions associated with an exposure.	Possible bias toward the null because the frequency of exposure is greater than is anticipated in the reference group.
Matching.	Selection bias may be introduced by either frequency or individual matching.	Bias toward the null may occur because of overmatching, when matching is undertaken on nonconfounding factors, which are associated with the exposure but not the disorder. Can be controlled by statistical analyses that adjust for these factors used to match.
Inappropriate definition of eligible population.		
In systematic reviews and meta-analyses:		
Language bias (systematic reviews and meta-analyses).	There may be a bias to exclude reports in languages other than English.	In this case of an "inappropriate definition of the eligible population," the "population" consists of the articles accepted for review and analysis.
Lack of accuracy of sampling frame.		
Nonrandom sampling bias.		
Telephone random sampling bias.	Some households (e.g., without cellular telephones) in a survey may be systematically excluded, resulting in coverage bias.	An example is a cell-phone or internet survey, which could result in undersampling of less socioeconomically advantaged households and dwellers. This effect may be more pronounced in developing economies.
Systematic reviews and meta-analyses/ Citation bias.	Citation of statistically significant findings and/or articles in the most readily available journals (e.g., those with highest impact factors, citation half-lives, and immediacy indices).	

(Continued)

Table 3.4 (Continued) Examples of bias. Part 1: Selection bias

Bias	Definition/Context	Example or effect (bias toward or away from null) and how to accommodate or neutralize
Systematic reviews and meta-analyses.		
Dissemination bias.	The entire publication process may be influenced by different patterns of information retrieval.	
Post hoc analysis.	Excessive reliance on *post hoc* subgroup analyses, which may be less methodically planned than initial experiments, may result in "data dredging," "cherry picking," "salami slicing," or "fishing expeditions."	*Post hoc* analyses are by nature only hypothesis generating, not rejecting or confirming. Bias away from the null can occur because multiple comparisons increase the likelihood of finding statistically significant differences on the basis of random probability alone. Bonferroni, Breslow–Day, and other statistical tests can adjust or control such effects.
Publication bias.	Published reports may not accurately represent all studies because certain trials are more likely to be reported: those with statistically significant, positive (not negative or null) findings, large sample sizes, study design, study quality, funding body, and the reputation of the authors/institution.	Studies with smaller sample populations may need to report wider (and lower p value) intergroup disparities (effect sizes) to be published. Funnel plots, which graph precision (SE or N) on the y-axis (e.g., odds ratios) (ordinate) versus treatment effect size on the x-axis (abscissa) can help to assess and exclude this form of bias.
Imbalanced diagnostic procedures in the target population.	Detection bias may occur in case-control studies if an exposure influences disease diagnosis (i.e., detection bias).	
Diagnostic-suspicion bias.	Exposure may be misconstrued as another diagnostic standard.	Exposure can elicit greater exploration for an illness, biasing results away from the null.
Unmasking-detection signal bias.	Exposure may result in a disease manifestation that favors making a diagnosis of a disorder.	
Mimicry bias.	Exposure elicits a disease manifestation that favors making a diagnosis of a disorder, especially a benign condition that is otherwise similar to the disease being studied	

(Continued)

Table 3.4 (Continued) Examples of bias. Part 1: Selection bias

Bias	Definition/Context	Example or effect (bias toward or away from null) and how to accommodate or neutralize
During-study implementation.		
Losses/Withdrawals to follow-up.	In both experimental and cohort studies, imbalanced attrition can influence the statistical validity of the results and conclusions.	
Missing information in multivariable analysis.	Chart reviews and other retrospective analyses may include only patients with complete data across all variables in prespecified multivariable analyses.	Patients with complete data may not exemplify the entire population. Patients with more clinical data may stay longer in hospital, have more serious conditions, or both.
Nonresponse bias.	Study subjects (e.g., survey respondents) may differ systematically compared to nonparticipants.	Surveys on medication adherence and other health-seeking behaviors, especially when fielded in patient-advocacy groups, may bias these factors away from the null because less socioeconomically disadvantaged persons are not included.
Healthy volunteer effect.	Subjects may have superior health status compared to the general population.	

Source: Selected data from Delgado-Rodriguez M, Llorca J. Bias. *J Epidemiol Community Health* 2004;58:635–41.[20]
Abbreviations: N, total number of subjects; SE, standard error.

Simpson's Paradox results because of a failure to recognize and control for covariates, often in epidemiologic research. A covariate may influence predictive relationships between exposures (e.g., treatments) and outcomes (e.g., disease events). In the aforementioned example, the covariate was an increased incidence of cigarette smoking, which paralleled the rise in car sales, during the 1950s. Performing an ANCOVA to control for cigarette smoking would largely abolish or neutralize the spurious association between car sales and lung cancer.

The importance of ANCOVA in controlling for potentially important baseline covariates is supported by an example from the endocrinology literature.[21] In a 1993 thyroid-eye clinic study of 101 visits (20 by men; 81 by women), men had

significantly worse ophthalmic function than women, as measured by log ophthalmic index (OI) ($p < 0.01$ by Student *t*-test). However, plotting OI versus age suggested that men were older than women, and OI declined (ophthalmic function deteriorated) as a function of advancing age.

Named after Frederick M. Lord, Lord's Paradox occurs when introduction of an additional continuous covariate reverses the apparent relationship between an outcome that is continuous and an exposure that is categorical. Tu and co-workers offer the example of an evident association between the exposure of birth weight expressed as a binary variable (*BWb*) in categorical strata and the outcome of BP (*BP*; assessed as a continuous variable). When assessing this association in isolation, we might find that higher (vs. lower) *BWb*

Table 3.5 Examples of bias. Part 2: Information bias

Bias	Definition/Context	Effect (bias toward or away from null) and how to accommodate or neutralize
Misclassification bias.	A procedure to detect either an exposure or an effect has suboptimal specificity or sensitivity.	Exposed/ill subjects can be misclassified as unexposed/healthy or vice versa. May result from random errors, including data entry/capture, end-digit preference, rounding, and/or missing data.
Differential misclassification bias.	Misclassification is unequal between groups being compared.	Can bias findings toward or away from the null.
Nondifferential misclassification bias.	Misclassification is equal between populations.	Binary variables may be biased toward the null, whereas polytomous (2+ categories) variables may be biased away from the null.
Causes of misclassification bias:		
Detection bias.	May operate in studies with long-term follow-up, including cohort studies and clinical trials.	
Observer/ interviewer bias.	Knowledge of disease status and/or interventions can introduce bias. Interviewers can introduce error by "helping" respondents in subtle ways.	May bias away from the null. Can be neutralized or reduced by blinding the observer or interviewer.
Observer expectation bias.	The fact that the observer knows the subject's illness, exposure, and/or interventions can affect the way she records data.	May bias away from the null.
Apprehension bias.	Measuring an exposure can affect its estimated value.	"White-coat hypertension" is an example.
Recall bias.	Intercurrent disease events can influence the overall perception of a disease, exposure, or treatment.	
Rumination bias.	May result when the presence of a disease affects the way its causes are interpreted.	
Exposure-suspicion bias.	May result when the presence of a disease affects exploration of its causes.	

(Continued)

Table 3.5 (Continued) Examples of bias. Part 2: Information bias

Bias	Definition/Context	Effect (bias toward or away from null) and how to accommodate or neutralize
Participant-expectation bias.	May result when a subject in a clinical trial knows that the treatment or other exposure received may influence their answers.	
Reporting bias. Obsequiousness bias.	Investigator and subject may "conspire" to yield the responses that are desired by, or of interest to, the investigator.	Can be neutralized or reduced by observer and/or participant blinding.
Family aggregation bias.	Detection of a case of a disease may result in further testing, detection, and/or reporting of the condition by relatives.	
Under-reporting bias.	Potential survey participants may refuse to answer potentially embarrassing questions about a socially or otherwise unacceptably risky health behavior.	
Mode-for-mean bias.	When certain frequency-quantity surveys of health behaviors are used, respondents may report the most frequent, rather than average, behaviors.	Potential bias toward the null, with underestimation of average intakes.
Ecological fallacy.	May result when analyses at the group level (i.e., ecological) are used to inform data interpretation at the individual level.	May be triggered by within-group biases, including misclassification, confounding, selection bias, and effect modification.
Regression to the mean.	Occurs when an initial, extreme datum is followed by values closer to the middle of the distribution (mean or median).	

(Continued)

Table 3.5 (Continued) Examples of bias. Part 2: Information bias

Bias	Definition/Context	Effect (bias toward or away from null) and how to accommodate or neutralize
Regression dilution bias.	Also termed "regression attenuation," regression dilution bias may occur in longitudinal trial assessing associations between changes from baseline levels in a continuous variable (e.g., serum cholesterol) and a disease outcome (e.g., incidence of ischemic stroke).	Potential bias toward the null when evaluating associations between exposure and outcome. May be neutralized or reduced by including many (rather than one or a few) observations, especially during baseline screening periods.
Hawthorne effect (responder bias).	A form of responder bias initially observed in the 1920s at the Hawthorne (Chicago) plant of Western Electric Co., in which productivity increased among plant workers who were cognizant that they were under observation.	An example is in clinical trials. Medication adherence and other health-seeking behaviors may be exaggerated (i.e., biased away from the null) by subjects' interest in continuing to be included in the study (and hence receive potentially advanced care).
Lead-time bias.	Diagnosis of a condition during its latency period because of a study increases the effective duration of the condition.	
Protopathic bias.	Associations between disorders may be biased by observations in patients with prodromal or early-stage illness. Latent onset of the target outcome influences measured exposure status.	Bias away from the null, suggesting a causal effect of treatment, can be adjusted by a "lag-time" approach that excludes exposures in a certain interval before diagnosis. Another example may occur when a medication is prescribed for an early sign or symptom of a condition that has yet to be diagnosed.
Sick-quitter bias.	Patients with high-risk health behaviors (e.g., alcoholism) may cease them once an organic disease (e.g., alcoholic hepatitis) manifests.	Bias toward the null in studies attempting to trace associations between behavioral risk factors and diseases when patients who have quit the risky behavior are erroneously classified as unexposed.
Temporal ambiguity.	May occur in cross-sectional or ecological studies, when it is not clear if the exposure precedes the effect or outcome.	

(Continued)

Table 3.5 (Continued) Examples of bias. Part 2: Information bias

Bias	Definition/Context	Effect (bias toward or away from null) and how to accommodate or neutralize
Will Rogers phenomenon.	Enhanced diagnostic tests ameliorate staging of an illness.	May result in migration to more advanced stages and be observed when comparing survival rates over time or across clinics.
Work-up bias (verification bias).	When assessing the validity of a diagnostic test, the current criterion standard is performed less frequently if results of the newly assessed test are negative.	May be exacerbated when disease manifestations affect results of tests.
Confounding (susceptibility bias).	May occur when an exposure to disease risk factors is especially likely in persons susceptible to experience an outcome.	Can be neutralized or reduced by study designs using randomization or matching.
Confounding by group.	May ensue when occurrence of an exposure in each group is associated with the risk of disease among unexposed persons within the same population.	Can result in ecological fallacy when the rate of disease is regressed on the prevalence of exposure in different communities.
Confounding by indication.	May occur when a perceived elevated disease risk, manifestations, or poor prognosis evidently indicate a more advanced level or kind of intervention; the indication is associated with both the disease risk factors and the selected therapeutic modality.	The confounding factor is the indication, which reflects the risk or severity of a disease and is also related to the treatment administered.
Specific biases in trials.		
Allocation of intervention bias.	May occur when interventions (or their sequences) are differentially allocated to a population, especially in studies that are not randomized.	May bias treatment effects away from the null. In prospective randomized trials, it can be neutralized or reduced by concealing the allocation sequence.
Compliance bias.	May occur in trials that mandate treatment adherence, when the extent of adherence also affects evaluations of efficacy.	

(Continued)

Table 3.5 (Continued) Examples of bias. Part 2: Information bias

Bias	Definition/Context	Effect (bias toward or away from null) and how to accommodate or neutralize
Contamination bias.	May occur when interventions (or versions of them) being assessed in the active treatment group "drop into" the placebo or usual-care control group.	
Differential maturation.	This term relates to imbalanced secular trends among groups in a group-randomized trial, favoring one condition versus another. Instead of individuals, identifiable groups are randomized to interventions to assess an intervention.	
Lack of intention-to-treat analysis.	In analyses of RCTs, data from participants need to remain in the group (e.g., treatment or placebo) to which they were initially allocated, in order to avoid selection bias and confounding.	If nonadherent study subjects or individuals receiving an incorrect treatment are excluded, the experimental arms of an RCT may not be comparable.

Source: Selected data from Delgado-Rodriguez M, Llorca J. Bias. *J Epidemiol Community Health* 2004;58:635–41.[20]
Abbreviation: RCT, randomized controlled trial.

is associated with higher current BP. Now let us introduce another continuous variable: the covariate of current body weight (*CBW*). Using a linear regression model that adjusts for the continuous confounding variable, while including a group-allocating variable that is categorical, Tu's group found that patients with higher *BWb* actually have a significantly *lower BP* than those with lower *BWb*.[22]

3.7.3 Regression to the mean (RTM) and maturation effects

Also termed "regression artifact," RTM may occur in a nonrandom population sample with incompletely correlated data when repeated measurements are made on the same individuals. When sampling data from such a population and setting, one might find an extreme variable (one that

is far from the population mean); however, the next observation is likely to be closer to the mean or center of the distribution.[23,24] Conversely, if observations are not made at random, or the data are correlated, the observation after the extreme one may be equally or more extreme! As the statistical adage would have it: "the trend is your friend!"

RTM can be interpreted as a special example of Gauss's Central Limit Theorem. The term "RTM" was coined by the father of linear regression, polymath, psychologist, and many other admirable things, Sir Francis Galton.

In broad terms, RTM can also be viewed as a form of information bias, as can a related concept, regression dilution bias.[20,25] This phenomenon occurs in longitudinal studies when the association between a single baseline data point (e.g., a continuous risk factor) which, after all, represents only one observation among many values fluctuating around a mean, and a time-related outcome (e.g., disease event 5 years later), is underestimated, potentially attenuating a linear relationship.

One way to adjust for or even neutralize the effects of RTM is to randomly assign patients to comparative treatment groups (e.g., active treatment vs. placebo) because both treatment groups will be affected by RTM. Another study design that may help to minimize RTM and regression dilution bias would be to include a run-in period during which several baseline measures (rather than a single measure) are taken and then averaged. This sort of design reduces the variability or spread (i.e., dispersion, error) of the data and hence the likelihood of RTM from extreme data points at baseline to after treatment (when, by nature of improved control of surrogate endpoints or risk factors in the active-treatment group, the "spread" of the data is likely to be reduced). A third approach to minimize RTM is to include an untreated "natural-history" treatment arm.

Other potential threats to internal data validity may occur for nonstatistical reasons, including maturation and practice effects. Suppose that we are studying long-term effects of a treatment for attention deficit–hyperactivity disorder (ADHD) on educational achievement. We conduct a study with a "before-after" design and assess performance on the same standardized test at baseline and after 3 years of treatment. Unless we include a well-matched control group that receives usual care or some other intervention, and/or undergoes similar tests and retests over time, we cannot rule out maturation, or test-retest practice, effects as causes of (or contributors to) enhanced performance on the test over time.

3.8 COMPREHENSIVE REVIEW OF PRECISION, REPRODUCIBILITY, RELIABILITY, VALIDITY, EFFECT MODIFICATION, INTERACTION, AND BIAS

We state that a measure is precise when the relative amount of error or dispersion of a measurement or series of measurements is small. When repeated under the same or very similar conditions, precise measurements return more consistent findings than imprecise ones. In an unbiased system, precision can be increased by taking more and more observations.

Related concepts include "repeatability" and "reproducibility."[26] We say that an assessment instrument or other measure is repeatable when results are very similar after a single study participant is assessed using the same measure, by the same investigator (or other rater), under identical or very similar circumstances, and during a short window during which the measured variable is not likely to change on its own. An assessment measure is termed reproducible when the relative dispersion in values returned when a single subject is assessed *under changing circumstances* is small.[26]

We classify an assessment measure as reliable when the degree of dispersion (error) in observed measurements associated with intrinsic variation between study participants in the quantity being measured according to an error-free or true level is small. On repetition under unchanged experimental circumstances, reliable assessments return very similar results. Measures of height are typically reliable. Examples include intrarater, inter-rater, and test-retest reliability. When data are categorical (nominal), the κ (kappa) coefficient can be used to determine reliability.[27]

Reliability is mathematically defined as[26]:

$$\text{Reliability} = \frac{(\text{SD of subject's true values})^2}{(\text{SD of subjects' true values})^2 + (\text{SD of measurement error})^2}$$

In general, the reliability of measurements of continuous variables can be quantified using Cronbach's α as well as the intraclass correlation coefficient (ICC) and Cohen's κ for nominal data.[28] The former may be taken as an example of internal consistency as applied to tests or scales. Cronbach's α reflects the situation when a set of test questions measures the same quantity: the underlying principle (latent construct) is singular and unidimensional.

Suppose that we have a very precise measurement of some biological endpoint. Will such an index necessarily suit our experimental needs?

Measurements can be reliable and precise but have little clinical utility because the measurements must also approximate some "real-world" external value. "Accuracy" relates to the relative proximity of an assessment to some true or "reference" value.

Consequently, measurements must be not only precise but also valid: close to some external "target" measure, close to what they purport to assess, and consistent with both statistical laws and prevailing biological and clinical theories and disease or pharmacodynamic mechanisms.

3.8.1 Effect modification[29]

In this example, an association between an exposure E and a disease D is "modified" by a third variable; the effect on an outcome of an exposure differs because of the presence of the third factor.[30] Unlike interaction and confounding, which have mainly statistical meanings, effect modification refers to disease biology and mechanisms. The classical case occurs when study participants from different baseline sociodemographic or clinical strata experience distinct outcomes in response to the same exposure, be it a risk factor or a treatment. In fact, we term as "moderators" factors that affect the direction or strength of an association between an exposure variable (or independent variables; IV) and an outcome (dependent variable; DV).[31] Gender is said to be a moderator of the association between diabetes and major depressive disorder (MDD); women with diabetes mellitus (type 1 or 2) are more likely to experience MDD compared to their male counterparts with diabetes.[32]

Another example from the literature is the association between exposure (Cesarian birth [C/B]) and disease (childhood atopic sensitization). This association is modified by a third variable: family history of allergy. Another way to summarize this form of effect modification is that children with a family history of allergy who are born by C/B are at greater risk of atopy compared to those born by C/B who have no family history. Although the p value for effect modification in a study of these factors was 0.06, the odds ratio (OR compared to children with vaginal births) was significantly elevated (OR = 2.62; 95% CI = 1.38 − 5.00) for children with a family allergy history but not for those without such a history (OR = 1.16; 95% CI = 0.64 − 2.11), after adjusting for potential confounders.[30]

Unlike moderators, "mediators" may explain a disease or treatment mechanism. Mediators "identify why and how treatments have effects," whereas moderators "identify on whom and under what circumstances treatments have different effects."[31]

Another example from the published literature is the finding that smokers and study participants with diabetes mellitus have a significant association of relative telomere length (RTL) with progression of chronic kidney disease (CKD), whereas their nonsmoking counterparts without diabetes have no significant association (the hazard ratio [HR] overlaps 1.0).[33] When DNA telomere length approaches Hayflick limits, renal cells undergo senescence and apoptosis, rendering them less able to proliferate, repair, and regenerate. Each 0.1-U decrease in RTL is significantly associated with an increased relative risk of CKD progression, in both smokers (HR = 1.44; 95% CI = 1.16–1.81; p = 0.001) and patients with diabetes (HR = 1.16; 95% CI = 1.01–1.34; p = 0.03), after adjustment for gender, glomerular filtration rate, proteinuria, and baseline age.[33]

Studying effect modification enables us to: (1) adjust or otherwise augment the precision of our measurements of associations (e.g., HRs adjusted for effect modifiers); (2) identify special populations who may derive especially marked benefits from different interventions; and (3) help to formulate hypotheses related to etiologic pathways from exposure to disease.

3.8.2 Interaction

Interaction may occur when the observed joint effects of risk factors are either markedly lower (biased toward the null) or higher (biased away from the null) than expected based on their independent, additive effects.[29]

In this context, another way to (operationally) define interaction is that the joint effects of risk factors—expressed as a sum in additive statistical models such as linear regression or as a product in multiplicative models such as logistic regression models—exceed or fall below what we would expect based on the individual components. In short, the whole exceeds the sum or product of the parts in positive interaction or synergy and falls short in negative interaction or antagonism (or "dyssynergy").[34]

3.8.3 Prominent forms of bias

3.8.3.1 OVERVIEW

Instrumental in the process of developing a sober, even-handed, evidence-based (fair-balanced) overall argument or Discussion is to understand, disclose, and consider the likely effects of study limitations. As depicted in Figure 3.2, retrospective and epidemiologic (observational) studies, such as case-control trials, are generally more susceptible to biases than RCTs.

Table 3.6[35] presents issues in the design of Likert and other rating scales that may bias respondents' behaviors and hence skew survey data.

A very useful review of bias includes the following definition:

> The lack of internal validity or incorrect assessment of the association between an exposure and an effect in the target population. In contrast, external validity conveys the meaning of [generalization] of the results observed in one population to others. There is [no] external validity without internal validity, but the presence of the second does not guarantee the first. Bias should be distinguished from random error or lack of precision. Sometimes, the term ['bias' refers] to the mechanism that produces lack of internal validity.[20]

In broad terms, there are two forms of bias: selection bias[36] (SB; Table 3.4) and information bias (IB; Table 3.5). Major forms of SB include self-selection bias, sampling bias, ascertainment bias, and Berkson's bias (Berkson's fallacy).[20,37,38] Other forms include:

- Medical surveillance bias;
- Neyman's bias;
- Survivor treatment selection bias;
- Duration-biased sampling;
- Health-care access bias; and
- Spectrum bias (ascertainment bias applied to assessing diagnostic tests).

Major forms of IB include misclassification bias, ecological fallacy, and RTM (and the related regression dilution bias).

3.8.3.2 SELECTION BIAS

Cohort studies may be affected by either "emigrative" or "immigrative" SB. In the former, study participants are selected out of a cohort because of factors influenced by both the risk of an outcome (e.g., disease) and the exposure (or a factor contributing to the exposure). In the latter, enrollment into the cohort is influenced by these factors. To adjust for selection bias, inverse probability weighting is one potential approach.

One example of SB encountered in my own practice is self-selection bias. Examples include surveys of respondents via patient advocacy societies to determine treatment adherence. Suppose that a patient survey, conducted using a fancy application via the costliest cell phone and carrier, from a national disease society finds that adherence to biological medications for rheumatoid arthritis is significantly higher than adherence to an older medication (e.g., methotrexate [MTX]). Both self-selection bias and sampling bias may help to inflate adherence. First, respondents to a survey would be expected (on average) to be more health conscious and motivated to adopt health-promoting behaviors, such as adhering to medication regimens.

Heightening the concern, the special population of respondents in a patient advocacy society might be especially health conscious and occupy higher SES strata than nonmembers, given that they were reached via some newfangled and expensive "app." They may hence be better able to afford, and be more motivated to keep taking, the more expensive biological medications. Nonrespondents, including those in lower SES strata, may lack the financial resources and educational attainment to acquire such regimens, understand the need to take them, and then adhere despite a high acquisition or out-of-pocket cost (vs. MTX).

All sampling methods were not created equal, in terms of their potential to introduce bias. Least likely to be confounded or biased in most instances are studies using simple random sampling and stratified sampling. Conversely, "convenience sampling" relies mainly on data that happen to be available, and "snowball sampling" seeks to enrich enrollment by identifying and inviting individuals acquainted with those already enrolled.

Also termed ascertainment bias, unmasking bias, and detection-signal bias,[39] medical surveillance bias[40] results when an exposure (*E*; e.g.,

Table 3.6 Examples of bias and other issues in rating scales and respondent behaviors

Type of scale	Survey issues and respondent perceptions/Behaviors	Potential consequences
Interval.	Uneven intervals between response options. For example, response options of: "terrible, horrible, awful, fair, slightly good, all right, and reasonably good." The "perceived psychological distance"[35] between "awful and fair" is not equivalent to that between "fair and slightly good."	If gaps between response categories are unequal, parametric statistics may not be applicable.
Likert/Other.	Possible instance of social desirability bias: avoid extreme response options.	Central-tendency bias.
	Seek to satisfy the investigator by agreeing with statements as given.	Acquiescence bias. May occur in a setting of institutionalization.
Likert.	Seek to indicate strength.	"Faking-good" bias.
	Seek to indicate infirmity/disability.	"Faking-bad" bias.
	Seek to represent oneself in a more socially acceptable manner.	Social-desirability bias. Intersubjective version of "faking good" bias.
	Seek to represent oneself in a less socially acceptable manner.	Norm-defiance bias. Intersubjective version of "faking-bad" bias.
	Cross-cultural issues.	Persons from different cultures, both across and within countries, have distinct values, which can bias responses.
Other.	Respondents may be more likely to select positive (vs. negative) response options.	It may be important to use weaker modifiers (e.g., "not quite") rather than stronger ones (e.g., "totally") for negative response options.
	Implicit assumptions.	Questions worded as "How concerned are you about..." imply to the respondent that she should be concerned, leading to overstatement of concern. Using a screening question (e.g., "Are you concerned...") can neutralize this potential bias.
	Omit responses of "undecided" and "no opinion."	Forcing-choice bias. Overestimation of numbers (%) of respondents with opinions and may level/reduce outliers because undecideds may be more likely to choose middle ratings (e.g., fair, average).

(Continued)

Table 3.6 (Continued) Examples of bias and other issues in rating scales and respondent behaviors

Type of scale	Survey issues and respondent perceptions/ Behaviors	Potential consequences
Other.	Poor balance: rating scales with response options of (1) "good, average, poor, very poor, and awful" or (2) "excellent, very good, good, average, poor."	When confronted with such options, subjects may respond more negatively to scale 1 and more positively to scale 2.
	Order effects.	In Likert and other scales, respondents may show a bias toward response options listed to the left rather than the right. To avoid bias, it may be necessary to administer scales to respondents more than once, using "strongly agree" on the left and "strongly disagree" on the right in one test and the opposite in a second (in random sequence).
	Direction-of-comparison bias: respondents focus on and favor the entity that defines a comparison rather than the referent.	Presented with a question such as "When you think of sports, would you say that golf is more exciting, or tennis?" Respondents may be more likely to select "golf," and the pattern is reversed when the sequence of the sport names is reversed.

Source: Selected data from Friedman HH, Amoo T. Rating the rating scales. *J Marketing Management* 1999;9:114–23.[35]

screening, intervention) results in some symptom, sign, or other intermediate event or phenomenon that is on the causal path to, and triggers enhanced vigilance for, a disease (*D*), increasing its detection (and hence its incidence or frequency).

Related to this example but confined to studies of hospital inpatients is Berkson's bias or fallacy.[41] Formulated by Joseph Berkson,[42] the concept embodies the following premise:

Persons with two or more diseases have a higher probability [of being] hospitalized than persons with only one disease—even if these results are independent.[43]

In broad terms, Berkson's bias is a form of both SB and attrition bias. This bias may emerge in a setting of prevalent, hospitalized illnesses, because both exposure to risk and occurrence of disease increase the risk of hospitalization. If, for instance, hospitalized controls are less likely (vs. cases) to be exposed to certain risk factors, the strength of the association between the risk factor and the disease outcome in the cases may be inflated. Patients who have more than one disease are more likely to be admitted to hospital than individuals with one. Bias toward or away from the null is possible. Suppose that we conduct a retrospective hospital-based case-control study on the association between long-term (10+-year) nut and seed consumption and 5-year colon cancer mortality from 1995 through 2000. Cases hospitalized with colon cancer may have had low ingestion of nuts and seeds over a long period of time.

Many of the same gastroenterologist's hospitalized controls (on internal medicine wards) with diverticular disease might have been prohibited from diets high in nuts and seeds because such consumption was thought to be potentially harmful to patients with these conditions (although possibly protective vs. colon cancer).[44] Any inverse association between nut and seed consumption and cancer of the large bowel might be biased away from the null because inpatients without colon cancer were not exposed to high nut-seed diets, which might otherwise have reduced their cancer colon mortality rate. "But wait," you say, "high-fiber diets, including nuts and seeds, are now known to potentially *reduce* the risk of diverticulitis." True![45] However, we must study the problem "in situ": during a period (going back to the 1990s) when the prevailing wisdom was that patients with diverticulosis or diverticulitis should avoid eating nuts and seeds.

To minimize Berkson's bias in a case-control study, incident rather than prevalent cases could be sampled from outpatient clinics and other data sources (e.g., government registries), not only from hospitals. Population controls could be sampled from the community (e.g., using random-dialing telephone surveys).

3.8.3.3 INFORMATION BIAS

Misclassification bias may result in cases being categorized as controls, and vice versa. Causes include suboptimal test sensitivity or specificity, missing data, data entry or capture that is influenced by random errors, and rounding data to a 5 or 0 ("end-digit preference").[20] This type of bias can be nondifferential or differential. When exposure is misclassified to an equivalent degree in both cases and controls (or other compared groups), the bias is nondifferential. Cases and controls (or other groups) may not recall certain exposures or other clinical factors equally, leading to differential misclassification bias. Studies can limit this bias by prospectively observing and recording exposures as well as using objective biomarkers and self-administered scales for subjects; conversely, case-control studies may be more prone to misclassification bias when observations of exposure are retrospective.

Recall bias may result when patients who have certain diseases (e.g., cases) or who are aware of their treatment assignment in a clinical trial, think harder about (and recollect more effectively)

certain exposures compared to their healthier counterparts (e.g., controls). This example may involve a combination of rumination bias and exposure suspicion bias. One way to minimize recall bias is to measure and confirm exposure and overall medical history more objectively (e.g., via chart review or electronic medical record [EMR] analysis).

Another way to minimize recall bias is to more effectively blind subjects and confirm their recollections of exposures using objective markers, such as biological or toxicological assay values and genotypes (e.g., serum cotinine levels in former vs. current smokers). However, even these measures may be biased by different detection limits for exposure markers with longer or shorter plasma residences. A third approach would be to conduct a nested case-control study.[46]

Observer/interviewer bias, observer expectation bias, and reporting bias are types of IB that include the investigator or clinician, subject or patient, or some interaction between them. Blinding the observer and/or study participant can help to minimize these biases, although certain aspects of exposures (e.g., niacin-induced flushing) or patient status (e.g., wasted state in cancer or AIDS) may complicate such blinding. In addition to "stacking the deck" through construction of rating scales (Table 3.6), investigators may communicate a desired subject response nonverbally. Conversely, the well-documented "white-coat pressor effect," in which office BP measurement by a physician upwardly biases the observation, is a form of apprehension bias.

A subject's merely knowing that she is being studied—irrespective of which exposure or treatment she might be receiving—can alter her behaviors or other measured variables. This form of responder bias is often termed the Hawthorne effect, because it was initially observed in the Hawthorne plant of a Chicago utility company in the 1920s. Contemporary study participants may be incentivized to offer the "desired" response (or demonstrate the desired outcome) because they are receiving medications gratis or overall more conscientious care compared to *"extra-studium ex."*

Information biases also include the ecological fallacy, lead-time bias, protopathic bias, sick-quitter bias, and temporal ambiguity[20]:

- An ecological fallacy occurs when inferences about individual study participants are influenced by analyses at a larger group or ecological level.
- Lead-time bias refers to "the added time of illness produced by the diagnosis of a condition during its latency period."[20] A very broadly related concept is immortal-time bias,[47] which is strictly considered a form of misclassification bias or SB. Immortal-time bias can corrupt findings when cohorts are interrogated using time-fixed analyses that are inherently imbalanced. The study protocol may mandate a baseline, "look-back," or other observational period during which, by design, eligible subjects cannot die or experience a disease event. As an example, untreated patients may be monitored from diagnosis until death (or other disease event), whereas treated patients are followed from diagnosis until first treatment, and then until the same endpoint. The interval from diagnosis until first treatment in the treated (vs. untreated) patients may bias the former's life expectancy or duration of disease-free survival away from the null. Patients experiencing an event during the baseline period may also be excluded from the treated group, further biasing disease-free survival away from the null in this group.
- In protopathic bias, evidence of subclinical or early-stage disease (or treatments for these conditions) may falsely associate an exposure with an outcome. A treatment may be instituted to manage a distressing sign or symptom that is actually a manifestation of a disease or other emerging entity that has not yet been diagnosed or defined. A spurious association between the treatment and disease may emerge.
- Sick-quitter bias may conceal a true association between an exposure and a disease outcome. A study of the association between smoking and lung cancer might enroll ex-smokers who quit because they developed diseases, biasing the actual association toward the null.
- Temporal ambiguity often occurs in cross-sectional studies. Did the exposure precede the outcome, or vice versa? In observational/uncontrolled studies, one cannot be sure. Cross-sectional studies may be especially limited when evaluating certain

immune-mediated inflammatory diseases (IMIDs; e.g., psoriasis, rheumatoid arthritis) with relapsing-remitting disease trajectories.

Cross-sectional (and case-control) studies may also be susceptible to incidence-prevalence bias, which is also termed selective survival bias and Neyman's bias. This bias may occur when the presence of a disease exposure (e.g., prognostic factor) affects fatality. Suppose that we wish to evaluate the association between alcohol abuse and current (prevalent) hepatocellular carcinoma (HCC).[48] Because heavy drinkers are more likely to die of HCC, the association between alcohol abuse and prevalent HCC may be biased toward the null. However, the association between alcohol abuse and the incidence of HCC should be largely immune from this form of bias.

3.8.3.4 OTHER ISSUES

Index event bias (IEB) relates to a paradoxically inverted association between an exposure (IV; e.g., risk factor) and an outcome (DV; e.g., disease) in patients with a history of this outcome (disease).[49–51] Often conceived as a form of SB, IEB may result from a clustering of certain risk factors (or protective factors) in patients with a history of a certain condition; these extraneous variables may militate against recurrences of the condition. IEB includes the "obesity paradox" whereby a history of being overweight "protects" against recurrent coronary events.[52,53] According to Dahabreh and Kent, IEB may be partly explained by (the aforementioned) "collider effects":

> Because risk factors often have congruent effects on the index and recurrent events, [a] negative association will tend to bias [the effect of an exposure] on recurrence risk toward the null, unless there is a thorough accounting for all shared risk factors. For example, in a recent study, propensity score–matched analysis eliminated the obesity paradox.[51,54]

Perhaps the clearest example of IEB, offered by Dahabreh and Kent, is the paradoxical "protective effect (again, it is really an association and not an "effect") of a patent foramen ovale (PFO) on recurrent cryptogenic stroke.[55] Patients with cryptogenic stroke are about two times as likely to have PFO compared to the general population. The well-established pathological mechanism is right-to-left shunts via the PFO, which enable thromboemboli from the venous circulation to reach the arterial circulation, a phenomenon termed "paradoxical embolism."

Why should patients with a history of PFO experience an ostensible "protective effect" against recurrent stroke? The answer lies in an auspicious clustering of potentially salutary variables among cryptogenic stroke survivors with PFO: relative freedom from a number of otherwise vasculopathological exposures. Compared to their counterparts with stroke not ascribed to PFO, patients with this congenital defect are less likely to smoke or have elevated cholesterol, hypertension, or diabetes. They also tend to be younger. This favorable constellation of clinical variables, not the existence of PFO per se, explains the "paradoxical protective effect" of PFO against recurrent cryptogenic stroke.[51,55]

A type of allocation bias (or nonrandom assignment), channeling bias may result in a spurious association between treatment with a medication and an undesirable disease outcome.[56] According to Lobo and co-workers, "Channeling occurs when drug therapies with similar indications are preferentially prescribed to groups of patients with varying baseline prognoses."[57] Irrespective of potential health benefits demonstrable in clinical trials, observational studies may incorrectly associate a therapy with less favorable outcomes because recipients of a treatment are inherently less likely to respond. Purported (or putative) benefits of a new medication may "channel" it to patients with a different disease profile, leading investigators to ascribe morbidity to the treatment. Propensity score analysis is one statistical method to adjust for allocation bias and resulting channeling bias.[57]

Prospective studies that randomly allocate patients while stratifying on age, disease severity, number and severity of comorbidities, and other baseline sociodemographic or clinical factors can largely neutralize these potential biases. ANCOVAs must be structured in a thoughtful, methodical way, using published literature and other data to inform *a priori* (prespecified) decisions concerning which covariates to include in the models. Although constructing an effective ANCOVA can help to control for factors that might otherwise bias findings, doing so reduces the number of degrees of freedom of an analysis.

Finally, two major forms of bias that often plague RCTs, which are otherwise designed to minimize such effects, are contamination (or crossover) bias and lack of intention-to-treat (ITT) analysis. Examples of the former include "drop-in" effects, whereby study participants in the control arm receive the active treatment after some length of time, often out of a justifiable ethical concern that patients with a serious and treatable condition should not be denied active treatment. In this example, benefits of the active treatment compared to placebo might tend to be biased toward the null (underestimated). In the Fenofibrate Intervention and Event Lowering in Diabetes (FIELD) study of patients with type 2 diabetes mellitus and dyslipidemia who were not using a statin at baseline and were randomized to the fibric-acid derivative or placebo, many study participants initially randomized to placebo received more effective agents (vs. fenofibrate, i.e., statins), potentially biasing the findings to the null.[58]

One way to adjust for contamination bias is to conduct a Complier Average Causal Effect.[59] Other statistical methods include inverse probability weighting of censoring and rank-preserving structural failure time models.[60]

By including all subjects randomly allocated to one experimental group or another, ITT analyses tend to minimize SB and confounding more effectively.

3.9 STATISTICAL TESTS FOR CATEGORICAL DATA: EXAMPLES AND EXERCISES

3.9.1 Paired data

3.9.1.1 McNEMAR'S TEST[61]

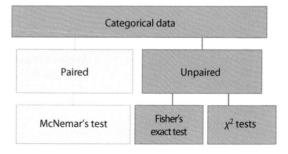

The dependence of categorical data that are paired or matched is evaluated using McNemar's test. One major application in biostatistics is to determine genetic linkage disequilibrium. McNemar's test is considered to be a special application of the χ^2 (chi-squared) test, which is reviewed in further detail below.

The McNemar test statistic is given as:

$$\chi^2_{1df} = \frac{\left(\left|b-c\right|\right)-1)^2}{b+c}$$

where χ^2_{1df} = McNemar's χ^2 with 1 degree of freedom.

For McNemar's test (and other statistical tests of potential associations or relationships among categorical data), we construct a contingency (often 2 × 2; see below) table (Table 3.7).

The variable a is the number of pairs with a "yes (case)-yes (control)" combination; b is "yes-no"; c is "no-yes"; and d is "no-no."

As an illustration, suppose that we have two groups of patients: cases with chronic obstructive pulmonary disease (COPD) and controls without. The NH and AH may be stated as follows:

H_0: Smoking history (expressed as a binary variable) is not statistically significantly associated with the presence or absence of COPD in a respiratory clinic.

H_1: Smoking history (expressed as a binary variable) is statistically significantly associated with the presence or absence of COPD in a respiratory clinic.

The contingency table structure is shown in Table 3.8, and hypothetical sets of paired data for smoking (yes/no) and COPD present (case) or absent (control) are summarized in Table 3.9. We are interested in concordant and discordant pairs.

$$\chi^2_{1df} = \frac{\left(\left|b-c\right|\right)-1)^2}{b+c}$$

$$\chi^2_{1df} = \frac{\left(\left|9-0\right|\right)-1)^2}{9+0}$$

$$\chi^2_{1df} = 7.1$$

For 1 degree of freedom, the χ^2_{1df} value of 7.1 (see Appendix 2) is significant at $\alpha < 0.01$.

The NH is rejected at p < 0.01, and the AH is accepted.

H_1: Smoking history (expressed as a binary variable) is statistically significantly associated with the presence or absence of COPD in a respiratory clinic.

As a second example, consider empirical treatment for a suspected outbreak of iatrogenic, expanded-spectrum β-lactamase (ESBL)–producing Gram-negative (Enterobacteriaceae) bacillary bacteremia in an adult intensive-care unit. The paired data might comprise a positive ("infection present") or negative ("infection

Table 3.7 Contingency table for categorical analyses

Biological factor present for:			
	Control member of pair	Control member of pair	
Diseased member of pair	Yes	No	Row totals
Yes	a	b	a + b
No	c	d	c + d
Column totals	a + c	b + d	
	Subject measure on variable B (present/absent)		
Subject measure on variable A (present/absent)	Yes	No	Row totals
Yes	a	b	a + b
No	c	d	c + d
Column totals	a + c	b + d	

Table 3.8 Contingency table for McNemar's test

Biological factor present for:	Control member of pair	Control member of pair
Diseased member of pair	Yes	No
Yes	a	b
No	c	d
Smoking present for		
	Controls	Controls
COPD cases	Yes	No
Yes	2	9
No	0	3

Table 3.9 Data for McNemar's test

Patient pair number	Smoking history?	
	COPD case	Control
1	Yes	No
2	No	No
3	Yes	Yes
4	Yes	No
5	Yes	No
6	No	No
7	Yes	Yes
8	No	No
9	Yes	No
10	Yes	No
11	Yes	No
12	Yes	No
13	Yes	No
14	Yes	No

absent") diagnosis before and after treatment of all patients with an investigational carbapenem. Our NH and AH follow:

H_0: There is no statistically significant association between treatment with the investigational carbapenem and the presence or absence of Enterobacteriaceae+ bacillary bacteremia.

H_1: There is a statistically significant association between treatment with the investigational carbapenem and the presence or absence of Enterobacteriaceae+ bacillary bacteremia.

Hypothetical data for 20 adults randomized to active treatment are presented in Table 3.10 and the appropriate 2 × 2 contingencies in Table 3.11.

$$\chi^2_{1df} = \frac{\left(|b-c|-1\right)^2}{b+c}$$

$$\chi^2_{1df} = \frac{\left(|11-3|-1\right)^2}{11+3}$$

$$\chi^2_{1df} = 3.5$$

For 1 degree of freedom, the χ^2 value of 3.5 is not significant at $\alpha = 0.05$. The NH is not rejected at $p < 0.05$.

H_0: There is no significant association between treatment with the investigational carbapenem and the presence or absence of Enterobacteriaceae+ bacillary bacteremia.

3.9.2 Unpaired Data

3.9.2.1 FISHER'S EXACT TEST (FET) OR FISHER'S EXACT TEST OF CONTINGENCY[62–64]

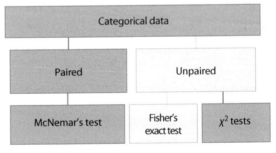

Sir Ronald Aylmer (R.A.) Fisher (February 17, 1890–July 29, 1962) was a mathematician and geneticist who, along with Karl Pearson (originally "Carl"; March 27, 1857–April 27, 1936), was among the most influential biostatisticians in history. Although the FET bears his name, we could also refer to his other tests and methods as "Fisher's ANOVA," "Fisher's ANCOVA," and "Fisher's randomization." He was also the first person to suggest (in 1926) that an α value of 0.05 might be a useful starting point to compare treatments for statistical significance; however, Sir Ronald was equally willing to consider varying this value according to prior expectation, suggesting that the great "frequentist" also had "Bayesian interests" and reminding us that the value of 0.05 and the 95% level of confidence are arbitrary.

Table 3.10 Data for McNemar's test

Patient number	Enterobacteriaceae[+] bacteremia present? Before treatment with investigational carbapenem	Enterobacteriaceae[+] bacteremia present? After treatment with investigational carbapenem
1	Yes	No
2	No	Yes
3	Yes	Yes
4	Yes	No
5	No	Yes
6	No	No
7	Yes	Yes
8	No	No
9	Yes	No
10	Yes	No
11	Yes	No
12	Yes	No
13	Yes	No
14	Yes	No
15	No	No
16	Yes	No
17	No	Yes
18	Yes	No
19	Yes	Yes
20	Yes	No

Table 3.11 Contingency table and data for McNemar's test

Before treatment	After treatment Disease present	After treatment Disease absent
Disease present	a	c
Disease absent	b	d
Before treatment	After treatment Disease present	After treatment Disease absent
Disease present	3	11
Disease absent	3	3

A brief historical digression may be instructive. In his book *Lady Tasting Tea: How Statistics Revolutionized Science in the Twentieth Century* (2002; Henry Holt), mathematician David Salsburg, PhD, chronicled a study reported by Fisher,[65] who is also the progenitor of randomization in contemporary clinical trials. (He also developed analysis of variance [ANOVA], which is discussed below. The corresponding progenitor of experimental blinding? That would

be America's Founding Father Benjamin Franklin, who used the procedure to debunk Mesmerism.)

As the story goes, Dr. Blanche Muriel Bristol, a psychologist and student of ways in which algae obtain nutrients, claimed that she could reliably discern the order in which the tea or milk was poured into her teacup. Sir Ronald seized on this premise as an opportunity for empirical testing, rather than the proverbial "tempest in a teapot."

Fisher devised an experiment in which 8 cups of tea would be prepared ($n = 8$ total cups): 4 each with the tea or milk added first ($k = 4$). Eight cups were put before Dr. Bristol in a randomized sequence unknown to her (although she was informed that she was being tested), after which she was asked to ply her purportedly keen gastronomical and olfactory talents. In other words, she would sample each of the 8 cups and needed to determine which 4 were prepared by one or the other method. Fisher computed the total number of permutations of choices, according to random probability, as

$$\frac{n!}{(n-k!)k!}$$

$$= \frac{8!}{(8 - 4!)4!} = 70$$

Sir Fisher's NH and AH can be summarized as follows:

H_0: Dr. Bristol cannot reliably discern the true sequence in which tea or milk is added to her cup.

H_1: Dr. Bristol can reliably discern the true sequence in which tea or milk is added to her cup.

When Dr. Bristol proved herself able to categorize all 8 cups, the NH was rejected at a p value of < 5% because the likelihood of doing so entirely by chance was 1/70 (1.43%).

In this case, Fisher was testing the dependence of two categorical variables: (1) whether tea or milk was actually poured first into Dr. Bristol's cup and (2) whether Dr. Bristol correctly judged that tea or milk was poured first. In a manner of speaking, William Sealy Gosset was the author of Student's t-test, but "the Fisher King" and knighted mathematician was the author of "**Fisher's 'Tea-Test!'**"

In truth, the mathematician J.O. Irwin developed a similar formulation in parallel, although Fisher reported his findings in 1935 and Irwin in 1936. (The FET is hence also often referred to as the Fisher–Irwin Test).

The FET evaluates the independence of categorical variables, typically in relatively small sample sizes, and yields an "exact" p value (rather than e.g., p < 0.05) befitting its name. Conversely, FET also provides the probability that an observed level of dependence occurs more frequently than might be expected by chance. In modern biostatistics, FET is often used to compare categorical descriptive data across treatment or other groups (e.g., baseline sociodemographic or clinical characteristics). Typically, FET is used with smaller samples, including cell values of ≤5 to 10.

FET statistics are given as:

$$p = \frac{(a+b)!(c+d)!(a+c)!(b+d)!}{a!b!c!d!n!}$$

(The symbol "!" signifies "factorial," where, for example, 4! [factorial] = 4 × 3 ×2 ×1.)

The hypergeometric formula applies to a contingency table such as is shown in Table 3.12. Tabulated are the likelihoods of successful surgical outcomes (let us say, appendectomy without infectious or other complications) by surgeons trained in a community hospital (A) or a tertiary-care, academic hospital (B).

Let us now introduce the observed data for a total of 20 surgical procedures (Table 3.13). The NH and AH may be stated as follows:

H_0: There is no statistically significant difference in surgical outcome between Hospitals A and B.

H_1: There is a statistically significant difference in surgical outcome between Hospitals A and B.

Table 3.12 Contingency table for Fisher's exact test (FET)

Surgical outcome	Hospital A	Hospital B	Row totals
No complications	a	b	a + b
Complications	c	d	c + d
Column totals	a + c	b + d	a + b + c + d (= n)

Table 3.13 Data for FET

Surgical outcome	Hospital A	Hospital B	Row totals
No complications	1	9	10
Complications	9	1	10
Column totals	10	10	20

$$p = \frac{(a+b)!(c+d)!(a+c)!(b+d)!}{a!b!c!d!n!}$$

$$p = \frac{(1+9)!(9+1)!(1+9)!(9+1)!}{1!9!9!1!20!}$$

$$p = 5.41 \times 10^{-4}$$

The NH is rejected at p = 0.000541 and we accept the AH:

H_1: There is a significant difference in surgical outcome between Hospitals A and B.

3.9.2.2 χ^2 (CHI-SQUARED) TEST[66]

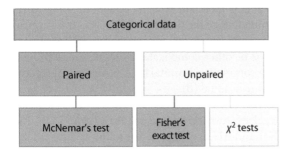

To determine whether observed differences between unpaired categorical data from large samples can be attributed to random probability, the χ^2 test is appropriate. The χ^2 test is used when there is at least one category of frequency data involving a simple random sample ($N \geq 10$, as mentioned above) comprising independent observations.

The χ^2 test statistics is given as follows:

$$\chi^2 = \sum_{i}^{2} \sum_{j}^{2} \frac{\left(\left|n_{ij} - e_{ij}\right|\right)^2}{e_{ij}}$$

In the above equation, i is the row value and j is the column value in a contingency table with two rows and two columns; the two "sigmas" (Σs) with the digit 2 above them instruct us to sum across these i rows and j columns. (If there were three columns and three rows, the digit above the sigma would be 3.) n_{ij} signifies the count (total) n in row i and column j that is observed, whereas e_{ij} signifies the numbers in row i and column j that would be expected based on random probability alone if the data summarized (or tabulated) in the columns were independent of those in the rows. The e_{ij} (expected) value can be calculated from the observed values, as we will demonstrate in the exercise below.

The number of degrees of freedom (df) for the above equation with r number of rows and c number of columns in the contingency table is given as

$$df = (r-1)(c-1)$$

When the numbers inside rows (r) and columns (c) in a contingency table evaluating associations between (or among) categorical variables exceed 10, it becomes inefficient (even for a computer) to calculate the FET. Instead we turn to the χ^2 test, which provides an approximate, rather than an exact, p value because the computed sampling distribution approximates the theoretical χ^2 distribution when the NH is not false. For this reason, although we typically prefer to report exact p values, with the χ^2 test we must accept values such as p < 0.0001.

As an example, let us say that we wish to determine whether the presence of either a 1 $\log_{10}$ increase in RNA viral load or a 100-cell/mm^3 decrease in CD4$^+$ T lymphocytes in a 1-year period is associated with conversion from HIV to AIDS in patients who have not been treated with highly active antiretroviral therapies. The NH and AH may be stated as follows:

H_0: There is no statistically significant association between the presence of increased viral load and/or decreased T-cell counts over 1 year and the likelihood of converting from HIV to AIDS.

H_1: There is a statistically significant association between the presence of increased viral load and/or decreased T-cell counts over 1 year and the likelihood of converting from HIV to AIDS.

Table 3.14 presents the contingency table and Table 3.15 the hypothetical data.

We compute the expected value for each cell from the observed values:

$$e_{ij} = \frac{ni \times nj}{n}$$

Expected values are calculated as:

$$\text{Expected} = \frac{\text{row sum} \times \text{column sum}}{\text{total sum}}$$

e_{11} (expected value for row 1, column 1)

$$= \frac{177\,(\text{row 1 total}) \times 153\,(\text{column 1 total})}{318} = 85.2$$

e_{12} (expected value for row 1, column 2)

$$= \frac{177\,(\text{row 1 total}) \times 165\,(\text{column 2 total})}{318} = 91.8$$

e_{21} (expected value for row 2, column 1)

$$= \frac{141\,(\text{row 2 total}) \times 153\,(\text{column 1 total})}{318} = 67.8$$

e_{22} (expected value for row 2, column 2)

$$= \frac{141\,(\text{row 2 total}) \times 165\,(\text{column 2 total})}{318} = 73.2$$

$$\chi^2 = \sum_i^2 \sum_j^2 \frac{\left(\left|n_{ij} - e_{ij}\right|\right)^2}{e_{ij}}$$

$$\chi^2 = \frac{\left[\left|110 - 85.2\right|\right]^2}{85.2} + \frac{\left[\left|67 - 91.8\right|\right]^2}{91.8}$$

$$+ \frac{\left[\left|43 - 67.8\right|\right]^2}{67.8} \frac{\left[\left|98 - 73.2\right|\right]^2}{73.2}$$

$$\chi^2 = 7.2 + 6.7 + 9.1 + 8.4 = 31.4$$

Table 3.14 Contingency table for χ^2 test

Numbers of patients with conversion from HIV to AIDS			
Viral load/CD4 criteria	Yes	No	Total
Either criteria met	n_{11}	n_{12}	ni_1
Neither criteria met	n_{21}	n_{22}	ni_2
Total	nj_1	nj_2	n_{ij} (n)

n_{11} = First row (i_1), first column (j_1); n_{12} = first row (i_1), second column (j_2); n_{21} = second row (i_2), first column (j_1); and n_{22} = second row (i_2), second column (j_2). ni_1 and ni_2 = Totals of rows 1 and 2; nj_1 and nj_2 = totals of columns 1 and 2; and n_{ij} = totals of columns and rows.

Table 3.15 Data for χ^2 test

Viral load/CD4 criteria	Patients converted from HIV to AIDS — Yes	Patients converted from HIV to AIDS — No	Total
Either criteria met	110	67	177
Neither criteria met	43	98	141
Total	153	165	318

There are 2 rows (r) and 2 columns (c); hence, $df = (r - 1)(c - 1) = (2 - 1)(2 - 1) = 1$.

In the χ^2 distribution for 1 df, 31.4 > 3.84 (critical significance value; Appendix 2).

The association is significant at a two-tailed $\alpha < 0.0005$.

The NH is rejected at p < 0.0005, and the AH is accepted.

H_1: There is a statistically significant association between the presence of increased viral load and/or decreased T-cell counts over 1 year and the likelihood of converting from HIV to AIDS.

3.9.2.2.1 Cochran–Mantel–Haenszel (CMH) χ^2_{MH} test[67,68]

Also known simply as the Mantel–Haenszel test, the CMH allows us to evaluate the conditional independence of binary (categorical) variables by testing associations in a total of k 2 × 2 contingency tables. Such associations include measures taken in two groups at more than one time or setting. We might have three nominal variables, such as treatment with a certain medication (binary variable 1; yes or no), improvement in a biological parameter (binary variable 2; yes or no), and a third nominal variable concerning the independence of these variables in different clinical trials, at different times, or in distinct clinical settings (i.e., repeat nominal variable). The CMH test can also generate a common odds ratio (OR_{MH}) to assess effect sizes when pooled across these different studies, with an NH of conditional independence assuming that all conditional OR_{MH} values across the k tables = 1.0. The CMH test also enables us to evaluate potential effects of confounding variables on associations between variables.

The test statistic is given as:

$$\chi^2_{MH} = \frac{\sum |[a-(a+b)(a+c)/n]|-0.5]]^2}{\sum (a+b)(a+c)(b+d)(c+d)/(n^3-n^2)}$$

where the numerator comprises the square of the sum of absolute values of differences between observed and expected nominal variables in cells, and the denominator comprises the variance of these squared differences.

As suggested above, if we fail to consider potentially confounding variables, which are associated with both the dependent variable (e.g., treatment or exposure) and the independent variable (e.g., outcome), "the results do not reflect the actual relationship between the variables under study."[69]

The following example is informed by a cross-sectional study of asthma prevalence among 14,244 children in disadvantaged communities.[70] Suppose that we define one nominal variable as Non-Hispanic White (NHW) or Non-Hispanic Black (NHB) race. The second nominal variable is the presence or absence of asthma symptoms in youngsters. Table 3.16 presents the contingency table and Tables 3.17 and 3.18 present the hypothetical data. The prevalence of asthma symptoms in NHB and NHW children is approximately 15%. Is this the entire story?

Alas, no. The confounding factor (again) is SES, which was associated with both the exposure (race) and the outcome (asthma symptoms) in the study population.[70] NHBs in this study were more likely to occupy lower SES strata, and residence in these strata was in turn related to exposure to poorer air quality (a risk factor for asthma symptoms) and reduced economic resources to afford asthma care (another risk factor for prevalent asthma symptoms). Let us now set up revised contingency tables according to SES as a binomial, nominal variable: either <50% or ≥50% of the federal poverty level (FPL).

When broken out by SES, the data reveal that similar proportions of both NHB and NHW youngsters in lower strata had asthma symptoms. The disparity in data derived from the fact that, in this population, higher numbers (%) of NHB youngsters resided in disadvantaged circumstances. Residence in lower SES strata was in turn associated with both the exposures (poor air

Table 3.16 Contingency table for Cochran–Mantel–Haenszel (CMH) test

Exposure	Treatment outcome (improved)	Treatment outcome (not improved)	Row totals
Treatment	a	b	$a + b$
No treatment	c	d	$c + d$
Column totals	$a + c$	$b + d$	$a + b + c + d (= n)$

Table 3.17 Contingency table and data for CMH test

SES	Disease status Asthma symptoms present	Disease status Asthma symptoms absent	Row totals
<50% × FPL (Exposure 2)	d_{1i}	h_{1i}	n_{1i}
≥50% × FPL (Exposure 1)	d_{0i}	h_{0i}	n_{0i}
Column totals	d_i	h_i	n_i

Stratum 1 (NHBs)

SES	Disease status Asthma symptoms present	Disease status Asthma symptoms absent	Row totals
<50% × FPL (Exposure 2)	200 (22.2%)	700 (77.8%)	900
≥50% × FPL (Exposure 1)	31 (5.5%)	536 (94.5%)	567
Column totals	231 (15.7%)	1,236 (84.3%)	1,467

Stratum 2 (NHWs)

SES	Disease status Asthma symptoms present	Disease status Asthma symptoms absent	Row totals
<50% × FPL (Exposure 2)	152 (22.1%)	536 (77.9%)	688
≥50% × FPL (Exposure 1)	28 (5.5%)	484 (94.5%)	512
Column totals	180 (15.0%)	1,020 (85.0%)	1,200

Table 3.18 Contingency table and data for CMH test

Race	Disease status Asthma symptoms present	Disease status Asthma symptoms absent	Row totals
NHB (1)	d_{1i}	h_{1i}	n_{1i}
NHW (0)	d_{0i}	h_{0i}	n_{0i}
Column totals	d_i	h_i	n_i

Race	Disease status Asthma symptoms present	Disease status Asthma symptoms absent	Row totals
NHB race	231 (15.7%)	1,236 (85.0%)	1,467
NHW race	180 (15.0%)	1,020 (85.0%)	1,200
Column totals	411	2,256	2,667

The variable d denotes presence of disease and h absence of disease (healthy).

quality, fewer health-care resources) and outcome (presence of asthma symptoms).

The relationship described above meets the definition of confounding. In this population, the confounding variable (C) of SES relates to both the exposure (E; race) and outcome or disease (D; asthma symptoms). This situation is likely not explained by effect modification because there is no evidence that race alone modified the association between SES and the presence of asthma symptoms: in each race, the risk of asthma symptoms was nearly 4-fold greater in the lower (vs. upper) SES stratum.

Let us use the CMH test to evaluate whether asthma symptoms (present or absent) are associated with SES (<50% or ≥50% × FPL), each expressed as nominal variables.

The NH and AH may be stated as follows:

H_0: There is no statistically significant association between SES (<50% or ≥50% × FPL) and the presence or absence of asthma symptoms.

H_1: There is a statistically significant association between SES (<50% or ≥50% × FPL) and the presence or absence of asthma symptoms.

We apply the following equations to compute the CMH summary OR (Table 3.19):

$$OR_{MH} = \frac{Q}{R}$$

where:

$$Q = \sum \frac{(d_{1i} \times h_{0i})}{n_i}$$

$$R = \sum \frac{(d_{0i} \times h_{1i})}{n_i}$$

where d_{1i} is the number of observed outcomes (disease = D = youngsters with asthma symptoms) among those exposed to low SES (exposure = E; e_{1i}) across both racial subgroups.

O is the sum of observed numbers with asthma = 411.
E is the sum of expected numbers.
V is the sum of variances.

$$V = \sum \frac{d_i \times h_i \times n_{0i} \times n_{1i}}{n_i^2 \times (n_i - 1)}$$

The OR for asthma symptoms according to lower versus higher SES is computed as:

$$OR_{MH} = \frac{Q}{R} = 134.4 \div 27.3 = 4.92$$

Youngsters in the lower (vs. higher) SES stratum are nearly 5 times more likely to experience asthma symptoms. The value is midway between the OR values in the NHW (4.90) and NHB (4.94) groups.

To compute the 95% CI around the OR_{MH} = 4.92
95% CI = OR_{MH}/EF to OR_{MH} × EF
where EF = error factor = exp(1.96 × s.e.$_{MH}$)

In the case of the OR_{MH}, we compute s.e.$_{MH}$ as follows:

$$s.e._{MH} = \sqrt{\frac{V}{(Q \times R)}}$$

From Table 3.19, we have:

$$V = 83.6; Q = 134.4; R = 27.3$$

$$s.e._{MH} = \sqrt{\frac{83.6}{(134.4 \times 27.3)}} = 0.151$$

Table 3.19 Calculations for the CMH test

Stratum i (by SES)	OR_i	$\dfrac{R}{\dfrac{d_{0i} \times h_{1i}}{n_i}}$	$\dfrac{Q}{\dfrac{d_{1i} \times h_{0i}}{n_i}}$	V_i	d_{1i}	$E_{1i} = \dfrac{d_i \times n_{1i}}{n_i}$
NHBs (i =1)	4.94	$\frac{31 \times 700}{1,467} = 14.8$	$\frac{200 \times 536}{1,467} = 73.1$	46.1	200	$\frac{231 \times 900}{1,467} = 141.7$
NHWs (i = 2)	4.90	$\frac{28 \times 536}{1,200} = 12.5$	$\frac{152 \times 484}{1,200} = 61.3$	37.5	152	$\frac{180 \times 688}{1,200} = 103.2$
Totals		R = 27.3	Q = 134.4	V = 83.6 (sum of variances)	O =352 (sum of observed values)	E = 244.9 (sum of expected values)

$$95\% \text{ CI} = \text{OR}_{MH}/\text{EF (lower limit) to OR}_{MH}$$
$$\times \text{EF (upper limit)}$$

$$\textbf{EF} = \textbf{exp}(\textbf{1.96} \times \textbf{s.e.}_{MH})$$

$$\text{EF} = \exp(1.96 \times 0.15)0.151$$

$$95\% \text{ CI} = 4.92/\exp(1.96 \times 0.151) \text{ to } 4.92$$
$$\times \exp(1.96 \times 0.151)$$
$$4.92/1.35 \text{ to } 4.92 \times 1.35 =$$
$$\times$$
$$= 3.64 \text{ to } 6.64$$
$$95\% \text{ CI} = 3.64 \text{ to } 6.64$$

$$U = O - E = 352.0 - 244.9 = 107.1$$

$$\chi^2_{MH} = \frac{(U)^2}{V} = \frac{(107.1)^2}{83.6}$$

$$\chi^2_{MH} = 136.9, df = 1$$

This value far exceeds the critical value.

$$\chi^2_{MH} = 136.9, df = 1, p < 0.0005$$

We reject the NH and accept the AH:

H_1:   There is a statistically significant association between SES (<50% or ≥50% × FPL) and the presence or absence of asthma symptoms.

The CMH test can also assess the effects of at least two confounders.[13] Other statistical tests (aside from CMH) to control for confounding in observational studies include PSM and ANCOVA.

3.9.2.2.2 χ^2 Test of heterogeneity

Effect modification was discussed earlier in this chapter. One example would be a finding that diabetes (exposure, or E) is a stronger risk factor for incident coronary heart disease (CHD; disease, or D) in one gender compared with another: for example, the relative risk for coronary events

might be higher in women (stratum 1) compared to men (stratum 2).[71]

Regression models are effective and flexible strategies to test for effect modification.[13] However, performing the χ^2 test of heterogeneity can also meet this need (Table 3.20). Building on the prior example, the NH and AH may be expressed as follows:

H_0:   Racial identity does not modify the association between SES and the risk of asthma symptoms. The OR in each stratum does not differ significantly from the overall summary OR_{MH} (4.92 in the above example).

H_1:   Racial identity modifies the association between SES and the risk of asthma symptoms. The OR in each stratum does differ significantly from the overall summary OR_{MH} (4.92 in the above example).

The χ^2 test of heterogeneity statistic is given as

$$\chi^2 = \sum \frac{(d_{1i} \times h_{0i} - \text{OR}_{MH} \times d_{0i} \times h_{1i})^2}{\text{OR}_{MH} \times V_i \times n_i^2}$$

$df = c$ **(number of strata)** $- 1 = 1$ **(in this example)**

For calculations, see Table 3.20. For $df = 1$, $\chi^2_{MH} = 0.00067$ is much less than the critical value. The NH is not rejected.

H_0:   Racial identity does not significantly modify the association between SES and the risk of asthma symptoms. There is no effect modification.

3.10 STATISTICAL TESTS FOR CONTINUOUS DATA: EXAMPLES AND EXERCISES

3.10.1 Parametric tests

3.10.1.1 STUDENT'S (GOSSET'S) t-TEST (SMALLER SAMPLES)[72] OR z-TEST (LARGER SAMPLES) (PAIRED)

Student's t-test compares population means of continuous variables between two groups, such as active treatment versus placebo or before versus after treatment. For tests of continuous

Table 3.20 Data for χ^2 test of heterogeneity (for CMH test)

SES	Disease status — Asthma symptoms present (j_1)	Disease status — Asthma symptoms absent (j_2)	Row totals
<50% × FPL (Exposure 2) (i_1)	d_i	h_i	n_i
≥50% × FPL (Exposure 1) (i_2)	d_{0i}	h_{0i}	n_{0i}
Column totals	d_{1i}	h_{1i}	n_{1i}

Stratum i	$(d_{1i} \times h_{0i} - OR_{MH} \times d_{0i} \times h_{1i})^2$	$OR_{MH} \times V_i \times n_i^2$	$\dfrac{\Sigma(d_{1i} \times h_{01} - OR_{MH} \times d_{0i} \times h_{1i})^2}{OR_{MH} \times V_i \times n_i^2}$
NHBs ($i = 1$)	$(200 \times 536 - 4.92 \times 31 \times 700)^2 = 1.90 \times 10^5$	$4.92 \times 46.2 \times 1,467^2 = 4.89 \times 10^8$	$\dfrac{1.91 \times 10^5}{4.89 \times 10^8} = 3.91 \times 10^{-4}$
NHWs ($i = 2$)	$(152 \times 484 - 4.92 \times 28 \times 536)^2 = 7.36 \times 10^4$	$4.92 \times 37.5 \times 1,200^2 = 2.66 \times 10^8$	$\dfrac{7.36 \times 10^4}{2.66 \times 10^8} = 2.77 \times 10^{-4}$
			Total = $6.7 \times 10^{-4} = 0.00067$

data among three or more populations, refer to ANOVA.

Student's t-test statistic is given as:

$$t = \frac{\bar{x}}{SE}$$

$$SE = \frac{s}{\sqrt{n}}$$

$$= \frac{\bar{x}}{s\sqrt{n}}$$

where $\bar{x}$ = the mean of the paired difference in data; SE = the standard error of the difference between the means; s = the SD of this difference, and n = the number of pairs.

The "Student" in Student's t-test was the pseudonym of agrostatistician William Sealy Gosset, who was an employee of Guinness around the turn of the twentieth century. (Yes, *that* Guinness: the beer maker!) While applying statistical methods to identify high-yielding barleys, Gosset collaborated with the aforementioned Karl Pearson. A prior

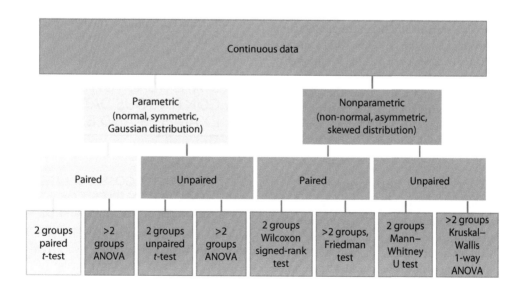

Guinness researcher had reported trade secrets, leading the company to forbid its employees to publish further papers, irrespective of their content. Gosset exhorted his employer to allow publication of his findings, which were of interest to mathematicians and not necessarily other breweries. Guinness acquiesced but mandated use of the pseudonym.

To honor the progenitor of this influential test, henceforth this text will refer to "Student's *t*-test" as "Gosset's *t*-test." I urge wider adoption of this name—unless, of course, my urging this might result in reduced access to a nice glass of stout!

As a hypothetical example, let us suppose that an investigational antidiabetic medication is being compared to placebo in a randomized, controlled crossover trial ($N = 10$; where each subject receives active treatment or placebo in a randomized sequence and hence serves as his or her own control). The data are presented in Table 3.21.

The NH and AH may be stated as follows:

H_0: There is no statistically significant difference between the effects of active treatment and placebo on hemoglobin A1c (HbA1c).

H_1: There is a statistically significant difference between the effects of active treatment and placebo on HbA1c.

Table 3.21 Data for Student's (Gosset's) *t*-test

Patient no.	HbA1c,% Active treatment	HbA1c,% Placebo	Difference
1	6.3	7.2	−0.9
2	6.2	7.4	−1.2
3	6.5	7.3	−0.8
4	6.8	7.8	−1.0
5	6.1	7.3	−1.2
6	6.3	7.5	−1.2
7	7.0	8.0	−1.0
8	6.9	7.8	−0.9
9	7.2	7.6	−0.4
10	6.4	7.9	−1.5
Mean ($\bar{x}$)=	6.57	7.58	1.01
SD (*s*) =	0.38	0.28	0.28

Table 3.21 summarizes continuous paired data for 10 subjects.

$$t = \frac{1.01}{0.28\sqrt{10}}$$

$$t = 1.14 \; df = 9(10-1)$$

For 9 *df*, the *t* value for a two-tailed $\alpha = 0.05 = 2.262$. We are not able to reject the NH.

The NH is not rejected at p < 0.05

H_0: There is no statistically significant difference between the effects of active treatment and placebo on hemoglobin A1c (HbA1c).

Figure 3.10 shows how to conduct Gosset's *t*-test using Microsoft Excel. The two distributions are significantly different at $p = 9.55 \times 10^{-6}$ ($p = 0.00000955$, or, by convention, p < 0.0001).

3.10.1.2 ONE-WAY ANALYSIS OF VARIANCE (ANOVA); *F* TEST[73,74]

As mentioned above, ANOVA partitions variation due to treatment effects (in the numerator) versus variation due to random probability and/or biological variation (in the denominator). In statistical terminology, ANOVA partitions sums of squares (SS) into different elements: SS due to group mean differences (SSM) and SS due to within-group differences between data (i.e., residual SS due to error [SSE]). Assumptions of ANOVA and the *F* test include a normally distributed outcome and a population SD value between individuals that is identical in each exposure group.[13]

ANOVA enables the analyst to evaluate the equality of more than two groups. In this manner, ANOVA extends Gosset's *t*-test to three or more populations. Hence, ANOVA and Gosset's *t*-test have similar assumptions: (1) a normal (i.e., symmetrical, Gaussian) distribution of results in each group (i.e., normally distributed residuals), (2) independent (i.e., not correlated) observations, and (3) equal variances in each group. This final condition is also known as "homogeneity of variances" or homoscedasticity in certain cases.

However, compared to Gosset's *t*-test, ANOVA is less frequently associated with Type 1 Error.

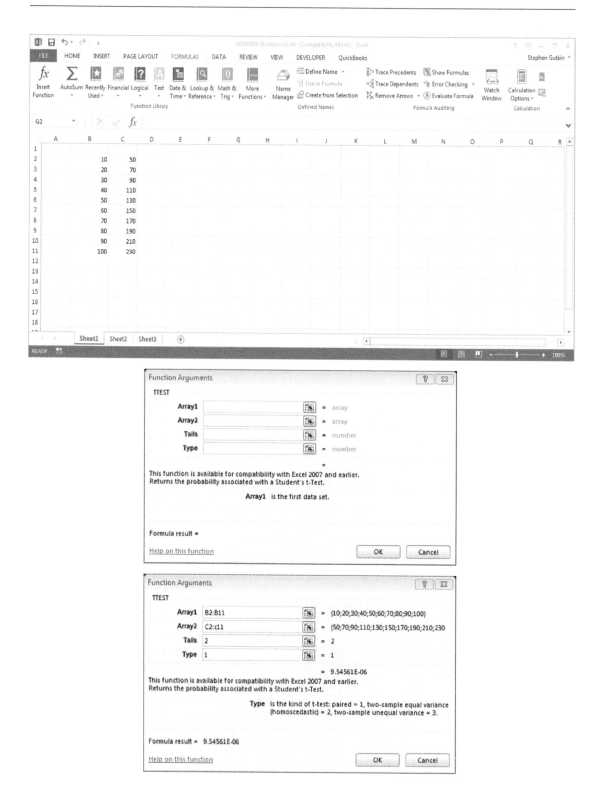

Figure 3.10 Using Microsoft Excel to conduct two-tailed Student's (Gosset's) *t*-test between two distributions of paired data.

The *F* test ANOVA statistic (also known as the variance ratio test) is given as:

$$F = \frac{\text{Between-group MS}}{\text{Within-group MS}} = \frac{\text{MSM}}{\text{MSE}} = \frac{sm^2}{se^2}$$

where *MS* = mean square.

The numerator may also be expressed as variance due to mean treatment effects, or MSM. The denominator may also be expressed as variance due to random probability and biological variation (error), or MSE.

Sum of squares of mean treatment effects (i.e., sum of squares of means, or SSM) are computed as

$$\text{SSM} = \sum_{}^{k} n_i (m_1 - m)^2$$

$$sm^2 = \text{MSM} = \frac{\text{SSM}}{(k-1)} \sum n_i \frac{(m_1 - m)^2}{k-1}$$

where *k* = the number of treatment groups and $m_i - m$ = the differences between each of *k* different treatment group means (m_i) and the overall mean (*m*), and *n* is the number of observations.

The sum of squares due to differences between observations (and mean) within each group (i.e., sum of squares of error, SSE, or residual sum of squares) =

$$\text{SSE} = \text{SST} - \text{SSM} = \sum_{}^{n} (m_1 - m)^2 - \sum_{}^{k} (m_1 - m)^2$$

$$\text{SSE} = \sum_{}^{k} (n_i - 1) s_i^2$$

$$se^2 = \text{MSE} = \sum_{}^{k} \frac{(n_i - 1) s_i^2}{n - k}$$

where SST is the total sum of squares; s_i is the SD of each group's mean; *n* is the overall number of observations or patients; and *k* is the number of different treatment groups.

As an example, let us suppose that we wish to determine if the effects on hemoglobin (Hgb) levels differ significantly across three daily doses of an investigational erythropoietin-stimulating agent (ESA) (compound TF-1844 [2, 3, and 4 mg]) in 3 (= *k*) separate (independent, unpaired) treatment groups of women (Hgb reference range = 12.0 – 15.5 mg/dL; Table 3.22). Eligible patients had anemia associated with chronic kidney disease (CKD; baseline values not shown).

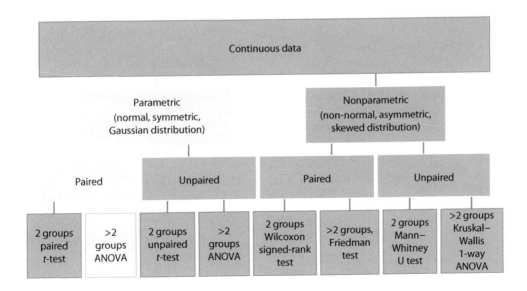

Table 3.22 Data for ANOVA

TF-1844 (2 mg)	On-treatment Hgb, mg/dL	On-treatment Hgb, mg/dL	
	TF-1844 (3 mg)	TF-1844 (4 mg)	Overall
11.8	12.5	15.2	
11.6	15.6	16.2	
12.2	12.4	15.8	
10.7	12.5	15.7	
13.8	13.2	16.5	
12.9	11.8	15.5	
11.7	12.4	14.9	
10.8	12.0	16.9	
11.5	12.5	15.0	
10.6	12.3	15.1	
12.1	12.2	15.4	
12.2	12.9	15.5	
10.4	12.7	15.9	
10.5	11.9	15.3	
11.2	12.9	14.1	
11.4	12.1	16.1	
11.3		15.1	
11.1		15.6	
10.9		15.5	
10.7			
Mean = 11.47	Mean = 12.62	Mean = 15.54	Total mean (pooled data) = 13.17
SD = 0.86	SD = 0.88	SD = 0.63	Overall SD = 1.90
$n = 20$	$n = 16$	$n = 19$	$N = 55$

The NH and AH are stated below.

H_0: There is no statistically significant difference among the effects of three daily doses of TF-1844 on hemoglobin levels in women with anemia associated with CKD.

H_1: There is a statistically significant difference among the effects of three daily doses of TF-1844 on hemoglobin levels in women with anemia associated with CKD.

$$F = \frac{\text{Between-group MS}}{\text{Within-group MS}} = \frac{\text{MSM}}{\text{MSE}} = \frac{sm^2}{se^2}$$

$$\text{MSM} = \sum_{i}^{k} n_i \frac{(m_i - m)^2}{k - 1}$$

$$\text{MSM} = \frac{20\left(11.47 - 13.17\right)^2 + 16\left(12.62 - 13.17\right)^2 + 19\left(15.54 - 13.17\right)^2}{3 - 1}$$

$$\text{MSM} = 84.68$$

$$\text{MSE} = \sum^{k} \frac{(n_i - 1)s_i^2}{n - k}$$

$$\text{MSE} = \frac{(19 \times 0.86^2) + (15 \times 0.88^2) + (18 \times 0.63^2)}{55 - 3}$$

$$\text{MSE} = 0.63$$

$$F = \frac{\text{Between-group MS}}{\text{Within-group MS}} = \frac{84.68}{0.63} = 134.4$$

For numerator $df = 2$ and denominator $df = 52$, the critical F value ranges from 3.15 to 3.18.

$$F = 134.4 > 3.15 - 3.18;\ p < 0.05$$

The NH is rejected at $p < 0.05$ and the AH is accepted.

H_1: There is a statistically significant difference among the effects of three daily doses of TF-1844 on hemoglobin levels in women with anemia associated with CKD.

One limitation of this ANOVA is that variances (SD^2) were similar across the 2- and 3-mg, but not the 4-mg, treatment group. This disparity might warrant further statistical testing (e.g., sensitivity analyses) or discussion in the study report manuscript. Figure 3.11 shows how to conduct a one-way ANOVA using Microsoft Excel.

We test whether there is a significant difference in outcomes among three different groups: study participants receiving Treatment A, B, or placebo.

H_0: There is no statistically significant difference in outcomes among the three treatment groups.
H_1: There is a statistically significant difference in outcomes among the three treatment groups.

First, we populate the spreadsheet and list the data. Note "Data Analysis" tab at extreme right. Highlight the data, right click, and then select "Copy." Next, we need to manage the inputs and outputs. The inputs will be the criteria of the ANOVA, will identify the data as ranging from B2 through D11, and will also include "One-way ANOVA or F test" in the "Data Analysis" drop-down menu. We will check the box indicating that the first row = headers. We will then specify the output: in which cells we want our summary ANOVA table to appear. In this example, we will choose K1.

Next, we click on "OK" to open windows that will enable us to enter inputs (data arrays and analyses) and outputs: where we want the summary ANOVA table to appear in the spreadsheet (in this case, row K1). By convention, we will accept $\alpha = 0.05$ as our significance level. We click "Labels in First Row," because our top rows include a heading for each group, and then indicate where we want the summary ANOVA table output to go (cell K1).

The input range is generated by holding the cursor over cells B2 through D11 or using the "up" arrows within the Data Analysis ANOVA menu. These arrows easily allow us to specify cells for both the inputs and outputs, including the summary data table for the F test. We have specified that the output needs to appear in cell K1. Now, when we click on "OK" our ANOVA summary table will appear in that cell. (Further instructions to conduct ANOVA using Microsoft Excel are provided in the legend to Figure 3.12).

3.10.1.2.1 Further background on, and implications of, ANOVA: Regression analysis, general linear model, two-factor ANOVA, repeated-measures ANOVA, and ANCOVA

ANOVA can also be considered to be an example of multiple regression analysis.[7] It is a versatile, "computationally elegant" test that has been applied in numerous experimental designs, enables comparisons of multiple samples, and is also robust to violations of assumptions (e.g., independence, normality, equal variances).[13] The ANOVA F test limits statistical error and hence augments power.

ANOVA may also be seen as a form of general linear model. When two categorical explanatory variables are included in a multiple-regression model, the results are identical to those from a two-way ANOVA.

3.10.1.3 ANCOVA[75]

Lowry aptly termed ANCOVA "a felicitous marriage between [ANOVA] and... concepts and procedures of linear correlation and regression..."[76] When seeking to adjust associations of IVs and DVs for the effects of one or more continuous variables, which are often termed "covariates," (CVs), "codeviates" (CDs), or "nuisance variables," one can often resort to ANCOVA.

One aim of ANCOVA is to increase statistical power by decreasing error variance when trial participants are studied under several independent experimental settings. In nonrandomized studies, ANCOVA can be employed to offset biases in samples.[77]

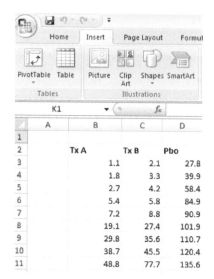

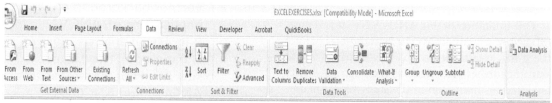

Figure 3.11 Using Microsoft Excel to conduct a one-way analysis of variance (ANOVA). *(Continued)*

Examples of CVs (or CDs) commonly encountered in RCTs and their analyses include treatment center, gender, and baseline values for age, disease severity, and comorbidities, which are often expressed as a continuous variable using the Charlson Comorbidity Index.[78] (The following exercise is informed by Lowry's example, which can be accessed at http://vassarstats.net/textbook/ch17pt2.html.[76])

ANCOVAs assess the effects of variation in a continuous variable (covariate) on variation in a categorical variable.[76] Let us suppose that we are interested in evaluating whether two methods of weight loss in 20 overweight patients differ in effectiveness (Table 3.23). (The ANOVA is completed via Excel in the latter panels of Figure 3.11.) Treatment A (categorical variable) comprises high-protein solid foodstuffs in 10 study participants, whereas

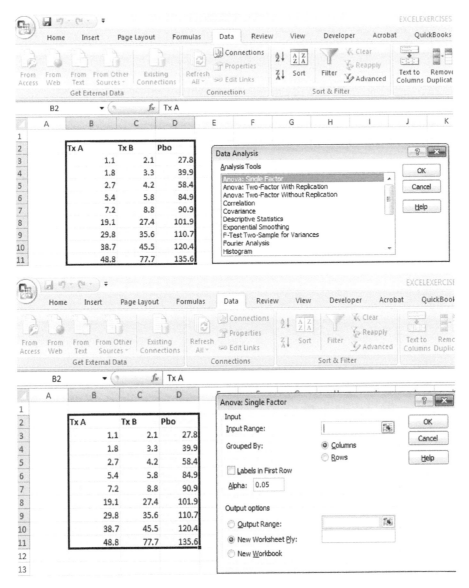

Figure 3.11 (Continued) Using Microsoft Excel to conduct a one-way ANOVA. *(Continued)*

Treatment B (categorical variable) is composed of isocaloric prepackaged nutrient drinks ("shakes") in the remaining 10.

Before we administer either of these regimens, however, we assess each subject's level of interest in carbohydrates on the Craving Scale, which ranges from 1 to 30. A response of 1 = extreme cravings and 30 = no cravings.

The independent variable X is the level of craving as scored continuously from 1 to 30, whereas the dependent variable Y is also a continuous variable: the number of pounds lost over 3 months. In a straightforward ANOVA, we might state the NH and AH as follows:

H_0: There is no statistically significant difference between Treatments A and B in their effects on weight loss after 3 months.

H_1: There is a statistically significant difference between Treatments A and B in their effects on weight loss after 3 months.

To perform the single-factor ANOVA, we list the hypothetical data according to the outcome variable

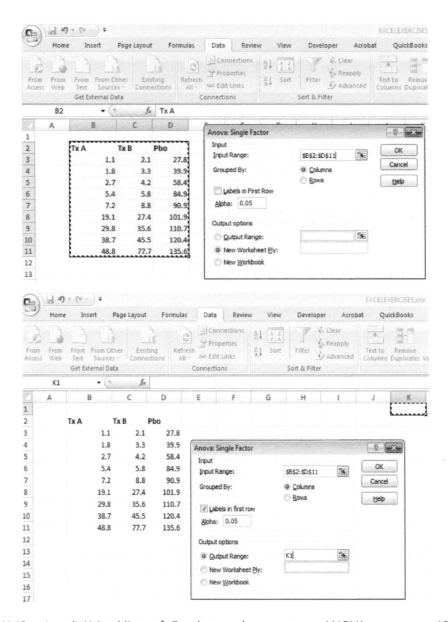

Figure 3.11 (Continued) Using Microsoft Excel to conduct a one-way ANOVA.   (Continued)

Y (weight lost in 3 months, in pounds) in Treatment A (Y_a) and Treatment B (Y_b) groups (Table 3.23). Figure 3.11 shows how to conduct an ANOVA of the data using Microsoft Excel. Treatment Group A has a mean (SD) weight loss of 30.8 (7.3). Treatment Group B has a mean (SD) weight loss of 29.8 (6.0).

The summary ANOVA table appears in Figure 3.11. The F value (0.112613) is well below the critical value (4.413873), meaning that weight loss did not differ significantly (p = 0.741069) in Treatment Groups A and B.

To assess whether weight loss in the two treatment groups covaries with carbohydrate cravings, we plot scores on the Craving Scale in the two groups (Tables 3.23–3.25). As mentioned above, the scale is scored from 1 (extreme cravings) to 30 (no cravings). The mean (SD) Craving Score is 13.2 (5.8) in Group A and 18.0 (7.5) in Group B.

Following steps explained in Figure 3.11, we conduct a one-way ANOVA of the craving scores (X_{ab}) using Microsoft Excel, resulting in data presented in Table 3.24. The F value (2.561265) is well below

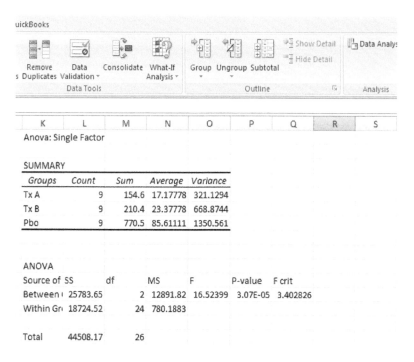

Figure 3.11 (Continued) Using Microsoft Excel to conduct a one-way ANOVA.

the critical value (4.413873), meaning that craving scores did not differ significantly (p = 0.126915) in Treatment Groups A and B.

Data to conduct an ANCOVA, in order to determine if carbohydrate cravings covary with weight loss in the two treatment groups, are presented in Table 3.25. (This example is informed by work by Richard Lowry, Vassar College, with calculations posted at http://vassarstats.net/textbook/ch17pt2.html. Last accessed November 1, 2017.) In an ANCOVA, the sum of the codeviates (SC) represents the raw measure of covariance between two variables and is computed as:

Table 3.23 Data for ANOVA

Subject no.	Weight lost in 3 mo, lb Treatment group A (Ya)	Subject no.	Weight lost in 3 mo, lb Treatment group B (Yb)
a1	22	b1	20
a2	24	b2	28
a3	32	b3	35
a4	26	b4	36
a5	33	b5	29
a6	42	b6	33
a7	28	b7	36
a8	44	b8	34
a9	27	b9	26
a10	30	b10	21
	$\Sigma Y_a = 308$		$\Sigma Y_b = 298$

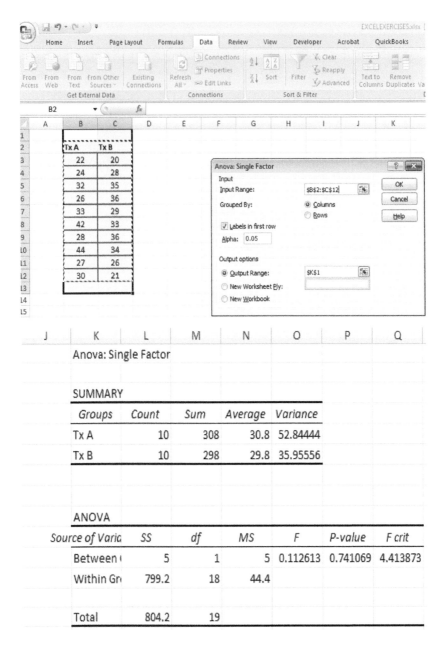

Figure 3.12 Using Microsoft Excel to conduct a one-way ANOVA. You may have to begin by loading, as an "Add-In," an "Analysis ToolPak." You can do this from the "File," "Options" drop-downs. If your version of Excel includes this function (or you have loaded it successfully), you will see the tab "Data Analysis" to the extreme right of your Excel toolbar. If not, click on File, Options, and "Manage Add-Ins," then add the Analysis ToolPak. Once completed, click on the "Data" tab to find the "Data Analysis" option to the extreme right of the task bar. Clicking on this brings up "Single-factor ANOVA" as the first option. After selecting this, follow the "up" arrow prompts to select your cells for data inputs and outputs (the summary table to compute *F*). *(Continued)*

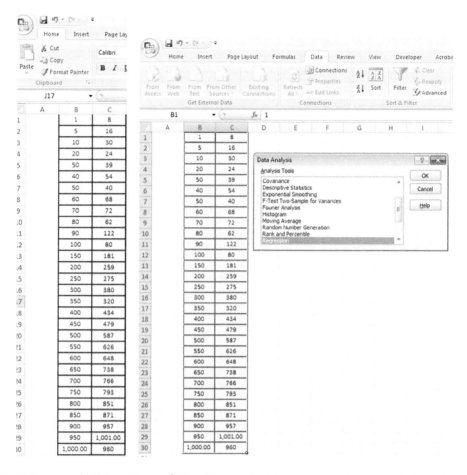

Figure 3.12 (Continued) Using Microsoft Excel to conduct linear regression analysis. The data set is from Table 3.33. (*Continued*)

$$SC = \sum (X_i - M_x)(Y_i - M_y) =$$

$$SC = \sum (X_i Y_i) - \frac{(\sum X_i)(\sum Y_i)}{N}$$

where:

$$(X_i - M_x) = \text{deviate}_x$$
$$(Y_i - M_y) = \text{deviate}_y$$
$$(X_i - M_x)(Y_i - M_y) = \text{codeviate}_{xy}$$

Two values are computed for SC: one for covariance of X and Y within each group (SC_{wg}) and the other for covariance within the total data array

(SC_T). We need to compute cross-products of Xi and Yi for each study participant in each treatment group (Table 3.26), as follows:

$$SC_T = \sum (X_i Y_i) - \frac{(\sum X_i)(\sum Y_i)}{N}$$

$$SC_T = 10,124 - \frac{(312)(606)}{20}$$

$$= 10,124 - 9,453.6 = 670.4$$

Above is the SC_T for the total array of data. Below are within-group SC (SC_{wg}) computations for each treatment arm.

Treatment Group A (High-Protein Solid Foodstuffs)

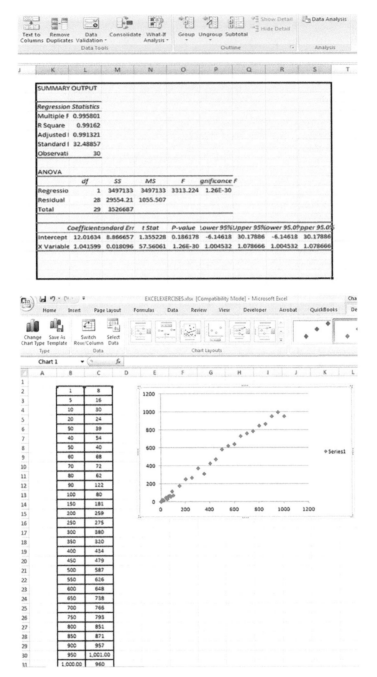

Figure 3.12 (Continued) Using Microsoft Excel to conduct linear regression analysis. The data set is from Table 3.33. *(Continued)*

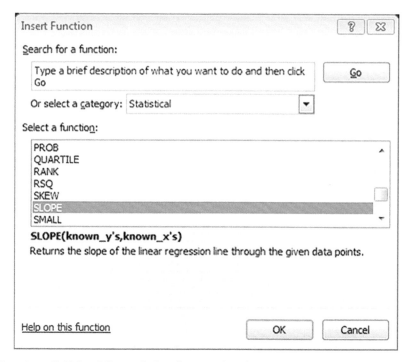

Figure 3.12 (Continued) Using Microsoft Excel to conduct linear regression analysis. The data set is from Table 3.33. (*Continued*)

$$SC_{wg(a)} = \sum (X_{ai}Y_{ai}) - \frac{(\sum X_{ai})(\sum Y_{ai})}{N_a}$$

$$SC_{wg(a)} = 4,374 - \frac{(132)(308)}{10}$$

$$= SC_{wg(a)} = 4,374.0 - 4,065.6 = 308.4$$

Treatment Group B (High-Protein Shakes)

$$SC_{wg(b)} = \sum (X_{bi}Y_{bi}) - \frac{(\sum X_{bi})(\sum Y_{bi})}{N_b}$$

$$SC_{wg(b)} = 5,750 - \frac{(180)(298)}{10} = 5,750 - 5,364 = 386$$

$$SC_{wg} = 308.4 + 386.0 = 694.4$$

From the above data and results summarized Table 3.26 and Figure 3.12 (ANOVA), we can now populate our summary table, including both ANOVA and covariance (SC) values (Table 3.27).

Next, we examine the correlation between X and Y to determine the total variability of Y that can be ascribed to covariance with X:

$$r_T = \frac{SC_T}{\sqrt[2]{SS_{T(x)} \times SS_{T(y)}}} = \frac{670.4}{\sqrt[2]{924.8 \times 804.2}}$$

$$SS_{Tx} = \sum x^2 - \frac{(\sum x)^2}{n}$$

$$SS_{Ty} = \sum y^2 - \frac{(\sum y)^2}{n}$$

$$r_T = \frac{670.4}{862.4} = 0.777$$

We compute the proportion of variance in weight lost in the two treatment groups in 3 months (Y) that can be ascribed to covariance with craving scores (X) using r^2:

$$(r_T)^2 = (0.777)^2 = 0.604$$

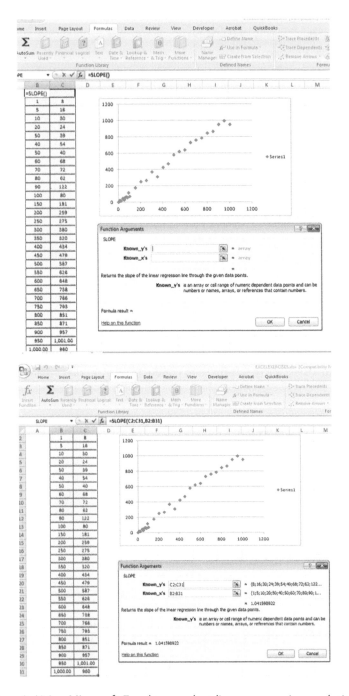

Figure 3.12 (Continued) Using Microsoft Excel to conduct linear regression analysis. The data set is from Table 3.33. (*Continued*)

Now we need to adjust the $SS_{T(Y)}$ value by removing the above proportion of covariance.

$$SS_{T(Y)} = 804.2 \times 0.604 = 485.7$$

$$\text{Adjusted } SS_{T(Y)} = 804.2 - 485.7 = 318.5$$

Additional needed data are from the original ANOVA for changes in weight on the two diets (without ANCOVA on craving scale), which can be found in Table 3.26 and Figure 3.12. We wish to adjust the $SS_{wg(Y)}$ value. However, we must first

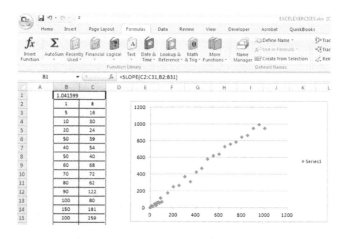

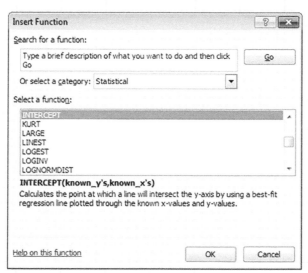

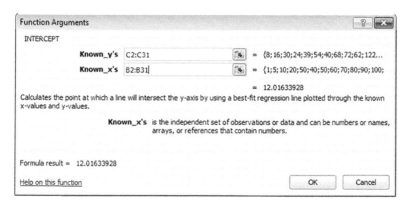

Figure 3.12 (Continued) Using Microsoft Excel to conduct linear regression analysis. The data set is from Table 3.33.   (*Continued*)

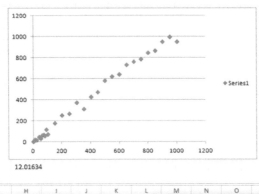

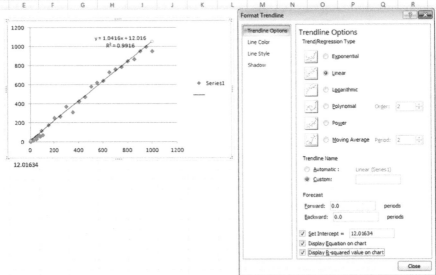

Figure 3.12 (Continued) Using Microsoft Excel to conduct linear regression analysis. The data set is from Table 3.33. The regression coefficient of 0.996 and r^2 value of 0.992 indicate very strong agreement (and $p = 1.26 \times 10^{-30}$). Using Microsoft Excel to plot data and determine parameters for the regression line (slope and intercept). The slope is 1.04 and the y intercept, 12.02. Another method in Powerpoint is to select "Insert Chart" and then "XY Scatter." Select the data in the Microsoft Excel spreadsheet and then "Add Trendline." Trendline options will include "linear" and allow you to set the intercept and display both the $y = mx + b$ equation and r^2 value on the chart.

determine the proportion of within-group variance in Y that can be ascribed to covariance with X, in a similar manner as above.

$$r_T = \frac{SC_{wg}}{\sqrt{SS_{wg(x)} \times SS_{wg(y)}}} = \frac{694.4}{\sqrt{809.6 \times 799.2}} = 804.4$$

$$r_T = \frac{694.4}{804.4} = 0.863$$

$$r_T^2 = 0.745$$

We also need to adjust the $SS_{wg(Y)}$ value by removing/adjusting for the above proportion of covariance.

$$SS_{wg(Y)} = 799.2 \times 0.745 = 595.4$$

$$Adjusted\ SS_{wgT(Y)} = 799.2 - 595.4 = 203.8$$

$$Adjusted\ SS_{bg(Y)} = Adjusted\ SS_{T(Y)} - Adjusted\ SS_{wg(Y)}$$

$$= Adjusted\ SS_{BG(Y)} = 318.5 - 203.8 = 114.7$$

$$F = \frac{Adj(\text{Between-group MS})}{Adj(\text{Within-group MS})} = \frac{Adj\ SS_{bg}/df_{bg}}{Adj\ SS_{wg}/df_{wg}}$$

Adjusted degrees of freedom for within group

$$= N_T - k - 1 = 20 - 2 - 1 = 17$$

Table 3.24 ANOVA: Single factor

SUMMARY

Groups	Count	Sum	Average	Variance
Tx A	10	132	13.2	33.51111
Tx B	10	180	18	56.44444

ANOVA

Source of variation	SS	df	MS	F	p value	F crit
Between Groups	115.2	1	115.2	2.561265	0.126915	4.413873
Within Groups	809.6	18	44.97778			
Total	924.8	19				

where: N_T = the total number of observations (20), k is the number of groups (2), and the 1 is subtracted to reflect the fact that we have removed the covariance aspect of within-group variability. The number of degrees of freedom for the between-group remains as

$$k - 1 = 2 - 1 = 1$$

$$F = \frac{Adj(\text{Between-group MS})}{Adj(\text{Within-group MS})} = \frac{Adj\,SS_{bg}/df_{bg}}{Adj\,SS_{wg}/df_{wg}}$$

$$F = \frac{114.7/1}{203.8/17} = \frac{114.7}{12.0} = 9.6(df = 1,17)$$

$F = 9.6$ exceeds the critical F of 8.4 (p = 0.01) with $df = 1,17$. Differences in body weight lost (y) significantly covary with differences in craving scores (x). Although the original mean values for weight lost between Groups A and B did not differ according to ANOVA, the adjusted mean values do differ significantly. After subtraction of the covariance of body weight lost (Y) with craving scores (X), the two intervention groups are significantly different.

3.10.1.4 SPECIAL EXAMPLES OF ANOVA

3.10.1.4.1 Factorial ANOVA

One assumption of this test is that the designs are balanced: all combinations of variables are equal. For example, if we have a study in which six patients are treated with one of two medications, each at one of three doses, over four time points (e.g., monthly visits), this would be a $2 \times 3 \times 4$ three-way factorial ANOVA in which each patient has 24 values × 6 = 144 total values.

3.10.1.4.2 Multivariate ANOVA (MANOVA)

This analysis extends ANOVA to a setting of two or more outcome measures or response variables. Suppose that obese patients received each of three interventions for 3 months: dietary modification only, increased physical activity only, and a single daily dose of an investigational agent. MANOVA would allow us to assess differences in changes in body weight across the three treatments and any interaction effects between them.

3.10.1.4.3 Repeated-Measures ANOVA (rmANOVA)

Suppose that we have a longitudinal trial in which each patient is randomized to more than one treatment, and we wish to assess effects over time. In this setting of matched data (i.e., each patient has a value for each treatment and observation time point), rmANOVA may be appropriate because it enables evaluation of random variability in both nonrepeated and repeated factors. An example might be a 12-month study of oral antidiabetic drugs (OADs) in 10 patients with four observations each: at quarterly clinic visits. Are mean changes in hemoglobin A1c (HbA1c) from baseline to 12 months different across the two treatments? Do changes in HbA1c differ over time in the same patient? To test these interactions, we can employ rmANOVA to account for variability within each patient, over time, between patients, and between treatments.

Assumptions of rmANOVA include: (1) sphericity/compound symmetry, which requires equal correlations between repeated measures, irrespective of the time between observations, and equal variances in the endpoint at each observation; (2) a normal (Gaussian) distribution of DVs for each level of variables within

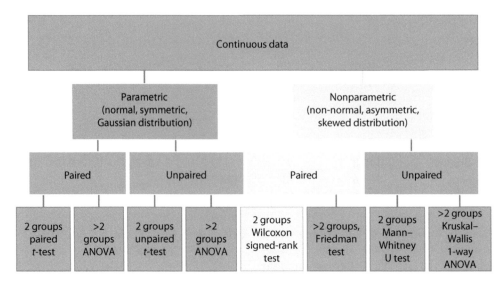

Table 3.25 Data for ANCOVA: Craving scores

Subject no.	X_{ai} score	Subject no.	X_{bi} score
a1	6	b1	8
a2	9	b2	11
a3	14	b3	28
a4	9	b4	24
a5	22	b5	17
a6	20	b6	21
a7	15	b7	27
a8	19	b8	22
a9	6	b9	14
a10	12	b10	8
	$\Sigma X_a = 132$		$\Sigma X_b = 180$

Scores and response options range from 1 ("extreme cravings") to 30 ("no cravings").

subject random variability, in that SDs do not differ markedly between treatments or individual patients; and (3) independent observations across patients with data drawn from randomly selected subjects or cases. To avoid violating the assumption of sphericity/circularity, it is important to randomize treatment sequences and space out observations adequately, such that the effect of a treatment on an outcome in a patient at one time point does not "carry over" to the next observation.

Potential limitations of rmANOVA include the fact that it (1) treats time as a categorical variable, meaning that all patients must be assessed at the same visits/times and over equal intervals between these observations; (2) cannot be used for covariates that are time dependent; (3) may result in a need to impute missing data; and (4) has restrictive assumptions concerning correlational structures.[79]

Most of these assumptions are not violated by the typical RCT but may very well be in patient registries and other cohort studies. In this setting, mixed (random- and fixed-effect) models may have advantages over rmANOVA in discriminating between-group differences in longitudinal studies with intracorrelated (within-patient) data. Mixed models: (1) retain maximal patient data, limiting the need to impute missing information; (2) function satisfactorily even if observations are not evenly spaced over time; (3) are effective irrespective of whether study designs are balanced or imbalanced; (4) do not require sphericity; and (5) enable computational flexibility. (For further information, see Howell DC. Overview of mixed models. Available at https://www.uvm.edu/dhowell/StatPages/More_Stuff/Mixed-Models-Repeated/Mixed-Models-for-Repeated-Measures1.html. Last accessed November 1, 2017.)

3.10.2 Nonparametric tests

3.10.2.1 WILCOXON SIGNED-RANK (WSR) AND RANK SUM (WRS) TESTS[80]

Rank-order methods are appropriate when[4]:

- Sample sizes are insufficient to draw conclusions about probability distributions.
- Primary data are ranked.

Rank-order tests are not sensitive to asymmetry (i.e., "skew") in population distributions. In short, such methods involve more liberal assumptions

Table 3.26 Data and calculations for ANCOVA

| Treatment group A | | | | Treatment group B | | | |
Subject	Craving score X_a	Weight lost, lb Y_a	X_aY_a product	Subject	Craving score X_b	Weight lost, lb Y_b	X_bY_b product
a1	6	22	132	b1	8	20	160
a2	9	24	216	b2	11	28	308
a3	14	32	448	b3	28	35	980
a4	9	26	234	b4	24	36	864
a5	22	33	726	b5	17	29	493
a6	20	42	840	b6	21	33	693
a7	15	28	420	b7	27	36	972
a8	19	44	836	b8	22	34	748
a9	6	27	162	b9	14	26	364
a10	12	30	360	b10	8	21	168
Sums	$\Sigma X_a = 132$ $(\Sigma X_a)^2 = 17{,}424$ $\Sigma X_a^2 = 2{,}044$	$\Sigma Y_a = 308$ $(\Sigma Y_a)^2 = 94{,}864$ $\Sigma Y_a^2 = 9{,}962$	$\Sigma (X_aY_a) = 4{,}374$		$\Sigma X_b = 180$ $(\Sigma X_b)^2 = 32{,}400$ $\Sigma X_b^2 = 3{,}748$	$\Sigma Y_b = 298$ $(\Sigma Y_b)^2 = 88{,}804$ $\Sigma Y_b^2 = 9{,}204$	$\Sigma (X_bY_b) = 5{,}750$
						Total array: Σ $(X_{Ti}Y_{Ti}) =$ $10{,}124$	
Sums					$\Sigma X_{T1} = 312$	$\Sigma Y_{T1} = 606$	

Table 3.27 Summary ANOVA and ANCOVA tables

X	Y	Adjusted Y	Covariance
$SS_{T(X)} = 924.8$	$SS_{T(Y)} = 804.2$	318.5	$SC_T = 670.4$
$SS_{wg(X)} = 809.6$	$SS_{wg(Y)} = 799.2$	203.8	$SC_{wg} = 694.4$
		114.7	

about underlying population distributions. Rank-order methods may also find application when sample size is small and the data distribution is not normal or amenable to transformation.

3.10.2.1.1 Wilcoxon signed-rank (WSR) test[80]

Is the median of differences between paired data in a population of asymmetrically distributed data equal to 0? The nonparametric WSR test addresses this question. One way to consider this test is as an extension of a paired Gosset's t-test to asymmetrical data distributions for ordered categorical data that are ranked. Data need to be interval or ordinal, derived from the same sample, and paired, with each pair selected independently and at random.

Consider hypothetical findings in Table 3.28: paired data from 16 subjects who have a history of CHD and are enrolled in an actively controlled crossover trial of a proprotein convertase subtilisin/

Table 3.28 Data for Wilcoxon signed-rank test: Levels of LDL-C (mg/dl) in patients according to treatment group

	Treatment			
Patient #	PCSK9I	UC	Difference	Rank of differences (ignoring sign), low to high
1	78	85	−7	4
2	57	71	−14	11
3	78	78	0	Do not rank differences = 0
4	61	69	−8	5
5	80	75	5	2
6	73	73	0	Do not rank differences = 0
7	67	77	−10	7
8	122	119	3	1
9	61	72	−11	8
10	49	61	−12	9
11	42	78	−26	14
12	74	87	−13	10
13	54	69	−15	12
14	41	64	−23	13
15	55	64	−9	6
16	80	74	6	3
	Mean = 67.0	Mean = 76.0		
	Median = 64.0	Median = 74.5		

Abbreviations: LDL-C, low-density lipoprotein cholesterol; PCSK9I, proprotein convertase subtilisin/kexin type 9 inhibitor; UC, usual care.

kexin type 9 (PCSK9) inhibitor. Each subject has two observations: a low-density lipoprotein cholesterol (LDL-C) level when receiving the PCSK9 inhibitor for 12 weeks and another when receiving usual care (UC), including an HMG-CoA reductase inhibitor (statin) at a maximum tolerated dose plus an American Heart Association (AHA) Step I diet, over the same interval. Hence, the data are paired (PCKS9 vs. UC in the same patients). The NH and AH may be stated as follows:

H_0: There is no statistically significant difference in the effects on LDL-C of PCSK9 inhibitors compared to usual care.

H_1: There is a statistically significant difference in the effects on LDL-C of PCSK9 inhibitors compared to usual care.

Each data distribution is skewed (the mean is greater than the median). We rank the data in ascending order according to the magnitude of each difference between groups, without regard to the sign (positive or negative) of these differences. We exclude paired data that do not differ (i.e., difference = 0).

T_+ = sum of ranks of positive differences

T_- = sum of ranks of negative differences

n = number of observations (*non*-0 ranks) = 14

$T_+ = 1 + 2 + 3 = 6$

$T_- = 4 + 5 + 6 + 7 + 8 + 9 + 10 + 11 + 12 + 13 + 14 = 99$

W = the smaller of T_+ and $T_- = 6$

If the effects of PCSK9 on LDL-C differed significantly from those of UC, we would expect the two sums of ranks (T_+ and T_-) to diverge sharply, as the above data certainly do. The lower the value of W, the lower the p value.

For $N = 14$ non-0 observations of ranked paired data, our value of 6 is much smaller than the threshold value for a two-tailed $\alpha = 0.010$.

∴ We reject the NH at $p < 0.010$ and accept the AH. The median of the paired differences ≠ 0.

H_1: There is a statistically significant difference in the effects on LDL-C of PCSK9 inhibitors compared to usual care.

3.10.2.1.2 Wilcoxon rank sum (WRS) test

Does the median difference between pairs of data in two populations equal 0? Do two data distributions share a single median? The WRS test addresses these types of questions. The WRS may be considered a nonparametric analogue of the two-sample Gosset's *t*-test.[13]

Our next example, for WRS, derives from the European Precocious Coronary Artery Disease (PROCARDIS) study, which examined levels of lipoprotein(a) (Lp[a]) and the risk of CHD.[81] The PROCARDIS Consortium reported that genetic differences at three chromosomal regions (especially 6q26-27) of the *LPA* gene were associated with increases in both circulating Lp(a) levels and CHD risk. In this case-control study, cases had either a personal and family (sibling) history of premature CHD, whereas population-matched controls had no such history. The presence of single-nucleotide polymorphisms (SNPs) rs3798220 and rs10455872 together explained 36% of the variance in Lp(a) levels (i.e., $r^2 = 0.36$).

Let us suppose that we wish to compare Lp(a) levels in individuals with (vs. without) the rs3798220 or rs10455872 SNP. In essence, we are comparing continuous variables (Lp[a] levels) across two categorical variables: the presence or absence of the rs3798220 or rs10455872 SNP. Table 3.29 shows hypothetical data concerning Lp(a) concentrations in cases and controls. The NH and AH may be stated as follows:

H_0: There is no statistically significant difference in Lp(a) levels between individuals with (vs. without) genetic variation at the *LPA* gene locus (i.e., with or without one of the two SNPs [or both] rs3798220 and rs10455872).

H_1: There is a statistically significant difference in Lp(a) levels between individuals with (vs. without) genetic variation at the *LPA* gene locus (i.e., with or without one of the two SNPs [or both] rs3798220 and rs10455872).

First, we aggregate the data and rank them in ascending order of Lp(a) level: within the entire population ($N = 27$; cases and controls), not within each cohort (Table 3.29). We then sum the ranks in each group. If the two populations were similar, we would expect the sum of their ranks (T) to differ minimally.

Table 3.29 Data for the Wilcoxon rank sum test

LPA SNP group (with rs3798220/ rs10455872 SNP; $n_2 = 14$)		"Wild-type" LPA group (without rs3798220/ rs10455872; $n_1 = 13$)	
Lp(a), mg/dL	Rank	Lp(a), mg/dL	Rank
48	14	33	8
94	24	40	11.5*
40	11.5*	26	5
62	19	32	7
50	15.5*	35	9
58	17	11	2
59	18	42	13
68	21	27	6
95	25	14	3
97	26	10	1
72	22	50	15.5*
64	20	16	4
77	23	36	10
100	27		
Mean = 70.3	**Sum = 283**	**Mean = 28.6**	**Sum = 95**
Median = 66.0		**Median = 32.0**	

Abbreviation: SNP, single-nucleotide polymorphism.
*Average of identically ranked data.

In fact, the data differ markedly: the T value (sum of ranks) of study participants with the lower Lp(a) levels (controls; $T = 95$) is much smaller than that of persons with higher Lp(a) levels (cases; $T = 283$). For the pair of 13 observations [lower Lp(a) levels, n_1 group, controls] and 14 observations [higher Lp(a) levels, n_2 group, cases], the range of values for a two-tailed $\alpha = 0.001$ is 116 (for the smaller group) and 248 (for the larger group). Our value of 95 is below the critical value for the lower limit of statistical significance, and the value of 283 is above the critical value of 248.

The NH is rejected at p < 0.001, and the AH is accepted.

H_1: There is a statistically significant difference in Lp(a) levels between individuals with (vs. without) genetic variation at the *LPA* gene locus (i.e., with or without one of the two SNPs [or both] rs3798220 and rs10455872).

3.10.2.2 FRIEDMAN TEST[82]

Developed by Nobel laureate economist Milton Friedman, the eponymous nonparametric test evaluates differences in paired ranked data. An example would be a total of n patients rating their satisfaction with k different treatments. The Friedman test can tell us not only which treatment ranked higher or lower, but also whether patients' ratings are consistent. Another application in clinical science is block randomization of three or more treatments of each patient.

The test statistic is given as:

$$F_r = \frac{12}{nk(k+1)} \times (T_1^2 + T_2^2 \dots T_k^2) - 3n(k+1)$$

where n = the number of patients with paired data; k = the number of different exposures or treatments to which each patient is subjected; and T_1, $T_2 \dots T_k$ = the sums of ranked data in each of the k groups (T_1 for first, T_2 for second....T_k for k[th]).

Our next example is informed by a clinical trial evaluating the effects of an anthelmintic treatment against *Schistosoma mansoni* in pregnant women by examining levels of antibodies and cytokines against this parasite in

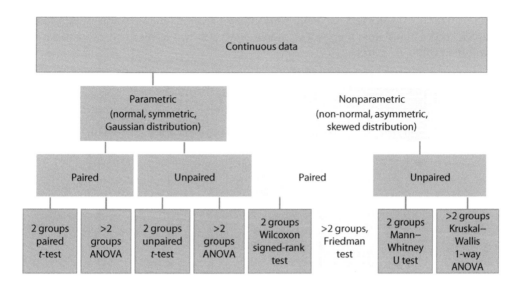

umbilical-cord and 1-year blood samples.[83] One way to minimize skewed data is to logarithmically transform them, such that 100 becomes 2 ($\log_{10} 100 = 2$ because $10^2 = 100$), 1,000 becomes 3, and so on. Even after this log transformation, many data distributions in the above study remained skewed.

Suppose that we wish to measure the effect of two different daily doses of an anthelmintic (or placebo) on cord blood antischistosomal antibodies when administered to each pregnant woman. The NH and AH may be stated as follows:

H_0: There is no statistically significant difference between maternal treatment with placebo and either of two doses of an investigational anthelmintic (TF-4418) and levels of antischistosomal antibodies in the cord blood of pregnant women with *S. mansoni* infection.

H_1: There is a statistically significant difference between maternal treatment with placebo and either of two doses of an investigational anthelmintic (TF-4418) and levels of antischistosomal antibodies in the cord blood of pregnant women with *S. mansoni* infection.

Hypothetical data are presented in Table 3.30.

$$F_r = \frac{12}{nk(k+1)} \times (T_1^2 + T_2^2 \ldots T_k^2) - 3n(k+1)$$

We rank data for each patient, proceeding across rows of three different treatment blocks (1 = placebo, 2 TF-4418 5 mg, 3 = TF-4418 10 mg), such that each rank must be 1, 2, or 3. We have $n = 10$ (number of patients); $k = 3$ (number of blocks, or rank levels compared); $T_1 = 27$; $T_2 = 20$; and $T_3 = 13$.

$$F_r = \frac{12}{10 \times 3(3+1)} \times (27^2 + 20^2 + 13^2) - (3 \times 10)(3+1) =$$

$$F_r = \frac{12}{120} \times (1,298) - 120 = 9.8$$

Examining the χ^2 distribution data in Appendix 2 for $3 - 1$ (2) *df*, we see that the value of 9.8 is consistent with a $p < 0.01$.

∴ The NH is rejected at $p < 0.01$ and the AH is accepted.

H_1: There is a statistically significant difference between maternal treatment with placebo and either of two doses of an investigational anthelmintic (TF-4418) and levels of antischistosomal antibodies in cord blood of pregnant women with *S. mansoni* infection.

3.10.2.3 MANN–WHITNEY U TEST[84]

Also termed the Mann–Whitney–Wilcoxon (MWW), Wilcoxon–Mann–Whitney (WMW), and WRS test, the Mann–Whitney U test can be used when the symmetry or asymmetry of a data distribution is unknown.

Table 3.30 Data for Friedman's test. Geometric mean Log_{10} levels of antibody against schistosome worm antigen in cord blood from pregnant women treated with two doses of an investigational anthelmintic medication or placebo

Patient	Cord blood Log_{10} IgG_2 (µg/mL) Placebo	Rank	Cord blood Log_{10} IgG_2 (µg/mL) TF-4418, 5 mg	Rank	Cord blood Log_{10} IgG_2 (µg/mL) TF-4418, 10 mg	Rank
1	5.4	3	2.8	2	2.1	1
2	5.9	3	2.5	2	1.9	1
3	1.1	2	1.0	1	5.1	3
4	3.8	3	3.1	2	3.0	1
5	3.9	3	2.1	1	3.2	2
6	3.2	3	2.0	2	1.9	1
7	3.0	3	2.7	2	2.2	1
8	3.0	3	2.5	2	1.6	1
9	2.4	2	5.6	3	1.8	1
10	3.4	2	5.9	3	2.1	1
Mean	3.51		3.02		2.49	
Median	3.30		2.60		2.10	
Column totals (ranks)		27		20		13

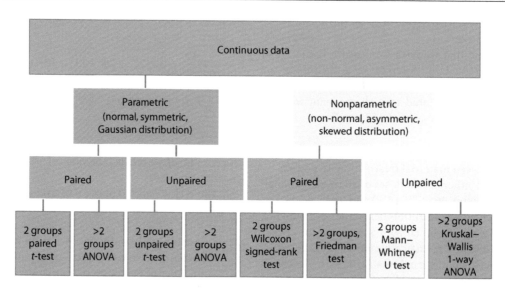

The Mann–Whitney U test statistic is given as:

$$U = (n_1 \times n_2) + \frac{n_1(n_1+1)}{2} - T_1$$

where n_1 is the size of sample 1; n_2 is the size of sample 2; and T_1 is the sum of the ranks in sample 1.

Suppose that a surgeon is studying outcomes between 14 obese patients randomized to a laparoscopic gastric band or gastrectomy sleeve. The primary outcome measure is body mass index (BMI). He ranks BMI data at 6 month's postop across two independent groups: patients receiving the band (0; $n = 7$) or the sleeve (1; $n = 7$).

The NH and AH may be stated as follows:

H_0: There is no statistically significant difference in BMI outcomes 6 months after laparoscopic placement of a gastric band or gastrectomy sleeve in obese patients.

Table 3.31 Data for the Mann–Whitney U test

BMI, kg/m²	Rank	Band (0) vs. Sleeve (1)	BMI, kg/m²	Rank	Band (0) vs. Sleeve (1)
27.8	1	1	31.7	7.5	1
28.0	2	0	38.9	9	1
28.9	3	1	39.8	10	0
29.7	4	0	40.1	11	0
30.0	5	1	42.2	12	1
31.4	6	0	43.3	13	0
31.7	7.5	0	44.0	14	1

H_1:   There is a statistically significant difference in BMI outcomes 6 months after laparoscopic placement of a gastric band or gastrectomy sleeve in obese patients.

We rank the data in ascending order (Table 3.31).

The mean and median BMI in the band group are 34.9 and 31.7 kg/m.² Corresponding values in the sleeve group are 34.8 and 31.7 kg/m.² The distributions are asymmetrical.

Summing the BMI ranks in the two groups, we find 53.5 for the band group and 51.5 for the sleeve group. Either can be used as the T value in the following equation:

$$U = (n_1 \times n_2) + \frac{n_1(n_1+1)}{2} - T_1$$

$$U = (7 \times 7) + \frac{7(7+1)}{2} - 53.5 = 23.5$$

For $n_1 = n_2 = 7$, a U value between 23 and 24 corresponds to a two-tailed p value between 0.902 and 1.00.

∴ The NH is not rejected at p < 0.05.

H_0:   There is no statistically significant difference in BMI outcomes 6 months after laparoscopic placement of a gastric band or gastrectomy sleeve in obese patients.

3.10.2.4 KRUSKAL–WALLIS (K–W) TEST[85]

Also termed the one-way ANOVA on ranks, the K–W test is a nonparametric statistical assessment of ranked data. This method can be used to assess differences between at least two experimental arms of an IV or a DV that is either ordinal or continuous. In some ways, it can be interpreted as (1) the Wilcoxon RST extended to at least three groups; and (2) a nonparametric analogue of a one-way ANOVA. The K–W test may also be useful when one-way ANOVA assumptions are not met.[13]

The test statistic is given as

$$H = \frac{12}{n(n+1)} \times \left(\frac{T_1^2}{n_1} + \frac{T_2^2}{n_2} \cdots \frac{T_k^2}{n_k} \right) - 3(n+1)$$

where n_1 is the size of sample 1; n_2 is the size of sample 2; n is the sum (all patients in k groups); k is the number of groups (populations); and T_1, T_2, and T_k are the sums of ranks in groups 1 and 2 through k.

A hypothetical example informed by the published literature is instructive (Table 3.32).[86] Pulse pressure (PP) is the mmHg difference between systolic and diastolic blood pressure (SBP, DBP). Suppose that a group of nephrologists seek to determine if PP differs significantly in 21 patients with three different forms of largely subclinical target-organ damage (TOD):

- Microalbuminuria [fasting AM urinary albumin: creatinine ratio (ACR) = 2.38–20.00; $n = 7$];
- Left-ventricular hypertrophy (LVH; echocardiographic LV motion index > 51 g/m$^{2.7}$; $n = 8$);
- Carotid intima media thickness (CIMT; ≥1.3 mm; $n = 6$).

The distribution of hypothetical PP values is asymmetrical (see Table 3.32), calling for a nonparametric test.

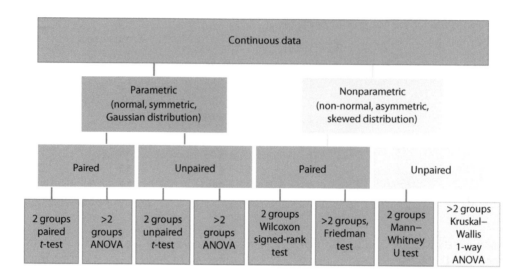

Table 3.32 Data for Kruskal–Wallis test/One-way ANOVA on ranks

Pulse pressure, mmHg	Rank for patients with IMT (Group 1)	Rank for patients with ACR (Group 2)	Rank for patients with LVH (Group 3)
21.8			1
27.5	2		
34.9			3
40.8			4
48.0			5
48.5	6		
52.1		7	
53.2			8
54.4			9
58.6			10
60.7		11	
64.3		12	
67.5			13
68.7	14		
98.1		15	
104.4	16		
108.2		17	
109.3		18	
113.1	19		
114.2		20	
114.7	21		
Mean = 69.7			
Median = 60.7			
Group rank totals (T)	$T_1 = 78$	$T_2 = 100$	$T_3 = 53$

The NH and AH may be stated as follows:

H_0: There is no statistically significant difference in PP values among patients with subclinical target-organ damage (TOD): microalbuminuria, LVH, or CIMT.

H_1: There is a statistically significant difference in PP values among patients with subclinical TOD: microalbuminuria, LVH, or IMT.

We rank the hypothetical PP data in ascending order (Table 3.32) according to group of origin.

$$H = \frac{12}{21(21+1)} \times \left(\frac{78^2}{6} + \frac{100^2}{7} + \frac{53^2}{8} \right) - 3(21+1) =$$

$$H = 0.026 \times [1,014.0 + 1,428.6 + 351.1] - 66 = 6.6$$

For χ^2 with $k - 1$ (3 −1) = 2 df, the critical value for p = 0.05 is 5.99.

The H value is greater than this value.

∴ The NH is rejected at p < 0.05. The AH is accepted:

H_1: There is a statistically significant difference in PP values among patients with subclinical TOD: microalbuminuria, LVH, or IMT.

3.11 SELECTED STATISTICAL TESTS ORGANIZED IN ASCENDING ALPHABETICAL ORDER

3.11.1 ANCOVA. See above (as an extension of ANOVA)

The aims of ANCOVA are to increase precision of comparisons between groups by accounting for variation on important covariates, which may have prognostic value. ANCOVA adjusts comparisons between groups for imbalances in these variables (i.e., "covariates," "codeviates," "nuisance variables"): often baseline characteristics that might interact with and otherwise modify treatment effects. It may apply when continuous covariates are introduced into an ANOVA.

In theory, ANCOVA represents a combination of ANOVA and regression. ANOVA partitions effects due to treatment (the mean square [MS]

of between-group variance) in the numerator by effects due to random probability or biological variation (MS of within-group variance) in the denominator. In statistical terms, ANCOVA partitions variance in DV into variance associated with a categorical IV, variance associated with covariates, and residual variance.

Potential shortcomings of ANCOVA included the fact that no set of prespecified covariates is ever complete/exhaustive. In most RCTs, covariates controlled for in ANCOVAs include treatment and study center. Somewhat less frequently controlled are patient age, duration of disease, and degree of comorbidity, which are often clinically important. Each covariate controlled reduces the overall power of the statistical analysis (degrees of freedom).

3.11.2 Bayesian statistics[87]

Riffenburgh aptly summarized the practical differences between the traditional, frequentist (*a priori*) and the Bayesian (*a posteriori* or *ex ante*) statistical orientations[4]:

> The frequentist says, "I believe in my data — if I can't show a result with data, I can't believe the result." The Bayesian says, "If you have information beyond your data, specifically a prior probability, it should be used. Both views can be argued convincingly."

Bayes' theorem is given as[13]:

$$\text{prob}[P](B \text{ given } A) = P \frac{(B \text{ given } A) \times P(A)}{\text{prob}(B)}$$

Bayes' theorem projects the probability of events according to "conditional probabilities": the likelihood of observing outcome or event A given the presence of outcome or event B (and vice versa).[88] It allows us to integrate new observations with previous beliefs (*a posteriori* approach). It is formally expressed as:

$$P(A|B) = \frac{P(B|A)P(A)}{P(B)}$$

where:

- A and B = events;
- P = probability or likelihood;
- $P(A)$ = likelihood of observing event A irrespective of event B (marginal probability);
- $P(B)$ = likelihood of observing event B irrespective of event A (marginal probability)
- $P(A|B)$ = likelihood of observing event A given B (conditional or posterior probability); and
- $P(B|A)$ = likelihood of observing event B given A (conditional probability).

In Bayesian models, it is important to begin with an accurate "base case," especially before setting in motion any probabilistic Markov "chains."

Suppose that we wish to estimate the probability of developing incident oral cancer within 1 year in a cohort of randomly sampled US adults. The annual number of new cases of oral cancer in the US population is approximately 50,000.[89] Given that the American population is approximately 325,000,000, the annual incidence is 0.0154%. Half of all incident cases of oral cancers occur in patients aged $\geq$ 65 years (0.008%). Assuming that 5,000 patients aged exactly 65 develop oral cancer in 1 year, we compute P (B/A) as 5,000/50,000 (10%).

Now let us suppose that we want to know the probability of an individual in this cohort developing oral cancer in 1 year but know only that he or she is 65 years old. We will assume that there are 5 million Americans aged 65.

$$P(A|B) = \frac{P(B|A)P(A)}{P(B)}$$

- $P(A/B)$ = likelihood of developing oral cancer in 1 year given that a patient is age 65 (conditional probability);
- $P(B|A)$ = likelihood of being 65 given that a patient develops oral cancer in 1 year (conditional probability; 10%);
- $P(A)$ = likelihood of a patient developing oral cancer in 1 year, irrespective of age (marginal probability; 0.0154%);
- $P(B)$ = likelihood of being exactly 65 years old, irrespective of developing oral cancer (marginal probability; we assume this to be 5 million; 5 million/325 million = 1.54%);

$$P(A|B) = \frac{P(B|A)P(A)}{P(B)}$$

$$P(A|B) = \frac{10.0000\% \times 0.0154\%}{1.5400\%}$$

$$P(A|B) = 0.001(0.1\%)$$

Being 65 is associated with a 1 in 1,000 absolute risk of developing incident oral lung cancer in the next year. If the 65-year-old person was a long-time (~50-year) smokeless-tobacco user, the likelihood of developing oral cancer would increase 50-fold because such habitual users are at markedly increased probability compared to age-matched nonusers.[90] The probability of developing oral cancer in the next year could be estimated at 0.001 × 50 = 50 × 0.001 = 5.0%. The smokeless-tobacco user would hence have a 1 in 20 (5%) absolute risk of developing oral cancer in the next year.

One special application of Bayesian principles to simulate uncertain events via successive random sampling from a conditional data distribution is Markov Chain Monte Carlo (MCMC) modeling.[91] The successive random selections comprise a Markov chain. These methods are used frequently in cost-effectiveness, cost-utility, and other forms of health economics and outcomes research (HEOR).[4] MCMC modeling is a so-called stochastic simulation process, in that its models are dynamic and project changes in random values over time. Markov chains can treat time as either a continuous or categorical (discrete) variable.

In health care and HEOR, MCMC models often project disease progression and events based on initial conditions and transition probabilities. A Markov chain is a stochastic-systems model in which transition probabilities govern continuous or discrete states.[92]

Conditional probability is also at the heart of Kaplan–Meier survival analysis (see below).

3.11.3 Bland–Altman (B–A) Plot[93,94]

Can quantitative measures from two independent diagnostic methods be correlated but not in agreement? They can, as the next exercise will demonstrate. The B–A plot is a straightforward, graphical way to assess bias between two sets of data. To construct it, we plot differences between paired values over the average of these values (mean difference line). We then introduce horizontal lines representing the lower and upper limits of the 95% CI: one above and the other below the mean difference line.[4] These are termed limits of agreement. We are then able to assess bias between the mean differences.[95] Four types of anomalies in data can be discerned[4]:

1. "Systematic error (mean offset);
2. Proportional error (trend);
3. Inconsistent variability; and
4. Excessive or erratic variability."

Correlation coefficients characterize relationships between two data sets but not their agreement. The clinical or biological meaning of the difference or concordance between two entities (e.g., diagnostic methods) cannot be informed by B–A plots: only the degree of bias. Bias occurs when the "line of equality is not within the CI of the mean difference."[95] By statistical convention when dealing with normally distributed data, we use the 95% CI, but, to enrich the meaning of B–A plots, it may be advisable to construct more "biologically informed" precision limits, as is also done in noninferiority analyses.

Suppose that we wish to determine agreement between two laboratory methods (A and B).[95] Visually inspecting the paired data for Methods A and B (columns 1 and 2 of Table 3.33), we can infer that the two sets of continuous data are broadly in agreement. We can use Microsoft Excel to determine the degree of association between the two data sets by conducting a linear regression analysis and/or by scatter-plotting the data and determining the regression equation (Figures 3.12 and 3.13).

What more can the B–A plot tell us? A horizontal line intersecting 0 signifies an absence of bias between the two measurements: any differences between them can be ascribed to analytical variability alone.

Examining data in Table 3.33, we observe potential bias between Methods: the mean difference is –27.2 (not 0), which implies that Method A measures 27.2 units below Method B, on average. Expressed as a percent, the bias is –17.4% (in the same direction; Method A measures below Method B). B–A plots show the difference between Methods A and B (or the difference expressed as a percentage) on the ordinate

(y-axis) and the mean of Methods A and B on the abscissa (x-axis).

In a B–A plot of these data, we would observe that low values for Method A – Method B and the mean of Methods A and B are grouped closely together, whereas higher values have a wider spread or dispersion. If we can determine that the data are normally distributed—either by plotting the data or analyzing them by the Shapiro–Wilk (S–W) or Kolmogorov–Smirnov (K–S) test,[96,97] we can construct 95% confidence limits around the mean difference of –27.2 using the paired data in Table 3.33:

$$SE = \sqrt{\frac{s^2}{n}} = \sqrt{\frac{34.8^2}{30}} = 6.35$$

For 30 observations, we have $30 - 1$ df. The t value for 29 degrees of freedom is 2.05.

$$\text{Confidence} = SE^*t = 6.35 \times 2.05 = 13.0$$

The 95% CI around the mean difference = $-27.2 - 13.0$ (lower limit) and $-27.2 + 13.0$ (upper limit), or -40.2 to -14.2. Clearly, the line of equality drawn horizontally from 0 would not lie within these limits.

Although Methods A and B are clearly not in agreement, Figure 3.12 (using the same values as Table 3.33) shows that data from these methods are correlated.

3.11.4 Bootstrapping[13]

This iterative form of statistical analysis seeks to simulate the true population mean (i.e., μ) from data in the sample population. The name of this test is related to the sense of "pulling oneself up from one's bootstraps." In a statistical sense, bootstrapping implies an *a-posteriori* process of repeatedly resampling from a data set. Doing so enables one to generate new characteristics for the data, such as SDs and CIs. Each data point from the generated data set is selected at random, and in an independent manner, until the new set has the same number of data points as the original. The new (bootstrapped) data set can vary from the original *a-priori* set because some observations from the original set may be chosen twice, or not at all, in the bootstrapped set.

Table 3.33 Paired data for a Bland–Altman plot

Method A (units)	Method B (units)	Mean (A + B)/2 (units)	(A − B) (units)	(A − B)/Mean (%)
1.0	8.0	4.5	−7.0	−155.6
5.0	16.0	10.5	−11.0	−104.8
10.0	30.0	20.0	−20	−100.0
20.0	24.0	22.0	−4.0	−18.2
50.0	39.0	44.5	11.0	24.7
40.0	54.0	47.0	−14.0	−29.8
50.0	40.0	45.0	10.0	22.2
60.0	68.0	64.0	−8.0	−12.5
70.0	72.0	71.0	−2.0	−2.8
80.0	62.0	71.0	18.0	25.4
90.0	122.0	106.0	−32.0	−30.2
100.0	80.0	90.0	20.0	22.2
150.0	181.0	165.5	−31.0	−18.7
200.0	259.0	229.5	−59.0	−25.7
250.0	275.0	262.5	−25.0	−9.5
300.0	380.0	340.0	−80.0	−23.5
350.0	320.0	335.0	30.0	9.0
400.0	434.0	417.0	−34.0	−8.2
450.0	479.0	464.5	−29.0	−6.2
500.0	587.0	543.5	−87.0	−16.0
550.0	626.0	588.0	−76.0	−12.9
600.0	648.0	624.0	−48.0	−7.7
650.0	738.0	694.0	−88.0	−12.7
700.0	766.0	733.0	−66.0	−9.0
750.0	793.0	771.5	−43.0	−5.6
800.0	851.0	825.5	−51.0	−6.2
850.0	871.0	860.5	−21.0	−2.4
900.0	957.0	928.5	−57.0	−6.1
950.0	1001.0	975.5	−51.0	−5.2
1000.0	960.0	980.0	40.0	4.1
Mean			−27.2	−17.4
SD			34.8	−12.6

Source: Reproduced with permission from Giavarina D. Understanding Bland Altman analysis. *Biochem Med (Zagreb)* 2015;25:141–51.[95] Copyright ©2015 Croatian Society for Medical Biochemistry and Laboratory Medicine.

3.11.5 Correlation

Assessing the extent of associations between two variables (often in a linear array) using a bivariate analysis falls within the domain of correlation. Ranging from −1 (perfect inverse association) to 0 (no association) to +1.0 (perfect direct association), correlation coefficients include the Pearson's product-moment correlation coefficient (*r*), Spearman's ρ (rho), and Kendall's τ (tau). Unlike the case with typical hypothesis testing, two variables may be statistically significantly, but not necessarily strongly, correlated. Suppose that a bivariate analysis returns a Pearson's *r* = 0.189 (p = 0.04); the proximity of 0.189 to 0 indicates that the correlation is not strong. In fact, to determine the proportion of variance in the DV explained by the IV, we would take the square of this value: $r^2 = 0.189^2 = 0.036$.

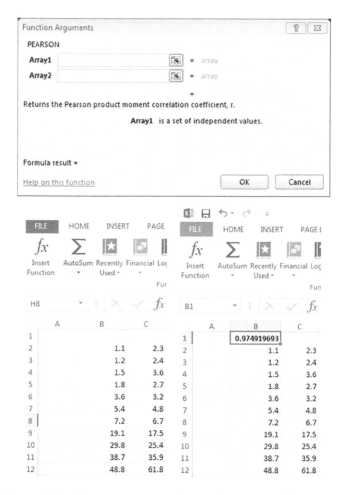

Figure 3.13 Using Microsoft Excel to compute correlations (Pearson's r) between two data sets. The r of 0.975 is consistent with a strong correlation. The r^2 value (0.975^2) of 0.950 signifies that 95% of the variance in one data set is explained by variance in the other.

Only about 4% of the variance in the DV can be explained by the IV.

3.11.6 Correlation 1: Pearson's product-moment correlation (coefficient = r)[66,98]

Correlations between two groups of continuous data (x,y) can be determined by the Pearson r coefficient. Data need to be continuous, distributed symmetrically around a regression line (i.e., be homoscedastic; with a "tube-like" rather than "cone-like" shape of points around the regression line), and there must be a linear relationship between the two sets of variables.

As discussed in the above ANCOVA exercise, Pearson's r is given as the ratio between covariance of x and y (in the numerator) to the product of their SDs (in the denominator). In regression models, this test statistic is equivalent to the product of the regression line's slope ($b1$) and the ratio of SDs in these two groups. That is:

$$r = \frac{SC_{xy}}{s_x \times s_y}$$

Another way to compute Pearson's r is as the product of the regression slope and the ratio of the SDs

$$b_1 \times \frac{s_x}{s_y}$$

between variables in the ith ranked pair.

Pearson's r indicates the degree of correlation between continuous variables that are symmetrically distributed and homoscedastic, such as daily sodium content (in grams) and waking BP (in mmHg) among patients with salt-sensitive hypertension. Spearman's ρ and Kendall's τ indicate the degree of correlation among paired ranked data in asymmetric data distributions. These tests can be thought of as nonparametric counterparts of Pearson's r.

Figure 3.13 shows how to compute Pearson's r for two data sets using Excel.

3.11.7 Correlation 2: Spearman's rank correlation (coefficient = ρ)[99]

Spearman's rank correlation is a nonparametric test used to measure the degree of association between two ranked (ordinal) variables, X and Y. Spearman's rank correlation test requires no assumptions about the distribution of the data (e.g., linearity). In addition to ordinal data, requirements include a monotonic relationship between one variable and the other.

The test statistic is given as

$$\rho = 1 - \frac{6 \sum d_i^2}{n(n^2 - 1)}$$

where d_i = the difference between variables in the ith ranked pair and n = the total number of data pairs.

The next example is also loosely based on published literature, in this case as related to patients with rheumatoid arthritis (RA). Let us suppose that distribution of rheumatoid factor (RF; IgG, IgM, IgA) is skewed to the right.[100] Treatment with a tumor necrosis factor α inhibitor (TNFα-I) for 3 months significantly decreased RF and anti-cyclic citrullinated protein antibody (ACPA) in patients with RA.

Table 3.34 lists hypothetical RF data before and after treatment with the TNFα-I. Each distribution (for RF data before and after treatment) is positively skewed (has a rightward tail): each mean exceeds the population median.

$$\rho = 1 - \frac{6 \sum d_1^2}{n(n^2 - 1)}$$

$$\rho = 1 - \frac{6(52)}{11(11^2 - 1)} =$$

$$\rho = 1 - \frac{312}{1,320} = 0.76$$

$$\rho = 0.76$$

3.11.8 Correlation 3: Kendall's correlation (coefficient = τ)[101]

Another nonparametric method of assessing the strength of dependence between paired, ranked data that are asymmetrically distributed is to examine the ratio of concordant (C) and discordant (D) pairs. If paired ranks of each set of data both increase or decrease when proceeding from one pair to the next, these are designated as concordant pairs.

Although it requires ranked values, Kendall's τ test is flexible enough to analyze data that are not normally distributed and/or have a monotonic but not linear relationship. Unlike Spearman's test, Kendall's τ test can also accommodate ties in ranked data.

Kendall's τ test statistic is given as:

$$\tau = \frac{2(C - D)}{n(n - 1)}$$

See Table 3.34 to understand how to compute C and D.

$$\tau = \frac{2(45 - 9)}{11(11 - 1)} = 0.65$$

If the populations were distributed normally, the Pearson product moment correlation (r), Spearman coefficient (ρ), and Kendall coefficient (τ) would be related as follows[13]:

$$r = \sin\left(\frac{\pi}{2} \times \tau\right) = 2\sin\left(\frac{\pi}{6} \times \rho\right)$$

Table 3.34 Hypothetical data to compute correlation: Kendall's τ[a]

Subject #	RF (IgM) level, IU/mL Baseline	Rank	RF (IgM) level, IU/mL 3-months (post-TNF-α inhibitor)	Rank	d_i^2	Concordant	Discordant
1	104.2	1	88.9	3	4	8	2
2	109.7	2	101.8	5	9	6	3
3	127.7	3	168.9	7	16	4	4
4	148.9	4	74.1	1	9	7	0
5	160.9	5	87.3	2	9	6	0
6	201.9	6	97.6	4	4	5	0
7	358.8	7	148.3	6	1	4	0
8	367.3	8	278.0	8	0	3	0
9	398.3	9	322.9	9	0	1	0
10	399.9	10	358.2	10	0	1	0
11	402.2	11	376.6	11	0		
Mean	252.7		191.1		52	$\sum C = 45$	$\sum D = 9$
Median	201.9		148.3				

[a] Concordant pairs are indicated when numbers below each subject's rank on 3-month data (second set of ranks) are larger than that number. For instance, 8 numbers below the rank of 3 are larger than 3 and are hence concordant. Discordant pairs are indicated by decreasing numbers below each subject's rank. For instance, 2 numbers below the rank of 3 are smaller than 3 and are hence discordant. d_i^2, square of difference in ranks.

3.11.9 Funnel plot[102]

The major aim of systematic literature reviews (SLRs) and meta-analyses is to pool published study data and hence increase statistical power compared to analyzing each study population separately. Frequently, such reviews display relative risks of an outcome, including odds ratios (ORs) or hazard ratios (HRs), with typically 95% CIs, in a forest plot. Ninety-five percent confidence intervals for ORs or HRs that overlap 1.0 indicate that they are not statistically significant.

Though frequently the most effective barometer of the "state of science" in terms of the relative effectiveness of various health interventions, SLRs and meta-analyses are not immune from bias. According to statistician Martin Bland, reporting via the University of York ("Meta-analysis: publication bias"; March 6, 2006. Available at: https://www-users.york.ac.uk/~mb55/msc/systrev/week7/pub_text.pdf. Last accessed December 18, 2015):

> One of the great problems with systematic review is that not all studies carried out are published. Those which are published may be different from those which are not…Combining only

published studies may lead to an [overly] optimistic conclusion.

Publication bias may result from the fact that many peer-reviewed journals (PRJs) are more likely to publish clinical trials with larger (vs. smaller) sample sizes; smaller trials hence must report greater effect sizes to be published. Many PRJs are also somewhat prejudiced against publishing reports of studies with "negative" (null; p > 0.05) results.[103] Well-designed and well-conducted studies may not be published because they are less likely to show statistically significant differences between groups compared to poorly designed and conducted trials. Publication and other forms of bias in SLRs may be indicated by skewed distribution when plotting variability or study sample size on the ordinate against effect size on the abscissa.[104]

Language bias may interact with publication bias. In a study of 62 paired English and German RCTs, researchers were nearly 4 times more likely to publish statistically significant findings in an English- (vs. German-) language journal. Hence, the conclusions of meta-analyses and SLRs involving only English RCT reports may, on average, be biased away from the null.[105]

Unless censoring is employed, the character of an SLR or meta-analysis and the strengths of their conclusions will be consistent with the quality of the studies analyzed.

Methods to test or adjust for publication bias include (1) Begg and Egger's test, (2) trim and fill, (3) selection models, (4) meta-regression, and (5) funnel plots.[106]

To construct a funnel plot, graph the SE or sample size (measure of imprecision) on the ordinate (y-axis) and the OR or percent mean difference (effect size) on the abscissa (x-axis). According to certain authorities, the most advantageous approach is to plot SE (not sample size) on the ordinate, in part because a symmetrical funnel will ensue when bias is absent, and such plots may more effectively represent smaller studies that are more prone to bias.[104] To evaluate differences in conclusions between small trials and larger trials, one may choose to plot the inverse of the variance on the ordinate. The plot will often approximate an inverted funnel. If asymmetrical, the funnel plot may suggest publication bias. The finding of a symmetrical funnel plot reduces the possibility of publication bias.

Guidelines for the use of funnel plots[107] include the fact that: (1) publication bias is only one possible explanation of funnel plot asymmetry; (2) a "contour-enhanced" funnel plot may help to identify disproportionate influences of certain trials (e.g., missing data) on the conclusions concerning publication bias; (3) "small-study effects" suggest but do not prove that publication bias is present; (4) the investigator or MW should consider using methods other than the funnel plot when the total number of studies is below 10 because the test's performance in discriminating true asymmetry from random effects is typically insufficient (i.e., funnel plots have inadequate statistical power); and (5) caution should be exercised (or another test considered) when analyzing studies with similar SEs for effect sizes and similar sample population sizes.

As shown in Chapter 2, software to assist in funnel plotting is available online from the Cochrane Collaboration (Review Manager [Rev Man 5]; http://community.cochrane.org/tools/review-production-tools/revman-5).

3.11.10 General linear model (including regression models), generalized linear model, generalized linear mixed model (GLMM), and generalized estimating equation (GEE)[108,109]

3.11.10.1 GENERAL LINEAR MODELS

"General linear model" is a broad term that refers to a program formulated to encompass various types of analyses, including multiple regression, ANOVA, ANCOVA, and MANOVA.[4] In fact, the test statistic for simple and multiple linear regression models represents an example of general linear models:

$$y = \beta_0 + \beta_{1x1} + \beta_{2x2} + \ldots \beta_{pxp}$$

where y = a numerical outcome; x = exposure variable; and β = regression coefficients related to the exposure variables (total = p).[13]

In contrast, the term "generalized linear model" is very specific and relates to models developed to accommodate correlated data; generalized linear models represent extensions of linear regression to cases in which response variables have non-normally distributed errors. GEEs and GLMMS enable assessment of clustered or intracorrelated data. In patient registry and other longitudinal data, each observation in the same registrant or study participant over time is not entirely independent; the data are intracorrelated within each individual.

Generalized linear models associate exposure variables, or independent variables (IVs) to outcomes, or dependent variables (DVs), by means of a linear link function. This link function is logarithmic in Poisson and Cox regression models and log odds ("logit") in logistic regression models.[13] Poisson models, which relate to infrequent events, including rare genetic disorders, and Cox models, which may include survival analyses, consider a transformed DV rather than the DV per se. According to Kirkwood and Sterne, "multiple regression is a special case of generalized linear model in which the link function is the identity function $f(y) = y$."[13]

Apart from the data transformation, the statistic for logistic regression is similar to that above for general linear models:

$$\log \textbf{odds of outcome}(y) = \log\left(\frac{\pi}{1-\pi}\right) = \boldsymbol{\beta}_0$$
$$+ \boldsymbol{\beta}_{1x1} + \boldsymbol{\beta}_{2x2} + \boldsymbol{\beta}_{pxp}$$

where π is the probability of the event.

Special examples of generalized linear models are conditional regression models. These include Cox regression and conditional logistic regression. In these models, distributions of exposures of study participants within certain risk sets or case-control strata are used as the basis for estimation.[13]

Classes of generalized linear models include[110]:

- Linear mixed models, which are appropriate for correlated responses partly modeled by random effects.
  - GEEs are appropriate for intracorrelated responses that are binary or otherwise categorical (rather than continuous); and
  - GLMMs are extensions of generalized linear models that include both fixed and random effects.

Typically, GLMMs are used for patient-specific inferences and GEEs for average population inferences.[110] GLMMs, which take the perspective of a single patient, characterize changes in each patient's mean Y that are conditional on her random effect (b). However, GEEs, which take the perspective of the overall population, for health providers and policymakers, characterize differences in mean Y across a total population.[110] Data from GEEs may inform formulary decision making, which requires that treatment responses be optimized for an entire population (e.g., hospital, clinic, or health plan).

The mathematics of these models is complex, involving matrices and vectors. For the record, the mathematical form of GLMMs, written in matrix notation, is given as follows:

$$y = X\boldsymbol{\beta} + Zu + \boldsymbol{\varepsilon} = X\boldsymbol{\beta} + Zy + \boldsymbol{\varepsilon}$$

where:

- y = a $N \times 1$ column vector, the outcome variable;
- X = a $N \times p$ matrix of the p predictor values;
- β = a $p \times 1$ column vector of fixed-effects regression coefficients (the "betas");
- Z = the $N \times q$ design matrix for the q random effects (a random complement to the fixed X);
- y = a $q \times 1$ vector of the random effects (the random alternative to the fixed β); and
- ε = a $N \times 1$ column vector of the residuals, the aspect of y that is not explained by the model $X\beta + Zy$.[111]

Rather than attempt to master (or even fathom!) the mathematics, it is more important for MWs to understand the applications of these models in clinical studies. Extensions of the generalized linear model to correlated observations, which occur in longitudinal studies and cluster study designs, include GEEs.[108] When analyzing longitudinal data, GEEs are appropriate for population-averaged models, which characterize the ways in which average responses across subjects change with covariates.[112] GEEs are typically employed with binary data, such as an increase or decrease in variability as an IV and either a decrease or an increase in an outcome as a DV.[108,109] However, GEEs may require large sample sizes to ensure adequate accuracy and are not robust to nonrandom missing data. GEEs do not include a probability model for the origin of correlations. Consequently, GEE models are acceptable when random effects and their variances are not of interest. They determine correlations among data but not the origins of these correlations.

GLMMs can help to explain the origins of correlations, in part by providing a probability model that considers random effects as a linear predictor. GLMMs can provide subject-specific estimates when the investigator wishes to model the effects of changing one component (or more) of an IV on responses or outcome (DV) in a given individual. GLMMs are a type of mixed model (also known as a multilevel model). One limitation of GLMMs is that they are more demanding to construct and fit to data (vs. GEEs).

Three types of general linear models include fixed-effects models (i.e., Class I ANOVA), random-effects models (i.e., Class II ANOVA), and mixed models. What do we mean by fixed and random effects? Gender is a fixed effect. In most (but not all) studies, treatment group assignment is also not varied and hence is a fixed effect. For a study without a long duration of follow-up, baseline age or age group is also typically considered a fixed effect. Random effects include each study participant, who can be viewed as a random sample of the study population.

Mixed models incorporate both fixed and random effects. An example of a mixed model might apply to an HEOR study assessing the effects of different depressor medications on BP in a large number of patients, such as enrollees in a health-care plan. A fixed-effects model might compare the BP effects of three angiotensin$_{II}$ receptor blockers (ARBs) that are on the plan's formulary. A random-effects model might compare the BP effects of three randomly selected medications. A mixed-effects model might compare the BP effects of fixed (formulary) medications to those of the randomly selected medications.

Another example of a mixed-effects model was discussed by Magezi.[113] Suppose that we wished to determine participant reaction time (RT) to the human voice as a function of various explanatory variables. These might include:

- Language of the test's voice: e.g., English, French, or German
- Sound volume in decibels (dB)
- Study participant
- Study participant's native language

Fixed effects might include language, sound volume, and the participant's native language, whereas random effects might include each study participant.

Mixed models also need to account for interactions between fixed and random variables. In the above examples, RT might decrease as a function of increasing sound volume, but the relationship (e.g., slope of regression line) may differ in each participant. In the full mixed-model repeated-measures (MMRM) analysis, a random slope term for RT would need to be introduced to account for possible interactions between participant (random) and sound volume (fixed) effects. Similarly, the full model might need to introduce a random slope term for RT to account for interactions between participant (random) and language (fixed).

As mentioned elsewhere, MMRM analyses may be well suited to intracorrelated or clustered data. Such analyses are also "data conserving" in that all observations of a subject are not lost in the event of consent withdrawal or attrition.

Open-source coding to facilitate some of these calculations include "R" and GLIMMPSE (Available at: https://glimmpse.samplesizeshop.org/#/. Last accessed March 25, 2018).[114] GLIMMPSE 2.2.8 is a user-friendly interface designed for both applied scientists and biostatistical specialists.

There are certain reasons to prefer a GEE over a fixed-effects model. First, GEEs offer greater computational efficiency and stability. Second, a less restrictive correlational structure can be employed with GEEs. One reason to prefer a mixed model is that the coefficients have a subject-specific interpretation.

3.11.11 Heterogeneity

In our earlier exercise on the CMH test, we explored the χ^2 to test heterogeneity, which also ruled out effect modification in a hypothetical example. Excessive methodologic or other forms of heterogeneity (e.g., statistical; heterogeneity of variance) can undermine attempts to pool data from different studies. DerSimonian and Laird[115,116] put forth an elegant statistical assessment: the τ^2 test of between-study variance. Other forms of heterogeneity may relate to disparities in sample populations, interventions, definitions of endpoints, and other clinical aspects, such as variability in direction or magnitude of the effects of risk factors or treatments.[106] Methods and results may be heterogeneous in that individual studies are seeking to measure different parameters, in different ways, and in patients who are dissimilar to each other. These considerations militate against pooling data.

Statistical tests for heterogeneity include[106]

- Galbraith plots;
- Meta-regression analysis;
- Random-effects modeling;
- Cochran's Q test statistic; and
- I^2 test statistic.

In the Cochran Q statistic, the analyst sums the squared SDs of each trial's effects estimate (i.e., dispersion from the overall estimate in the meta-analysis), weighting the contribution of each trial by the inverse of the variance.[117] By convention,

75% is considered high; 50%, moderate; and 25%, low heterogeneity.

The I^2 test characterizes the contribution to the total variation across summarized trials that can be ascribed to heterogeneity rather than random probability. It is computed as:

$$I^2 = 100\% \times \left(\frac{Q - df}{Q} \right)$$

where df = degrees of freedom and Q = Cochran's (or χ^2) heterogeneity statistic. Results range from 0 (no heterogeneity) to 100% (all variation between studies attributable to heterogeneity).

What can we do if studies in a pooled-data analysis (e.g., meta-analysis) are (or are likely to be) heterogeneous? Strategies include (1) allowing for the heterogeneity by employing a random-effects meta-analysis, which models and incorporates between-study heterogeneity into the meta-analysis; (2) deciding not to pool the findings, instead generating a more descriptive "narrative review"; (3) using a fixed-effects model, which essentially ignores the heterogeneity but might be biased and result in pooled estimates that are difficult to interpret; and (4) exploring and attempting to account for potential causes of between-study heterogeneity (e.g., using a sensitivity analysis that either includes or excludes the most divergent studies [those with ORs most distant from the summary OR for the meta-analysis]).[106]

As shown in Chapter 2, software to assist in evaluating heterogeneity (by I^2) is available on-line from the Cochrane Collaboration (RevMan; http://community.cochrane.org/tools/review-production-tools/revman-5). I^2 values exceeding 0.75 are thought to be consistent with unacceptable heterogeneity and do not support data pooling.

3.11.12 Hosmer and Lemeshow's test[118,119] (goodness of fit in predictive models)

This test statistic determines goodness of fit for prognostic (e.g., risk prediction) models: especially logistic regression models. When projected probabilities (expected frequencies of events) match observed frequencies, we say that the prognostic model is adequately calibrated. In general, this test statistic conforms to a χ^2 distribution in an asymptotic manner, with df equal to the number of groups $(G) - 2$.

The Hosmer–Lemeshow test statistic is given as:

$$H = \sum_{g=1}^{G} \frac{(O_{g1} - E_{g1})^2}{N_{g1} \pi_{g1} (1 - \pi_{g1})}$$

In addition to G, E_g = the expected events; O_g = observed events; N_g = total number of observations; and π_g = predicted risk ("Pi" for "predicted") in the gth decile risk group.

Other useful terms when working with predictive models[120] include sensitivity, specificity, negative predictive value (NPV), positive predictive value (PPV), receiver-operator characteristics (ROC) curve, and the c-statistic (area under curve [AUC] for the ROC plot).

Sensitivity (true-positive rate) is calculated as the ratio of true positives divided by the sum of true positives and false negatives. It signifies the probability that a test result will be positive when a patient has a disease (or some other predicted quantity is being observed/measured).

Also termed the true-negative rate, specificity is computed as the ratio of true negatives divided by the sum of false positives and true negatives. It constitutes the probability that a test result will not be positive when a patient does not have a disease (or other predicted entity).

Negative predictive value (NPV) is calculated as the ratio of the number of patients who do not have the disease and also have negative test results (true negatives) divided by the sum of false negatives and true negatives; in other words, the proportion of patients who have a negative test result and do not have the disease.

Positive predictive value (PPV) is computed as the ratio of the number of patients who have the disease and also positive test results (true positives) divided by the sum of false positives and true positives; in other words, the proportion of patients who have a positive test result and have the disease.

ROC curves plot sensitivity (true-positive rate) on the ordinate against 1 – specificity (true-negative rate) on the abscissa and enable the analyst to determine the discriminative ability or performance of the prognostic model. ("ROC" stands for "receiver operating characteristics.")

The *c*-statistic, or the computed area under curve (AUC) of the ROC curve, determines the discriminative performance of the predictive model. In general, a *c*-statistic > 0.70 is considered to be acceptable; however, as with Cronbach's α, such cut-points are somewhat arbitrary and continue to be debated.[121]

3.11.13 Imputation

In the words of Dr. Paul Allison (University of Pennsylvania):

> Sooner or later (usually sooner), anyone who does statistical analysis runs into problems with missing data.[122]

Given that Professor Allison wrote an entire book on the subject, imputation methods largely exceed the purview of the "Gutkin Manual." However, a few points can be made. The concept includes substituting one value for a missing observation. Use of mixed-effects models can reduce problems associated with missing data. Such models essentially treat discrete observations as exactly that: single data points. If a single observation is missing, remaining data from the subject at other time points (e.g., clinic visits in RCTs) are not lost. Mixed-effects models are also often useful in RWE studies with irregular visit schedules or observation points in time. In terms of comparing subjects or groups, it does not matter if one individual has her second assessment at 3 weeks and the next at 3 months, while another has his at 3 months and the next at 6 months.

Common forms of imputation are last observation carried forward (LOCF), regression imputation, and "hot-deck imputation." Others include[122]:

- Listwise deletion, which typically functions more effectively, and with a lower bias if data are missing completely at random (MCAR) rather than missing at random (MAR) only;
- Pairwise deletion (available-case analysis), which is appropriate for linear models, such as factor analysis and linear regression, and which (like listwise deletion), can result in biased estimates if data are MAR rather than MCAR;
- Dummy variable adjustment, finds application in regression analysis, when one IV or more is missing, by assigning a constant dummy variable (*D*) and then regressing the dependent variable on both IV and *D* (however, this method may lead to biased estimates of coefficients);

- Maximum-likelihood (ML) method, including the example of least-squares linear regression, enables the analyst to "choose as estimates … values that, if true, would maximize the probability of observing what has, in fact, been observed."[122] (ML functions effectively for certain models—linear and log-linear—but not for others, such as ordered logistic regression or Cox proportional hazards); and
- Multiple imputation (MI) method, which surmounts many of the above limitations of ML, is considered to be variable rather than deterministic, in that the MI process includes and embraces random variation and hence is less likely to underestimate the values of covariances and variables with missing information. The MI method includes
  - Single random imputation, which "[makes] random draw from the residual distribution of each imputed variable and [adds] …random numbers to the imputed values. Then, conventional formulas can be used to calculate variances and covariances."[122]
  - Multiple random imputation, which "[repeats] the imputation process more than once, producing multiple 'completed' data sets. Because of the random component, estimates of the parameters of interest will be slightly different in each imputed data set. This variability across imputations can be used to adjust [SE values] upward."[122]

The LOCF convention of data imputation is restrictive because it assumes that there is no (systematic) relationship between either the observed or unobserved outcomes on the variable being analyzed and the probability of dropout. Hence, it assumes that data from lost patients are MCAR. LOCF also assumes that there is no change in data from the last available visit or observation to the end of study. MAR is usually more plausible and applicable than MCAR because "MAR is valid in every case when MCAR is valid, but MCAR is not always valid when MAR is valid."[123] Mixed-model repeated-measures (MMRM) analyses allow for the possibility that observed outcomes are indeed related to the probability of dropout and are consistent with MAR, not MCAR.

3.11.13.1 KOLMOGOROV AND SMIRNOV'S (K–S) AND SHAPIRO AND WILK'S (S–W) TESTS[96,97] AND DATA NORMALITY

Because the mathematics of the K–S and S–W tests are complex, and the computational burden is typically handled by software packages, we will not rigorously present the formal test statistics but rather summarize them qualitatively. One value of the K–S test, which is a nonparametric analysis, is that it does not require that a data distribution be either Gaussian (normal, symmetrical) or skewed (asymmetrical). In fact, like the S–W test, which is more powerful and less conservative, the K–S test can be used to test the normality of a distribution by comparing it to a reference distribution. In this manner, it can be interpreted as a type of goodness-of-fit test (broadly similar to the Hosmer–Lemeshow test). The K–S test can be used for distributions of continuous variables only, and it tends to be more sensitive to a small number of values in the tails of the distribution.

Initially intended for sample sizes of <50, the S–W test is considered to be a less conservative and more powerful test of normality; normality. Both the one-sample K–S and the χ^2 goodness-of-fit test are more conservative tests.[4] One potential practical limitation of the S–W test is that some statistical software programs allow the analyst to enter, as the reference (normal) population for comparison, only the mean and SD of a sample population (i.e., $\bar{x}$ and s) rather than the true or theoretical population values (i.e., μ and σ).[4]

3.11.14 Propensity score matching (PSM)

Prospective RCTs minimize bias via allocation concealment, randomization, and blinding. These procedures tend to result in experimental groups that are well balanced at baseline. Conversely, retrospective cohort studies and others with observational (RWE) designs are inherently unable to include such protocols and are hence not immune from bias, which may result from baseline imbalances between groups. PSM seeks to neutralize such between-group imbalances by matching subjects in each group according to a number of potentially influential baseline factors that might otherwise bias the findings (covariates). In fact, PSM can

result in different groups that are more effectively balanced compared to randomization.[124]

PSM represents an attempt to simulate randomization or realize its "leveling" effect on bias. Through a process that is, on the surface, somewhat akin to bootstrapping (at least to a non–full-time-statistician!), the analyst reviews a data set and seeks to match patients according to certain important sociodemographic or clinical characteristics at baseline. After matching, each of the (now more similar) matched pairs is "allocated" (retrospectively) to one group or another (e.g., active treatment vs. placebo; cases vs. controls). In this way, a better balance can be achieved between the two groups. In more formal, statistical terms, PSM represents the likelihood of treatment allocation conditional on observed baseline characteristics. Limitations of matching controls to cases include incomplete and inexact matching, including loss of data from cases and a relative inability to balance unmeasured confounding variables.

Neither PSM nor regression analysis can control for confounding on unmeasured variables. In Glynn and co-workers' systematic review of RWE studies that used both PSM and regression analysis, most (>80%) returned similar results; in some cases, PSM biased findings toward the null compared to regression analysis. Glynn's group[124] identified the following potential advantages of PSM over multivariate analysis (MVA) and other more conventional methods:

- PSM can neutralize confounding by indication because PSM focuses on drug use and nonuse in a study.
- More conventional forms of modeling cannot accommodate/compare patients who were, versus were not, exposed to treatment (e.g., patients with contraindications), whereas PSM can.
- Matching methods do not strongly assume linearity, eliminate data from patients with no comparable controls, and allow for a relatively transparent and simple analysis.
- PSM is more effective for use when there are relatively few outcomes as against the number of covariates, "[reducing] the dimensionality of the covariates"[124] before modeling. Cepeda's "Rule of Eight" suggests that PSM can be used when there are fewer than eight outcomes per covariate.
- PSM is more useful to determine whether the effectiveness of a drug is related to the strengths of its indication for use.

- RWE studies have shown that some patients with weak indications or even contraindications (i.e., low propensity to receive drug) do not benefit from treatment, or are actually harmed by it, compared to those with stronger indications to receive treatment. Other methods that use propensity scores include covariate adjustment, stratification, and inverse probability weighting.

There are two major PSM algorithms (calculations are typically performed using SAS/STAT® LOGISTIC procedural code): greedy and optimal matching.[125] The greedy algorithm is often used to match cases (set X) and controls (set Y) in a set of decisions; the matching decisions are final and not revisited when matching the next pair. The optimal algorithm allows the analyst to revisit prior case-control matches before matching the next pair (i.e., "break" prior matches to enhance the overall match).

3.11.15 Principal component analysis (PCA)

In theory and practice, PCA is a form of exploratory data analysis (EDA). Its progenitor was the very same Karl Pearson whom we have mentioned previously.[126] Perhaps the best way to summarize PCA is that it constitutes a complex mathematical method (an eigenvalue-based orthogonal transformation) of reducing a set of complex data to a few "principal components"; the number of original variables is always larger than that of principal components. PCA reduces an array of variables that may be correlated into a new set that are linearly uncorrelated: these are the principal components. Related analyses include cluster analysis and factor analysis. Cluster analysis seeks to group individuals into certain natural systems (e.g., numerical taxonomy). Factor analysis may be applied to reduce the complexity of certain psychometric tests to a set of more basic constructs (e.g., general intelligence).

In a study report on which I served as a contributor, PCA reduced responses to questions on three indices of sexual function (among >4,000 respondents) into three discrete principal components of sexual satisfaction. Taken together, these components accounted for >90% of the variance in scores on the various indices.[127] Most of the factors were correlated with Spearman ρ values

exceeding 0.60, except for responses to one question on the International Index of Erectile Function (IIEF–question 6), which related to the frequency of attempts at sexual intercourse ($\rho < 0.35$). The analysis suggested that this "frequency" construct represented a different dimension of sexual satisfaction.

3.11.16 Regression analyses

We have considered regression analysis above, as a form of a general linear model. This "associational and not causal" form of analysis is widely used to predict or estimate a DV according to the presence of certain IVs. Regression models may include comparisons of (1) different levels of a treatment response (DV) across two intervention (or other exposure; IV) groups and (2) three or more exposure groups, estimating associations between discrete levels of a categorical value (vs. baseline) by using indicator variables.[13] Logistic regression analyses estimate associations between predictor variables (IVs) and a categorical (e.g., binary/dichotomous) DV. These tests estimate associations between continuous IVs and DVs (and potentially a random term).

To consider regression analyses in detail would exceed the purview of the "Gutkin Manual." (Dr. Allison has written entire volumes on both logistic regression[128] and multiple regression.[129]) However, there are a few nuances that we can better understand, including the often interchangeable—but incorrect—usage of the terms "multivariate" and "multivariable" linear regression.[130]

Multiple regression in general segregates associations related to IVs on a DV, enabling analysis of each variable separately. Linear regression models analyze a single predictor (or IV) and a continuous outcome (or DV). The equation is given as[130]:

$$y = \alpha + x\beta + \varepsilon$$

where x is a single IV, y a single DV, and β and ε are vector quantities.

The conditional probability of a continuous DV and either a categorical or continuous IV is evaluated using linear regression models when the association between variables is known or likely to be linear. Simple linear regression models include a single IV (explanatory variable or predictor), whereas multiple linear regression models include two or more IVs. An example might include the association between the number of hours spent reading the "Gutkin Manual" and first-journal target acceptance rates (continuous IV and DV). An example of a multiple linear regression analysis might involve seeking to determine associations (with the same continuous DV of first-journal target % acceptance rate) of several IVs, including hours spent reading the "Gutkin Manual," annual number of professional congresses attended, and number of subscriptions to high-tier multispecialty journals.

Logistic regression analyses are often useful when associations between IV and DV are not (or are unlikely to be) linear; in many cases the associations are exponential. It evaluates the conditional probability of a continuous or categorical IV and a categorical (e.g., binary) DV, where the relationship is not known to be linear. An example might comprise numbers of hours spent reading the "Gutkin Manual" (continuous IV) and whether a student passes or fails her writing accreditation test (categorical [binary] DV: pass/fail).

To model multiple predictors (IVs), which may be either categorical or continuous, a multivariable linear regression model may be appropriate. The equation is given as[130]:

$$y = \alpha + x_1\beta_1 + x_2\beta_2 + \ldots x_k\beta_k + \varepsilon$$

where x is a single predictor (IV) in the simple model and $x_1, x_2 \ldots x_k$ are multiple predictors (IVs) in the multivariable model; y is the continuous DV; and β and ε are vector quantities.

How does a MVA differ? This form of analysis evaluates the joint probability distribution of IV and DV: how several outcomes vary together. MVA can also be used to handle data from either repeated measures in a single person (i.e., multiple observations) over time or from clustered or nested settings, in which there are two or more persons within each cluster. The equation for a multivariate linear regression analysis is given as[130]:

$$Y_{n \times p} = X_{n \times (k+1)}\ \beta_{(k+1) \times p} + \varepsilon$$

where $X_{n \times (k+1)}$ is the single set of IV or predictor variables and $Y_{n \times p}$ signifies associations between multiple sets of DVs or outcome variables. Multivariate analysis can determine a number of independent risk factors for a single DV (e.g., independent risk factors for developing adhesions after operative procedures).

3.11.17 Risk concepts: Toward a more nuanced understanding

Risk of disease is the probability of experiencing an adverse disease event over time, including different levels of potential magnitude. Contributing to the likelihood of developing a disease are genetic and other forms of vulnerability (genotype/phenotype); hazard, the pathogenic (e.g., biologic, pharmacologic) or other substrate or substance that can cause disease events; and the duration and intensity of exposure to these hazards (Figure 3.14).

The incidence rate of disease is its likelihood in an at-risk population over a prespecified time interval:

$$\text{Incidence rate} = \frac{\text{No. of new cases of a disease during a time period}}{\text{Total no. of persons at risk who are followed during this period (in person-years)}}$$

Dividing the number of new cases in the numerator by the number of initially healthy persons within the population in the denominator yields the incidence proportion. If 100 of 10,000 initially healthy individuals experience new disease events, the incidence proportion is expressed as 100 per 10,000 population (1%).

Absolute (global) risk can be defined as the probability of experiencing a disease event over a specified interval, typically expressed as a small decimal (and often across a long time horizon such 5 years).

Using data in Table 3.35, we compute the 1-year absolute risk of the disease outcome with the intensive treatment as 6 out of 100 or 6% (0.06). In contrast,

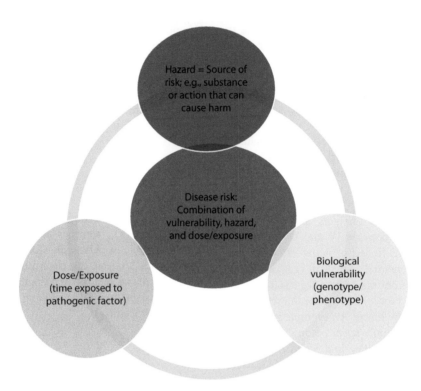

Figure 3.14 Concepts of risk. Selected data from http://www.zerobreastcancer.org. Last accessed November 1, 2017.

the 1-year absolute risk with the moderate therapy is 13% (0.13). The risk of events can also be calculated over different time frames, including a 10-year or annual risk.

Other measures of differences in risk between A and B include absolute risk reduction (excess risk, risk difference) or the relative risk.

$$\text{Absolute risk reduction} = [\textbf{Absolute risk in exposed (e.g., control / moderately treated)}]$$

$$- [\textbf{Absolute risk in unexposed (e.g., actively / intensively treated)}]$$

In the above hypothetical example:

Absolute risk reduction (ARR) = 0.13 – 0.06 = 0.07. Another way to express this difference is that 7 fewer patients receiving the intensive treatment will experience a disease event in every 100 treated.

Relative risk is the ratio of the risk of experiencing a disease event in the exposed (intensively treated) group divided by the risk in the unexposed (moderately treated) group.

$$\text{Relative risk} = \frac{\textbf{Absolute risk of disease in the actively or intensively treated group}}{\textbf{Absolute risk of disease in the moderately treated or control group}}$$

Table 3.35 Data to compute absolute risk reductions and numbers needed to treat to benefit (NNT_B)

Treatment	N	Absolute risk
A (Intensive)	100	6/100 = 0.06
B (Moderate)	100	13/100 = 0.13

In the hypothetical example:

$$\text{Relative risk} = 0.06/0.13 = 0.46$$

Patients receiving the intensive treatment were nearly half (46.2%) as likely to experience a disease event as those receiving moderate therapy.

Relative risk (i.e., the ratio of risks in those receiving moderate vs. intensive treatment) should not be confused with relative risk reduction, which compares the absolute risk reduction to a reference or background rate.

As an example, to communicate the difference between relative and absolute risk, consider the following scenario. The absolute risk of a person experiencing a plane crash is minuscule: 1 in 1.2 million to 1 in 11 million. Without this intuition, it would be difficult for any of us to fly. Now imagine that you are in the terminal lounge and see your flight's pilot and copilot enjoying a few "preflight rounds." Compared to a passenger on a plane whose navigators and navigatrixes are teetotalers, you are at a greatly elevated relative risk. In short, one "terminal event" may lead to another!

Relative risk reduction (RRR) can be computed as[131]:

$$\textbf{Relative risk reduction}$$
$$= 1 - \text{relative risk (e.g., OR, RR)}$$

or:

$$\frac{(ARC - ART)}{ARC}$$

where ARC = absolute risk of events in the control (or moderately treated) group and ART = absolute risk of events in the treated (or intensively treated) group.

Relative risk reduction is considered to be a reliable measure of treatment effect because it does not vary substantially in patients at distinct levels of baseline absolute risk.[132–134] The lower the disease event rate in the control (or unexposed) group, the higher the disparity between RRR and ARR.[135]

Number needed to treat to benefit (NNT_B) is the number of patients who would need to receive one treatment (e.g., the active or intensive treatment above) to prevent a single disease event compared to a second treatment (e.g., the control or moderate treatment above), over a given time frame (typically 5–10 years).

NNT_B is computed as the inverse of the absolute risk reduction between two therapies (risk difference = RD) over a given time frame[136]:

$$\textbf{NNT} = \frac{1}{\textbf{ARR}} = \frac{1}{\textbf{RD}}$$

or

$$NNT_B = 100 \div ARR \text{ (expressed as a percentage)}$$

To compute NNT_B from the above hypothetical example:

$$NNT_B = \frac{1}{[0.13 - 0.06]} = 14.3$$

A total of 15 patients would need to be treated with the intensive therapy, compared to the moderate therapy, to avoid a single disease event over the same treatment interval. NNT values can be further adjusted by treatment adherence. If the ARR between an intensive and moderate lipid therapy regimen administered over 5 years is 0.04 in the entire population (consistent with an $NNT_B = 25$), and the medication adherence rate is computed as 0.85, then the ARR in the 100% adherent group is computed as 0.040 ÷ 0.85 = 0.047, which is consistent with an $NNT_B = 21$ in 100% adherent patients.

At a population level, baseline absolute risk may drive both the outcomes and justifications for treatments. If treatments have similar efficacy in reducing disease event risk, treatment of patients at high baseline absolute risk is likely to confer larger absolute risk reductions and hence result in lower NNT_B values.

This is one reason why the most intensive therapies are often targeted toward patients at highest absolute risk (e.g., those who have already experienced a disease event). One reason why (primary) preventive therapies may not be reimbursed (shortsightedly, in many observers' opinions) as liberally as more "interventional approaches" in persons with disease is that healthier individuals are at much lower absolute risk. On a population basis, a larger number of healthier individuals may need to be screened or treated to avoid a single disease event; in other words, NNT_B values are higher.

For those receptive to likelihood as "odds," the odds ratio (OR) is computed as follows. In a 2×2 contingency table, place "Standard Treatment" atop the first column and "New Treatment" atop the second. As row heading 1, introduce "Event Happens" and row heading 2 (row 2), "Event does not happen. Now populate the cells from left to right as a, b, c, and d; OR $= (a \times d)/(b \times c)$. An OR of 5.0 for syncope might mean that the odds are 5 times higher in the presence (vs. absence) of chronic volume depletion. In the world of diagnostics, a salient measure is the likelihood ratio (LR). The LR for a test result is the probability that it is positive in a patient with (vs. without) disease, or the likelihood of correctly (vs. incorrectly) predicting disease.

3.11.18 Number needed to treat to harm

The number needed to treat to harm (NNT_H) is the number of patients who would need to receive one treatment (vs. another) for 1 of them to experience an adverse effect. It is calculated in the same manner as NNT_B. Suppose that the 1-year event rate for severe gastric bleeding is 3% for Treatment A compared to 7% for Treatment B. NNT_H is computed as

$$NNT_H = \frac{1}{ARR}$$

$$NNT_H = \frac{1}{0.07 - 0.03} = 25$$

On average, 25 patients would need to receive Treatment B (vs. Treatment A) to experience a single case of bleeding over 1 year.

NNT is not difficult to calculate; however, there are some limitations with respect to bias and precision. NNTs should not be computed from numbers of events and subjects across studies because such calculations are not robust to different assumptions about randomization (especially imbalances).[135] Like willingness-to-pay thresholds in HEOR cost-effectiveness analyses, thresholds for acceptable NNTs may have a subjective component and be estimated differently by different stakeholders (e.g., patients, physicians, and consensus treatment guideline panels).

Time horizons are important with NNTs. In a large outcome study comparing an intensive and a moderate therapy, very few disease events may be observed in the first year of treatment; both absolute risk and ARRs in disease events may be small, resulting in a large NNT_B. Over a longer time horizon, however, many more disease events will occur, resulting in larger absolute risks and ARRs, and hence smaller NNT_Bs. These considerations may inform the benefit:risk calculus for using a medication (Figure 3.15).

For example, consider HMG-CoA reductase inhibitors (statins) for lipid lowering in cardiovascular prevention (especially secondary prevention, in persons who have already experienced cardiovascular disease). The NNT_B to avert a single cardiovascular disease event over 5 years is on the order of 50, with lower values in secondary prevention. In contrast, the absolute risk of serious adverse events such as myopathy and the often-fatal rhabdomyolysis are exceedingly low; given that statins elevate these absolute risks modestly, the ARRs are small and NNT_H values exceedingly large. Millions of prescriptions may need to be written to observe a single case of rhabdomyolysis.

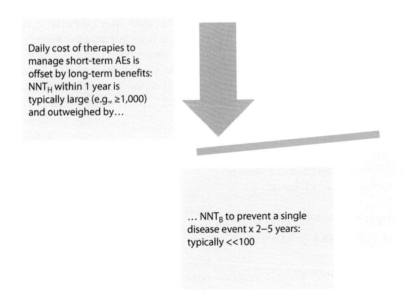

Near term (first treatment year)

Absolute risk of medication AEs is higher, but most AEs are mild and tolerable.

NNT_H is computed over a short time horizon because many AEs occur early and then dissipate and/or resolve.

Long term (2–5 treatment years)

Absolute risk of major disease events increases over time.

Costs of disease events (human and economic) are high and need to be avoided.

NNT_B is computed over a longer time horizon.

Absolute risk of major disease events is relatively low.

Overall costs of medications to prevent disease events and manage AEs over time are typically more than offset by preventing costly disease events.

NNT thresholds and treatment decisions

Daily cost of therapies to manage short-term AEs is offset by long-term benefits: NNT_H within 1 year is typically large (e.g., ≥1,000) and outweighed by…

… NNT_B to prevent a single disease event x 2–5 years: typically <<100

Figure 3.15 Concepts of risk. Short- and long-term benefit:risk considerations in determining an NNT threshold (NNTT), which is defined as the inverse value of absolute risk reduction at which therapeutic benefits equal therapeutic risks. The NNT to harm (NNT_H) may include serious or life-threatening events (e.g., rhabdomyolysis with statins or QTc prolongation or *torsades de pointes* with other therapies).
Abbreviations: AE, adverse event; NNT, number needed to treat.

It is important to distinguish between ORs and risk ratios (RRs). We typically appreciate the OR as a link between exposure and outcome. The RR is simply the ratio of disease risk in one group (e.g., cases) compared to (or, actually, divided by) another (e.g., controls).

An RR value of 1.28 means that cases are at a 28% higher relative risk of disease compared to controls. (The 95% CI must not overlap 1.0 if the RR value is significant at p < 0.05.) When the outcome is observed in >10% of the control (unexposed) group, the OR overestimates the RR.[137]

If we know an assumed control risk (ACR) in a meta-analysis of studies involving risk ratios, we can compute the NNT.[136] Suppose that the summary or aggregate RR in patients receiving Treatment A (intensive) compared to another therapy (e.g., moderate Treatment B or placebo + usual care) is 0.88, and the ACR is 240 events per 1,000 (0.24). We can compute the NNT_B as follows:

$$NNT_B = \frac{1}{ACR \times |(1 - RR)|}$$

$$NNT_B = \frac{1}{0.24 \times |(1 - 0.88)|} =$$

$$NNT_B = \frac{1}{0.24 \times 0.12} = 34.7$$

A total of 35 patients must be treated with Treatment A (vs. Treatment B) to avoid a single adverse clinical event. The effect of Treatment A (vs. Treatment B) in terms of numbers of disease events averted can be computed as follows:

Number fewer events per 1,000 = 1,000 × 0.24 (ACR)

$$\times (1 - 0.88) = 28.8$$

Treatment A prevents about 29 disease events per 1,000 population.

Finally, it is also possible to compute the risk ratio from a summary odds ratio in a meta-analysis in which we know or can project ACR[136]:

$$RR = \frac{OR}{1 - ACR \times (1 - OR)}$$

Table 3.36 summarizes concepts of risk.

3.11.19 Survival analyses: Kaplan–Meier[138] (K–M) and proportional hazards (PH)[139] (or Cox regression) methods

K–M plots enable us to determine the probability of surviving from a fixed starting point over time intervals that are divided into smaller, discrete segments.[140] K–M plots are useful to compare cumulative survival between two treatments, given the vicissitudes of patient participation in a study. The segments are often defined by a number of clinic visits over the lifetime of a study. Also termed the "product limit estimate," the K–M test does not determine exactly when an event (e.g., death) occurs; only that it happened between two clinic visits (or other prespecified intervals). The K–M method results in a cumulative estimate of survival over time, because the probability of survival at each observation point (e.g., clinic visit) is multiplied by that of the next time point, the one after that, and so on. The probability of survival at one observation point is computed as follows[139]:

$$S(t) = \pi \left(1 - \frac{d_i}{n_i} \right)$$

Survival at time t is related to the number of events (d_i) divided by the number of individuals known to have survived (n_i).

Over time, some study participants are uncooperative or lose contact with study personnel (or vice versa). Observations from these subjects are censored (not included in the denominator for interval survival calculations). K–M analysis requires that subjects enrolled early and late in the study have identical probabilities of survival and that, at any

Table 3.36 Concepts of relative risk

Concept	Definition
Hazard ratio (HR)	Ratio of event incidence in one group (e.g., active treatment) compared to another (e.g., placebo + usual care). Unlike odds ratio (OR), HR provides a time-specific risk rather than a cumulative risk over time. HR is used in Kaplan–Meier survival analyses, which show disease incidences at each of several observation points (visits) during a clinical trial.
Odds ratio (OR)	OR provides the ratio of odds of a disease when predicted (e.g., in the presence of widely recognized risk factors or precipitants), to the odds when it is not predicted (i.e., when in the absence of these factors). It is typically expressed as ratios such as 1:100. When diseases are infrequent, the OR is close to the relative risk.
Risk difference (RD)	The difference in absolute risk of an event in two groups (e.g., risk in placebo control minus risk in active treatment). The number needed to treat to benefit or harm one patient is computed as the reciprocal of RD (or of the absolute risk reduction).

observation point (e.g., clinic visit) when a study participant's data are censored, the subject has the same likelihood of survival as those who continue in the study.[140] In K–M plots, numbers of available subjects (i.e., those who have not died, experienced another event, or been censored) at each clinic visit are typically listed below the x-axis for time (in a grid).

Preliminarily, K–M survival plots for two different treatments can be compared by visual inspection. The likelihood of an event (e.g., death, survival, disease-free survival) at each clinic visit is plotted on the y-axis and time on the x-axis. Researchers speak of "separation" as the time (observation point, on the abscissa) at which curves diverge or depart. One way to evaluate the difference is to compute the log rank test statistic:

$$\text{Log rank test statistic} = \frac{(O_1 - E_1)^2}{E_1} + \frac{(O_2 - E_2)^2}{E_2}$$

where O_1 and O_2 represent the total numbers of observed events in each group and E_1 and E_2 signify the expected numbers.

Let us suppose that, in Group 1, at clinic visit 1 (2 weeks), 100 subjects were alive, and 2 died by clinic visit 2 (4 weeks). The observed risk of the event in Group 1 (O_1) is 0.02. Now let us say that 50 subjects were alive at clinic visit 1 (2 weeks) in Group 2. The expected number of deaths at clinic visit 2 in this group (E_2) would be 50 × 0.02 = 1. E_2 (the total number of expected deaths in Group 2) is computed as the sum of expected events at all observation points (clinic visits).

Another way to analyze survival data is via Cox PH regression models. The test statistic is given as

$$\text{Log}[h(t)] = \log[h_0(t)] + \beta_1 x_1 + \beta_2 x_2 + \dots \beta_p x_p$$

where $h_0(t)$ is the baseline hazard of an event (e.g., death) at time t; x signifies exposure variables, of which there are a total of p; and β denotes the regression coefficient related to each exposure variables.[13]

Figure 3.16 summarizes considerations relevant to computing hazards ratios and plotting a Kaplan–Meier survival curve using Microsoft Excel.

- In survival analysis, data are segregated into mutually exclusive treatment time intervals, which are plotted on the abscissa (x-axis). The probability of survival (or of not experiencing a disease event) is plotted on the ordinate (y-axis).
- During each interval, a study participant can survive, die (or have an event), or be lost to follow-up or have other events (e.g., protocol violations), which are censored.
- Such data need to be censored, in part because we don't know if they did or did not die or experience an event—i.e., should they contribute to the numerator, or denominator?
- In each interval, the probability of survival [$P(S)$] is conditional. It is the probability of surviving to the beginning of the treatment interval multiplied by the probability of surviving during the interval, given survival to the beginning of the interval.

Interval, mo.	Begin	Died	Lost/ Censored	End	$P(S_B) \times P(S_E)$	S
Survival: Active treatment						
0 (outset)	350	0	0	350	1.0000	1.000
3	350	10	0	340/350 (0.9714)	1.0000 × 0.9714	0.9714
6	340	21	1	318/340 (0.9353)	0.9714 × 0.9353	0.9085
9	318	2	1	315/318 (0.9904)	0.9085 × 0.9904	0.8998
12	315	25	2	288/315 (0.9143)	0.8998 × 0.9143	0.8226
15	288	40	5	280/288 (0.9728)	0.8226 × 0.9728	0.8002
18	280	11	3	266/280 (0.9500)	0.8002 × 0.9500	0.7600

The survival probabilities can be computed in MS Excel, but the Kaplan–Meier equation/function may not be on standard versions; hence, you may need to load an online add-in (File/Options).

(a)

Figure 3.16 Considerations relevant to computing hazard ratios and plotting a Kaplan–Meier survival curve using Microsoft Excel. Data for active treatment (a).   (Continued)

Interval, mo.	Begin	Died	Lost/ Censored	End	$P(S_B) \times P(S_E)$	S
Survival: Placebo control						
0	370	0	0	370	1.0000	1.000
3	370	22	2	336/370 (0.9085)	1.0000 × 0.9085	0.9085
6	336	82	0	254/336 (0.7570)	0.9085 × 0.7570	0.6877
9	254	21	4	229/254 (0.8998)	0.6877 × 0.8998	0.6188
12	229	6	2	221/229 (0.9669)	0.6188 × 0.9669	0.5983
15	221	10	5	206/221 (0.9303)	0.5983 × 0.9303	0.5566
18	206	5	7	194/206 (0.9439)	0.5566 × 0.9439	0.5254

(b)

The survival probabilities can be computed in MS Excel, but the Kaplan–Meier equation/function may not be on standard versions; hence, you may need to load an online add-in (File/Options).

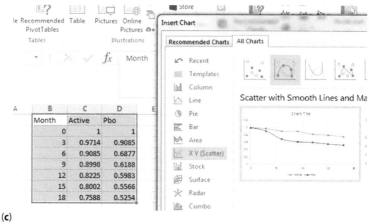

(c)

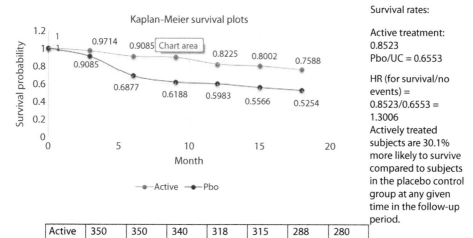

Survival rates:

Active treatment: 0.8523
Pbo/UC = 0.6553

HR (for survival/no events) =
0.8523/0.6553 =
1.3006
Actively treated subjects are 30.1% more likely to survive compared to subjects in the placebo control group at any given time in the follow-up period.

Active	350	350	340	318	315	288	280
Pbo/UC	370	370	336	254	229	221	206

Figure 3.16 (Continued) Considerations relevant to computing hazard ratios and plotting a Kaplan–Meier survival curve using Microsoft Excel. Data for control **(b)**, and final output **(c)**. K–M curves can also be graphed using SigmaPlot. (Available at: https://systatsoftware.com/. Last accessed March 25, 2018.)

REFERENCES

1. Jaynes ET. In: *Probability Theory: The Logic of Science*. St. Louis: Washington University, 1995: 101–18.

2. Pólya G. *Mathematics and Plausible Reasoning*. Princeton, NJ: Princeton University Press, 1954.

3. Strasak AM, Zaman Q, Pfeiffer KP et al. Statistical errors in medical research: a review of common pitfalls. *Swiss Med Wkly* 2007;137:44–9.

4. Riffenburgh RH. *Statistics in Medicine*. 3rd ed. Academic Press, 2012.

5. Perez-Ruiz F, Schlesinger N. Management of gout. *Scand J Rheumatol* 2008;37:81–9.

6. du Prel JB, Rohrig B, Hommel G et al. Choosing statistical tests: part 12 of a series on evaluation of scientific publications. *Dtsch Arztebl Int* 2010;107:343–8.

7. Bulmer MG. *Basic Statistics*. Cambridge, MA: MIT University Press, 1968.

8. Westfall PH. Kurtosis as peakedness, 1. *Am Stat* 2014;68:191–5.

9. Barretto H, Howland F. *Introductory Econometrics: Using Monte Carlo Simulation with Microsoft Excel*. New York: Cambridge University Press, 2006.

10. Lane DM. History of the Normal Distribution. Available at: http://online statbook.com/2/normal_distribution/history_normal.html. Last accessed November 1, 2017.

11. Watier NN, Lamontagne C, Chartier S. What does the mean mean? *J Stat Educ* 2011;19:1–12.

12. Bharmal M, Payne K, Atkinson MJ et al. Validation of an abbreviated Treatment Satisfaction Questionnaire for Medication (TSQM-9) among patients on antihypertensive medications. *Health Qual Life Outcomes* 2009;7:36.

13. Kirkwood BR, Sterne JAC. *Essential Medical Statistics*. 2nd ed. Malden, MA: Blackwell Science, 2007.

14. Richland J. *Stats: Measures of Variation*. Available at: people.richland.edu/james/lecture/m170/ch03-var.html. Last accessed November 1, 2017.

15. Noordzij M, Tripepi G, Dekker FW et al. Sample size calculations: basic principles and common pitfalls. *Nephrol Dial Transplant* 2010;25:1388–93.

16. Motulsky HM. *Prism 5 Statistics Guide*. Available at www.graphpad.com. Last accessed November 1, 2017. La Jolla, CA: GraphPad Software Inc., 2007.

17. Regieli JJ, Jukema JW, Doevendans PA et al. Paraoxonase variants relate to 10-year risk in coronary artery disease: impact of a high-density lipoprotein-bound antioxidant in secondary prevention. *J Am Coll Cardiol* 2009;54:1238–45.

18. Shahar E. Causal diagrams for encoding and evaluation of information bias. *J Eval Clin Pract* 2009;15:436–40.

19. Salas M, Hofman A, Stricker BH. Confounding by indication: an example of variation in the use of epidemiologic terminology. *Am J Epidemiol* 1999;149:981–3.

20. Delgado-Rodriguez M, Llorca J. Bias. *J Epidemiol Community Health* 2004; 58:635–41.

21. Perros P, Crombie AL, Matthews JN et al. Age and gender influence the severity of thyroid-associated ophthalmopathy: a study of 101 patients attending a combined thyroid-eye clinic. *Clin Endocrinol (Oxf)* 1993;38:367–72.

22. Tu YK, Gunnell D, Gilthorpe MS. Simpson's Paradox, Lord's Paradox, and Suppression Effects are the same phenomenon—the reversal paradox. *Emerg Themes Epidemiol* 2008;5:2.

23. Bland JM, Altman DG. Some examples of regression towards the mean. *BMJ* 1994;309:780.

24. Davis CE. The effect of regression to the mean in epidemiologic and clinical studies. *Am J Epidemiol* 1976;104:493–8.

25. MacMahon S, Peto R, Cutler J et al. Blood pressure, stroke, and coronary heart disease. Part 1, Prolonged differences in blood pressure: prospective observational studies corrected for the regression dilution bias. *Lancet* 1990;335:765–74.

26. Bartlett JW, Frost C. Reliability, repeatability and reproducibility: analysis of measurement errors in continuous variables. *Ultrasound Obstet Gynecol* 2008;31:466–75.

27. Gwet KL. In: D'Agostino RB, Sulivan L, Massaro J, eds. *Wiley Encyclopedia of Clinical Trials*. London: Wiley Interscience, 2008.

28. Bravo G, Potvin L. Estimating the reliability of continuous measures with Cronbach's alpha or the intraclass correlation coefficient: toward the integration of two traditions. *J Clin Epidemiol* 1991;44:381–90.

29. VanderWeele TJ. On the distinction between interaction and effect modification. *Epidemiology* 2009;20:863–71.

30. Kolokotroni O, Middleton N, Gavatha M et al. Asthma and atopy in children born by caesarean section: effect modification by family history of allergies—a population based cross-sectional study. *BMC Pediatr* 2012;12:179.

31. Kraemer HC, Wilson GT, Fairburn CG et al. Mediators and moderators of treatment effects in randomized clinical trials. *Arch Gen Psychiatry* 2002;59:877–83.

32. Anderson RJ, Freedland KE, Clouse RE et al. The prevalence of comorbid depression in adults with diabetes: a meta-analysis. *Diabetes Care* 2001;24:1069–78.

33. Raschenberger J, Kollerits B, Ritchie J et al. Association of relative telomere length with progression of chronic kidney disease in two cohorts: effect modification by smoking and diabetes. *Sci Rep* 2015;5:11887.

34. Szklo M, Nieto FJ. *Epidemiology: Beyond the Basics*. Sudbury, MA: Jones & Bartlett Publishers, 2007.

35. Friedman HH, Amoo T. Rating the rating scales. *J Marketing Management* 1999;9:114–23.

36. Hernan MA, Hernandez-Diaz S, Robins JM. A structural approach to selection bias. *Epidemiology* 2004;15:615–25.

37. Westreich D, Daniel RM. Commentary: Berkson's fallacy and missing data. *Int J Epidemiol* 2014;43:524–6.

38. Pearce N, Richiardi L. Commentary: Three worlds collide: Berkson's bias, selection bias and collider bias. *Int J Epidemiol* 2014;43:521–4.

39. Sackett DL. Bias in analytic research. *J Chronic Dis* 1979;32:51–63.

40. Haut ER, Pronovost PJ. Surveillance bias in outcomes reporting. *JAMA* 2011;305:2462–3.

41. Conn HO, Snyder N, Atterbury CE. The Berkson bias in action. *Yale J Biol Med* 1979;52:141–7.

42. Berkson J. Limitations of the application of the fourfold table analysis to hospital data. *Biometrics Bull.* 1946;2:47–53.

43. Snoep JD, Morabia A, Hernandez-Diaz S et al. Commentary: A structural approach to Berkson's fallacy and a guide to a history of opinions about it. *Int J Epidemiol* 2014;43:515–21.

44. Granlund J, Svensson T, Granath F et al. Diverticular disease and the risk of colon cancer—a population-based case-control study. *Aliment Pharmacol Ther* 2011;34:675–81.

45. National Institute of Diabetes and Digestive and Kidney Diseases. Diverticular Disease. Available at: https://www.niddk.nih.gov/health-information/digestive-diseases/diverticulosis-diverticulitis. Last accessed November 1, 2017.

46. Hassan E. Recall bias can be a threat to retrospective and prospective research designs. *Internet J Epidemiol* 2005(3).

47. Levesque LE, Hanley JA, Kezouh A et al. Problem of immortal time bias in cohort studies: example using statins for preventing progression of diabetes. *BMJ* 2010;340:b5087.

48. Hassan MM, Hwang LY, Hatten CJ et al. Risk factors for hepatocellular carcinoma: synergism of alcohol with viral hepatitis and diabetes mellitus. *Hepatology* 2002;36:1206–13.

49. Jarvinen TL, Michaelsson K, Jokihaara J et al. Overdiagnosis of bone fragility in the quest to prevent hip fracture. *BMJ* 2015;350:h2088.

50. Smits LJ, van Kuijk SM, Leffers P et al. Index event bias-a numerical example. *J Clin Epidemiol* 2013;66:192–6.

51. Dahabreh IJ, Kent DM. Index event bias as an explanation for the paradoxes of recurrence risk research. *JAMA* 2011;305:822–3.

52. Lavie CJ, Milani RV, Ventura HO. Obesity and cardiovascular disease: risk factor, paradox, and impact of weight loss. *J Am Coll Cardiol* 2009;53:1925–32.

53. Gruberg L, Weissman NJ, Waksman R et al. The impact of obesity on the short-term and long-term outcomes after percutaneous coronary intervention: the obesity paradox? *J Am Coll Cardiol* 2002;39:578–84.

54. Adamopoulos C, Meyer P, Desai RV et al. Absence of obesity paradox in patients with chronic heart failure and diabetes mellitus: a propensity-matched study. *Eur J Heart Fail* 2011;13:200–6.

55. Kent DM, Thaler DE. Is patent foramen ovale a modifiable risk factor for stroke recurrence? *Stroke* 2010;41:S26–S30.

56. Petri H, Urquhart J. Channeling bias in the interpretation of drug effects. *Stat Med* 1991;10:577–81.

57. Lobo FS, Wagner S, Gross CR et al. Addressing the issue of channeling bias in observational studies with propensity scores analysis. *Res Social Adm Pharm* 2006;2:143–51.

58. Keech A, Simes RJ, Barter P et al. Effects of long-term fenofibrate therapy on cardiovascular events in 9795 people with type 2 diabetes mellitus (the FIELD study): randomised controlled trial. *Lancet* 2005;366:1849–61.

59. Keogh-Brown MR, Bachmann MO, Shepstone L et al. Contamination in trials of educational interventions. *Health Technol Assess* 2007;11:iii, ix-iii, 107.

60. Ishak KJ, Proskorovsky I, Korytowsky B et al. Methods for adjusting for bias due to crossover in oncology trials. *Pharmacoeconomics* 2014;32:533–46.

61. McNemar Q. Note on the sampling error of the difference between correlated proportions or percentages. *Psychometrika* 1947;12:153–7.

62. Fisher RA. On the interpretation of χ^2 from contingency tables, and the calculation of P. *J Royal Stat Soc* 1922;85:87–94.

63. Fisher RA. *Statistical Methods for Research Workers*. Edinburgh: Oliver & Boyd, 1954.

64. Fisher RA, Yates F. *Statistical Tables for Biological, Agricultural and Medical Research*. 6th ed. Edinburgh: Oliver & Boyd, 1963.

65. Fisher RA. In: Newman JR, ed. *The World of Mathematics*. Courier Dove Publications, 1956.

66. Pearson K. On the criterion that a given system of deviations from the probable in the case of a correlated system of variables is such that it can be reasonably supposed to have arisen from random sampling. *Philosophical Magazine Series 5* 1900;50:150–75.

67. Cochran WG. Some methods for strengthening common χ^2 tests. *Biometrics* 1954;10:417–51.

68. Mantel N, Haenszel W. Statistical aspects of the analysis of data from retrospective studies of disease. *J Natl Cancer Inst* 1959;22:719–48.

69. Pourhoseingholi MA, Baghestani AR, Vahedi M. How to control confounding effects by statistical analysis. *Gastroenterol Hepatol Bed Bench* 2012;5:79–83.

70. Smith LA, Hatcher-Ross JL, Kahn RS. Rethinking race/ethnicity. income and childhood asthma: racial/ethnic disparities concentrated among the very poor. *Public Health Rep* 2005;120:109–16.

71. Penn State University Eberly School of Science. Stat 507 Epidemiological Research Methods.5 Bias, Confounding and Effect Modification. 2015.

72. Student. The probable error of a mean. *Biometrika* 1908;6:1–25.

73. Fisher RA. On the "probable error" of a coefficient of correlation deduced from a small sample. *Metron* 1921;1:3–32.

74. Fisher RA. The correlation between relatives on the supposition of Mendelian inheritance. *Philosophical Transactions of the Royal Society of Edinburgh.* 1918;52:399–433.

75. Fisher RA. *Statistical Methods for Research Workers,* 4th ed. Edinburgh: Oliver & Boyd, 1932.

76. Lowry R. Chapter 17: One-Way Analysis of Covariance for Independent Samples. In: *Concepts and Applications of Inferential Statistics*. Vassar College. Available at: http://vassarstats.net/textbook/ch17pt2.html. Last accessed November 1, 2017.

77. Owen SV. Uses and abuses of the analysis of covariance. *Res Nursing Health* 1998;21:557–62.

78. Charlson M, Szatrowski TP, Peterson J et al. Validation of a combined comorbidity index. *J Clin Epidemiol* 1994;47:1245–51.

79. Sainani K. GEE and Mixed Models for Longitudinal Data. *Available at: www.pitt.edu.* 2015; accessed November 15, 2015.

80. Wilcoxon F. Individual comparisons by ranking methods. *Biometrics Bulletin* 1945;1:80–3.

81. Clarke R, Peden JF, Hopewell JC et al. Genetic variants associated with Lp(a) lipoprotein level and coronary disease. *N Engl J Med* 2009;361:2518–28.

82. Friedman M. The use of ranks to avoid the assumption of normality implicit in the analysis of variance. *J Am Stat Assoc* 1937;32:675–701.

83. Tweyongyere R, Mawa PA, Kihembo M et al. Effect of praziquantel treatment of *Schistosoma mansoni* during pregnancy on immune responses to schistosome antigens among the offspring: results of a randomised, placebo-controlled trial. *BMC Infect Dis* 2011;11:234.

84. Mann HB, Whitney DR. On a test of whether one of two random variables is stochastically larger than the other. *Ann Math Statistics* 1947;1:50–60.

85. Kruskal W, Wallis WA. Use of ranks in one-criterion variance analysis. *J Am Stat Assoc* 1952;47:583–621.

86. Viazzi F, Leoncini G, Parodi D et al. Pulse pressure and subclinical cardiovascular damage in primary hypertension. *Nephrol Dial Transplant* 2002;17:1779–85.

87. Bayes T, Price R. An essay towards solving a problem in the doctrine of chance. doi:10.1098/rstl.1763.0053. *Philosophical Transactions Roy Soc London* 1763;53:370–418.

88. Geyer C. Introduction to Markov Chain Monte Carlo. Available at: http://www.mcmchandbook.net/HandbookChapter1.pdf. 2016; accessed January 4, 2016.

89. Centers for Disease Control and Prevention. Fact Sheet: Smokeless Tobacco Use in the United States. Available at: http://www.cdc.gov/tobacco/data_statistics/fact_sheets/smokeless/use_us/#national. Last accessed November 1, 2017.

90. Illinois Department of Public Health. Cancer in Illinois: Oral Cancer. Available at: www.idph.state.il.us/cancer/statistics.htm. Last accessed November 1, 2017.

91. Metropolis N, Rosenbluth AW, Rosenbluth MN et al. Equation of state calculations by fast computing machines. *J Chemical Phys* 1953;21:1087–92.

92. Cook JR, Yin D, Alemao E et al. Development and validation of a model to project the long-term benefit and cost of alternative lipid-lowering strategies in patients with hypercholesterolaemia. *Pharmacoeconomics*. 2004;22 Suppl 3:37–48.

93. Altman DG, Bland JM. Measurement in medicine: the analysis of method comparison studies. *The Statistician* 1983;307–17.

94. Bland JM, Altman DG. Statistical methods for assessing agreement between two methods of clinical measurement. *Lancet* 1986;1:307–10.

95. Giavarina D. Understanding Bland Altman analysis. *Biochem Med (Zagreb)* 2015;25:141–51.

96. Shapiro SS, Wilk MB. An analysis of variance test for normality (complete samples). *Biometrika* 1965;52:591–611.

97. Kolmogorov A. *Sulla determinazione empirica di una legge di distribuzione. G Ist Ital Attuari* 1933;4:83–91.

98. Pearson K. Notes on regression and inheritance in the case of two parents. *Proc Royal Soc London* 1895;58:240–32.

99. Spearman C. The proof and measurement of association between two things. *Am J Psychology* 1904;15:72–101.

100. Chen HA, Lin KC, Chen CH et al. The effect of etanercept on anti-cyclic citrullinated peptide antibodies and rheumatoid factor in patients with rheumatoid arthritis. *Ann Rheum Dis* 2006;65:35–9.

101. Kendall M. *Rank Correlation Methods.* London: Charles Griffin & Company Limited, 1948.

102. Light RJPDB. *Summing up: The Science of Reviewing Research.* Cambridge, MA: Harvard University Press, 1984.

103. Juni P, Holenstein F, Sterne J et al. Direction and impact of language bias in meta-analyses of controlled trials: empirical study. *Int J Epidemiol* 2002;31:115–23.

104. Sterne JA, Egger M. Funnel plots for detecting bias in meta-analysis: guidelines on choice of axis. *J Clin Epidemiol* 2001;54:1046–55.

105. Egger M, Zellweger-Zahner T, Schneider M et al. Language bias in randomised controlled trials published in English and German. *Lancet* 1997;350:326–9.

106. Bland M. Meta-analysis: heterogeneity and publication bias. Available at: https://www-users.york.ac.uk/~mb55/msc/systrev/week7/hetpub-compact.pdf. Last accessed November 1, 2017.

107. Sterne JAC, Sterne JAC, Sutton AJ, Ioannidis JPA. Recommendations for examining and interpreting funnel plot asymmetry in meta-analyses of randomised controlled trials. *BMJ* 2011;342:d4002.

108. Johnson PE. Generalized estimating equations. 2004;1–7. Available at: http://pj.freefaculty.org/guides/stat/Regression/TimeSeries-Longitudinal-CXTS/CXTS-GEE_v1.pdf. Last accessed November 1, 2017.

109. Hanley JA, Negassa A, Edwardes MD et al. Statistical analysis of correlated data using generalized estimating equations: an orientation. *Am J Epidemiol* 2003;157:364–75.

110. Greene T. GEE and Generalized Linear Mixed Models. Available at: http://slideplayer.com/slide/6106341/ Last accessed November 1, 2017.

111. Institute for Digital Research and Education (IDRE). Introduction to Generalized Linear Mixed Models. Available at: http://www.ats.ucla.edu/stat/mult_pkg/glmm.htm. 2015; accessed October 18, 2015 (Introduction to SAS. UCLA: Statistical Consulting Group).

112. Zeger SL, Liang KY. Longitudinal data analysis for discrete and continuous outcomes. *Biometrics* 1986;42:121–30.

113. Magezi DA. Linear mixed-effects models for within-participant psychology experiments: an introductory tutorial and free, graphical user interface (LMMgui). *Front Psychol* 2015;6:2.

114. Guo Y, Logan HL, Glueck DH et al. Selecting a sample size for studies with repeated measures. *BMC Med Res Methodol* 2013;13:100.

115. DerSimonian R, Laird N. Meta-analysis in clinical trials revisited. *Contemp Clin Trials* 2015;45:139–45.

116. DerSimonian R, Laird N. Meta-analysis in clinical trials. *Control Clin Trials* 1986;7:177–88.

117. Higgins JP, Thompson SG, Deeks JJ et al. Measuring inconsistency in meta-analyses. *BMJ* 2003;327:557–60.

118. Hosmer DW, Lemeshow S. *Applied Logistic Regression*. New York: Wiley, 2013.

119. Hosmer DW, Taber S, Lemeshow S. The importance of assessing the fit of logistic regression models: a case study. *Am J Public Health* 1991;81:1630–5.

120. Parikh R, Mathai A, Parikh S et al. Understanding and using sensitivity, specificity and predictive values. *Indian J Ophthalmol* 2008;56:45–50.

121. Dunn TJ, Baguley T, Brunsden V. From alpha to omega: a practical solution to the pervasive problem of internal consistency estimation. *Br J Psychol* 2014;105:399–412.

122. Allison PD. *Missing Data*. Sage University Papers Series on Quantitative Applications in the Social Sciences, series no. 07-136. ed. Thousand Oaks, CA: Sage Publications, Inc., 2002.

123. Prakash A, Risser RC, Mallinckrodt CH. The impact of analytic method on interpretation of outcomes in longitudinal clinical trials. *Int J Clin Pract* 2008;62:1147–58.

124. Glynn RJ, Schneeweiss S, Sturmer T. Indications for propensity scores and review of their use in pharmacoepidemiology. *Basic Clin Pharmacol Toxicol* 2006;98:253–9.

125. Parsons LS. Reducing bias in a propensity score matched-pair sample using greedy matching techniques. Paper 214-26. Available at: http://www2.sas.com/proceedings/sugi26/p214-26.pdf. 2015; accessed September 15, 2015.

126. Pearson K. On line and planes of closest fit to systems of points in space. *Philosophical Magazine* 1901;2:559–72.

127. Fugl-Meyer A, Althof S, Buvat J et al. Aspects of sexual satisfaction in men with erectile dysfunction: a factor analytic and logistic regression approach. *J Sex Med* 2009;6:232–42.

128. Allison PD. *Logistic Regression Using SAS®: Theory and Application*. 2nd ed. Cary, NC: SAS Institute Inc., 2012.

129. Allison PD. *Multiple Regression: a Primer*. Thousand Oaks, CA: Pine Forge Press, A Sage Publications Company, 1999.

130. Hidalgo B, Goodman M. Multivariate or multivariable regression? *Am J Public Health* 2013;103:39–40.

131. Furukawa TA, Guyatt GH, Griffith LE. Can we individualize the 'number needed to treat'? An empirical study of summary effect measures in meta-analyses. *Int J Epidemiol* 2002;31:72–6.

132. Schmid CH, Lau J, McIntosh MW et al. An empirical study of the effect of the control rate as a predictor of treatment efficacy in meta-analysis of clinical trials. *Stat Med* 1998;17:1923–42.

133. Barratt A, Wyer PC, Hatala R et al. Tips for learners of evidence-based medicine: 1. Relative risk reduction, absolute risk reduction and number needed to treat. *Can Med Assoc J* 2004;171:353–8.

134. Baigent C, Blackwell L, Emberson J et al. Efficacy and safety of more intensive lowering of LDL cholesterol: a meta-analysis of data from 170,000 participants in 26 randomised trials. *Lancet* 2010;376:1670–81.

135. Sinclair JC, Cook RJ, Guyatt GH et al. When should an effective treatment be used? Derivation of the threshold number needed to treat and the minimum event rate for treatment. *J Clin Epidemiol* 2001;54:253–62.

136. Schünemann HJ, Oxman AD, Vist G. Interpreting results and drawing conclusions. In: *Cochrane Handbook for Systematic Reviews of Interventions*. Version 5.1.0 of the Cochrane Handbook. West Sussex, UK: The Cochrane Collaboration and Wiley-Blackwell, 2011: 12.1–12.24; pages 359–383. Available at: http://handbook-5-1.cochrane.org/ Last accessed November 1, 2017.

137. Viera AJ. Odds ratios and risk ratios: what's the difference and why does it matter? *South Med J* 2008;101:730–4.

138. Kaplan EL, Meier P. Nonparametric estimation from incomplete observations. *J Amer Statist Assn* 1958;53:457–81.

139. Cox DR. *Regression Models and Life-Tables.* London: Imperial College, 1972.

140. Goel MK, Khanna P, Kishore J. Understanding survival analysis: Kaplan–Meier estimate. *Int J Ayurveda Res* 2010;1:274–8.

4

Best practices: Consensus recommendations and standards to prepare high-quality, ethical, transparently disclosed manuscripts for journal publication

CONTENTS

CHAPTER OBJECTIVES

The aims of this chapter are to:

- Survey best practices to prepare high-quality manuscripts that are most likely to be accepted by your first journal targeted.
- Introduce quality-control (QC) checklists from consensus guidelines to prepare reports of most types of investigations, including CONSORT for randomized controlled trials (and extensions) and STROBE for observational studies (and extensions).
- Offer templates, forms, and figures to assist in preparing and submitting ethical, transparently disclosed manuscripts.

EXECUTIVE SUMMARY

Consensus guidelines for medical manuscript preparation have proliferated since the year 2000. Peer-reviewed journals are increasingly predicating acceptance of manuscripts on the extent to which they meet these recommendations.

The unique value of Chapter 4 in augmenting journal acceptance rates for medical writers (MWs) is twofold. For the first and only time to my knowledge, this textbook aggregates and advocates, in a single publication:

1. Consensus QC guideline checklists and forms (~60) to prepare most types of medical

manuscripts for journal publication, including (in descending order of medical evidence quality and influence):

- Systematic literature reviews;
- Meta-analyses;
- Randomized controlled trials (RCTs);
- Observational studies (including molecular epidemiology and genetic studies);
- Case reports and series; and
- In vivo and in vitro research. (Using these checklists and forms should help to optimize first-journal acceptance rates because many journals refer to them to discriminate the quality, and determine the disposition, of submitted manuscripts.)

2. Best practices for manuscript submission and publication informed and validated by my 23 years of successful practice as president of a global medical communications company. Most of these experiences are consistent with guidance from the International Committee of Medical Journal Editors (ICMJE). (Available at http://www.icmje.org/recommendations/browse/manuscript-preparation/preparing-for-submission.html. Last accessed January 27, 2018.) In particular:

- Tables 4.1–4.8 include my organization's internal guidelines, which overlap most consensus recommendations for manuscript preparation (these checklists also build on principles and practices detailed in Chapters 1 through 3 of this *User's Manual*).
- Forms 1–4 include templates and other documents to facilitate manuscript submission and ethical disclosures of authors' intellectual contributions and financial interests. (These are largely informed by guidance from the ICMJE, which are available at http://www.icmje.org, and the Committee on Publication Ethics [COPE], which are available at www.publicationethics.org.)
- Figure 4.1 is an example of a Consolidated Standards of Reporting Trials (CONSORT) patient disposition flow diagram. (www.consort-statement.org/consort-statement/flow-diagram. Last accessed October 28, 2017.) Figures 4.2–4.6 present flow diagrams for editors to handle plagiarism; fabricated

data; ghost, guest, or gift authorship; other ethical problems; and undisclosed conflicts of interest in submitted manuscripts or published articles, from COPE (Available at: https://publicationethics.org. Last accessed October 28, 2017). Plagiarism can be averted via both primary and secondary strategies. The paramount strategy advocated throughout this textbook (especially in Chapters 1 and 2) is to read critically and fashion your own analysis and/or synthesis: "appraise, then apprise." The secondary strategy is to submit written work for electronic checking by software systems. (See www.ithenticate.com, www.crossref.org, and www.grammarly.com.)

Other QC checklists and guidelines covered in this chapter include

- ICMJE for all manuscripts (Table 4.9)
- Good Publication Practice (GPP3) for all manuscripts (Tables 4.10–4.12)
- Medical Publishing Insights and Practices (MPIP) guidelines for all manuscripts (Table 4.13)
- Cochrane Collaboration guidelines for all manuscripts (Table 4.14)
- Preferred Reporting Items for Systematic Reviews and Meta-Analyses (PRISMA; Table 4.15)
- PRISMA protocols (PRISMA-P; Tables 4.16 and 4.17)
- Sampling strategy, Type of studies, Approaches, Range of years, Limits, Inclusions (Exclusions), Terms used, Electronic sources (STARLITE) for review articles (Table 4.18)
- Meta-analysis of Observational Studies in Epidemiology (MOOSE; Table 4.19)
- Improving the Quality of Reports of Meta-Analyses of Randomised Controlled Trials (QUOROM; Table 4.20)
- CONSORT (Tables 4.21–4.25)
- Strengthening the Reporting of Observational Studies in Epidemiology (STROBE; Tables 4.26–4.29)
- Guidelines for Treatment Reporting of Outbreak Reports and Intervention Studies of Nosocomial Infection (ORION; Table 4.30)

- Further STROBE QC checklists (Tables 4.31 and 4.32)
- Strengthening the Reporting of Genetic Risk Prediction Studies (GRIPS; Table 4.33)
- Consolidated Health Economic Evaluation Reporting Standards (CHEERS; Table 4.34)
- Transparent Reporting of Evaluations with Nonrandomized Designs (TREND; Table 4.35)
- Good Research Practices for Comparative Effectiveness Studies from the International Society for Pharmacoeconomics and Outcomes Research (ISPOR; Table 4.36)
- Standards for Quality Improvement Reporting Excellence (SQUIRE; Table 4.37)
- Pragmatic Explanatory Continuum Indicator Summary (PRECIS; Table 4.38)
- Rethinking Pragmatic Randomized Controlled Trials (cohort multiple randomized controlled trials; Table 4.39)
- CONSORT guidelines for pragmatic trials (Table 4.40)
- Consolidated Criteria for Reporting Qualitative Research (COREQ; Table 4.41)
- Guidelines for submitting adverse-event (AE) reports for publication (Table 4.42)
- Standard Protocol Items: Recommendations for Interventional Trials (SPIRIT; Table 4.43)
- Relevance, Appropriateness, Transparency, Soundness (RATS; Table 4.44)
- Standards for Reporting Studies of Diagnostic Accuracy (STARD; Table 4.45)
- Transparent Reporting of a Multivariable Prediction Model for Individual Prognosis or Diagnosis (TRIPOD; Table 4.46)
- Guidelines for Reporting Reliability and Agreement Studies (GRRAS; Table 4.47)
- Case Report (CARE) guidelines for clinical case reporting (Table 4.48)
- Further guidance to prepare reports of case series (Table 4.49)
- Animal Research: Reporting of *In Vivo* Experiments (ARRIVE) guidelines (Table 4.50)
- Publication planning insights (Table 4.51)
- Example of a publication/journal options grid (Table 4.52)
- COPE: how to spot authorship problems (Table 4.53)
- Differences between nonpromotional and promotional media (Table 4.54)

An emerging paradigm in medical journal publications links manuscript quality with proactive transparent disclosure (PROTRANSDISC, my term). Consistent with §801 of the Food and Drug Administration Amendments Act (FDAAA) of 2007, RCTs are registered at www.clinicaltrials.gov. Registering a study, then including its NCT ID number in your report, enables a reader (or journal editor or referee) to compare the methods and findings reported in the manuscript to those prospectively set forth. Other examples of Internet portals to enhance proactive disclosures of study methods and outcome measures include:

- World Health Organization's International Clinical Trials Registry (ICTR) Platform, which is available at: http://apps.who.int/trialsearch.
- University of York's (UK) International Prospective Register of Systematic Reviews (PROSPERO), which is available at: http://www.crd.york.ac.uk/PROSPERO.
- US NIH List of Registries, which is available at: http://www.nih.gov/health-information/nih-clinical-research-trials-you/list-registries.
- US Agency for Healthcare Research and Quality (AHRQ)'s Registry of Patient Registries (RoPR), which is available at https://patientregistry.ahrq.gov.

At this writing, prospective public registration of observational (noninterventional) studies is not typically required, but momentum is building to transform this disclosure landscape.[1] Recent work by a group from the European League Against Rheumatism (EULAR) enabled evaluation and comparison of European registrants initiating treatment with biological disease-modifying antirheumatic drugs (bio-DMARDs).[2] On the same continent, the EMA (European Medicines Agency) also enables registration of observational studies. To follow developments concerning these issues in particular, and remain up to date with consensus guidance for manuscript preparation in general, "stay tuned" to the Enhancing the Quality and Transparency of Health Research (EQUATOR) website: www.equator-network.org.

And now, without further ado, I give you everything you ever wanted to know about how to prepare almost every kind of biomedical study report but may have "lacked 95% confidence" to ask!

PART 1: QC CHECKLISTS AND OTHER TABLES TO OPTIMIZE MANUSCRIPT QUALITY

Table 4.1 QC checklist for all manuscripts. Part 1: By manuscript section (Title and abstract)

Item	Requirements	Comments 1	Comments 2
Title page (pg 1).	Title.	**Do:** • Name treatments or other interventions. • Name disease, population, and/or setting. • Briefly specify study design (e.g., "Randomized Controlled Trial").	**Do not:** • Include complete sentences. • "Give away" the findings. • Exceed 150 characters, including spaces (for most journals).
	Authors, affiliations.[3]	• Be consistent across author affiliations. Usually provide academic or hospital affiliation but not both. • Before or soon after kickoff meeting, distribute **Form 2** in this chapter to obtain author contact information needed for journal submission and **Form 3** to proactively notify authors of their roles.	**Check journal style (Author Guidelines [AGs] and online content) concerning whether to:** • Include degrees or "honorifics" (e.g., FACP), or not? • Use number or letter footnotes for affiliations?
	Funding statement.	**Provide name and contact information of sponsor** (i.e., funding source; e.g., life sciences company [LSC], government agency, patient advocacy society, philanthropic organization) for study and/or communication.	**Include role of funding source in:** • Study design. • Data acquisition and analysis. • Preparation of the manuscript. • Decision to report the findings.
	Running title.	**Do:** • Include running title as manuscript header.	**Do not:** • Include author (or sponsor) name in header (doing so complicates journal blinding for peer review). • Exceed 50 characters, including spaces (for most journals).
	Corresponding author contact information.	• Provide postal address, telephone (with country code if necessary), fax, e-mail of university or hospital (by journal/author preference). Distribute **Form 2** to obtain information.	When corresponding author information is not provided, research using Internet—Google Scholar will often have information in online published articles. (Avoid author queries.)

(Continued)

Table 4.1 (Continued) QC checklists for all manuscripts. Part 1: By manuscript section (Title and abstract)

Item	Requirements	Comments 1	Comments 2
Abstract. (pg 2)	Typically write a structured abstract (consult journal AGs for type of paper). See Box 2.1 in Chapter 2.	• **Introduction**: Study background, rationale, aims and any hypotheses (**unique/ incremental value of study**). • **Methods and Main Outcomes**: Study design, treatment (allocation), population/setting, outcome measures, and any statistical methods for results reported. • **Results**: One result for each outcome measure mentioned above. • **Conclusions**: Key "takeaway" messages (what your findings add to the literature).	**Abstract Conclusions do**: • Include 1 sentence on study limitations. **Abstract Conclusions don't**: • Copy Conclusions from body of essay.
	Key words (n = 3 – 6).	**If possible, include**: • Name of disease. • Type of therapy (but not the name of a particular drug). • Type of study/publication. • The term human, animal, in vitro, in vivo, or ex vivo (whichever is most accurate and descriptive).	• Use MeSH terms. • If possible, use the key words as a broad guide to organize your manuscript. Try not to drift too far from the general "script" provided by these terms.
Pg 3 (between abstract and text).	Define and aggregate all abbreviations.	If journal AGs allow, include a list of abbreviations and definitions. Consult journal AGs regarding abbreviations that do not need to be defined (e.g., DNA, RNA).	Minimize overall number of abbreviations. **Two rules of thumb**: • ≤0.5% × words of text (i.e., 5–10 abbreviations per 2,000 words). • Abbreviate multiple words but not a single word (e.g., coronary heart disease [CHD] but not triglyceride [TG]).
	Provide NCT # for study registered at www.clinical trials.gov.	Specify previous presentation of data (congress name, date, place, and any poster or abstract number).	Other study registries: International Clinical Trials Registry (WHO; ex-US RCTs); PROSPERO registry (systematic reviews).
	Provide manuscript statistics vs. journal maximums.	For example, "249/250 words Abstract; 2,498/2,500 words text; 23/25 references; 3/5 tables; 4/5 figures."	Obtain maximum values from journal AGs.

Abbreviations: FACP, Fellow of the American College of Physicians; MeSH, medical subject headings (search terms in MEDLINE/PubMed); WHO, World Health Organization.

Table 4.2 QC checklist for all manuscripts. Part 1: By manuscript section (Introduction)

Item	Requirements	Comments 1	Comments 2
Introduction.	Build to the rationale for the study, research questions, and objectives.	KEY QUESTIONS TO ASK YOURSELF AND OTHER AUTHORS (AT KICKOFF MEETING) WHAT IS THE SINGULAR, UNIQUE, OR INCREMENTAL VALUE OF OUR STUDY? WHAT EDUCATIONAL NEEDS OF READERS ARE UNIQUELY SERVED BY ITS REPORT? WHICH JOURNAL'S READERS WOULD BE MOST INTERESTED?	• Do not exceed 500 words.
	Gutkin 4 × 4 Structure (see Table 2.5 in Chapter 2): 1. Disease state overview and dimensions. 2. Pathophysiology/natural history. 3. Consensus guidelines, history of RCTs and further background to study rationale and unique/incremental value of study. 4. Study objectives.	• What is the clinical problem, and how does your study address it? • Why is the study/paper necessary? What knowledge gap(s) does it address? • Frame scientific background, study rationale, objectives, and/or hypotheses (null hypotheses [NHs] should be formally stated in form of "H_0: The NH was that…" in Introduction or Methods section). • Review online sources to determine if study was mandated by FDA or other regulatory body and, if so, how this mandate affected study objectives/methods.	• Maintain external fidelity: fact check to ensure faithfulness of text to referenced findings ("reference every number and number every reference"). • Be careful when citing epidemiologic statistics; they are often discrepant because of different definitions across studies. • Prefer to cite ranks (e.g., a disease is 3rd-ranked cause of disability or of total health costs and incidences/prevalences (%, cases/100,000) over millions of people with disease/billions of dollars in costs (forgettable). • Try to include "neat" data relations, e.g., "for every 1-mmol/L decrease in LDL-C, there is a 20% decline in 5-year CHD events." • Avoid patient-advocacy data such as "every 15 seconds, an American has a heart attack."

(Continued)

Table 4.2 (Continued) QC checklist for all manuscripts. Part 1: By manuscript section (Introduction)

Item	Requirements	Comments 1	Comments 2
	Objectives should be specific, meaningful, and actionable.	**Incentivize the reader.** Do not "give away" the findings in the Introduction. (It is remarkable how often one sees this guideline violated in the published literature. When authors do this, one might ask oneself, "Why read on?")	• Begin research with a recent review in a high-quality journal (*Ann Intern Med, BMJ, Lancet, JAMA, NEJM, Cochrane Database of Systematic Reviews http://www.cochranelibrary.com/cochrane-database-of-systematic-reviews/index.html*. • Obtain and cite consensus guidelines. • Cite references from past 5 years (most papers). • Remember that "aim" is used correctly as a noun ("the aim of this study") and not a verb ("we aimed to …"). • The aim of any study is to "evaluate" or "assess," not to "demonstrate." (The latter is "argumentative.")

Abbreviations: BMJ, *British Medical Journal*; CHD, coronary heart disease; FDA, Food and Drug Administration; JAMA, *Journal of the American Medical Association*; LDL-C, low-density lipoprotein cholesterol; NEJM, *New England Journal of Medicine*.

Table 4.3 QC checklist for all manuscripts. Part 1: By manuscript sections (Methods)

Item	Requirements	Comments 1	Comments 2

Methods.	Enable another researcher to repeat the study. Also provides "road map" to readers and peer reviewers.
	
	Components of most human studies
	Gutkin 4 × 4 Structure (see Chapter 2):
	1. Study design, setting, and participants.
	2. Interventions/ Comparisons.
	3. Assessments/ Outcome measures (endpoints).
	4. Statistical methods.
		"Rule of Chekhov's Gun" (Chapter 2) Part 1: Do not include any endpoint/test in the Methods without reporting corresponding data in Results.
		• Study design
		  • Controlled, randomized, blinded, open-label, preclinical, pharmacokinetic, phase 1–3, observational (including type), meta-analysis, systematic review, diagnostics/predictive model, health-economics and outcomes research (HEOR; e.g., cost-effectiveness or cost-utility analysis).
		• Eligibility (inclusion, exclusion) criteria.
		• Interventions: treatments (rules to titrate) and comparisons.
		• Assessments/outcome measures:
		  • Efficacy ("hard clinical" vs. physiologic/surrogate).
		  • Specify "endpoint hierarchy" (e.g., primary, secondary).
		  • Patient-reported outcomes (PROs; e.g., SF-36, disease-specific indices).
		  • Safety (e.g., 12-lead ECG, vital signs, laboratory results).
		  • Tolerability (define AEs, TEAEs, SAEs, and specify dictionary, e.g., MedDRA Version 17.1 [www. meddra.org] and preferred term [PT] or system organ class [SOC]).
			• The Methods section is the **"Rosetta Stone of Clarity"** for the entire manuscript" (Chapter 1).
			
			• Include a figure (schema) depicting study design and timeline, including efficacy and safety assessment dates (by week/month/visit) if allowed by journal and otherwise appropriate (consult journal AGs and online content).
			• Detail assessments/ instruments so that reader can understand Results
			  • Range of scores.
			  • Does an increase or decrease signify improved (or worsened) status?
			  • MCIDs (see Appendix 1 of the "Gutkin Manual").
			  • Normative data.
			  • Test properties/ predictive ability of indices (sensitivity, specificity, NPV, PPV).

(Continued)

Table 4.3 (Continued) QC checklist for all manuscripts. Part 1: By manuscript sections (Methods)

Item	Requirements	Comments 1	Comments 2
	RCTs.	• Ethics: Recruitment/ Enrollment/Ethics (DOH/ ICD/IRB). • Treatments (including rules for titration, e.g., to goal). • Randomization/Allocation concealment. • Blinding implementation (who was blinded/how?). • Protocol amendments/ Violations; DSMB, interim analyses, stopping rules.	**Types of randomization**[3]: • Simple. • Block. • Stratified. • Covariate adaptive.

	Observational studies.	Cohort study
		 • Type of database (e.g., administrative-claims, EMR).
		 • Method of case ascertainment: e.g., ICD-10 (Read codes [UK]).
		 • Precisely define cohorts, subcohorts, index date, look-back, and follow-up intervals. Focus on the index date, which often serves as a sort of "fulcrum" for the entire study timeline and data analysis.
		 • **Registry study** (representativeness ecological validity) of clinical setting.
		 • **Survey** (sampling method, interviewer training/ blinding, any translation or back-translation of survey questionnaire with validation).
			Ethics: If appropriate, specify that data were anonymized, add any HIPAA or other patient-privacy protections, and whether study conduct was consistent with guidance from the International Society for Pharmacoepidemiology Guidelines for Good Pharmacoepidemiology Practices.
			
			 Take steps to minimize bias related to
			 • Convenience samples.
			 • Surveys (e.g., recall bias, selection bias).
			 • **Registries**
			   • Intracorrelated longitudinal data.
			   • Missing data.
			   • Other biases in treatment (e.g., channeling).
			   • Test-retest reliability.[4]

Abbreviations: AE, adverse event; ANCOVA, analysis of covariance; DOH, Declaration of Helsinki; DSMB, data safety monitoring board; ECG, electrocardiogram (electrocardiography); EMR, electronic medical records; HIPAA, Health Insurance Portability and Accountability Act; ICD, Informed-consent document or International Classification of Disease; IRB, institutional review board; MCID, minimum clinically important difference; MedDRA, Medical Dictionary of Regulatory Activities; NPV, negative predictive value; PPV, positive predictive value; RCT, randomized controlled trial; SAE, serious adverse event; SF-36, Rand 36-Item Short Form Health Survey, generic quality-of-life instrument; TEAE, treatment-emergent adverse event.

Table 4.4 QC checklist for all manuscripts. Part 1: By manuscript section (Methods: Statistical)

Item	Requirements	Comments 1	Comments 2
Statistical methods.	Components of all studies.	• Measures of central tendency and dispersion. • Statistical analyses of categorical (e.g., χ^2 test) versus continuous (e.g., Student's t-test) data. • Outcome measures and comparisons. • NHs (for inferential statistics). • Paired vs. unpaired data analyses. • Parametric vs. nonparametric testing. • Decision criteria: *a priori* α and two- versus one-tailed testing (favor two-tailed) for p values and 95% CIs. • ANCOVA and other model structures. • Handling outliers, missing data, other issues. • Software (e.g., SAS, SPSS) and version #.	• State test to adjust for multiple comparisons (e.g., Bonferroni, Breslow–Day). • Prespecify any patient segments for subgroup analyses (try to avoid excessive *post hoc* analyses). • If unsure (from literature review) if data will be symmetrical (i.e., requiring parametric tests) or asymmetrical (i.e., requiring nonparametric tests), consider using the Shapiro–Wilk test of normality or the Microsoft Excel test of skew. (See Chapter 3.)
	RCTs.	• Sample size calculations: need to know: α (significance level), β (and power = $1 - \beta$), effect size, and variance. • Analysis sets (e.g., ITT, safety, per-protocol). • Specific imputation methods for missing data (e.g., LOCF).[5] • Protocol violations. • Survival analysis (e.g., Kaplan–Meier).	**Special issues:** • Interim analyses. • Sample size calculations should be based on a published study or other database involving similar interventions and tests but should not be based on the population being studied.

(Continued)

Table 4.4 QC checklist for all manuscripts. Part 1: By manuscript section (Methods: Statistical)

Item	Requirements	Comments 1	Comments 2
	Observational studies.	Approaches to control or account for bias/ Confounding: • ANCOVA modeling/ covariate adjustment. • CMH Test (see Chapter 3). • Matching/propensity score matching. • Regression analyses. • Sensitivity analyses. • Stratification.	Approaches to control for missing and intracorrelated longitudinal data (e.g., registry): • Linear mixed models. • Generalized linear mixed models. • Generalized estimating equations[6]; specify correlational-matrix structures (autoregressive, exchangeable, independent, M-dependent, unstructured).
	Meta-analyses/ Systematic reviews.	Tests of publication bias: • Funnel plot. • Begg and Egger Test. • Meta-regression analysis. • Selection modeling. • Trim and fill.	Tests of heterogeneity: • I^2. • Galbraith plots. • Meta-regression analysis. • Random-effects model.
	HEOR.	• Base-case assumptions. • Sensitivity analyses versus these assumptions.	Challenge assumptions/Use sensitivity analyses: • Model structure, inputs, outputs. • Discount rate (e.g., 3% vs. 6%).
	Diagnostics/Predictive models.	• Bland–Altman plots. • Negative and positive predictive values. • Sensitivity and specificity. • Hosmer–Lemeshow Test (goodness of fit of regression models).	AUC for receiver operating characteristics (ROC) plot (i.e., C-statistic) should exceed 0.70.

Abbreviations: ANCOVA, analysis of covariance; AUC, area under curve; CI, confidence interval; CMH, Cochran–Mantel–Haenszel; DSMB, data monitoring safety board; HEOR, health economics and outcomes research; ITT, intent-to-treat; LOCF, last observation carried forward; NH, null hypothesis; SAS, Statistical Analysis System; SPSS, Statistical Package for the Social Sciences.

Table 4.5 QC checklist for all manuscripts. Part 1: By manuscript section (Results)

Item	Requirements	Comments 1	Comments 2
Results.	Gutkin 4 × 4 Structure (see Table 2.5 in Chapter 2). 1. Patient (data) disposition. 2. Baseline characteristics. 3. Efficacy/PRO outcomes. 4. Safety/tolerability outcomes.	• Report results approximately in sequence specified in Methods. • Present a result (effect size + precision) for each primary, secondary, sensitivity, or subgroup analysis in Methods. • Report both (+) and (−) findings. • Avoid "unanchored," (e.g., by MCID) qualitative descriptors (e.g., "good"), especially superlatives (e.g., "robust").	**"Rule of Chekhov's Gun" (Chapter 2). Part 2:** • Do not introduce any Result (especially with statistical tests) that was not "motivated" (described) in the Methods. • Designate any data derived from *post hoc* ("hypothesis-generating") analyses. • Do not overstate/speculate (e.g., "highly significant" or "borderline-significant").
	Most studies.	**Consider including:** • CONSORT flow diagram for patient disposition or other data flow (e.g., number [%] assessed, randomized, dropped out [with reasons], and completed): number of subjects in each data set (RCTs; e.g., ITT, safety). • Table of baseline characteristics (model outputs in HEOR), including sociodemographic and clinical factors. • Table of main efficacy or other data (one result for each endpoint specified in Methods), including clinical, PROs, forest plots (meta-analyses), model outputs (HEOR). • Table of TEAE frequencies in active versus control groups (total and by PT or SOC), exceeding prespecified %, e.g., 3% or 5%. • Safety (usually in text; SAEs = safety, not tolerability). • If off-label use of a medication is stated or implied, immediately flag for discussion with the corresponding author before finalizing or submitting the manuscript to the journal. Avoid "prelabel" issues by appropriately identifying any investigational agents or indications.	• If a graphic does not include specific numerical data (e.g., mean, SD, 95% confidence interval), consider including these numbers in narrative text or a separate table. • Ensure that results cited in Results narrative text agree with those in tables/figures and Abstract (**Chapter 2: "Internal Fidelity"**). • Ensure that results agree with raw or analyzed data, including tables, figures, and patient listings (e.g., CRFs, CIOMS) from CSR/other source documents (**Chapter 2: "External Fidelity"**). • Footnote inconsistencies (e.g., "percentages do not sum to 100 because of rounding," "percentages of subjects with adverse events sum to >100 because each subject could have more than one adverse event").

Abbreviations: CIOMS, Council for International Organizations of Medical Sciences; CRF, case report form; CSR, clinical study report; HEOR, health economics and outcomes research; ITT, intent-to-treat; MCID, minimum clinically important difference; PRO, patient-reported outcome; PT, preferred term; RCT, randomized controlled trial; SAE, serious adverse event; SD, standard deviation; SOC, system organ class.

Table 4.6 QC checklist for all manuscripts. Part 1: By manuscript section (Discussion)

Item	Requirements	Comments 1	Comments 2
Discussion.	**Gutkin 4 × 4 Structure (see Table 2.5 in Chapter 2):** 1. Restate key findings (e.g., minimum clinically important difference; $p < 0.05$ and $p > 0.05$); expected versus unexpected, and potential biological mechanisms. 2. Compare versus published literature. 3. Consider potential study limitations (+ strengths) and clinical implications. 4. Conclusions (+ future research). **Limitations subsection twofold objective:** 1. Consider reasonable (nonspeculative) sources of imprecision, bias, and confounding. 2. Explain how study dealt with these issues and why they most likely do not alter the prevailing conclusions. **Clinical implications subsection:** • After accounting for potential limitations, what unique or incremental "takeaway" can be derived from the findings as compared to the published literature and prevailing theory?	• Which NHs/endpoints were/were not rejected? Why or why not? • Generalizability: how do findings in the target population apply to the general population of readers' patients? • How do findings relate to previously reported data (expected/unexpected)? • Provide context for safety/tolerability (and efficacy) data. • Are there other plausible explanations of the findings? **Potential statistical issues and how they were addressed (and/or any effects on findings: toward or away from null):** • Type 1 or 2 error. • Multiple comparisons. • Intracorrelated longitudinal data from each patient/subject. • Nonrandom patient attrition. • Test-retest reliability. **Forms of bias (mainly in observational studies):** • Treatment by indication. • Selection. • Recall (survey). • Publication (systematic reviews). • Medical surveillance (ascertainment).	• **Internal validation:** review study objectives (Introduction) and targeted enrollment/randomization protocol (Methods). Were they met? Why or why not? See **Chapter 3: Biostatistics** for major limitations (and strengths) of different study designs and a comprehensive listing of study biases. **Summary: RCT versus observational study:** • **RCT:** High quality of individual data, homogeneous population, rigid treatment protocols, and limited follow-up intervals (high internal validity and quality of patient data designed to demonstrate efficacy of treatment for regulatory and other purposes). **versus** • **Observational study:** More relaxed patient entry criteria (heterogeneous populations), dynamic treatments, and longer follow-up intervals (high ecological validity designed to simulate or otherwise represent naturalistic practice milieus of most readers). *(Continued)*

Table 4.6 (Continued) QC checklist for all manuscripts. Part 1: By manuscript section (Discussion)

Item	Requirements	Comments 1	Comments 2

Discussion.	• Explain why findings are statistically sound and biologically plausible.
	• Explain how findings advance the field (e.g., disease diagnosis and management).
		• **Other issues:**
		  • Confounding due to unmeasured variables.
		  • Effect modification.
		  • Interaction.
		  • Heterogeneity (meta-analysis).
		• Causation (presence/direction) claimed or implied based on associational data.
		• Longitudinal perspective implied in report of cross-sectional study (e.g., survey).
			• **RCT:** Often not powered or of sufficient duration to detect intertreatment differences in safety/tolerability (especially infrequent AEs or signs [e.g., ECG QTc prolongation]).
			   versus
			• **Observational study:** May include higher number of patients followed up for a longer duration and hence have greater power to discern safety signals (pharmacovigilance).

Avoid Discussion pitfalls.		• What are the unique or incremental findings of the study (present in an objective, fair-balanced way)? • What does the study and its report add to the field (basic or applied science) and the literature? • What research is needed to advance the field?	
Conclusions.			• Include treatment or other recommendations based on findings. • Consider medical benefits and risks. • Do not exceed 100 words.

Abbreviations: AE, adverse event; ECG, electrocardiography; NH, null hypothesis; RCT, randomized controlled trial.

Table 4.7 QC checklist for all manuscripts. Part 1: By manuscript section (Remaining sections: Acknowledgment, References, Tables, Figures)

Item	Requirements	Comments 1	Comments 2
Disclosures.	**Twofold Disclosure Objective:** 1. **Author intellectual contributions** (including by nonauthors such as medical writers, statisticians, laboratory personnel, other technical personnel [e.g., CRAs], nonjournal peer reviewers). 2. **Author financial disclosures and potential conflicts of interests.**	**Use Form 3. Author Intellectual Contributions (below*) to:** • Confirm that each author qualifies for authorship by ICMJE criteria. • Specify each author's role (using initials) in meeting or participating in ICMJE criteria/categories. **Use Form 4. Author financial disclosures (below*) to disclose:** • Financial relationships with study sponsor and manufacturers/marketers of competing therapies or technologies. • Different forms of financial support, including serving as an investigator, receiving personal monies (e.g., speaker/faculty/ honoraria), holding intellectual property (e.g., patented inventions), and providing expert testimony. • Financial support in the broad (not narrow) therapeutic category, such as any antidiabetic therapy in a study of an injectable GLP-1 receptor agonist and not just other GLP-1 receptor agonists. • That there are no relevant financial interests to report (if this is the case).	• I have often found in my practice that the most fundamental financial relationship— between an investigator and study sponsor—is evidently "assumed" and hence unstated. Consider beginning by asking the investigator "in addition to any relationship with the sponsor [please detail these], what other industry, academic, or other forms of financial support do you disclose?" • If appropriate, it is important for authors to specify "no financial interests to disclose" and/or "I did not receive compensation from the study sponsor to participate as an investigator and/or author." • Medical writers and other personnel who made acknowledged contributions to the manuscript may consider disclosing their financial relationships with competing manufacturers/ marketers or other financial supporters in addition to the study sponsor.

(Continued)

Table 4.7 (Continued) QC checklists for all manuscripts. Part 1: By manuscript section (Remaining sections: Acknowledgment, References, Tables, Figures)

Item	Requirements	Comments 1	Comments 2
References.	• Accurate, in ascending numerical sequence, and not duplicated.	**External fidelity:** • Highlight references and other backup sources (e.g., USPI/SPC) for information cited. • Cite specific, consequential data; do not "overcite" (Please avoid, e.g., "the heart pumps blood."[1,2,4–26]) • Ensure consistency between your text and both the letter and overall spirit of the published reference (its denotation and connotation). • Avoid secondary referencing. If you reference a paper as identified in a review, obtain the original paper and check for veracity versus statement in review. • Ensure that any URL link to online reference is active.	**Internal fidelity:** • Duplication may occur when referencing software includes both pre- and post-publication citations. • 1-page citation may signal an abstract, requiring an abstract number (but try to avoid citing abstracts and seek a reported paper if available). • Page ranges with letters (especially "S") may signal a journal supplement, which needs to be included with issue data. • Exclude certain information from Reference list (Data on file, personal communication).
Tables/figures.	• Call out each table and figure in text. For non-English native speakers and when reporting highly complex data, consider introducing each sentence or paragraph with "Table 1/Figure 1 shows…"	• Treat each table and figure as "its own universe." Some readers apprehend most information from Abstract and Discussion text, and others from Abstract and tables/figures. • Based on Table title or Figure legend, define abbreviations, and statistical tests used to generate p values; ensure that reader can understand the table/figure with minimal reference to text.	• Logically present results, e.g., by patient group, endpoint hierarchy, continuous (mean ± SD) versus categorical (no. [%]) data. • Define each abbreviation (other than common ones such as DNA, RNA).

(Continued)

Table 4.7 (Continued) QC checklists for all manuscripts. Part 1: By manuscript section (Remaining sections: Acknowledgment, References, Tables, Figures)

Item	Requirements	Comments 1	Comments 2
Tables/figures.		• One acceptable approach is to define all abbreviations in one table/figure legend and refer reader to it in subsequent ones. • Include technical data, e.g., type of stain (e.g., H&E) and magnification. • Ensure that axes and labels are clear and complete (including defining any axis label abbreviations in legend). • Provide key/legend for, e.g., symbols and arrows. • In forest plot, any odds ratio whose 95% CI overlaps 1.0 is not significant at $p < 0.05$. • Any t-test comparison whose 95% CI overlaps 0 is not significant at $p < 0.05$.	• Footnote p values (with statistical test used to generate each) and account for missing data/items that do not "add up" (e.g., n values of subgroups do not sum to total N; percentages do not sum to 100). • Avoid temptation to "magnify" a modest difference (e.g., by shrinking y-axis of bar graph).

Abbreviations: CI, confidence interval; CRA, clinical research associate; GLP–1, glucagon-like peptide–1; H&E, hematoxylin and eosin; ICMJE, International Committee of Medical Journal Editors; SD, standard deviation; SPC, Summary of Product Characteristics; USPI, US full prescribing information (package insert).

*A fillable .pdf and other original forms for ethical disclosure are available at www.icmje.org.

Table 4.8 QC checklist for all manuscripts. Part 2: Writing style (refer to Chapters 1 and 2)

Item	Requirements	Comments 1	Comments 2
Writing style.	**External fidelity:** • Fidelity to data sources without using jargon or dehumanizing figures of speech. • *"Ma non troppo"*: "too much external fidelity" = plagiarism! See Figure 4.2 and use proprietary software to prevent it. • Accurate spelling, capitalization, and abbreviations of terminology in published references. **Internal fidelity:** • Stable essay structure (see Table 2.5 in Chapter 2; thesis statement at top; topic sentence at head of each paragraph derived from major line in outline [capital lettered items]). • Sound logic: Idea flow and connections between paragraphs/sections; consistent use of headings and subheadings; repetition and linkage by key words. • Correct and consistent syntax, semantics, and punctuation. Avoid the following: • Subject-predicate disagreement (see Chapter 2: "Plural Effusions") is one of the most prevalent defects in medical writing. • Run-on-sentence (ROS): Excess "ing" verbs/ subordinate clauses often set these in motion; two witches make a potion, but two "whiches" often make a ROS! • Sentence fragments, dangling modifiers, poor parallel structure.	• Write in a direct but not simple way, to convey data concisely and clearly. • Prose should be "learned" and well informed but not pompous or pedantic. • "Well-tempered" prose: 20–25 words per sentence with data (means, SDs, p values, 95% CIs) in parentheses. Organize logically and avoid verbal speed bumps/ interruptions and "respectively" constructions. • In most cases, "lead with the news" (outcomes) and follow with the background (e.g., study design). • Data in Introduction, Methods, and Conclusions in Abstract are consistent with those in text. • Data in Abstract match those in the Results narrative, which in turn match those in tables and figures (but do not excessively repeat them). • "Do the math" to ensure that data and conclusions are logically presented, statistically defensible, and biologically plausible (+ minutely accurate).	• For example, "The frequency of ALT elevation >3XULN was significantly higher in the active-treatment (11%) compared to the placebo (4%) arm (p = 0.004 by χ² test)." **Not:** • "The frequency of ALT elevation >3XULN was significantly (p = 0.004 by χ² test) higher in the active-treatment compared to the placebo arm, 11% vs. 4%, respectively." [A tough "read"] • Define abbreviations at first mention and use them consistently. • Define SI or English units of measure (and/or provide conversion factors). • Use abbreviations and units of measure consistently (e.g., do not switch between English and SI units) within the essay. • Use consistent spelling (e.g., all US or all UK) within the essay. • Use consistent tense (usually past, but Discussion may include present or future tense).

(Continued)

Table 4.8 (Continued) QC checklist for all manuscripts. Part 2: Writing style (refer to Chapters 1 and 2)

Item	Requirements	Comments 1	Comments 2
Writing style.		**Consistent:** • **Spacing** • After period (most journals now favor a single space). Use nonbreaking hyphen (insert special character) for, e.g., "Grade 1," "$p < 0.05$." • On either side of operator (typically 1 full space before and after operator). • **Hyphens and 1/N dashes** • A "well-informed essay" (conjoined adjective) or "the essay is well informed" (adverb). • Negative/minus signs are 1/N dashes (–), not hyphens (-). • 1/N dashes (–) in page/other ranges. • **Symbols** • Consistently use Greek symbols (in most journals).	**Consistent:** **Font:** Italics for only selected non-English phrases, book/journal names, and gene names (consult journal AGs); bold and bold italics for headings).
Other.	• Read the targeted journal's Aims/Scope, AGs, and online content, especially articles like your own, in order to discern readers' educational needs, including level of language, terminology, and sophistication. • For example, readers of a specialty journal may not need to be reminded of basic epidemiologic statistics, pathophysiology/natural history, and consensus management guidelines of a disease (e.g., in a study report on a diabetes therapy for readers of *Diabetes Care*). Proceed directly to the clinical problem and your study's (and its report's) role in addressing it.	• Avoid long parentheses or 1/M dashes (—) with words but not data. • Subordinate these as separate, second sentences. • Use headings to minimize redundant/wordy text (e.g., a heading of "RCTs" in a review organizes data and prevents repetition of phrases, such as "In one RCT. In another RCT. In a third RCT."	**Don't overdo internal consistency (in prose style):** • Vary sentence structure, terminology, and voice. • Try to mix in some active voice along with conventional passive. • Avoid skeins of "Subject-to-be-predicate dyads" ("HIV is this. HIV is that.")

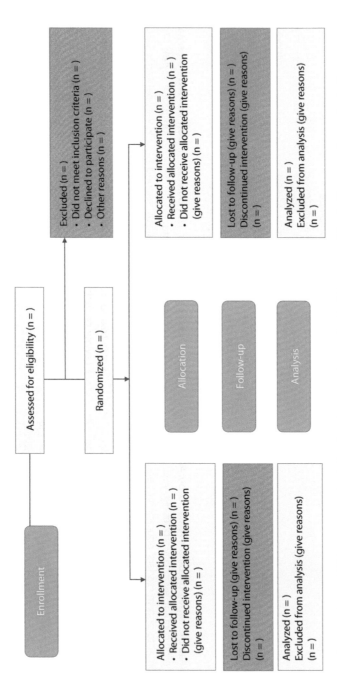

Figure 4.1 Reports of randomized controlled trials: Consolidated Standards of Reporting Trials (CONSORT) patient disposition flow diagram and pivotal analysis populations.[7]

Source: Reproduced with permission from Moher D, Schulz KF, Altman D. The CONSORT statement: revised recommendations for improving the quality of reports of parallel-group randomized trials. JAMA 2001;285:1987–91.

Analysis populations: ITT, intent-to-treat (typical analyses): every patient randomized. Ignores anything that happens after randomization (e.g., protocol deviation, nonadherence, consent withdrawal). PP, per-protocol (efficacy analyses): all patients who completed protocol (without e.g., protocol violation, nonadherence, consent withdrawal). Safety: subset of ITT that includes all patients who were randomized and received at least one dose of study treatment (including placebo or usual care/treatment as usual). Unlike the ITT, the safety population takes into account what happens after randomization.

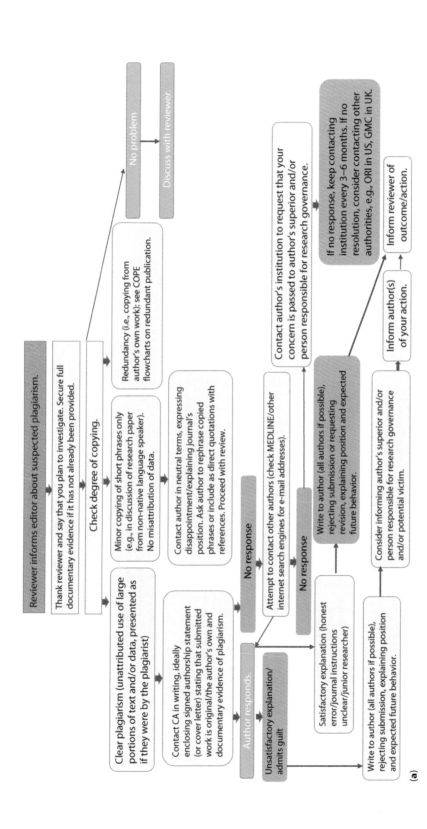

Figure 4.2 What to do if you suspect plagiarism in a submitted manuscript (a) or published article (b).

Source: Reproduced with permission from the Committee on Publication Ethics (COPE). Available at: www.publicationethics.org. Last accessed May 20, 2017.

Abbreviations: CA, corresponding author; GMC, General Medical Council; ORI, Office of Research Integrity.

(Continued)

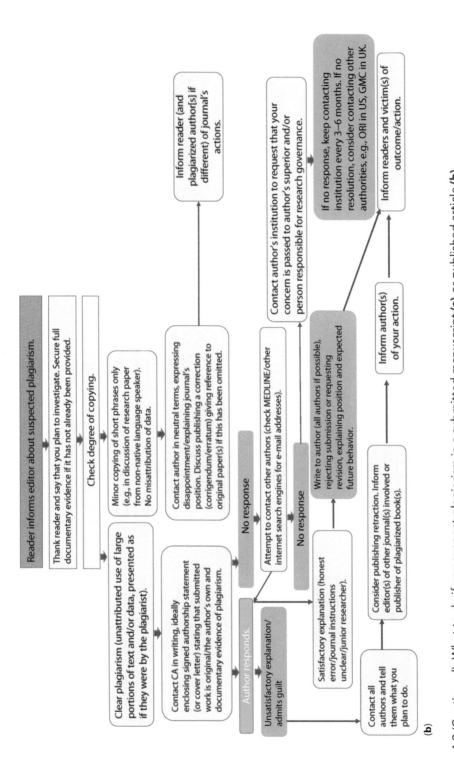

Figure 4.2 (Continued) What to do if you suspect plagiarism in a submitted manuscript **(a)** or published article **(b)**.

Source: Reproduced with permission from the Committee on Publication Ethics (COPE). Available at: www.publicationethics.org. Last accessed May 20, 2017.

Abbreviations: CA, corresponding author; GMC, General Medical Council; ORI, Office of Research Integrity.

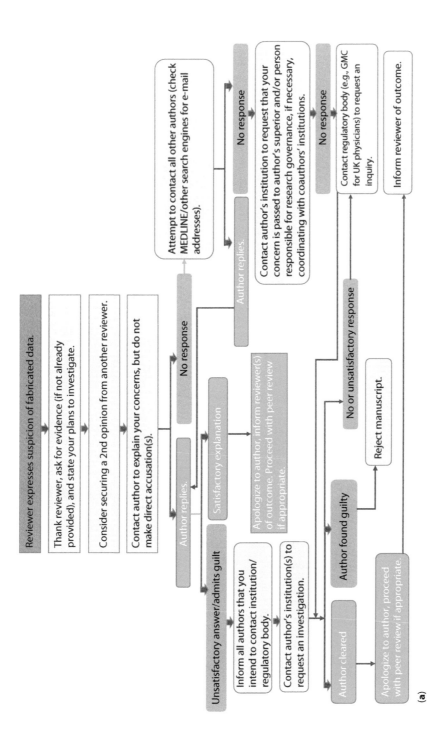

Figure 4.3 What to do if you suspect fabricated data in a submitted manuscript (**a**) or published article (**b**).

Source: Reproduced with permission from the Committee on Publication Ethics (COPE). Available at: www.publicationethics.org. Last accessed May 20, 2017.

Abbreviation: GMC, General Medical Council.

(Continued)

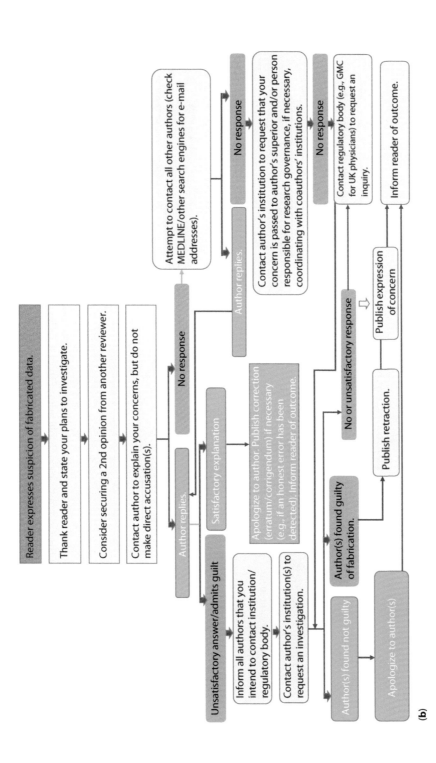

Figure 4.3 (Continued) What to do if you suspect fabricated data in a submitted manuscript (**a**) or published article (**b**).

Source: Reproduced with permission from the Committee on Publication Ethics (COPE). Available at: www.publicationethics.org. Last accessed May 20, 2017.

Abbreviation: GMC, General Medical Council.

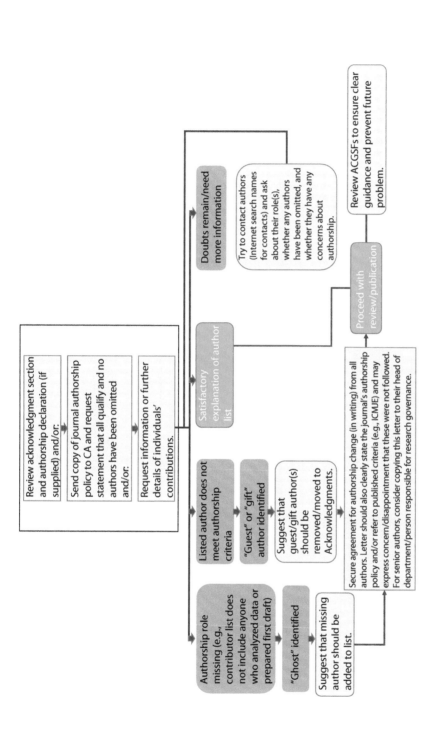

Figure 4.4 What to do if you suspect ghost, guest, or gift authorship. Use Form 3. Author Intellectual Contributions (original available at www.icmje.org) and retain all red-lined (tracked-changed) edited versions (or cover e-mails with comments) from all authors showing where they (1) drafted sections of the manuscript; (2) acquired data or analyses (e.g., by statisticians); (3) made substantive intellectual contributions in the form of line edits, additions, or deletions (Comments of "I approve" throughout [not just to approve the final draft, which is required] are not sufficient to qualify for ethical author status under criteria of ICMJE.); and (4) approved the final manuscript.

Source: Reproduced with permission from the Committee on Publication Ethics (COPE). Reference: Marusic A, Bates T, Anic A et al. How the structure of contribution disclosure statements affects validity of authorship: a randomized study in a general medical journal. *Curr Med Res Opin* 2006;22:1035–44.[27] Available at: www.publicationethics.org. Last accessed October 28, 2017.

Abbreviations: ACGSFs, author/contributor guidelines and submission forms; CA, corresponding author; ICMJE, International Committee of Medical Journal Editors.

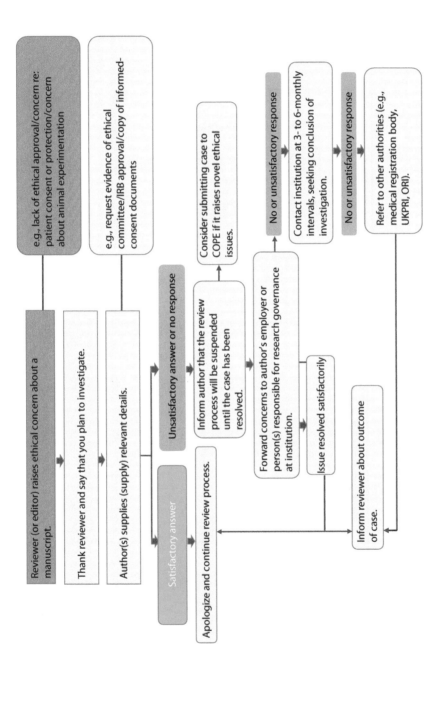

Figure 4.5 What to do if you suspect an ethical problem in a submitted manuscript.

Source: Reproduced with permission from the Committee on Publication Ethics. Available at: www.publicationethics.org. Last accessed October 28, 2017.

Abbreviations: COPE, Committee on Publication Ethics; IRB, institutional review board; ORI, Office of Research Integrity; UKPRI, United Kingdom Panel of Research Integrity.

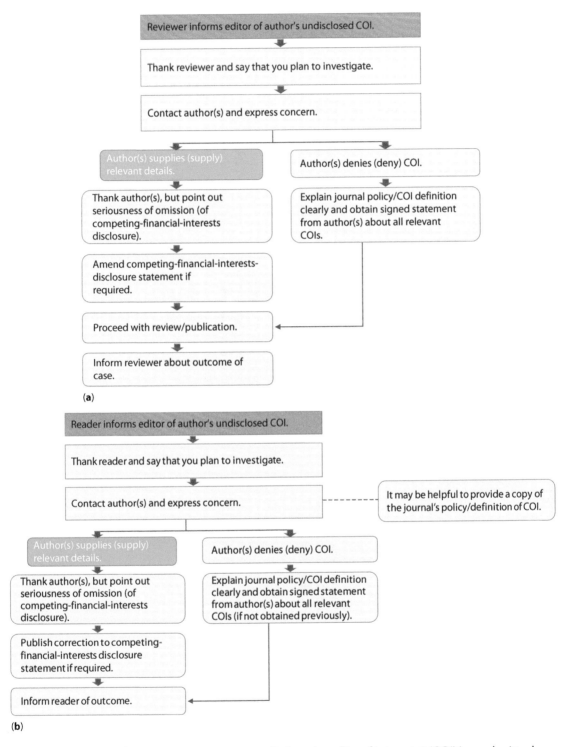

Figure 4.6 What do if a reviewer suspects an undisclosed conflict of interests* (COI) in a submitted manuscript **(a)**. What to do if a reader suspects an undisclosed COI in a published article **(b)**. * "Conflict of interests" (plural) is the accurate term; there is no conflict without more than one interest.
Source: Reproduced with permission from the Committee on Publication Ethics (COPE). Available at: www.publicationethics.org. Last accessed May 20, 2017.

Table 4.9 QC checklist for all manuscripts: Recent history of updates to recommendations for the conduct, reporting, editing, and publication of scholarly work in medical journals (ICMJE)

Section of document	(December 2014–2015) Former text	December 2016 text revision	December 2017 text revision
II. Roles and Responsibilities of Authors, Contributors, Reviewers, Editors, Publishers, and Owners. A. Defining the Role of Authors and Contributors; 1. Why authorship matters.	"Editors are strongly encouraged to develop and implement a contributorship policy, as well as a policy that identifies who is responsible for the integrity of the work as a whole."	"Editors are strongly encouraged to develop and implement a contributorship policy ~~as well as a policy that identifies who is responsible for the integrity of the work as a whole.~~"	
B. Author Responsibilities— Conflicts of Interest; 2. Reporting conflicts of interest; C. Responsibilities in the submission and peer-review process; 1. Authors.	"Authors should abide by all principles of authorship and declaration of conflicts of interest."	"A growing number of entities are advertising themselves as "medical journals" yet do not function as such ("predatory journals"). Authors have a responsibility to evaluate the integrity, history, practices and reputation of the journals to which they submit manuscripts. Further guidance is available at http://www.wame.org/."	"A growing number of entities are advertising themselves as 'scholarly medical journals' yet do not function as such. These journals ('predatory' or 'pseudo-journals') accept and publish almost all submissions and charge article processing (or publication) fees, often informing authors about this after a paper's acceptance for publication. They often claim to perform peer review but do not and may purposefully use names similar to well-established journals. They may state that they are members of ICMJE but are not (see www.icmje.org for current members of the ICMJE) and that they follow the recommendations of organizations such as the ICMJE, COPE, and WAME.

(Continued)

Table 4.9 (Continued) QC checklist for all manuscripts: Recent history of updates to recommendations for the conduct, reporting, editing, and publication of scholarly work in medical journals (ICMJE)

Section of document	(December 2014–2015) Former text	December 2016 text revision	December 2017 text revision
III. Publishing and Editorial Issues Related to Publication in Medical Journals. B. Scientific Misconduct, Expression of Concern, and Retraction; 2. Duplicate and prior publication.	2. Duplicate publication.	2. Duplicate and prior publication.	Researchers must be aware of the existence of such entities and avoid submitting research to them for publication. Authors have a responsibility to evaluate the integrity, history, practices, and reputation of the journals to which they submit manuscripts. Guidance from various organizations is available to help identify the characteristics of reputable peer-reviewed journals (http://www.wame.org/identifying predatory-or-pseudo-journals and http://www.wame.org/about/principlesof-transparency-and-best-practice)."

(Continued)

Table 4.9 (Continued) QC checklist for all manuscripts: Recent history of updates to recommendations for the conduct, reporting, editing, and publication of scholarly work in medical journals (ICMJE)

Section of document	(December 2014–2015) Former text	December 2016 text revision	December 2017 text revision
	"Duplicate publication is publication of a paper that overlaps substantially with one already published, without clear, visible reference to the previous publication."	"Prior publication may include release of information in the public domain."	
III. Publishing and Editorial Issues Related to Publication in Medical Journals. B. Scientific Misconduct, Expression of Concern, and Retraction; 2. Duplicate publication (continued).	"Authors should also consider how dissemination of their findings outside of scientific presentations at meetings may diminish the priority [that] journal editors assign to their work. An exception to this principle may occur when information that has immediate implications for public health needs to be disseminated, but when possible, early distribution of findings before publication should be discussed with and agreed upon by the editor in advance."	"Authors should also consider how dissemination of their findings outside of scientific presentations at meetings may diminish the priority [that] journal editors assign to their work." ~~An exception to this principle may occur when information that has immediate implications for public health needs to be disseminated, but when possible, early distribution of findings before publications should be discussed with and agreed upon by the editor in advance.~~	Clinical trials (i) Registration "The ICMJE expects authors to ensure that they have met the requirements of their funding and regulatory agencies regarding aggregate clinical trial results reporting in clinical trial registries, and encourages registry results reporting even when not required. It is the authors', and not the journal editors', responsibility to explain any discrepancies between results reported in registries and journal publications. The ICMJE will not consider as prior publication the posting of trial results in any registry

(Continued)

Table 4.9 (Continued) QC checklist for all manuscripts: Recent history of updates to recommendations for the conduct, reporting, editing, and publication of scholarly work in medical journals (ICMJE)

Section of document	(December 2014–2015) Former text	December 2016 text revision	December 2017 text revision
		"In the event of a public health emergency (as defined by public health officials), information with immediate implications for public health should be disseminated without concern that this will preclude subsequent consideration for publication in a journal."	that meets the above criteria if results are limited to a brief (500-word) structured abstract or tables (to include trial participants enrolled, baseline characteristics, primary and secondary outcomes, and adverse events)."
			(ii) Data sharing "1. As of July 1, 2018, manuscripts published in ICMJE journals that report the results of clinical trials must contain a data-sharing statement as described below. 2. Clinical trials that begin enrolling participants on or after January 1, 2019 must include a data-sharing plan in the trial's registration. The ICMJE's policy regarding trial registration is explained at: www.icmje.org/recommendations/browse/publishing-and-editorial-issues/clinical-trial-registration.html. If the data-sharing *(Continued)*

Table 4.9 (Continued) QC checklist for all manuscripts: Recent history of updates to recommendations for the conduct, reporting, editing, and publication of scholarly work in medical journals (ICMJE)

Section of document	(December 2014–2015) Former text	December 2016 text revision	December 2017 text revision
			plan changes after registration, this should be reflected in the statement submitted and published with the manuscript, and updated in the registry record." "Data-sharing statements must indicate the following: whether individual deidentified participant data (including data dictionaries) will be shared; what data in particular will be shared; whether additional, related documents will be available (e.g., study protocol, statistical analysis plan); when the data will become available and for how long; and by what access criteria data will be shared (including with whom, for what types of analyses, and by what mechanism)."
IV. Manuscript Preparation and Submission. A. Preparing a Manuscript for Submission to a Medical Journal; 3. Manuscript sections; a. Title page	Author information.	Add: "ICMJE encourages the listing of authors' Open Researcher and Contributor Identification (ORCID)."	

(Continued)

Table 4.9 (Continued) QC checklist for all manuscripts: Recent history of updates to recommendations for the conduct, reporting, editing, and publication of scholarly work in medical journals (ICMJE)

Section of document	(December 2014–2015) Former text	December 2016 text revision	December 2017 text revision
IV. A. 3. f. Discussion	~~Emphasize the new and important aspects of the study and the conclusions that follow from them in the context of the totality of the best available evidence. Do not repeat in detail data or other information given in other parts of the manuscript, such in the Introduction or the Results section. For experimental studies, it is useful to begin the discussion by briefly summarizing the main findings, then explore possible mechanisms or explanations for these findings, compare and contrast the results with other relevant studies, state the limitations of the study, and explore the implications of the findings for future research and for clinical practice.~~	Replace with: "It is useful to begin the discussion by briefly summarizing the main findings, and explore possible mechanisms or explanations for these findings. Emphasize the new and important aspects of your study and put your findings in the context of the totality of relevant evidence. State the limitations of your study, and explore the implications of your findings for future research for clinical practice or policy. Do not repeat in detail data or other information given in other parts of the manuscript, such as in the Introduction or the Results section."	

Source: Data available at www.icmje.org/recommendations/archives/. Selected data reported by Taichman DB, Backus J, Baethge C et al. Sharing clinical trial data: a proposal from the International Committee of Medical Journal Editors. *N Engl J Med* 2016;374:384–6.[8]
Abbreviations: COPE, Committee on Publication Ethics; WAME, World Association of Medical Editors.

Table 4.10 QC checklist for all manuscripts: GPP3. General guidance (Part 1)

Item	Recommendation
Study design and results.	• Should be reported in a complete, accurate, balanced, transparent, and timely manner.
Reporting and publication processes.	• Should follow applicable laws and consensus guidelines (e.g., FDAAA 2007, ICMJE, EQUATOR network).
Journal and congress requirements.	• Should be followed, especially ethical guidelines on originality and avoiding redundancy (i.e., duplicate publication).
Publication planning and development.	• Should be a collaboration among all persons involved, e.g., clinicians, statisticians, researchers, and publication professionals (e.g., medical writers) and reflect the collaborative nature of research and the range of skills required to conduct, analyze, interpret, and report research findings.
Rights, roles, requirements, and responsibilities of all contributors (authors and nonauthor contributors).	• Should be confirmed in writing, ideally at the start of the research and, in all cases, before publication preparation begins.
Author roles and integrity.	• All authors should have access to relevant aggregated study data and other information (e.g., study protocol) required to understand and report research findings. • The authors should take responsibility for the way in which research findings are presented and published, be fully involved at all stages of publication and presentation development, and be willing to take public responsibility for all aspects of the work.
Author lists and contributorship statements.	Should accurately reflect all substantial intellectual contributions to the research, data analyses, and publication or presentation development. Relevant contributions from persons who did not qualify as authors should also be disclosed.
The role of the sponsor in the design, execution, analysis, reporting, and funding (if applicable) of the research.	Should be fully disclosed in all publications and presentations of the findings.
	Any involvement by persons or organizations with an interest (financial or nonfinancial) in the findings should also be disclosed.
	All authors and contributors should disclose any relationships or potential competing interests related to the research and its publication or presentation.

Source: Reproduced from *Annals of Internal Medicine*, Battisti WP, Wager E, Baltzer L et al. Good Publication Practice for Communicating Company-Sponsored Medical Research: GPP3. vol. 163, pages 461–4. Copyright ©2015. American College of Physicians. All rights reserved. Reprinted with permission from the American College of Physicians, Inc.[9]

Abbreviations: EQUATOR, Enhancing the Quality and Transparency of Health Research; FDAAA, Food and Drug Administration and Amendments Act; GPP3, Good Publication Practice 3 guideline; ICMJE, International Committee of Medical Journal Editors.

Table 4.11 QC Checklist for all manuscripts: GPP3. Authorship criteria (Part 2)[9,10]

ICMJE 2013 criteria	GPP3 2015 guidance
Substantial contributions to the conception or design of the work or the acquisition, analysis, or interpretation of data for the work.	"A substantial contribution is an important intellectual contribution, rather than technical assistance, without which the work, or an important part of the work, could not have been completed or the manuscript could not have been written and submitted for publication." Simply collecting data (e.g., enrolling many patients) would not necessarily be considered a qualifying criterion for authorship.*
–	Some examples of what might represent a substantial intellectual contribution include actively guiding the scientific or medical content of the publication or presentation, statistical analysis and interpretation, crafting of the discussion, and developing the protocol.
Drafting the article or revising it critically for important intellectual content.	This criterion refers to revisions beyond minor corrections for grammar, language, formatting, or layout. The key is sustained intellectual contribution, the provision of substantial comments, and approval of the final version. Although preferred, it is not always feasible or necessary for authors to comment on every stage of manuscript development.
Final approval of the version to be published.	To give final approval, it is necessary to have carefully read the entire manuscript from start to finish.
Agreement to be accountable for all aspects of the work in ensuring that questions related to the accuracy or integrity of any part of the work are appropriately investigated and resolved.	Each author is accountable for the work and should have confidence in the integrity of the other authors' contributions. Each author should be able to identify who wrote each section.

Source: Reproduced from *Annals of Internal Medicine*, Battisti WP, Wager E, Baltzer L et al. Good Publication Practice for Communicating Company-Sponsored Medical Research: GPP3. vol. 163, pages 461–4. Copyright ©2015. American College of Physicians. All rights reserved. Reprinted with permission from the American College of Physicians, Inc.[9]

Abbreviations: GPP3, Good Publication Practice 3; ICMJE, International Committee of Medical Journal Editors.

*Use Form 3 (original available at www.icmje.org) to document intellectual contributions that meet ICMJE authorship criteria. To meet the second of three ICMJE authorship criteria, a prospective author needs to write pages of the draft (record page numbers on Form 3) or substantively revise the manuscript (record page numbers on Form 3). Approval of the final manuscript is a necessary, but not sufficient, condition of authorship. It is not adequate to state merely "I approve the manuscript" at each stage of development; one must make at least one substantive revision if he or she did not draft the manuscript or sections of it.

Table 4.12 QC checklist for all manuscripts: GPP3. Common issues about authorship (Part 3)

Item	GPP3 guidance
Number of authors.	Consideration should be given to the number of qualified authors needed to take responsibility for the publication. To some extent, this will depend on the complexity of the research and of the publication, but it would be unusual in biomedical research (with few exceptions) to require >10 authors to meet this need. A high number of authors calls into question whether they could all have provided "substantial intellectual contributions." Fewer authors are often preferable, and others can be acknowledged (e.g., as nonauthor contributors or collaborators). Some journals limit the number of authors allowed on a publication.
Author sequence.	Authors should decide how this will be determined at the initiation of the work, including the designation of the lead and corresponding authors, who may or may not be the same person. Final order, however, should be based on authors' actual roles and contributions in the development of the publication (and therefore cannot be agreed upon until this is complete). Those who made the greatest contribution are generally listed first, but alphabetical order may also be used. It may be useful to describe in the contributorship section of the publication whether alphabetical order or some other convention was used to determine author order.*
Addition or removal of an author.	In certain circumstances during the development of a publication, it may be necessary to add or remove an author (e.g., if an author fails to provide a substantial contribution or approve the final version of the work). In such cases, all authors should agree to the change. Only in rare cases, such as the work substantially changing in response to reviewer comments, should addition or removal of an author be considered after submission. For encore presentations of abstracts at local language congresses where presenters are required to be an author, an additional name may be added to the author list (with all authors' permission) for the purpose of presenting on behalf of the group in the local language. This person should be clearly identified as "Presenting on behalf of..." in the abstract author byline if possible but at least in the presentation.
Death or incapacity of an author.[†]	Should an author die after completing a major part of the work (i.e., fulfilling ICMJE criteria 1 and 2), posthumous authorship can be considered if agreed to by all other authors. We suggest, as a first step, seeking advice on correct attribution and process from journal instructions or the editorial office. If the journal agrees to posthumous authorship but requires submission forms to be signed, then in the case of a sponsor-employed author or a contractor, a supervisor may be the most appropriate proxy. Otherwise, a family member or person with power of attorney should be approached.[11] In all cases, efforts should be made to contact the family of the deceased author to inform them of the intention and request their consent to the listing or acknowledgment.

(Continued)

Table 4.12 (Continued) QC checklist for all manuscripts: GPP3. Common issues about authorship (Part 4)

Item	GPP3 guidance
Change of affiliation.	If an author changes affiliation before the work is published, his or her affiliation should reflect where the major part of the work was done. The current affiliation and contact details should be listed in a footnote or in the acknowledgment section. Change of affiliation alone is not a valid reason to remove an author from a publication if he or she meets authorship criteria.
Company- or sponsor-employed authors.	Sponsor-employed scientists and clinicians are often qualified to participate as authors of company-sponsored research publications and should have that opportunity. Such authors should not be denied authorship because of concerns about perception of bias. Whatever criteria are used to determine authorship should be applied equally to company employees, contractors, and others.
Professional writers as authors.	Professional medical writers who meet applicable authorship criteria should be listed as authors. If writers do not meet authorship criteria, their contribution should be disclosed (e.g., as a nonauthor contributor in the acknowledgment section). Writers who were not involved with study design, data collection, or data analysis and interpretation (e.g., those developing a primary publication from a clinical study report) generally do not meet ICMJE authorship criteria. However, professional writers working on other types of publication (e.g., literature reviews) may qualify as authors.

Source: Reproduced from *Annals of Internal Medicine*, Battisti WP, Wager E, Baltzer L et al. Good Publication Practice for Communicating Company-Sponsored Medical Research: GPP3. vol. 163, pages 461–4. Copyright ©2015. American College of Physicians. All rights reserved. Reprinted with permission from the American College of Physicians, Inc.[9]

Abbreviations: GPP3, Good Publication Practice 3 guideline; ICMJE, International Committee of Medical Journal Editors.

*Author order may be partly determined by the extent of data acquisition in terms of numbers of subjects enrolled and followed up in a clinical trial, in addition to the traditional contributions of obtaining funding; conceiving and designing the study; analyzing and interpreting data; drafting the manuscript; revising its intellectual content; and reviewing and approving the final version. The lead author is often the principal investigator, whereas the final author is often the senior investigator, e.g., sometimes a professor emeritus.

† The name of a deceased author typically is footnoted on the title page using a dagger.[11]

Table 4.13 QC checklist for all manuscripts: MPIP

Item	Recommendation
Title and abstract.	Ensure [that the] title and abstract are consistent with journal guidance regarding structure, form, word/character count.
	Ensure [that the] title and abstract match up and clearly relate to one another.
	Ensure [that the] abstract conclusions accurately represent outcomes and are consistent with study conclusions.
	As appropriate, include p values and absolute numbers for key findings in the abstract.
	Provide key words, as instructed by the journal, to enable database searching of the article.
Acknowledgments.	Make all required disclosures consistent with journal policy (i.e., for authorship, contributorship, funding, role of the sponsor, and competing interests) in appropriate format.
	Explicitly add a statement about what type of assistance, if any, was received from the sponsor (e.g., editorial support, graphics, statistical analysis) or sponsor's representatives (e.g., contract research organizations).
	Include the name(s) of any professional writer(s), editorial staff or other contributors, or any third-party associations that participated in manuscript development.
Introduction.	Clearly articulate the research question addressed by the study (e.g., journal editors mention that the conceptualization of the problem and approach is often not well conveyed), following journal's format for "hypothesis" if explicitly provided.
	State the importance of the research question to the field (e.g., is it new/relevant, and does it address an important research question?).
	Note relationships to other studies from the same or related datasets.
	Do not be afraid to acknowledge if a study has been conducted for regulatory purposes.
	Present the introduction in a straightforward manner, without excessive wordiness.
Methods.	Provide a full explanation of the study methodology, including study design, data collection and analysis principles, and underlying rationale, with special attention to:
	• Sample selection, including inclusion and exclusion criteria, and any ethical considerations that guided the study design.
	• Description of randomization or other group assignment methods used.
	• Description of the prespecified primary outcome measure(s), as well as secondary and other variables.
	Describe any unusual statistical methodologies, expressed so that nonexpert editors can understand deviations from standard approaches.
	Describe how subjects were recruited and compensated (if applicable).
	Describe how compliance (adherence) was measured (if applicable).
	For RCTs, follow journal's guidelines regarding adherence to the current version of the CONSORT statement relevant to the particular study type.
	Refer to journal instructions as to whether methods and results should remain as separate sections or be combined.

(Continued)

Table 4.13 (Continued) QC checklist for all manuscripts: MPIP

Item	Recommendation
Results.	Clearly report patient population characteristics, low response/study continuation rates, missing data, quality control issues or deviations from registered protocol (e.g., inconsistencies in recruiting, adherence).
	Report results for primary outcomes (and secondary, if appropriate) using tables and figures for additional clarity, with rationale for endpoint selection and explanation of why information was not collected on important unmeasured variables.
	Check if the journal allows excess text, figures, tables, or references to be included as online supplemental data, which is particularly important if the manuscript exceeds specified word limits.
	Check for consistency in reported data between text and tables/images.
	Thoroughly report the impact of unusual analytical methods.
	Explain any changes from the original hypothesis or objectives that occurred before, during, or after the study.
Discussion.	Structure the section so that it presents a natural flow of ideas—start with a simple statement of main findings, followed by strengths and limitations of the study, and what the study adds to previous knowledge.
	Describe briefly how the results are consistent or not consistent with other similar studies.
	Discuss any confounding factors [or biases] and their potential impact.
	Avoid excessive wordiness—editors and reviewers describe this section as one that is usually too wordy and often contains noncritical information.
Conclusions.	Address, but do not "over-sell," perceived significance of the study to the field and possible implications for practice policy.
	Ensure [that] conclusions relate directly to the stated a priori hypothesis (and not hypotheses from other studies or outside the area of the study).
	Avoid excessive generalizations of the implications, including unjustified extrapolations beyond the actual population(s).
	Remember that, except for RCTs, there can be only testable hypotheses and observed associations rather than rigorous proof of cause and effect.
	Address areas for improvement with future studies.
References.	Follow journal's policies and formatting instructions, including for web-based references, and obtain clarification from the journal as needed.
	In most cases, manuscripts "in submission" are not appropriate for inclusion in this section.
	Particularly note that some journals do not allow the use of unpublished "data on file" (DOF) statements from package inserts based solely on such data, or reviews that rely upon DOF as the only support for claims made; if DOF references are allowed by the journal, be sure to request the title, nature of the reference, and internal reference number for record-keeping purposes.

Source: Reproduced with permission from Chipperfield L, Citrome L, Clark J et al. Authors' Submission Toolkit: a practical guide to getting your research published. *Curr Med Res Opin* 2010;26:1967–82.[12]
Abbreviations: CONSORT, Consolidated Standards of Reporting Trials; RCT, randomized controlled trial.

Table 4.14 QC checklist for systematic reviews, research recommendations, and other documents

EPICOT mnemonic[13]	Factors that promote evidence quality	Factors that may erode evidence quality	Potential defects in reporting (reaching conclusions)
Evidence: What is the current evidence?	Large magnitude of effect.	Limited design and implementation of available studies (with bias).	Absence of evidence does not imply evidence of absence.
Population: Diagnosis, disease stage, comorbidity, risk factor, sex, age, ethnic group, specific inclusion or exclusion criteria, setting.	All plausible confounding would reduce a demonstrate effect or suggest a spurious effect when results show no effect.	Indirectness of evidence (indirect population, intervention, control, outcomes).	"Wishful thinking" I: A statement such as "the study was too small (or underpowered) to discern a significant effect" is misleading. If confidence intervals overlap 1.0 or 0, just state them and say that the results are incompatible with a statistically significant effect.
Intervention: Type frequency, dose, duration, prognostic factor.	Dose-response gradient.	Unexplained heterogeneity or inconsistency of results (e.g., problems with subgroup analyses).	"Wishful thinking" II: Statistically nonsignificant findings should not be reported as "trending" in a certain direction; positive effects should not be characterized as "promising." Avoid value judgments and simply report the data.
Comparison: Placebo, routine care, alternative treatment/ management.	–	Imprecision of results (e.g., wide confidence intervals).	Conclusions should not exceed the study parameters and evidence. This caveat applies especially when seeking to extend findings from study to normal practice settings (i.e., stating generalizability). Do so cautiously.
Outcome: Which clinical or patient-related outcomes will the researcher need to measure, improve, influence or accomplish? Which methods of measurement should be used?	–	High probability of publication bias.	–
Time (Time stamp): Date of literature search or recommendation.	–	–	–

Source: Selected data from Schünemann HJ, Oxman AD, Vist G et al. Chapter 12: Interpreting results and drawing conclusions. In Higgins JPT, Green S eds. *Cochrane Handbook for Systematic Reviews of Interventions*. Version 5.1.0 of the Cochrane Handbook. West Sussex, UK: The Cochrane Collaboration and Wiley-Blackwell, 2011: 12.1–12.24[14] and Brown P, Brunnhuber K, Chalkidou K et al. How to formulate research recommendations. *BMJ* 2006;333:804–6.[13] (Available at: http:// handbook-5-1.cochrane.org. Last accessed October 28, 2017.)

Table 4.15 QC checklist. PRISMA

Section/Topic	No.	Checklist item	On pg. no.
Title.			
Title.	**1**	Identify the report as a systematic review, meta-analysis, or both.	
Abstract.			
Structured summary.	**2**	Provide a structured summary including, as applicable: background; objectives; data sources; study eligibility criteria, participants, and interventions; study appraisal and synthesis methods; results; limitations; conclusions and implications of key findings; systematic review registration number.	
Introduction.			
Rationale.	**3**	Describe the rationale for the review in the context of what is already known.	
Objectives.	**4**	Provide an explicit statement of questions being addressed, with reference to Participants, Interventions, Comparisons, Outcomes, and Study Design (PICOS).	
Methods.			
Protocol and registration.	**5**	Indicate if a review protocol exists, if and where it can be accessed (e.g., web address), and, if available, provide registration information including registration number.	
Eligibility criteria.	**6**	Specify study characteristics (e.g., PICOS, length of follow-up) and report characteristics (e.g., years considered, language, publication status) used as criteria for eligibility, giving rationale.	
Information sources.	**7**	Describe all information sources (e.g., databases with dates of coverage, contact with study authors to identify additional studies) in the search and date last searched.	
Search.	**8**	Present full electronic search strategy for at least one database, including any limits used, such that it could be repeated.	
Study selection.	**9**	State the process for selecting studies (i.e., screening, eligibility, included in systematic review, and, if applicable, included in the meta-analysis).	
Data collection process.	**10**	Describe method of data extraction from reports (e.g., piloted forms, independently, in duplicate) and any processes for obtaining and confirming data from investigators.	
Data items.	**11**	List and define all variables for which data were sought (e.g., PICOS, funding sources) and any assumptions and simplifications made.	
Risk of bias in individual studies.	**12**	Describe methods used for assessing risk of bias of individual studies (including specification of whether this was done at the study or outcome level), and how this information is to be used in any data synthesis.	
Summary measures.	**13**	State the principal summary measures (e.g., risk ratio, difference in means).	

(Continued)

Table 4.15 (Continued) QC checklist. PRISMA

Section/Topic	No.	Checklist item	On pg. no.
Synthesis of results.	14	Describe the methods of handling data and combining results of studies, if done, including measures of consistency/heterogeneity (e.g., I^2) for each meta-analysis.	
Risk of bias across studies.	15	Specify any assessment of risk of bias that may affect the cumulative evidence (e.g., publication bias, selective reporting within studies).	
Additional analyses.	16	Describe methods of additional analyses (e.g., sensitivity or subgroup analyses, meta-regression), if done, indicating which were prespecified.	
Results.			
Study selection.	17	Give numbers of studies screened, assessed for eligibility, and included in the review, with reasons for exclusions at each stage, ideally with a flow diagram.	
Study characteristics.	18	For each study, present characteristics for which data were extracted (e.g., study size, PICOS, follow-up period) and provide the citations.	
Risk of bias within studies.	19	Present data on risk of bias of each study and, if available, any outcome level assessment (see item 12).	
Results of individual studies.	20	For all outcomes considered (benefits or harms), present, for each study: (a) simple summary data for each intervention group and (b) effect estimates and confidence intervals, ideally with a forest plot.	
Synthesis of results.	21	Present results of each meta-analysis done, including confidence intervals and measures of consistency.	
Risk of bias across studies.	22	Present results of any assessment of risk of bias across studies (see Item 15).	
Additional analysis.	23	Give results of additional analyses, if done (e.g., sensitivity or subgroup analyses, meta-regression [see Item 16]).	
Discussion.			
Summary of evidence.	24	Summarize the main findings, including the strength of evidence for each main outcome; consider their relevance to key groups (e.g., health-care providers, users, and policymakers).	
Limitations.	25	Discuss limitations at study and outcome level (e.g., risk of bias), and at review level (e.g., incomplete retrieval of identified research, reporting bias).	
Conclusions.	26	Provide a general interpretation of the results in the context of other evidence, and implications for future research.	
Funding.			
Funding.	27	Describe sources of funding for the systematic review and other support (e.g., supply of data); role of funders for the systematic review.	

Table 4.16 PRISMA-P 2015: Recommended items to include in a systematic review protocol.
Part 1: Terminology

Item	Definition
Systematic review.	A systematic attempt to collate all relevant evidence that fits prespecified study eligibility criteria to answer a specific research question. It uses explicit, systematic methods to minimize bias in the identification, selection, synthesis, and summary of studies. When done well, this provides reliable findings from which conclusions can be drawn and decisions made. The key characteristics of a systematic review are (a) a clearly stated set of objectives with an explicit, reproducible methodology; (b) a systematic search that attempts to identify all studies that would meet the eligibility criteria; (c) an assessment of the validity of the findings of the included studies (e.g., assessment of risk of bias and confidence in cumulative estimates); and (d) systematic presentation, and synthesis, of the characteristics and findings of the included studies.
Meta-analysis.	Meta-analysis is the use of statistical techniques to combine and summarize the results of multiple studies; they may or may not be contained within a systematic review. By combining data from several studies, meta-analyses can provide more precise estimates of the effects of health-care interventions than those derived from individual studies.
Protocol.	In the context of systematic reviews and meta-analyses, a protocol is a document that presents an explicit plan for a systematic review. The protocol details the rationale and *a priori* methodological and analytical approach of the review.

Source: Reproduced from *BMJ*, Shamseer L, Moher D, Clarke M et al. Preferred Reporting Items for Systematic Review and Meta-Analysis Protocols (PRISMA-P) 2015: elaboration and explanation. vol. 349, page g7647. Copyright ©2015 with permission from BMJ Publishing Group Ltd.[16]

Table 4.17 PRISMA-P 2015: Recommended items to include in a systematic review protocol. Part 2: QC checklist

Item	No.	Description
Administrative information.		–
Title.		–
Identification.	1a	Identify the report as a protocol of a systematic review.
Update.	1b	If the protocol is for an update of a previous systematic review, identify as such.
Registration.	2	If registered, provide the name of the registry (e.g., PROSPERO) and registration number.
Authors; contact.	3a	Provide name, institutional affiliation, and e-mail address of each protocol author, provide physical mailing address of the corresponding author.
Contributions.	3b	Describe contributions of protocol authors and identify the guarantor of the review.
Amendments.	4	If the protocol represents an amendment of a previously completed or published protocol, identify it as such and list changes; otherwise, state plan for documenting important protocol amendments.
Support; Sources.	5a	Indicate sources of financial or other support for the review.
Sponsor.	5b	Provide the name of the review funder and/or sponsor.
Role of sponsor or funder.	5c	Describe roles of funder(s), sponsor(s), and/or institution(s), if any, in developing the protocol.
Introduction.		
Rationale.	6	Describe the rationale for the review in the context of what is already known.
Objectives.	7	Provide an explicit statement of the question(s) the review will address, with reference to Participants, Interventions, Comparators, and Outcomes (PICO).
Methods.		
Eligibility criteria.	8	Specify the study characteristics (e.g., PICO, study design, setting, time frame) and report characteristics (e.g., years considered, language, publication status) to be used as criteria for eligibility for the review.
Information sources.	9	Describe all intended information sources (e.g., electronic databases, contact with study authors, trial registers, or other "gray" literature sources), with planned dates of coverage.
Search strategy.	10	Present draft of search strategy to be used for at least one electronic database, including planned limits, such that it could be repeated.
Study records; data management.	11a	Describe the mechanism(s) that will be used to manage records and data throughout the review.
Selection process.	11b	State the process that will be used for selecting studies (e.g., two independent reviewers) through each phase of the review (i.e., screening, eligibility, inclusion in meta-analysis).
Data collection process.	11c	Describe planned method of extracting data from reports (e.g., piloting forms, done independently, in duplicate), and processes for obtaining and confirming data from investigators.

(Continued)

Table 4.17 (Continued) PRISMA-P 2015: Recommended items to include in a systematic review protocol. Part 2: QC checklist

Item	No.	Description
Data items.	12	List and define all variables for which data will be sought (e.g., PICO items, funding sources), and preplanned data assumptions and simplifications.
Outcomes and prioritization.	13	List and define all outcomes for which data will be sought, including prioritization of main and additional outcomes, with rationale.
Risk of bias in individual studies.	14	Describe anticipated methods for assessing risk of bias in individual studies, including whether this will be done at the outcome or study level, or both; state how this information will be used in data synthesis.
Data synthesis.	15a	Describe criteria under which study data will be quantitatively synthesized.
	15b	If data are appropriate for quantitative synthesis, describe planned summary measures, methods of handling data, and methods of combining data from studies, including any planned exploration of consistency/heterogeneity (e.g., I^2 test or Kendall's τ).
	15c	Describe any proposed additional analyses (e.g., sensitivity or subgroup analyses, meta-regression).
	15d	If quantitative synthesis is not appropriate, describe the type of summary planned.
Meta-bias(es).	16	Specify any planned assessment of meta-bias(es) (e.g., publication bias across studies, selective reporting within studies).
Confidence in cumulative evidence.	17	Describe how the strength of the body of evidence will be assessed.

Source: Reproduced from *BMJ*, Shamseer L, Moher D, Clarke M et al. Preferred Reporting Items for Systematic Review and Meta-Analysis Protocols (PRISMA-P) 2015: elaboration and explanation. vol. 349, page g7647. Copyright ©2015 with permission from BMJ Publishing Group.[16]

Table 4.18 QC checklist. "STARLITE" mnemonic for reporting review articles

Element	Explanatory notes
S. Sampling strategy.	• Comprehensive: attempts to identify all relevant studies on the topic. • Selective: attempts to identify all relevant studies but only within specified limits. • Purposive: samples from specific disciplines, years, journals.
T. Type of studies.	• Fully reported: describes actual study types (e.g., grounded theory) or designs to be included. • Partially reported: uses an "umbrella" category such as "qualitative studies" without defining what this means.
A. Approaches.	• Approaches other than electronic subject searches. • Example: hand-searching. • Citation snowballing.
R. Range of years (start date–end date).	• Fully reported: includes start and end dates with justification for the period chosen. • Partially reported: includes start and end dates but only determined available coverage of databases.
L. Limits.	• Functional limits that are applied for logistic reasons but do not alter the topic conceptually (e.g., human, English).
I. Inclusion/exclusions.	• Conceptual limitations that mediate the scope of the topic area (e.g., geographical location, setting, or a specific focus of study).
T. Terms used.	• Fully present: example of a sample search strategy from one or more of the main databases. • Partially present: reports terminology used but without evidence of search syntax and operators.
E. Electronic sources.	Reports databases used and, optimally, search platforms and vendors to assist in replication.

Source: Reproduced with permission from Booth A. A brimful of "STARLITE": toward standards for reporting literature searches. *J Med Libr Assoc* 2006;94:421–9, e205.[17]

Table 4.19 QC checklist. MOOSE

Reporting of manuscript section ...	... Should include
Background.	Problem definition.
	Hypothesis statement.
	Description of study outcome(s).
	Type of exposure or intervention used.
	Type of study designs used.
	Study population.
Search strategy.	Qualification of searchers (e.g., librarians, investigators).
	Search strategy, including the period included in the synthesis and key words.
	Effort to include all available studies, including contact with authors.
	Databases and registries searched.
	Search software used, name and version, including special features used (e.g., explosion).
	Use of hand searching (e.g., reference lists of obtained articles).
	List of citations located and those excluded, including justification.
	Method of addressing articles published in languages other than English.
	Method of handling abstracts and unpublished studies.
	Description of any contact with authors.
Methods.	Description of relevance or appropriateness of studies assembled for assessing the hypothesis to be tested.
	Rationale for the selection and coding of data (e.g., sound clinical principles or convenience).
	Documentation of how data were classified and coded (e.g., multiple raters, blinding, and inter-rater reliability).
	Assessment of confounding (e.g., comparability of cases and controls in studies where appropriate).
	Assessment of study quality, including blinding of quality assessors; stratification or regression on possible predictors of study results.
	Assessment of heterogeneity.
	Description of statistical methods (e.g., complete description of fixed- or random-effects models, justification of whether the chosen models account for predictors of study results, dose-response models, or cumulative meta-analysis) in sufficient detail to be replicated.

(Continued)

Table 4.19 (Continued) QC checklist. MOOSE

Reporting of manuscript section ...	... Should include
Results.	Graphic summarizing individual study estimates and overall estimate.
	Table giving descriptive information for each study included.
	Results of sensitivity testing (e.g., subgroup analysis).
	Indication of statistical uncertainty of findings.
Discussion.	Quantitative assessment of bias (e.g., publication bias).
	Justification for exclusion (e.g., exclusion of non–English-language citations).
	Assessment of quality of included studies.
Conclusions.	Consideration of alternative explanations for observed results.
	Generalization of the conclusions (i.e., appropriate for the data presented and within the domain of the literature review).
	Guidelines for future research.

Source: Reproduced with permission from Stroup DF, Berlin JA, Morton SC et al. Meta-analysis of observational studies in epidemiology: a proposal for reporting. Meta-analysis of Observational Studies in Epidemiology (MOOSE) group. *JAMA* 2000;283:2008–12.[18]

Table 4.20 QC checklist. QUOROM

Heading	Subheading	Description	Reported? (Y/N)	Pg. no.
Title.		Identify the report as a meta-analysis [or systematic review] of RCTs.		
Abstract.		Use a structured format.		
	Objectives.	Describe the clinical question explicitly.		
	Data sources.	The databases (i.e., list) and other information sources.		
	Review methods.	Selection criteria (i.e., population, intervention, outcome, study design); methods for validity assessment, data abstraction, and study characteristics; and quantitative data synthesis in sufficient detail to permit replication.		
	Results.	Characteristics of the RCTs included and excluded; qualitative and quantitative findings (i.e., point estimates and confidence intervals); and subgroup analyses.		
	Conclusions.	The main results.		
Introduction.		The explicit clinical problem, biological rationale for the intervention, and rationale for review.		
Methods.	Searching.	The information sources, in detail (e.g., databases, registers, personal files, expert informants, agencies, hand-searching), and any restrictions (years considered, publication status, language of publication).[19,20]		
	Selection.	The inclusion and exclusion criteria (defining population, intervention, principal outcomes, and study design[21]).		
	Validity assessment.	The criteria and processes used (e.g., masked conditions, quality assessments, and their findings).[21–24]		
	Data abstraction.	The process(es) used (e.g., completed independently in duplicate).[24,25]		
	Study characteristics.	The type of study design, participants' characteristics, details of intervention, outcome definitions, and how clinical heterogeneity was assessed.		

(Continued)

Table 4.20 (Continued) QC checklist. QUOROM

Heading	Subheading	Description	Reported? (Y/N)	Pg. no.
	Quantitative data synthesis.	The principal measures of effect (e.g., relative risk), method of combining results (statistical testing and confidence intervals), handling of missing data; how statistical heterogeneity was assessed[26]; rationale for any *a priori* sensitivity and subgroup analyses; and any assessment of publication bias.[28]		
Results.	Trial flow.	Provide a meta-analysis profile summarizing trial flow.		
	Study characteristics.	Present descriptive data for each trial (e.g., age, sample size, intervention, dose, duration, follow-up interval).		
	Quantitative data synthesis.	Report agreement on the selection and validity assessment; present simple summary results (for each treatment group in each trial, for each primary outcome); present data needed to calculate effect sizes and confidence intervals in intention-to-treat analyses (e.g., 2 × 2 tables of counts, means, SDs, and proportions).		
Discussion.		Summarize key findings; discuss clinical inferences based on internal and external validity; interpret the results in light of the totality of available evidence; describe potential biases in review process (e.g., publication bias); and suggest a future research agenda.		

Source: Reprinted from *The Lancet*, Moher D, Cook DJ, Eastwood S et al. Improving the quality of reports of meta-analyses of randomised controlled trials: the QUOROM statement. vol. 354, pages 1896–1900. Copyright ©1999, with permission from Elsevier.[29]
Abbreviations: RCT, randomized controlled trial; SD, standard deviation.

Table 4.21 QC checklist for reports of randomized controlled trials: CONSORT

Section and topic	Item no.	Descriptor	Reported on pg. no.
Title and abstract.	1	How participants were allocated to interventions (e.g., "random allocation," "randomized," or "randomly assigned").	
Introduction.			
Background.	2	Scientific background and explanation of rationale.	
Methods.			
Participants.	3	Eligibility criteria for participants and the settings and locations where the data were collected.	
Interventions.	4	Precise details of the interventions intended for each group and how and when they were actually administered.	
Objectives.	5	Specific objectives and hypotheses.	
Outcomes.	6	Clearly defined primary and secondary outcome measures and, when applicable, any methods used to enhance the quality of measurements (e.g., multiple observations, training of assessors).	
Sample size.	7	How sample size was determined and, when applicable, explanation of any interim analyses and stopping rules.	
Randomization.			
Sequence generation.	8	Method used to generate the random allocation sequence, including details of any restrictions (e.g., blocking, stratification).	
Allocation concealment.	9	Method used to implement the random allocation sequence (e.g., numbered containers or central telephone), clarifying whether the sequence was concealed until interventions were assigned.	
Implementation.	10	Who generated the allocation sequence, who enrolled participants, and who assigned participants to their groups?	
Blinding (masking).	11	Whether participants, those administering the interventions, and those assessing the outcomes were blinded to group assignment. If done, how the success of blinding was evaluated.	

(Continued)

Table 4.21 (Continued) QC checklist for reports of randomized controlled trials: CONSORT

Section and topic	Item no.	Descriptor	Reported on pg. no.
Statistical methods.	12	Statistical methods used to compare groups for primary outcome(s); methods for additional analyses, such as subgroup analyses and adjusted analyses.	
Results.			
Participant flow.	13	Flow of participants through each stage (a diagram is strongly recommended; Figure 4.1). Specifically, for each group, report the numbers of participants randomly assigned,* receiving intended treatment, completing the study protocol, and analyzed for the primary outcome. Describe protocol deviations from study as planned, together with reasons.	
Recruitment.	14	Dates defining the periods of recruitment and follow-up.	
Baseline data.	15	Baseline demographic and clinical characteristics of each group.	
Numbers analyzed.	16	Number of participants (denominator) in each group included in each analysis and whether the analysis was by "intention-to-treat." State the results in absolute numbers when feasible (e.g., 10/20, not 50%).	
Outcomes and estimation.	17	For each primary and secondary outcome, a summary of results for each group, and the estimated effect size and its precision (e.g., 95% confidence interval).	
Ancillary analyses.	18	Address multiplicity by reporting any other analyses performed, including subgroup analyses and adjusted analyses; indicate those prespecified and those exploratory.	
Adverse events.	19	All important adverse events or side effects in each intervention group.	
Comment.			
Interpretation.	20	Interpretation of the results, taking into account study hypotheses, sources of potential bias or imprecision, and the dangers associated with multiplicity of analyses and outcomes.	
Generalizability.	21	Generalizability (external validity) of the trial findings.	
Overall evidence.	22	General interpretation of the results in the context of current evidence.	

Source: Reproduced with permission from Moher D, Schulz KF, Altman D. The CONSORT statement: revised recommendations for improving the quality of reports of parallel-group randomized trials. *JAMA* 2001;285:1987–91.[7]
*Ideally, a patient disposition flowchart (Figure 4.1) should also include the number of potential study participants screened as well as randomized. Including this information conveys the relative "selectedness" of the population and potential difficulties in recruiting and enrolling subjects.

Table 4.22 QC checklist for reports of randomized controlled trials: CONSORT update

Section/Topic	Item no.	Checklist item	Reported on pg. no.
Title and abstract.	**1a**	Identification as a randomized trial in the title.	
	1b	Structured summary of trial design, methods, results and conclusions (for specific guidance, see CONSORT for abstracts).	
Introduction.			
Background and objectives.	**2a**	Scientific background and explanation of rationale.	
	2b	Specific objectives or hypotheses.	
Methods.	**3a**	Description of trial design (e.g., parallel, factorial), including allocation ratio.	
Trial design.	**3b**	Important changes to methods after trial commencement (e.g., eligibility criteria), with reasons.	
Participants.	**4a**	Eligibility criteria for participants.	
	4b	Settings and locations where the data were collected.	
Interventions.	**5**	The interventions for each group, with sufficient details to allow replication, including how and when they were actually administered.	
Outcomes.	**6a**	Completely defined prespecified primary and secondary outcome measures, including how and when they were assessed.	
	6b	Any changes to trial outcomes after the trial commenced, with reasons.	
Sample size.	**7a**	How sample size was determined.	
	7b	When applicable, explanation of any interim analyses and stopping guidelines.	
Randomization.	**8a**	Method used to generate the random allocation sequence.	
Sequence generation.	**8b**	Type of randomization, details of any restriction (e.g., blocking and block size).	
Allocation concealment mechanism.	**9**	Mechanism used to implement the random allocation sequence (e.g., sequentially numbered containers), describing any steps taken to conceal the sequence until interventions were assigned.	
Implementation.	**10**	Who generated the random allocation sequence, who enrolled participants, and who assigned participants to interventions?	
Blinding (masking).	**11a**	If done, who was blinded after assignment to interventions (e.g., participants, care providers, those assessing outcomes) and how.	
	11b	If relevant, description of the similarity of interventions.	
Statistical methods.	**12a**	Statistical methods used to compare groups for primary and secondary outcomes.	
	12b	Methods for additional analysis, such as subgroup analyses and adjusted analyses.	

(Continued)

Table 4.22 (Continued) QC checklist for reports of randomized controlled trials: CONSORT update

Section/Topic	Item no.	Checklist item	Reported on pg. no.
Results.			
Participant flow (a diagram [Figure 4.1] is strongly recommended).	13a	For each group, the numbers of participants who were randomly assigned, received intended treatment, and were analyzed for the primary outcome.	
	13b	For each group, losses and exclusions after randomization, together with reasons.	
Recruitment.	14a	Dates defining the periods of recruitment and follow-up.	
	14b	Why the trial ended or was stopped.	
Baseline data.	15	A table showing baseline demographic and clinical characteristics for each group.	
Numbers analyzed.	16	For each group, number of participants (denominator) included in each analysis and whether the analysis was by original assigned groups.	
Outcomes and estimation.	17a	For each primary and secondary outcome, results for each group, and the estimated effect size and its precision (e.g., 95% confidence interval).	
	17b	For binary outcomes, presentation of both absolute and relative effect sizes is recommended.	
Ancillary analyses.	18	Results of any other analyses performed, including subgroup analyses and adjusted analyses, distinguishing prespecified from exploratory.	
Harms.	19	All important harms or unintended effects in each group (for specific guidance, see CONSORT for harms[32]).	
Discussion.			
Limitations.	20	Trial limitations; addressing sources of potential bias, imprecision, and, if relevant, multiplicity of analyses.	
Generalizability.	21	Generalizability (external validity, applicability) of the trial findings.	
Interpretation.	22	Interpretation consistent with results, balancing benefits and harms, and considering other relevant evidence.	
Other information.			
Registration.	23	Registration number and name of trial registry.	
Protocol.	24	Where the full trial protocol can be accessed, if available.	
Funding.	25	Sources of funding and other support (e.g., supply of drugs), role of funders.	

Source: Reproduced with permission from Moher D, Hopewell S, Schulz KF et al. CONSORT 2010 Explanation and Elaboration: Updated guidelines for reporting parallel group randomised trials. *J Clin Epidemiol* 2010;63:e1–37.[30] The article was published under the terms of the Creative Commons Attribution-NonCommercial-No Derivatives License (CC BY NC ND). Article available at: http://dx.doi.org/10.1016/j.jclinepi.2010.03.004. License available at: https://creativecommons.org/licenses/by-nc-nd/4.0.

Table 4.23 QC checklist for reports of randomized controlled trials: CONSORT—Cluster randomized controlled trials

Paper section and topic	Item	Descriptor
Title and abstract.		
Design.	1	How participants were allocated to interventions (e.g., random allocation, randomized, or randomly assigned), *specifying that allocation* was based on clusters.*
Introduction.		
Background.	2	Scientific background and explanation of rationale, *including the rationale for using a cluster design.*
Methods.		
Participants.	3	Eligibility criteria for participants *and clusters* and the setting and locations where the data were collected.
Interventions.	4	Precise details of the interventions intended for each group, *whether they pertain to individual level, the cluster level, or both*, and how and when they were actually administered.
Objectives.	5	Specific objectives and hypotheses *and whether they pertain to the individual level, the cluster level, or both.*
Outcomes.	6	Report clearly defined primary and secondary outcome measures, *whether they pertain to the individual level, the cluster level, or both*, and, when applicable, any methods used to enhance the quality of measurements (e.g., multiple observations, training of assessors).
Sample size.	7	How total sample size was determined (*including method of calculation, number of clusters, cluster size, a coefficient of intracluster correlation [ICC or k], and an indication of its uncertainty*) and, when applicable, explanation of any interim analyses and stopping rules.
Randomization.		
Sequence generation.	8	Method used to generate the random allocation sequence, including details of any restriction (e.g., blocking, stratification, *matching*).
Allocation concealment.	*9*	Method used to implement the random allocation sequence, *specifying that allocation was based on clusters rather than individuals* and clarifying whether the sequence was concealed until interventions were assigned.
Implementation.	10	Who generated the allocation sequence, who enrolled participants, and who assigned participants to their groups.
Blinding (masking).	11	Whether participants, those administering the interventions, and those assessing the outcomes were blinded to group assignment. If done, how the success of blinding was evaluated.

(Continued)

Table 4.23 (Continued) QC checklist for reports of randomized controlled trials: CONSORT—Cluster randomized controlled trials

Paper section and topic	Item	Descriptor
Statistical methods.	12	Statistical methods used to compare groups for primary outcome(s) *indicating how clustering was taken into account*, and methods for additional analyses, such as subgroup analyses and adjusted analyses.
Results.		
Participant flow.	13	Flow of *clusters* and individual participants through each stage (a diagram is strongly recommended). Specifically, for each group, report the numbers of *clusters* and participants randomly assigned, receiving intended treatment, completing the study protocol, and analyzed for the primary outcome. Describe protocol deviations from study as planned, together with reasons.
Recruitment.	14	Dates defining the periods of recruitment and follow up.
Baseline data.	15	Baseline information for each group *for the individual and cluster levels as applicable.*
Numbers analyzed.	16	Number of *clusters and* participants (denominator) in each group included in each analysis and whether the analysis was by intention to treat. State the results in absolute numbers when feasible (e.g., 10/20, not 50%).
Outcomes and estimation.	17	For each primary and secondary outcome, a summary of results *for each group for the individual or cluster level as applicable*, and the estimated effect size and its precision (e.g., 95% CI) *and a coefficient of intracluster correlation (ICC or k) for each primary outcome.*
Ancillary analyses.	18	Address multiplicity by reporting any other analyses performed, including subgroup analyses and adjusted analyses, indicating those prespecified and those exploratory.
Adverse events.	19	All important adverse events or side effects in each intervention group.
Discussion.		
Interpretation.	20	Interpretation of the results, taking into account study hypotheses, sources of potential bias or imprecision and the dangers associated with multiplicity of analyses and outcomes.
Generalizability.	21	Generalizability (external validity) *to individuals and/or clusters (as relevant)* of the trial findings.
Overall evidence.	22	General interpretation of the results in the context of current evidence.

Source: Reproduced with permission from *BMJ*, Campbell MK, Elbourne DR, Altman DG for the CONSORT Group. CONSORT statement: extension to cluster randomised trials. vol. 328, pages 702–8, ©2004 with permission from BMJ Publishing Group Ltd.[31]
Abbreviation: CI, confidence interval.
*Italics signify additions to the basic CONSORT 2010 guidelines.

Table 4.24 QC checklist for reports of randomized controlled trials: CONSORT—Reporting harms in randomized, controlled trials[a]

Standard CONSORT checklist paper section and topic	Standard CONSORT checklist item no.	Descriptor	Reported on pg. no.
Title and abstract.	1	If the study collected data on harms and benefits, the title or abstract should so state.	
Introduction/ Background.	2	If the trial addressed both harms and benefits, the introduction should so state.	
Methods.		–	
Participants.	3	–	
Interventions.	4	–	
Objectives.	5	–	
Outcomes.	6	List addressed adverse events with definitions for each (with attention, when relevant, to grading, expected vs. unexpected events, reference to standardized and validated definitions, and description of new definitions). Clarify how harms-related information was collected (mode of data collection, timing, attribution methods, intensity of ascertainment, and harms-related monitoring and stopping rules, if pertinent).	
Sample size.	7	–	
Randomization.	8	–	
Sequence generation.	9	–	
Allocation concealment.	10	–	
Implementation.	11	–	
Blinding (masking).	12	–	
Statistical methods.		Describe plans for presenting and analyzing information on harms (including coding, handling of recurrent events, specification of timing issues, handling of continuous measures, and any statistical analyses).	
Results.			
Participant flow.	13	Describe, for each arm, the participant withdrawals that are due to harms, and their experiences with the allocated treatment.	
Recruitment.	14	–	
Baseline data.	15	–	

(Continued)

Table 4.24 (Continued) QC checklist for reports of randomized controlled trials: CONSORT—Reporting harms in randomized controlled trials[a]

Standard CONSORT checklist paper section and topic	Standard CONSORT checklist item no.	Descriptor	Reported on pg. no.
Numbers analyzed.	16	Provide the denominators for analyses on harms.	
Outcomes and estimation.	17	Present the absolute risk per arm and per adverse event type, grade, and seriousness, and present appropriate metrics for recurrent events, continuous variables, whenever pertinent.[b]	
Ancillary analyses.	18	Describe any subgroup analyses and exploratory analyses for harms.[b]	
Adverse events.	19	–	
Discussion.		–	
Interpretation.	20	–	
Generalizability.	21	–	
Overall evidence.	22	Provide a balanced discussion of benefits and harms, with emphasis on study limitations, generalizability, and other sources of information on harms.[c]	

Source: Reproduced from *Annals of Internal Medicine*, Ioannidis JPA, Evans SJ, Gøtzsche PC et al. Better reporting of harms in randomized trials: an extension of the CONSORT statement. vol. 141, pages 781–8. Copyright ©2004. American College of Physicians. All rights reserved. Reprinted with permission from the American College of Physicians, Inc.[32]

[a] This proposed extension for harms includes 10 recommendations that correspond to the original CONSORT checklist.

[b] Descriptors refer to items 17, 18, and 19.

[c] Descriptor refers to items 20, 21, and 22.

Table 4.25 QC checklist for reports of randomized controlled trials: CONSORT—Abstracts

Item	Description
Title.	Identification of the study as randomized.
Authors.*	Contact details for the corresponding author.
Trial design.	Description of the trial design (e.g., parallel, cluster, noninferiority).
Methods.	
Participants.	Eligibility criteria for participants and the settings where the data were collected.
Interventions.	Interventions intended for each group.
Objective.	Specific objective or hypothesis.
Outcome.	Clearly defined primary outcome for this report.
Randomization.	How participants were allocated to interventions.
Blinding (masking).	Whether participants, care givers, and those assessing the outcomes were blinded to group assignment.
Results.	
Numbers randomized.	Number of participants analyzed in each group.
Recruitment.	Trial status.
Outcome.	For the primary outcome, a result for each group and the estimated effect size and its precision.
Harms.	Important adverse events or side effects.
Conclusions.	General interpretation of the results.
Trial registration.	Registration number and name of trial register.
Funding.	Source of funding.

Source: Reprinted from The Lancet, Hopewell S, Clarke M, Moher D et al. CONSORT for reporting randomised trials in journal and conference abstracts. vol. 371, pages 281–3. Copyright ©2008, with permission from Elsevier.[33]
*For conference abstracts.

Table 4.26 QC checklist. STROBE

Item	No.	Recommendation
Title and abstract.	1	(a) Indicate the study's design with a commonly used term in the title or the abstract.
		(b) Provide in the abstract an informative and balanced summary of what was done and what was found.
Introduction.		
Background/Rationale.	2	Explain the scientific background and rationale for the investigation being reported.
Objectives.	3	State specific objectives, including any prespecified hypotheses.
Methods.		
Study design.	4	Present key elements of study design early in the paper.
Setting.	5	Describe the setting, locations, and relevant dates, including periods of recruitment, exposure, follow-up, and data collection.
Participants.	6	(a) *Cohort study*—Give the eligibility criteria, and the sources and methods of selection of participants. Describe methods of follow-up.
		Case-control study—Give the eligibility criteria, and the sources and methods of case ascertainment and control selection. Give the rationale for the choice of cases and controls.
		Cross-sectional study—Give the eligibility criteria, and the sources and methods of selection of participants.
		(b) *Cohort study*—For matched studies, give matching criteria and number of exposed and unexposed.
		Case-control study—For matched studies, give matching criteria and the number of controls per case.
Variables.	7	Clearly define all outcomes, exposures, predictors, potential confounders, and effect modifiers. Give diagnostic criteria, if applicable.
Data sources/Measurement.	8*	For each variable of interest, give sources of data and details of methods of assessment (measurement). Describe comparability of assessment methods if there is more than one group.
Bias.	9	Describe any efforts to address potential sources of bias.
Study size.	10	Explain how the study size was arrived at.
Quantitative variables.	11	Explain how quantitative variables were handled in the analyses. If applicable, describe which groupings were chosen and why.
Statistical methods.	12	(a) Describe all statistical methods, including those used to control for confounding.
		(b) Describe any methods used to examine subgroups and interactions.
		(c) Explain how missing data were addressed.
		(d) *Cohort study*—If applicable, explain how loss to follow-up was addressed.
		Case-control study—If applicable, explain how matching of cases and controls was addressed.
		Cross-sectional study—If applicable, describe analytical methods, taking account of sampling strategy.
		(e) Describe any sensitivity analyses.

(Continued)

Table 4.26 (Continued) QC checklist. STROBE

Item	No.	Recommendation
Results.		
Participants.	13*	(a) Report numbers of individuals at each stage of study—e.g., numbers potentially eligible, examined for eligibility, confirmed eligible, included in the study, completing follow-up, and analyzed.
		(b) Give reasons for nonparticipation at each stage.
		(c) Consider use of a flow diagram.
Descriptive data.	14*	(a) Give characteristics of study participants (e.g., demographic, clinical, social) and information on exposures and potential confounders.
		(b) Indicate number of participants with missing data for each variable of interest.
		(c) *Cohort study*—Summarize follow-up time (e.g., average and total amount).
Outcome data.	15*	*Cohort study*—Report numbers of outcome events or summary measures over time.
		Case-control study—Report numbers in each exposure category, or summary measures of exposure.
		Cross-sectional study—Report numbers of outcome events or summary measures.
Main results.	16	(a) Give unadjusted estimates and, if applicable, confounder-adjusted estimates and their precision (e.g., 95% confidence interval). Make clear which confounders were adjusted for and why they were included.
		(b) Report category boundaries when continuous variables were categorized.
		(c) If relevant, consider translating estimates of relative risk into absolute risk for a meaningful time period.
Other analyses.	17	Report other analyses done—e.g., analyses of subgroups and interactions, and sensitivity analyses.
Discussion.		
Key results.	18	Summarize key results with reference to study objectives.
Limitations.	19	Discuss limitations of the study, taking into account sources of potential bias or imprecision. Discuss both direction and magnitude of any potential bias.
Interpretation.	20	Give a cautious overall interpretation of results, considering objectives, limitations, multiplicity of analyses, results from similar studies, and other relevant evidence.
Generalizability.	21	Discuss the generalizability (external validity) of the study results.
Other disclosures: funding.	22	Give the source of funding and the role of the funders for the present study and, if applicable, for the original study on which the present article is based.

Source: Reprinted from *The Lancet*, von Elm E, Altman DG, Egger M et al. The Strengthening the Reporting of Observational Studies in Epidemiology (STROBE) statement: guidelines for reporting observational studies. vol. 370, pages 1453–7. Copyright ©2007, with permission from Elsevier.[34]

*Give information separately for cases and controls in case-control studies and, if applicable, for exposed and unexposed groups in cohort and cross-sectional studies.

Table 4.27 QC checklist. REporting of studies Conducted using Observational Routinely collected health Data (STROBE–RECORD)

Item	No.	STROBE item	RECORD item
Title and abstract.	1	(a) Indicate study's design with a commonly used term in the title or the abstract.	**RECORD 1.1**: The type of data used should be specified in the title or abstract. When possible, the name of the databases used should be included.
		(b) Provide in the abstract an informative and balanced summary of what was done and what was found.	**RECORD 1.2**: If applicable, the geographic region and time frame within which the study took place should be reported in the title or abstract.
		–	**RECORD 1.3**: If linkage between databases was conducted for the study, this should be clearly stated in the title or abstract.
Introduction.			–
Background/ Rationale.	2	Explain the scientific background and rationale for the investigation being reported.	
Objectives.	3	State specific objectives, including any prespecified hypotheses.	–
Methods.			–
Study design.	4	Present key elements of study design early in the paper.	
Setting.	5	Describe the setting, locations, and relevant dates, including periods of recruitment, exposure, follow-up, and data collection.	–
Participants.	6	(a) *Cohort study*—Give the eligibility criteria and the sources and methods of selection of participants. Describe methods of follow-up.	**RECORD 6.1**: The methods of study population selection (e.g., codes or algorithms used to identify subjects) should be listed in detail. If this is not possible, an explanation should be provided.
		Case-control study—Give the eligibility criteria and the sources and methods of case ascertainment and control selection. Give the rationale for the choice of cases and controls.	**RECORD 6.2**: Any validation studies of the codes or algorithms used to select the population should be referenced. If validation was conducted for this study and not published elsewhere, detailed methods and results should be provided.
			RECORD 6.3: If the study involved linkage of databases, consider use of a flow diagram or other graphical display to demonstrate the data linkage process, including the number of individuals with linked data at each stage.

(Continued)

Table 4.27 (Continued) QC checklist. REporting of studies Conducted using Observational Routinely collected health Data (STROBE–RECORD)

Item	No.	STROBE item	RECORD item
		Cross-sectional study—Give the eligibility criteria and the sources and methods of selection of participants.	–
		(b) *Cohort study*—For matched studies, give matching criteria and number of exposed and unexposed.	–
		Case-control study—For matched studies, give matching criteria and the number of controls per case.	–
Variables.	7	Clearly define all outcomes, exposures, predictors, potential confounders, and effect modifiers. Give diagnostic criteria, if applicable.	**RECORD 7.1**: A complete list of codes and algorithms used to classify exposures, outcomes, confounders, and effect modifiers should be provided. If these cannot be reported, an explanation should be provided.
Data sources/ Measurement.	8	For each variable of interest, give sources of data and details of methods of assessment (measurement).	–
		Describe comparability of assessment methods if there is more than one group.	–
Bias.	9	Describe any efforts to address potential sources of bias.	–
Study size.	10	Explain how the study size was arrived at.	–
Quantitative variables.	11	Explain how quantitative variables were handled in the analyses. If applicable, describe which groupings were chosen and why.	–
Statistical methods.	12	(a) Describe all statistical methods, including those used to control for confounding.	–
		(b) Describe any methods used to examine subgroups and interactions.	–

(Continued)

Table 4.27 (Continued) QC checklist. REporting of studies Conducted using Observational Routinely collected health Data (STROBE–RECORD)

Item	No.	STROBE item	RECORD item
Statistical methods.		(c) Explain how missing data were addressed.	–
		(d) *Cohort study*—If applicable, explain how loss to follow-up was addressed.	–
		Case-control study—If applicable, explain how matching of cases and controls was addressed.	–
		Cross-sectional study—If applicable, describe analytical methods, taking account of sampling strategy.	–
		(e) Describe any sensitivity analyses.	–
Data access and cleaning methods.	12	–	RECORD 12.1: Authors should describe the extent to which the investigators had access to the database population used to create the study population. RECORD 12.2: Authors should provide information on the data cleaning methods used in the study.
Linkage.	12	–	RECORD 12.3: State whether the study included person-level, institutional-level, or other data linkage across two or more databases. The methods of linkage and methods of linkage quality evaluation should be provided.
Results. Participants.	13	(a) Report the numbers of individuals at each stage of the study (e.g., numbers potentially eligible, examined for eligibility, confirmed eligible, included in the study, completing follow-up, and analyzed).	RECORD 13.1: Describe in detail the selection of the persons included in the study (i.e., study population selection), including filtering based on data quality, data availability, and linkage. The selection of included persons can be described in the text and/or by means of the study flow diagram.
		(b) Give reasons for nonparticipation at each stage.	–
		(c) Consider use of a flow diagram.	–

(Continued)

Table 4.27 (Continued) QC checklist. REporting of studies Conducted using Observational Routinely collected health Data (STROBE–RECORD)

Item	No.	STROBE item	RECORD item
Descriptive data.	14	(a) Give characteristics of study participants (e.g., demographic, clinical, social) and information on exposures and potential confounders. (b) Indicate the number of participants with missing data for each variable of interest. (c) Cohort study: summarize follow-up time (e.g., average and total amount).	–
Outcome data.	15	*Cohort study*—Report numbers of outcome events or summary measures over time.	–
		Case-control study—Report numbers in each exposure category or summary measures of exposure.	–
		Cross-sectional study—Report numbers of outcome events or summary measures.	–
Main results.	16	(a) Give unadjusted estimates and, if applicable, confounder-adjusted estimates and their precision (e.g., 95% confidence interval). Make clear which confounders were adjusted for and why they were included.	–
		(b) Report category boundaries when continuous variables were categorized.	–
		(c) If relevant, consider translating estimates of relative risk into absolute risk for a meaningful time period.	–

(Continued)

Table 4.27 (Continued) QC checklist. REporting of studies Conducted using Observational Routinely collected health Data (STROBE–RECORD)

Item	No.	STROBE item	RECORD item
Other analyses.	17	Report other analyses done—e.g., analyses of subgroups and interactions and sensitivity analyses.	–
Discussion.			
Key results.	18	Summarize key results with reference to study objectives.	–
Limitations.	19	Discuss limitations of the study, taking into account sources of potential bias or imprecision. Discuss both direction and magnitude of any potential bias.	RECORD 19.1: Discuss the implications of using data that were not created or collected to answer the specific research question(s). Include discussion of misclassification bias, unmeasured confounding, missing data, and changing eligibility over time, as they pertain to the study being reported.
Interpretation.	20	Give a cautious overall interpretation of results, considering objectives, limitations, multiplicity of analyses, results from similar studies, and other relevant evidence.	–
Generalizability.	21	Discuss the generalizability (external validity) of the study results.	–
Funding.	22	Give the source of funding and the role of the funders for the present study and, if applicable, for the original study on which the present article is based.	–
Accessibility of protocol, raw data, and programming code.	–		RECORD 22.1: Authors should provide information on how to access any supplemental information such as the study protocol, raw data, or programming code.

Table 4.28 QC Checklist. Strengthening the Reporting of Observational Studies in Epidemiology/ Molecular Epidemiology (STROBE–ME)

Item	No.	STROBE guideline	Extension for STROBE–ME studies
Title and abstract.	1	(a) Indicate the study's design with a commonly used term in the title or the abstract.	ME-1 State the use of specific biomarker(s) in the title and/or in the abstract if they contribute substantially to the findings.
		(b) Provide in the abstract an informative and balanced summary of what was done and what was found.	–
Introduction. Background/ Rationale.	2	Explain the scientific background and rationale for the investigation being reported.	ME-2 Explain in the scientific background of the study how/ why the specific biomarker(s) have been chosen, potentially among many others (e.g., others studied but reported elsewhere, or not studied at all).
Objectives.	3	State specific objectives, including any prespecified hypotheses.	ME-3 *A priori* hypothesis: if one or more biomarkers are used as proxy measures, state the *a priori* hypothesis on the expected values of the biomarker(s).
Methods. Study design.	4	Present key elements of study design early in the paper.	ME-4 Describe the special study designs for molecular epidemiology (in particular nested case/control and case/ cohort) and how they were implemented.
Biological sample collection.		–	ME-4.1 Report on the setting of the biological sample collection; amount of sample; nature of collecting procedures; participant conditions; time between sample collection and relevant clinical or physiological endpoints.
Biological sample processing.		–	ME-4.2 Describe sample processing (centrifugation, timing, additives, etc.).
Biological sample storage.		–	ME-4.3 Describe sample storage until biomarker analysis (storage, thawing, manipulation, etc.).
Biomarker biochemical characteristics.		–	ME-4.4 Report the half-life of the biomarker, and chemical and physical characteristics (e.g., solubility).

(Continued)

Table 4.28 (Continued) QC checklist. Strengthening the Reporting of Observational Studies in Epidemiology/Molecular Epidemiology (STROBE–ME)

Item	No.	STROBE guideline	Extension for STROBE–ME studies
Setting.	5	Describe the setting, locations, and relevant dates, including periods of recruitment, exposure, follow-up, and data collection.	–
Participants.	6	(a) *Cohort study*—Give the eligibility criteria, and the sources and methods of selection of participants. Describe methods of follow-up.	**ME-6** Report any habit, clinical conditions, physiological factor, or working or living condition that might affect the characteristics or concentrations of the biomarker.
		Case-control study—Give the eligibility criteria, and the sources and methods of case ascertainment and control selection. Give the rationale for the choice of cases and controls.	–
		Cross-sectional study—Give the eligibility criteria, and the sources and methods of selection of participants.	–
		(b) *Cohort study*—For matched studies, give matching criteria and number of exposed and unexposed.	–
		Case-control study—For matched studies, give matching criteria and the number of controls per case.	
Variables.	7	Clearly define all outcomes, exposures, predictors, potential confounders, and effect modifiers. Give diagnostic criteria, if applicable.	–
Data source/measurement.	8	For each variable of interest, give sources of data and details of methods of assessment (measurement). Describe comparability of assessment methods if there is more than one group.	**ME-8** Laboratory methods: report type of assay used, detection limit, quantity of biological sample used, outliers, timing in the assay procedures (when applicable) and calibration procedures or any standard used.
Bias.	9	Describe any efforts to address potential sources of bias.	–

(Continued)

Table 4.28 (Continued) QC checklist. Strengthening the Reporting of Observational Studies in Epidemiology/Molecular Epidemiology (STROBE–ME)

Item	No.	STROBE guideline	Extension for STROBE–ME studies
Study size.	10	Explain how the study size was arrived at.	–
Quantitative variables.	11	Explain how quantitative variables were handled in the analyses. If applicable, describe which groupings were chosen, and why.	–
Statistical methods.	12	(a) Describe all statistical methods, including those used to control for confounding.	ME-12 Describe how biomarkers were introduced into statistical models.
		(b) Describe any methods used to examine subgroups and interactions.	–
		(c) Explain how missing data were addressed.	–
		(d) *Cohort study*—If applicable, explain how loss to follow-up was addressed.	–
		Case-control study—If applicable, explain how matching of cases and controls was addressed.	–
		Cross-sectional study—If applicable, describe analytical methods, taking account of sampling strategy.	
		(e) Describe any sensitivity analyses.	–
Validity/reliability of measurement and internal/ external validation.			ME-12.1 Report on the validity and reliability of measurement of the biomarker(s) coming from the literature and any internal or external validation used in the study.
Results.	13		ME-13 Give reason for loss of biological samples at each stage.
Participants.		(a) Report the numbers of individuals at each stage of the study–e.g., numbers potentially eligible, examined for eligibility, confirmed eligible, included in the study, completing follow-up, and analyzed.	
		(b) Give reasons for nonparticipation at each stage.	–
		(c) Consider use of a flow diagram.	–

(Continued)

Table 4.28 (Continued) QC checklist. Strengthening the Reporting of Observational Studies in Epidemiology/Molecular Epidemiology (STROBE–ME)

Item	No.	STROBE guideline	Extension for STROBE–ME studies
Descriptive data.	14	(a) Give characteristics of study participants (e.g., demographic, clinical, social) and information on exposures and potential confounders.	–
		(b) Indicate the number of participants with missing data for each variable of interest.	–
		(c) *Cohort study*—Summarize follow-up time (e.g., average and total amount).	–
Distribution of biomarker measurement.			**ME-14.1** Give the distribution of the biomarker measurement (including mean, median, range, and variance).
Outcome data.	15	*Cohort study*—Report numbers of outcome events or summary measures over time.	–
		Case-control study—Report numbers in each exposure category, or summary measures of exposure.	–
		Cross-sectional study—Report numbers of outcome events or summary measures.	–
Main results.	16	(a) Give unadjusted estimates and, if applicable, confounder-adjusted estimates and their precision (e.g., 95% confidence interval). Clarify which confounders were adjusted for and why they were included.	–
		(b) Report category boundaries when continuous variables were categorized.	–
		(c) If relevant, consider translating estimates of relative risk into absolute risk for a meaningful time period.	–

(Continued)

Table 4.28 (Continued) QC checklist. Strengthening the Reporting of Observational Studies in Epidemiology/Molecular Epidemiology (STROBE–ME)

Item	No.	STROBE guideline	Extension for STROBE–ME studies
Other analyses.	17	Report other analyses done—e.g., analyses of subgroups and interactions, and sensitivity analyses.	–
Discussion.			–
Key results.	18	Summarize key results with reference to study objectives.	
Limitations.	19	Discuss limitations of the study, taking into account sources of potential bias or imprecision. Discuss both direction and magnitude of any potential bias.	**ME-19** Describe main limitations in laboratory procedures.
Interpretation.	20	Give a cautious overall interpretation of results, considering objectives, limitations, multiplicity of analyses, results from similar studies, and other relevant evidence.	**ME-20** Give an interpretation of results in terms of *a priori* biological plausibility.
Generalizability.	21	Discuss the generalizability (external validity) of the study results.	–
Other information.	22		–
Funding.		Give the source of funding and the role of the funders for the present study and, if applicable, for the original study on which the present article is based.	
Ethics.			**ME-22.1** Describe informed consent and approval from ethical committee(s). Specify whether samples were anonymous, anonymized, or identifiable.

Source: Reproduced with permission from Gallo V, Egger M, McCormack V et al. STrengthening the Reporting of OBservational studies in Epidemiology–Molecular Epidemiology (STROBE–ME): an extension of the STROBE Statement. *PLoS Med* 2011;8:e1001117. Copyright ©2011 Gallo et al.[36] This is an open-access article distributed under the terms of the Creative Commons Attribution License, which permits unrestricted use, distribution, and reproduction in any medium, provided that the original author and source are credited.

Table 4.29 QC checklist. Strengthening the Reporting of Molecular Epidemiology for Infectious Diseases (STROME–ID): An extension of the STROBE statement

Item	No.	STROBE guideline	STROBE–STROME–ID extension
Title and abstract.	1	(a) Indicate the study's design with a commonly used term in the title or abstract. (b) Provide in the abstract an informative and balanced summary of what was done and what was found.	STROME–ID 1.1 The term "molecular epidemiology" should be applied to the study in the title or abstract and the key words when molecular and epidemiological methods contribute substantially to the study.
Introduction. Background/ Rationale.	2	Explain the scientific background and rationale for the investigation being reported.	STROME–ID 2.1 Provide background information about the pathogen population and the distribution of pathogen strains within the host population at risk.
Objectives.	3	State specific objectives, including any prespecified hypotheses.	STROME–ID 3.1 State the epidemiological objectives of using molecular typing.
Methods. Study design.	4	Present key elements of study design early in the paper.	
Molecular terminology.		–	STROME–ID 4.1 Define or cite definitions for key molecular terms used with the study (e.g., strain, isolate, clone).
Molecular markers.		–	STROME–ID 4.2 Clearly define the molecular markers that were used, with a standard nomenclature.
Infectious-disease case definition.		–	STROME–ID 4.3 Clearly state the infectious-disease definitions.
Laboratory methodology.			STROME–ID 4.4 Describe sample collection and laboratory methods, including any methods used to minimize and measure cross-contamination, and give the criteria used to interpret strain classification.
Setting.	5	Describe the setting, locations, and relevant dates, including periods of recruitment, exposure, follow-up, and data collection.	STROME–ID 5.1 Clearly state the timeframe of the study, consider and appropriately reference the molecular clock of markers if known, and the natural history of the infection.
Participants.	6	(a) *Cohort study*—Give the eligibility criteria and the sources and methods of selecting participants. Describe methods of follow-up.	STROME–ID 6.1 State the sources of participants and clinical specimens, and clearly describe sampling frame and strategy.

(Continued)

Table 4.29 (Continued) QC checklist. Strengthening the Reporting of Molecular Epidemiology for Infectious Diseases (STROME–ID): An extension of the STROBE statement

Item	No.	STROBE guideline	STROBE–STROME–ID extension
Participants.		*Case-control study*—Give the eligibility criteria, and the sources and methods of case ascertainment and control selection. Give the rationale for choosing cases and controls.	–
		Cross-sectional study—Give the eligibility criteria and sources and methods to select participants.	–
		(b) *Cohort study*—For matched studies, give matching criteria and number of exposed and unexposed.	–
		Case-control study—For matched studies, give matching criteria and number of controls per case.	–
Variables.	7	Clearly define all outcomes, exposures, predictors, potential confounders, and effect modifiers. Give diagnostic criteria (if applicable).	–
Data sources/ measurement.	8*	For each variable of interest, give sources of data and details of methods of assessment (measurement). Describe comparability of assessment methods if there is more than one group.	
Multiple-strain infections.			STROME–ID 8.1 Describe any methods used to detect multiple strain infections and measure their effect on the study findings.
Bias.	9	Describe any efforts to address potential sources of bias.	STROME–ID 9.1 Describe any effects made to address discovery or ascertainment bias.
Study size.	10	Explain how the study size was arrived at.	STROME–ID 10.1 Describe any unique restrictions placed on the study sample size.
Quantitative variables.	11	Explain how quantitative variables were handled in the analyses. If applicable, describe which groupings were chosen and why.	–

(Continued)

Table 4.29 (Continued) QC checklist. Strengthening the Reporting of Molecular Epidemiology for Infectious Diseases (STROME–ID): An extension of the STROBE statement

Item	No.	STROBE guideline	STROBE–STROME–ID extension
Statistical methods.	12	(a) Describe all statistical methods, including those used to control for confounding.	–
		(b) Describe any methods used to examine subgroups and interactions.	STROME–ID 12.1 State how the study took account of the nonindependence of sample data, if appropriate.
		(c) Explain how missing data were addressed.	STROME–ID 12.2 State how the study dealt with missing data.
		(d) *Cohort study*—If applicable, explain how loss to follow-up was addressed.	–
		Case-control study—If applicable, explain how matching of cases and controls was addressed.	–
		Cross-sectional study—If applicable, describe analytical methods taking account of sampling strategy.	–
		(e) Describe any sensitivity analyses.	–
Results.			–
Participants.	13*	(a) Report numbers of individuals at each stage of the study (e.g., numbers potentially eligible, examined for eligibility, confirmed eligible, included in the study, completing follow-up, and analyzed).	STROME–ID 13.1 Report numbers of participants and samples at each stage of the study, including the number of samples obtained, the number typed, and the number yielding data.
		(b) Give reasons why individuals did not participate at each stage.	STROME–ID 13.2 If the study investigates groups of genetically indistinguishable pathogens (molecular clusters), state the sampling fraction, the distribution of cluster sizes, and the study population turnover, if known.
		(c) Consider use of a flow diagram.	
Descriptive data.	14*	(a) Give characteristics of study participants (e.g., demographic, clinical, social) and information on exposures and potential confounders.	STROME–ID 14.1 Give information by strain type if appropriate, with use of standardized nomenclature.

(Continued)

Table 4.29 (Continued) QC checklist. Strengthening the Reporting of Molecular Epidemiology for Infectious Diseases (STROME–ID): An extension of the STROBE statement

Item	No.	STROBE guideline	STROBE–STROME–ID extension
		(b) Indicate the number of participants with missing data for each variable of interest.	–
		(c) *Cohort study*—Summarize follow-up time (e.g., average and total).	–
Outcome data.	15*	*Cohort study*—Report numbers of outcome events or summary measures over time.	–
		Case-control study—Report numbers in each exposure category or summary measures of exposure.	–
		Cross-sectional study—Report numbers of outcome events or summary measures.	–
Main results.	16	(a) Give unadjusted estimates and, if applicable, confounder-adjusted estimates and their precision (e.g., 95% confidence interval). Make clear which confounders were adjusted for and why they were included.	STROME–ID 16.1 Consider showing molecular relatedness of strain types by means of a dendrogram or phylogenetic tree.
		(b) Report category boundaries when continuous variables were categorized.	–
		(c) If relevant, consider translating estimates of relative risk into absolute risk for a meaningful time period.	–
Other analyses.	17	(a) Report other analyses done (e.g., analyses of subgroups and interactions and sensitivity analyses).	
Discussion.			
Key results.	18	Summarize key results with reference to study objectives.	
Limitations.	19	Discuss limitations of the study, taking into account sources of potential bias or imprecision. Discuss both direction and magnitude of any potential bias.	STROME–ID 19.1 Consider alternative explanations for findings when transmission chains are being investigated, and report the consistency between molecular and epidemiological evidence.

(Continued)

Table 4.29 (Continued) QC checklist. Strengthening the Reporting of Molecular Epidemiology for Infectious Diseases (STROME–ID): An extension of the STROBE statement

Item	No.	STROBE guideline	STROBE–STROME–ID extension
Interpretation.	20	Give a cautious overall interpretation of results, considering objectives, limitations, multiplicity of analyses, results from similar studies, and other relevant evidence.	
Generalizability.	21	Discuss the generalizability (external validity) of the study results.	
Other information.			
Funding.	22	Give the source of funding and the role of the funders for the present study and, if applicable, for the original study on which the present article is based.	
Ethics.	23		**STROME–ID 23.1** Report any ethical considerations with specific implications for infectious-disease molecular epidemiology.

Source: Reprinted from *The Lancet Infectious Disease*, Field N, Cohen T, Struelens MJ et al, Strengthening the Reporting of Molecular Epidemiology for Infectious Diseases (STROME–ID): an extension of the STROBE statement. vol. 14, pages 341–52. Copyright ©2014, with permission from Elsevier.[37]
*Give information separately for cases and controls in case-control studies and, if applicable, for exposed and unexposed groups in cohort and cross-sectional studies.

Table 4.30 QC checklist. ORION guidelines

Item	No.	Descriptor
Title and abstract.	1	Description of paper as an outbreak report or intervention study.
		Design of intervention study (e.g., Interrupted Time Series [ITS] with or without control group, crossover study).
		Brief description of intervention and main outcomes.
Introduction.		
Background.	2	Scientific and/or local clinical background and rationale.
		Description of organism as epidemic, endemic, or epidemic becoming endemic.
Type of paper.	3	Description of paper as intervention study or outbreak report. If an outbreak report, report the number of outbreaks.
Dates.	4	Start and finish dates of the study or report.
Objectives.	5	Objectives for outbreak reports. Hypotheses for intervention studies.
Methods.		Study design. Use EPOC classification, available at http://epoc.cochrane.org/epoc-taxonomy for ITS; or controlled before and after (CBA) study design.
Design.	6	Whether study was retrospective, prospective, or ambidirectional.
		Whether decision to report or intervene was prompted by any outcome data.
		Whether study was formally implemented with predefined protocol and endpoints.
Participants.	7	Number of patients admitted during the study or outbreak. Summaries of distributions of age and lengths of stays. If possible, proportion admitted from other wards, hospitals, nursing homes, or from abroad. Where relevant, potential risk factor for acquiring the organism. Eligibility criteria for study. Case definitions for outbreak report.
Setting.	8	Description of the unit, ward, or hospital and, if a hospital, the units included.
		Number of beds, the presence and staffing levels of an infection control team.
Interventions.	9	Definition of phases by major change in specific infection control practice (with start and stop dates). A summary table is strongly recommended, with precise details of interventions, how and when administered in each phase.
Culturing and typing.	10	Details of culture media, use of selective antibiotics, and local and/or reference typing. Where relevant, details of environmental sampling.
Infection-related outcomes.	11	Clearly defined primary and secondary outcomes (e.g., incidence of infection, colonization, bacteremia) at regular time intervals (e.g., daily, weekly, monthly) rather than as totals for each phase, with at least three data points per phase and, for many, two-phase studies, 12 or more monthly data points per phase. Denominators (e.g., numbers of admissions or discharges, patient bed days). If possible, prevalence of organism and incidence of colonization on admission at the same time intervals. Criteria for infection, colonization on admission, and directly attributable mortality. All-cause mortality.

(Continued)

Table 4.30 (Continued) QC checklist. ORION guidelines

Item	No.	Descriptor
		For short studies or outbreak reports, use of charts with duration patient stay and dates organisms detected may be useful.
Economic outcomes.	12	If a formal economic study was done, definition of outcomes to be reported, description of resources used in interventions, with costs broken down to basic units, stating important assumptions.
Potential threats to internal validity.	13	Which potential confounders were considered, recorded, or adjusted for (e.g., changes in length of stay, case mixture, bed occupancy, staffing levels, hand-hygiene compliance; antibiotic use, strain type, processing of isolates, seasonality).
		Description of measures to avoid bias, including blinding and standardization of outcome assessments and provision of care.
Sample size.	14	Details of power calculations, where appropriate.
Statistical methods.	15	Description of statistical methods to compare groups or phases. Methods for any subgroup or adjusted analyses, distinguishing between planned and unplanned (exploratory) analyses. Unless outcomes are independent, statistical approaches able to account for dependencies in the outcome data should be used, adjusting, where necessary, for potential confounders.
Description.		For outbreak reports, statistical analysis may be inappropriate.
Results. Recruitment.	16	For relevant designs, such as crossover studies, or where there are exclusions of groups of patients, the dates defining the periods of recruitment and follow-up, with a flow diagram describing participant flow in each phase.
Outcomes and estimation.	17	For the main outcomes, the estimated effect size and its precision (usually using confidence intervals). A graphical summary of the outcome data is often appropriate for dependent data (e.g., most time series).
Ancillary analyses.	18	Any subgroup analyses should be reported, and it should be stated whether or not it was planned (i.e., specified in the protocol) and adjusted for possible confounders.
Harms.	19	Prespecified categories of adverse events and occurrences of these in each intervention group. This might include drug side effects, crude or disease-specific mortality in antibiotic policy studies or opportunity costs in isolation studies.
Discussion. Interpretation.	20	
		For intervention studies, an assessment of evidence for/against hypotheses, accounting for potential threats to validity of inference, including regression to mean effects and reporting bias.
		For outbreak reports, consider the clinical significance of observations and hypotheses generated to explain them.
Generalizability.	21	External validity of the findings of an intervention study; i.e., to what degree can the results be expected to generalize to different target populations or settings. Feasibility of maintaining an intervention long term.
Overall evidence.	22	General interpretation of the results in context of current evidence.

Source: Reproduced with permission from Stone SP, Cooper BS, Kibbler CC et al. The ORION statement: guidelines for transparent reporting of outbreak reports and intervention studies of nosocomial infection. *J Antimicrob Chemother* 2007;59:833–40, by permission of the British Society for Antimicrobial Chemotherapy (BSAC).[38]
Abbreviations: EPOC, Effective Practice and Organisation of Care.

Table 4.31 QC checklist. STrengthening the REporting of Genetic Association studies (STROBE–STREGA)

Item	No.	STROBE guideline	STROBE–STREGA extension
Title and abstract.	1	(a) Indicate the study's design with a commonly used term in the title or abstract. (b) Provide in the abstract an informative and balanced summary of what was done and what was found.	–
Introduction.			
Background/ Rationale.	2	Explain the scientific background and rationale for the investigation being reported.	–
Objectives.	3	State specific objectives, including any prespecified hypotheses.	State if the study is the first report of a genetic association, a replication effort, or both.
Methods.			
Study design.	4	Present key elements of study design early in the paper.	–
Setting.	5	Describe the setting, locations, and relevant dates, including periods of recruitment, exposure, follow-up, and data collection.	–
Participants.	6	(a) *Cohort study*—Give the eligibility criteria and the sources and methods of selection of participants. Describe methods of follow-up.	Give information on the criteria and methods for selection of subsets of participants from a larger study, when relevant.
		Case-control study—Give the eligibility criteria and the sources and methods of case ascertainment and control selection. Give the rationale for the choice of cases and controls.	–
		Cross-sectional study—Give the eligibility criteria and the sources and methods of selection of participants.	–
		(b) *Cohort study*—For matched studies, give matching criteria and number of exposed and unexposed.	–
		Case-control study—For matched studies, give matching criteria and number of controls per case.	–

(Continued)

Table 4.31 (Continued) QC checklist. STrengthening the REporting of Genetic Association studies (STROBE–STREGA)

Item	No.	STROBE guideline	STROBE–STREGA extension
Variables.	7	(a) Clearly define all outcomes, exposures, predictors, potential confounders, and effect modifiers. Give diagnostic criteria, if applicable.	(b) Clearly define genetic exposures (genetic variants), using a widely used nomenclature system. Identify variables likely to be associated with population stratification (confounding by ethnic origin).
Data sources/ measurement.	8*	(a) For each variable of interest, give sources of data and detail methods of assessment (measurement). Describe comparability of methods of assessment methods if there is more than one group.	(b) Describe laboratory methods, including source and storage of DNA, genotyping methods and platforms (e.g., the allele-calling algorithm used and its version), error rates, and call rates. State the laboratory/center where genotyping was done. Describe comparability of laboratory methods if there is more than one group. Specify whether genotypes were assigned using all of the data from the study simultaneously or in smaller batches.
Bias.	9	(a) Describe any efforts to address potential sources of bias.	(b) For quantitative outcome variables, specify if any investigation of potential bias resulting from pharmacotherapy was undertaken. If relevant, describe the nature and magnitude of the potential bias and explain what approach was used to deal with this.
Study size.	10	Explain how the study size was arrived at.	–
Quantitative variables.	11	Explain how quantitative variables were handled in the analyses. If applicable, describe which groupings were chosen and why.	If applicable, describe how effects of treatment were dealt with.
Statistical methods.	12	(a) Describe all statistical methods, including those used to control for confounding.	State software version used and options (or settings) chosen.
		(b) Describe any methods used to examine subgroups and interactions.	–
		(c) Explain how missing data were addressed.	–

(Continued)

Table 4.31 (Continued) QC checklist. STrengthening the REporting of Genetic Association studies (STROBE–STREGA)

Item	No.	STROBE guideline	STROBE–STREGA extension
		(d) *Cohort study*—If applicable, explain how loss to follow-up was addressed.	–
Results.		*Case-control study*—If applicable, explain how matching of cases and controls was addressed.	–
		Cross-sectional study—If applicable, describe analytical methods, taking account of sampling strategy.	–
		(e) Describe any sensitivity analyses.	(f) State whether Hardy–Weinberg equilibrium was considered and, if so, how.
		–	(g) Describe any methods used to infer genotypes or haplotypes.
			(h) Describe any methods used to assess or address population stratification.
		–	(i) Describe any methods used to address multiple comparisons or to control risk of false-positive findings.
		–	(j) Describe any methods used to address and correct for relatedness among subjects.
Participants.	13*	(a) Report the numbers of individuals at each stage of the study—e.g., numbers potentially eligible, examined for eligibility, confirmed eligible, included in the study, completing follow-up, and analyzed.	Report numbers of individuals in whom genotyping was attempted and numbers of individuals in whom genotyping was successful.
		(b) Give reasons for nonparticipation at each stage.	–
		(c) Consider use of a flow diagram.	–
Descriptive data.	14*	(a) Give characteristics of study participants (e.g., demographic, clinical, social) and information on exposures and potential confounders.	Consider giving information by genotype.
		(b) Indicate the number of participants with missing data for each variable of interest.	–

(Continued)

Table 4.31 (Continued) QC checklist. STrengthening the REporting of Genetic Association studies (STROBE–STREGA)

Item	No.	STROBE guideline	STROBE–STREGA extension
Results.		(c) *Cohort study*—Summarize follow-up time e.g., average and total amount.	–
Outcome data.	**15***	*Cohort study*—Report numbers of outcome events or summary measures over time.	Report outcomes (phenotypes) for each genotype category over time.
		Case-control study—Report numbers in each exposure category or summary measures of exposure.	Report numbers in each genotype category.
		Cross-sectional study—Report numbers of outcome events or summary measures.	Report outcomes (phenotypes) for each genotype category.
Main results.	**16**	(a) Give unadjusted estimates and, if applicable, confounder-adjusted estimates and their precision (e.g., 95% confidence intervals). Make clear which confounders were adjusted for and why they were included.	–
		(b) Report category boundaries when continuous variables were categorized.	–
		(c) If relevant, consider translating estimates of relative risk into absolute risk for a meaningful time period.	–
		–	(d) Report results of any adjustments for multiple comparisons.
Other analyses.	**17**	(a) Report other analyses done—e.g., analyses of subgroups and interactions and sensitivity analyses.	–
		–	(b) If numerous genetic exposures (genetic variants) were examined, summarize results from all analyses undertaken.
		–	(c) If detailed results are available elsewhere, state how they can be accessed.
Discussion. Key results.	**18**	Summarize key results, with reference to study objectives.	–

(Continued)

Table 4.31 (Continued) QC checklist. STrengthening the REporting of Genetic Association studies (STROBE–STREGA)

Item	No.	STROBE guideline	STROBE–STREGA extension
Limitations.	19	Discuss limitations of the study, taking into account sources of potential bias or imprecision. Discuss both direction and magnitude of any potential bias.	–
Interpretation.	20	Give a cautious overall interpretation of results, considering objectives, limitations, multiplicity of analyses, results from similar studies, and other relevant evidence.	–
Generalizability.	21	Discuss the generalizability (external validity) of the study results.	–
Other information.			
Funding.	22	Give the source of funding and the role of the funders for the present study and, if applicable, for the original study on which the present article is based.	–

Source: Reproduced with permission from Little J, Higgins JPA, Ioannidis JPA et al. STrengthening the REporting of Genetic Association Studies (STREGA): an extension of the STROBE statement. *PLoS Med* 2009;6:e1000022.[39] This is an open-access article distributed under the terms of the Creative Commons Public Domain declaration, which stipulates that, once placed in the public domain, this work may be freely reproduced, distributed, transmitted, modified, built upon, or otherwise used by anyone for any lawful purpose. Copyright ©2009 Little J et al. Article available at: https://doi.org/10.1371/journal.pmed.1000022.

*Give information separately for cases and controls in case-control studies and, if applicable, for exposed and unexposed groups in cohort and cross-sectional studies.

Table 4.32 QC checklist. STrengthening the REporting of Immunogenomic Studies (STROBE–STREIS) statement

Item	No.	STROBE guideline	STROBE–STREGA extension	STROBE–STREGA–STREIS extension for immunogenomic studies
Methods. Variables.	7	Clearly define all outcomes, exposures, predictors, potential confounders, and effect modifiers. Give diagnostic criteria, if applicable.	Clearly define genetic exposures (genetic variants), using a widely used nomenclature system. Identify variables likely to be associated with population stratification (confounding by ethnic origin).	Describe HLA alleles in accordance with WHO Nomenclature Committee for Factors of the HLA System.
		–	–	Identify the IMGT/HLA database release number pertinent to the data.
		–	–	Describe KIR alleles in accordance with the IPD-KIR database.
		–	–	Identify the IPD-KIR database release number pertinent to the data.
Data sources/ Measurement.	8	For each variable of interest, give sources of data and details of methods of assessment (measurement). Describe comparability of assessment methods if there is more than one group.	Describe laboratory methods, including source and storage of DNA, genotyping methods and platforms (e.g., allele calling algorithm used and its version), error rates, and call rates.	Provide access to the primary, ambiguous genotype data for each individual.

(Continued)

Table 4.32 (Continued) QC checklist. STrengthening the REporting of Immunogenomic Studies (STROBE–STREIS) statement

Item	No.	STROBE guideline	STROBE–STREGA extension	STROBE–STREGA–STREIS extension for immunogenomic studies
Data sources/ measurement.	8	–	State the laboratory/ center where genotyping was done. Describe comparability of laboratory methods if there is more than one group.	Describe the system(s) used to store, manage, and validate genotype and allele data, and to prepare data for analysis.
		–	Specify whether genotypes were assigned using all of the data from the study simultaneously, or in smaller batches.	Use objective terms, identifying features assessed for each gene, to describe genotyping systems and genotyping results. Avoid using subjective terms (e.g., low, intermediate, high, or allele resolution), that may change over time, to describe genotyping systems and results.
		–	–	Document all methods applied to resolve ambiguity.
		–	–	Define any codes used to represent ambiguities.
		–	–	Describe any binning or combining of alleles into common categories that were performed.
Statistical methods.	12	Describe all statistical methods, including those used to control for confounding.	State software version used and options (or settings) chosen.	Discuss any modifications made to the data to have them comport to the expectations of a method for the purpose of analysis.

(Continued)

Table 4.32 (Continued) QC checklist. STrengthening the REporting of Immunogenomic Studies (STROBE–STREIS) statement

Item	No.	STROBE guideline	STROBE–STREGA extension	STROBE–STREGA–STREIS extension for immunogenomic studies
Statistical methods.	12	–	–	Document any caveats associated with each analysis as they pertain to immunogenic data.
Discussion. Limitations.	19	Discuss limitations of the study, taking into account sources of potential bias or imprecision.	–	Discuss the impact of any modifications made to the data for analysis.
		Discuss both the direction and magnitude of any potential bias.	–	Discuss any caveats associated with each analysis as they pertain to immunogenomic data.
			–	Discuss any potential impact of ambiguity resolution on the results.

Source: Reproduced from Hollenbach JA, Mack SJ, Gourraud PA et al. A community standard for immunogenomic data reporting and analysis: proposal for a STrengthening the REporting of Immunogenomic Studies statement. *Tissue Antigens* 2011;78:333–44. Copyright ©2011 Hollenbach JA et al. With permission from John Wiley & Sons, Inc.[40]

Abbreviations: HLA, human leukocyte antigen; IMGT, International ImMunoGeneTics database; IPD, Immuno Polymorphism Database; KIR, killer-cell immunoglobulin-like receptors; WHO, World Health Organization.

Table 4.33 QC checklist. GRIPS

Item	No.	Recommendation
Title and abstract.	1	(a) Identify the article as a study of risk prediction using genetic factors.
		(b) Use recommended key words in the abstract: genetic or genomic, risk, prediction.
Introduction.		
Background/ Rationale	2	Explain the scientific background and rationale for the prediction study.
Objectives	3	Specify the study objectives and state the specific model(s) that is/are investigated. State if the study concerns the development of the model(s), a validation effort, or both.
Methods.		
Study design and setting.	4*	Specify the key elements of the study design and describe the setting, locations, and relevant dates, including periods of recruitment, follow-up, and data collection.
Participants.	5*	Describe eligibility criteria and sources and methods of selection of participants.
Variables definition.	6*	Clearly define all participant characteristics, risk factors, and outcomes. Clearly define genetic variants, using a widely used nomenclature system.
Variables assessment.	7*	(a) Describe sources of data and details of methods of assessment (measurement) for each variable.
		(b) Give a detailed description of genotyping and other laboratory methods.
Variables coding.	8	(a) Describe how genetic variants were handled in the analyses.
		(b) Explain how other quantitative variables were handled in the analyses. If applicable, describe which groupings were chosen, and why.
Analysis: risk model construction.	9	Specify the procedure and data used for the derivation of the risk model. Specify which candidate variables were initially examined or considered for inclusion in models. Include details of any variable selection procedures and other model-building issues. Specify the time horizon of risk prediction (e.g., 5-year risk).
Analysis: validation.	10	Specify the procedure and data used for the validation of the risk model.
Analysis: missing data.	11	Specify how missing data were handled.
Analysis: statistical methods.	12	Specify all measures used for the evaluation of the risk model, including, but not limited to, measures of model fit and predictive ability.
Analysis: other.	13	Describe all subgroups, interactions, and exploratory analyses that were examined.
Results.		
Participants.	14*	Report the numbers of individuals at each stage of the study. Give reasons for nonparticipation at each stage. Report the number of participants not genotyped, and reasons why they were not genotyped.

(Continued)

Table 4.33 (Continued) QC checklist. GRIPS

Item	No.	Recommendation
Descriptives: population.	15*	Report demographic and clinical characteristics of the study population, including risk factors used in the risk modeling.
Descriptives: model estimates.	16	Report unadjusted associations between the variables in the risk model(s) and the outcome. Report adjusted estimates and their precision from the full risk model(s) for each variable.
Risk distributions.	17*	Report distributions of predicted risks and/or risk scores.
Assessment.	18	Report measures of model fit and predictive ability, and any other performance measures, if pertinent.
Validation.	19	Report any validation of the risk model(s).
Other analyses.	20	Present results of any subgroup, interaction, or exploratory analyses, whenever pertinent.
Discussion.		
Limitations.	21	Discuss limitations and assumptions of the study, particularly those concerning study design, selection of participants, and measurements and analyses, and discuss their impact on the results of the study.
Interpretation.	22	Give an overall interpretation of results, considering objectives, limitations, multiplicity of analyses, results from similar studies, and other relevant evidence.
Generalizability.	23	Discuss the generalizability of the findings and, if pertinent, the health care relevance of the study results.
Supplementary information.	24	State whether databases for the analyzed data, risk models, and/or protocols are or will become publicly available and, if so, how they can be accessed.
Funding.	25	Give the source of funding and the role of the funders for the present study. State whether there are any conflicts of interests.

Source: Reproduced with permission from Janssens ACJW, Ioannidis JPA, van Duijn CM et al. Strengthening the reporting of Genetic RIsk Prediction Studies: the GRIPS Statement. *PLoS Med* 2011;8:e1000420.[41] This is an open-access article distributed under the terms of the Creative Commons Public Domain declaration, which stipulates that, once placed in the public domain, this work may be freely reproduced, distributed, transmitted, modified, built upon, or otherwise used by anyone for any lawful purpose. Copyright ©2011. Janssens ACJW et al. Article available at: https://doi.org/10.1371/journal.pmed.1000420.

*Items with asterisks should be reported for every population in the study.

Table 4.34 QC checklist. CHEERS: Items to include when reporting economic evaluations of health interventions

Item	No.	Recommendation	On pg no.
Title.	1	Identify the study as an economic evaluation or use more specific terms such as "cost-effectiveness analysis," and describe the interventions compared.	
Abstract.	2	Provide a structured summary of objectives, perspective, setting, methods (including study design and inputs), results (including base-case and uncertainty analyses), and conclusions.	
Introduction. Background/ Objectives.	3	Provide an explicit statement of the broader context for the study. Present the study question and its relevance for health policy or practice decisions.	
Methods. Target population and subgroups.	4	Describe characteristics of the base-case population and subgroups analyzed, including why they were chosen.	
Setting and location.	5	State relevant aspects of the system(s) in which the decision(s) need(s) to be made.	
Study perspective.	6	Describe the perspective of the study and relate this to the costs being evaluated.	
Comparators.	7	Describe the interventions or strategies being compared and state why they were chosen.	
Time horizon.	8	State the time horizon(s) over which costs and consequences are being evaluated and say why appropriate.	
Discount rate.	9	Report the choice of discount rate(s) used for cost and outcomes, and say why appropriate.	
Choice of health outcomes.	10	Describe what outcomes were used as the measure(s) of benefit in the evaluation and their relevance for the type of analysis performed.	
Measurement of effectiveness.	11a	*Single study-based estimates*: Describe fully the design features of the single effectiveness study and why the single study was a sufficient source of clinical effectiveness data.	
	11b	*Synthesis-based estimates*: Describe fully the methods used for identification of included studies and synthesis of clinical effectiveness data.	
Measurement and valuation of preference-based outcomes.	12	If applicable, describe the population and methods used to elicit preferences for health outcomes.	

(Continued)

Table 4.34 (Continued) QC checklist. CHEERS: Items to include when reporting economic evaluations of health interventions

Item	No.	Recommendation	On pg no.
Estimating resources and costs.	13a	*Single study–based economic evaluation*: Describe approaches used to estimate resource use associated with the alternative interventions. Describe primary or secondary research methods for valuing each resource item in terms of its unit cost. Describe any adjustments made to approximate to opportunity costs.	
	13b	*Model-based economic evaluation*: Describe approaches and data sources used to estimate resource use associated with model health states. Describe primary or secondary research methods for valuing each resource item in terms of its unit cost. Describe any adjustments made to approximate to opportunity costs.	
Currency, price date, and conversion.	14	Report the dates of the estimated resource quantities and unit costs. Describe methods for adjusting estimated unit costs to the year of reported costs if necessary. Describe methods for converting costs into a common currency base and the exchange rate.	
Choice of model.	15	Describe and give reasons for the specific type of decision-analytic model used. Providing a figure to show model structure is strongly recommended.	
Assumptions.	16	Describe all structural or other assumptions underpinning the decision-analytic model.	
Analytical methods.	17	Describe all analytical methods supporting the evaluation. This could include methods for dealing with skewed, missing, or censored data; extrapolation methods; methods for pooling data; approaches to validate or make adjustments (such as half-cycle corrections) to a model; and methods for handling population heterogeneity and uncertainty.	
Results.			
Study parameters.	18	Report the values, ranges, references, and, if used, probability distributions for all parameters. Report reasons or sources for distributions used to represent uncertainty where appropriate. Providing a table to show the input values is strongly recommended.	

(Continued)

Table 4.34 (Continued) QC checklist. CHEERS: Items to include when reporting economic evaluations of health interventions

Item	No.	Recommendation	On pg no.
Incremental costs and outcomes.	19	For each intervention, report mean values for the main categories of estimated costs and outcomes of interest, as well as mean differences between the comparator groups. If applicable, report incremental cost-effectiveness ratios.	
Characterizing uncertainty.	20a	*Single study–based economic evaluation*: Describe the effects of sampling uncertainty for the estimated incremental cost and incremental effectiveness parameters, together with the impact of methodological assumptions (such as discount rate, study perspective).	
	20b	*Model-based economic evaluation*: Describe the effects on the results of uncertainty for all input parameters, and uncertainty related to the structure of the model and assumptions.	
Characterizing heterogeneity.	21	If applicable, report differences in costs, outcomes, or cost-effectiveness that can be explained by variations between subgroups of patients with different baseline characteristics or other observed variability in effects that are not reducible by more information.	
Discussion.	22	Summarize key study findings and describe how they support the conclusions reached. Discuss limitations, the generalizability of the findings, and how they fit with current knowledge.	
Study findings, limitations, generalizability, and current knowledge.			
Other.			
Source of funding.	23	Describe how the study was funded and the role of the funder in the identification, design, conduct, and reporting of the analysis. Describe other nonmonetary sources of support.	
Conflicts of interests.	24	Describe any potential for conflict of interests among study contributors, in accordance with journal policy. In the absence of a journal policy, we recommend that authors comply with International Committee of Medical Journal Editors' recommendations.	

Source: Reproduced from *BMJ*, Husereau D, Drummond M, Petrou S et al. Consolidated Health Economic Evaluation Reporting Standards (CHEERS) statement. vol. 346, page f10149. Copyright ©2013 with permission from BMJ Publishing Group Ltd.[42]

Table 4.35 QC checklist. TREND

Item	No.	Description	Examples from HIV behavioral prevention research
Title and abstract.	1	Information on how units were allocated to interventions.	Example (title): A nonrandomized trial of a clinic-based HIV counseling intervention for African American female drug users.
		Structured abstract recommended.	–
		Information on target population or study sample.*	–
Introduction/ Background.	2	Scientific background and explanation of rationale.	Example (theory used): The community-based AIDS intervention was based on social learning theory.
		Theories used in designing behavioral interventions.	
Methods. Participants.	3	Eligibility criteria for participants, **including criteria at different levels in recruitment/sampling plan (e.g., cities, clinics, subjects).**	–
		Method of recruitment (e.g., referral, self-selection), including the **sampling method** if a systematic sampling plan was implemented.	Example (sampling method): Using an alphanumeric sorted list of possible venues and times for identifying eligible subjects, every tenth venue-time unit was selected for the location and timing of recruitment.
		Recruitment setting.	Example (recruitment setting): Subjects were approached by peer opinion leaders during conversations at gay bars.
		Settings and location where the data were collected.	–
Interventions.	4	Details of the interventions intended for each study condition and how and when they were actually administered, specifically including:	–
		Content: What was given?	–
		Delivery method: How was the intervention given?	–
		Unit of delivery: How were subjects grouped during delivery?	Example (unit of delivery): The intervention was delivered to small groups of 5 to 8 subjects.
		Deliverer: Who delivered the intervention?	–

(Continued)

Table 4.35 (Continued) QC checklist. TREND

Item	No.	Description	Examples from HIV behavioral prevention research
Interventions.	4	**Setting: Where was the intervention delivered?**	Examples (setting): The intervention was delivered in bars; the intervention was delivered in the waiting rooms of sexually transmitted disease clinics.
		Exposure quantity and duration: How many sessions or episodes or events intended to be delivered? How long were they intended to last?	Examples (exposure quantity and duration): The intervention was delivered in five 1-hour sessions: the intervention consisted of standard HIV counseling and testing (pretest and post-test counseling sessions, each about 30 minutes).
		Time span: How long was it intended to take to deliver the intervention to each unit?	Examples (time span): Each intervention session was to be delivered (in five 1-hour sessions) once a week for 5 weeks; the intervention was to be delivered over a 1-month period.
		Activities to increase adherence (e.g., compliance or incentives).	Example (activities to increase adherence): Bus tokens and food stamps were provided.
Objectives.	5	Specific objectives and hypotheses.	–
Outcomes.	6	Clearly defined primary and secondary outcome measures.	–
		Methods used to collect data and any methods used to enhance the quality of measurements.	Examples (method used to collect data): Self-report of behavioral data using a face-to-face interviewer-administered questionnaire; audio-computer-assisted self-administered instrument.
		Information on validated instruments such as psychometric and biometric properties.	–
Sample size.	7	How sample size was determined and, when applicable, explanation of any interim analyses and stopping rules.	–

(Continued)

Table 4.35 (Continued) QC checklist. TREND

Item	No.	Description	Examples from HIV behavioral prevention research
Assignment method.	8	**Unit of assignment (the unit being assigned to study condition, e.g., individual, group, community).**	Example 1 (assignment method): Subjects were assigned to study conditions using an alternating sequence wherein every other individual enrolled (e.g., 1,3,5) was assigned to the intervention condition and the alternate subjects enrolled (e.g., 2,4,6) were assigned to the comparison condition.
		Method used to assign units to study conditions, including details of any restriction (e.g., blocking, stratification, minimization).	–
		Inclusion of aspects employed to help minimize potential bias induced by nonrandomization (e.g., matching).	–
			Example 2 (assignment method): For odd weeks (e.g., 1,3,5), subjects attending the clinic on Monday, Wednesday, and Friday were assigned to the intervention condition, and those attending the clinic on Tuesday and Thursday were assigned to the comparison condition; this assignment was reversed for even weeks.
Blinding (masking).	9	Whether or not participants, those administering the interventions, and those assessing the outcomes were blinded to study condition assignment; if so, statement regarding how the blinding was accomplished and how it was assessed.	Example (blinding): The staff member performing the assessments was not involved in implementing any aspect of the intervention and knew the participants only by their study identifier numbers.
Unit of analysis.	10	**Description of the smallest unit that is being analyzed to assess intervention effects (e.g., individual, group, or community).**	Example 1 (unit of analysis): Since groups of individuals were assigned to study conditions, the analyses were performed at the group level, where mixed-effects models were used to account for random subject effects within each group.

(Continued)

Table 4.35 (Continued) QC checklist. TREND

Item	No.	Description	Examples from HIV behavioral prevention research
Unit of analysis.	10	**If the unit of analysis differs from the unit of assignment, the analytical method used to account for this (e.g., adjusting the standard error estimates by the design effect or using multilevel analysis).**	Example 2 (unit of analysis): Since analyses were performed at the individual level, and communities were randomized, a prior estimate of the intraclass correlation coefficient was used to adjust the standard error estimates before calculating confidence intervals.
Statistical methods.	11	Statistical methods used to compare study groups for primary outcome(s), including complex methods for correlated data.	–
		Statistical methods used for additional analyses, such as subgroup analyses and adjusted analysis.	–
		Methods for imputing missing data, if used.	–
		Statistical software or programs used.	–
Results.			–
Participant flow.	12	Flow of participants through each stage of the study: enrollment, assignment, allocation, and intervention exposure, follow-up, analysis (a diagram is strongly recommended).	
		Enrollment: the numbers of participants screened for eligibility, found to be eligible or not eligible, declined to be enrolled, and enrolled in the study.	–
		Assignment: the numbers of participants assigned to a study condition.	–
		Allocation and intervention exposure: the number of participants assigned to each study condition and the number who received each intervention.	–
		Follow-up: the number of participants who completed the follow-up or did not complete the follow-up (i.e., lost to follow-up), by study condition.	–

(Continued)

Table 4.35 (Continued) QC checklist. TREND

Item	No.	Description	Examples from HIV behavioral prevention research
Results. Participant flow.	12	Analysis: The number of participants included in or excluded from the main analysis, by study condition.	–
		Description of protocol deviations from study as planned, along with reasons.	–
Recruitment.	13	Dates defining the periods of recruitment and follow-up.	–
Baseline data.	14	Baseline demographic and clinical characteristics of participants in each study condition.	–
		Baseline characteristics for each study condition relevant to specific disease prevention research.	Example (baseline characteristics specific to HIV prevention research): HIV serostatus and HIV testing behavior.
		Baseline comparisons of those lost to follow-up and those retained, overall and by study condition.	–
		Comparison between study population at baseline and target population of interest.	–
Baseline equivalence.	15	**Data on study group equivalence at baseline and statistical methods used to control for baseline differences.**	Example (baseline equivalence): The intervention and comparison groups did not statistically differ with respect to demographic data (gender, age, race/ethnicity: $p > 0.05$ for each), but the intervention group reported a significantly greater baseline frequency of injection drug use ($p = 0.03$); all regression analyses included baseline frequency of injection drug use as a covariate in the models.
Numbers analyzed.	16	Number of participants (denominator) included in each analysis for each study condition, particularly when the denominators change for different outcomes; statement of the results in absolute numbers when feasible.	Example (number of participants included in the analysis): The analysis of condom use included only those who reported at the 6-month follow-up having had vaginal or anal sex in the past 3 months (75/125 for intervention group and 35/60 for standard group).

(Continued)

Table 4.35 (Continued) QC checklist. TREND

Item	No.	Description	Examples from HIV behavioral prevention research
Numbers analyzed.	16	Indication of whether the analysis strategy was "intention to treat," or, if not, description of how noncompliers were treated in the analyses.	Example ("intention to treat"): The primary analysis was intention to treat and included all subjects as assigned with available 9-month outcome data (125 of 176 assigned to the intervention and 110 of 164 assigned to the standard condition).
Outcomes and estimations.	17	For each primary and secondary outcome, a summary of results for each study condition, and the estimated effect size and a confidence interval to indicate the precision.	–
		Inclusion of null and negative findings.	–
		Inclusion of results from testing prespecified causal pathways through which the intervention was intended to operate, if any.	–
Ancillary analyses.	18	Summary of other analyses performed, including subgroup or restricted analyses, indicating which are prespecified or exploratory.	Example (ancillary analyses): Although the study was not powered for this hypothesis, an exploratory analysis shows that the intervention effect was greater among women than men (although not statistically significant).
Adverse events.	19	Summary of all important adverse events or unintended effects in each study condition (including summary measures, effect size estimates, and confidence intervals).	Example (adverse events): Police cracked down on prostitution, which drove the target population, commercial sex workers, to areas outside the recruitment/sampling area.
Discussion. Interpretation.	20	Interpretation of the results, taking into account study hypotheses, sources of potential bias, imprecision of measures, multiplicative analyses, and other limitations or weaknesses of the study.	–

(Continued)

Table 4.35 (Continued) QC checklist. TREND

Item	No.	Description	Examples from HIV behavioral prevention research
Discussion. Interpretation.	20	**Discussion of results, taking into account the mechanism by which the intervention was intended to work (causal pathways) or alternative mechanisms or explanations.**	–
		Discussion of the success of and barriers to implementing the intervention, fidelity of implementation.	–
		Discussion of research, **programmatic, or policy implications.**	–
Generalizability.	21	Generalizability (external validity) of trial findings, taking into account the study population, the characteristics of the intervention, length of follow-up, **incentives, compliance rates, specific sites/ settings involved in the study,** and other contextual issues.	–
Overall evidence.	22	General interpretation of the results in the context of current evidence and theory.	–

Source: Reproduced from Des Jarlais DC, Lyles C, Crepaz N. Improving the reporting quality of nonrandomized evaluations of behavioral and public health interventions: the TREND statement. *Am J Public Health* 2004;94:361–6.[43]

*Descriptors appearing in boldface are specifically added, modified, or further emphasized from the CONSORT statement. Boldface topic/descriptors are not included in the CONSORT statement but are relevant for behavioral interventions using nonrandomized experimental designs.

Public domain: The TREND 22-item checklist is made available on a US government (Centers for Disease Control and Prevention) website. Available at http://www.cdc.gov/trendstatement. Last accessed October 28, 2017.

Table 4.36 QC checklist. Good research practices for comparative effectiveness research (ISPOR Good Research Practices for Retrospective Database Analysis Task Force Report—Part 1)—Adaptation of CONSORT and STROBE recommendations to reporting of observational (comparative effectiveness) studies

Section and topic	Item no.	Descriptor
Study design.	1	Description of study design.
Introduction.		
Background.	2	Scientific background and explanation of rationale, including discussion of the suitability of the database employed.
Methods. • Defining the question. • Objectives. • Selection of study design. • Selection of data source. • Definition of treatment cohorts.	3	Clearly defined goals of the study with description of specific subquestions. Description of study design and why it was chosen. Description of strengths and weaknesses of data source and how study groups were identified, including description of critical variables: diagnostic criteria, exposures, and potential confounders.
Measurements of treatment effects; classification bias.	4	Discuss how treatment effects were measured and how classification bias was addressed.
Measurement of outcomes; classification bias.	5	Discuss how outcomes were measured and how classification bias was addressed.
Confounding: • By indication. • Measured vs. unmeasured variables. • Time dependent. Analytic plan to address confounding.	6	Discuss the potential for confounding, both measured and unmeasured, and how this was assessed and addressed.
Discussion. • Internal validity.	7	Interpretation of results, taking into account confounding and imprecision of results.
• Generalizability.	8	Generalizability (external validity) of the study findings.
• Overall evidence.	9	General interpretation of the results in the context of current evidence.

Source: Reprinted from Berger ML, Mamdani M, Atkins D et al. Good research practices for comparative effectiveness research: defining, reporting and interpreting nonrandomized studies of treatment effects using secondary data sources: the ISPOR Good Research Practices for Retrospective Database Analysis Task Force Report—Part I. *Value Health.* vol. 12, pages 1044–52. Copyright ©2009 with permission from the International Society for Pharmacoeconomics and Outcomes Research (ISPOR).[44]

Table 4.37 QC checklist. SQUIRE

Text section	Section or item description
Title and abstract.	Did you provide clear and accurate information for finding, indexing, and scanning your paper?
1. Title.	(a) Indicates that the article concerns the improvement of quality (broadly defined to include the safety, effectiveness, patient-centeredness, timeliness, efficiency, and equity of care).
	(b) States the specific aim of the Intervention.
	(c) Specifies the study method used (e.g., "A qualitative study" or "A randomized cluster trial").
2. Abstract.	Summarizes precisely all key information from various sections of the text using the abstract format of the intended publication.
Introduction.	Why did you start?
3. Background knowledge.	Provides a brief, nonselective summary of current knowledge of the care problem being addressed and characteristics of organizations in which it occurs.
4. Local problem.	Describes the nature and severity of the specific local problem or system dysfunction that was addressed.
5. Intended improvement.	(a) Describes the specific aim (changes/improvements in care processes and patient outcomes) of the proposed intervention.
	(b) Specifies who (champions, supporters) and what (events, observations) triggered the decision to make changes and why now (timing).
6. Study question.	States precisely the primary improvement-related question and any secondary questions that the study of the intervention was designed to answer.
Methods.	What did you do?
7. Ethical issues.	Describes ethical aspects of implementing and studying the improvement, such as privacy concerns, protection of participants' physical well-being, and potential author conflicts of interest, and how ethical concerns were addressed.
8. Setting.	Specifies how elements of the local care environment considered most likely to influence change/improvement in the involved site or sites were identified and characterized.
9. Planning the intervention.	(a) Describes the intervention and its components in sufficient detail that others could reproduce it.
	(b) Indicates main factors that contributed to choice of the specific intervention (e.g., analysis of causes of dysfunction; matching relevant improvement experience of others with the local situation).
	(c) Outlines initial plans for how the intervention was to be implemented: *what* was to be done (initial steps; functions to be accomplished by those steps; how tests of change would be used to modify intervention) and *by whom* (intended roles, qualifications, and training of staff).

(Continued)

Table 4.37 (Continued) QC checklist. SQUIRE

Text section	Section or item description
Methods.	
10. Planning the study of the intervention.	(a) Outlines plans for assessing how well the intervention was implemented (dose or intensity of exposure).
	(b) Describes mechanisms by which intervention components were expected to cause changes, and plans for testing whether those mechanisms were effective.
	(c) Identifies the study design (e.g., observational, quasi-experimental, experimental) chosen for measuring impact of the intervention on primary and secondary outcomes, if applicable.
	(d) Explains plans for implementing essential aspects of the chosen study design, as described in publication guides for specific designs, if applicable (see, e.g., www.equator-network.org).
	(e) Describes aspects of the study design that specifically concerned internal validity (integrity of the data) and external validity (generalizability).
11. Methods of evaluation.	(a) Describes instruments and procedures (qualitative, quantitative, or mixed) used to assess the effectiveness of implementation, the contributions of intervention components and context factors to effectiveness of the intervention and primary and secondary outcomes.
	(b) Reports efforts to validate and test reliability of assessment instruments.
	(c) Explains methods used to assure data quality and adequacy (e.g., blinding; repeating measurements and data extraction; training in data collection; collection of sufficient baseline measurements).
12. Analysis.	(a) Provides details of qualitative and quantitative (statistical) methods used to draw inferences from the data.
	(b) Aligns unit of analysis with level at which the intervention was implemented, if applicable.
	(c) Specifies degree of variability expected in implementation, change expected in primary outcome (effect size), and ability of study design (including size) to detect such effects.
	(d) Describes analytic methods used to demonstrate effects of time as a variable (e.g., statistical process control).
Results.	What did you find?
13. Outcomes.	(a) Nature of setting and improvement intervention.
	i. Characterizes relevant elements of setting or settings (e.g., geography, physical resources, organizational culture, history of change efforts), and structures and patterns of care (e.g., staffing, leadership) that provided context for the intervention.
	ii. Explains the actual course of the intervention (e.g., sequence of steps, events or phases; type and number of participants at key points), preferably using a timeline diagram or flowchart.
	iii. Documents degree of success in implementing intervention components.

(Continued)

Table 4.37 (Continued) QC checklist. SQUIRE

Text section	Section or item description
Results.	
13. Outcomes.	*iv.* Describes how and why the initial plan evolved, and the most important lessons learned from that evolution, particularly the effects of internal feedback from tests of change (reflexiveness).
	(b) Changes in processes of care and patient outcomes associated with the intervention.
	i. Presents data on changes observed in the care delivery process.
	ii. Presents data on changes observed in measures of patient outcomes (e.g., morbidity, mortality, function, patient/staff satisfaction, service utilization, cost, care, disparities).
	iii. Considers benefits, harms, unexpected results, problems, failures.
	iv. Presents evidence regarding the strength of association between observed changes/improvements and intervention components/context function.
	v. Includes summary of missing data for intervention and outcomes.
Discussion.	What do the findings mean?
14. Summary.	(a) Summarizes the most important successes and difficulties in implementing intervention components, and main changes observed in care delivery and clinical outcomes.
	(b) Highlights the study's particular strengths.
15. Relation to other evidence.	Compares and contrasts study results with relevant findings of others, drawing on broad review of the literature; use of a summary table may be helpful in building on existing evidence.
16. Limitations.	(a) Considers possible sources of confounding, bias, or imprecision in design, measurement, and analysis that might have affected study outcomes (internal validity).
	(b) Explores factors that could affect generalizability (external validity), for example, representativeness of participants; effectiveness of implementation; dose-response effects; and features of local care setting.
	(c) Addresses the likelihood that observed gains may weaken over time and describes plans, if any, for monitoring and maintaining improvement; explicitly states if such planning was not done.
	(d) Reviews efforts made to minimize and adjust for study limitations.
	(e) Assesses the effect of study limitations on interpretation and application of results.

(Continued)

Table 4.37 (Continued) QC checklist. SQUIRE

Text section	Section or item description
Discussion.	
17. Interpretation.	(a) Explores possible reasons for differences between observed and expected outcomes.
	(b) Draws inferences consistent with the strength of the data about causal mechanisms and size of observed changes, paying particular attention to components of the intervention and context factors that helped determine the intervention's effectiveness (or lack thereof), and types of settings in which this intervention is most likely to be effective.
	(c) Suggests steps that might be modified to improve future performance.
	(d) Reviews issues of opportunity cost and actual financial cost of the intervention.
18. Conclusions.	(a) Considers overall practical usefulness of the intervention.
	(b) Suggests implications of this report for further studies of improvement interventions.
Other information.	Were there other factors relevant to the conduct and interpretation of the study?
19. Funding.	Describes funding sources, if any, and the role of the funding organization in design, implementation, interpretation, and publication of the study.

Source: Reproduced from *BMJ*, Davidoff F, Batalden P, Stevens D et al. Publication guidelines for improvement studies in health care: evolution of the SQUIRE Project. vol 338, page a3152. Copyright ©2009 with permission from BMJ Publishing Group Ltd.[45]

Table 4.38 QC checklist. PRECIS: A tool to help trial designers—Pragmatic and explanatory approaches to each domain

Domain	Pragmatic trial	Explanatory trial
Participants.		
Participant eligibility criteria.	All participants who have the condition of interest are enrolled, regardless of their anticipated risk, responsiveness, comorbidities, or past compliance.	Stepwise selection criteria are applied that: (a) Restrict study individuals to just those previously shown to be at highest risk of unfavorable outcomes. (b) Further restrict these high-risk individuals to those who are thought likely to be highly responsive to the experimental intervention. (c) Include just those high-risk, highly responsive study individuals who demonstrate high compliance with pretrial appointment keeping and a mock intervention.
Interventions and expertise. Experimental intervention—flexibility	Instructions on how to apply the experimental intervention are highly flexible, offering practitioners considerable leeway in deciding how to formulate and apply it.	Inflexible experimental intervention, with strict instructions for every element.
Experimental intervention—practitioner expertise.	The experimental intervention typically is applied by the full range of practitioners and in the full range of clinical settings, regardless of their expertise, with only ordinary attention to dose setting and side effects.	The experimental intervention is applied only by seasoned practitioners previously documented to have applied that intervention with high rates of success and low rates of complications, and in practice settings where the care delivery system and providers are highly experienced in managing the types of patients enrolled in the trial. The intervention often is closely monitored so that its "dose" can be optimized and its side effects treated; cointerventions against other disorders often are applied.

(Continued)

Table 4.38 (Continued) QC checklist. PRECIS: A tool to help trial designers—Pragmatic and explanatory approaches to each domain

Domain	Pragmatic trial	Explanatory trial
Comparison intervention—flexibility	"Usual practice" or the best alternative management strategy available, offering practitioners considerable leeway in deciding how to apply it.	Restricted flexibility of the comparison intervention; may use a placebo rather than the best alternative management strategy as the comparator.
Comparison intervention—practitioner expertise.	The comparison intervention typically is applied by the full range of practitioners, and in the full range of clinical settings, regardless of their expertise, with only ordinary attention to their training, expertise, and performance.	Practitioner expertise in applying the comparison intervention(s) is standardized to maximize the chances of detecting comparative benefit the experimental intervention might have.
Follow-up and outcomes. Follow-up intensity.	No formal follow-up visits of study individuals. Instead, administrative databases (e.g., mortality, registries) are searched for the detection of outcomes.	Study individuals are followed with many more frequent visits and more extensive data collection than would occur in routine practice, regardless of whether patients had experienced any events.
Primary trial outcome.	The primary outcome is an objectively measured, clinically meaningful outcome to the study participants. The outcome does not rely on central adjudication and is one that can be assessed under usual conditions: for example, special tests or training are not required.	The outcome is known to be a direct and immediate consequence of the intervention. The outcome is often clinically meaningful but may sometimes (e.g., early dose-finding trials) be a surrogate marker of another downstream outcome of interest. It may also require specialized training or testing not normally used to determine outcome status or central adjudication.
Compliance/adherence. Participant compliance with "prescribed" intervention.	There is unobtrusive (or no) measurement of participant compliance, and no special strategies to maintain or improve compliance are used.	Study participants' compliance with the intervention is monitored closely, may be a prerequisite for study entry, and both prophylactic strategies (to maintain) and "rescue" strategies (to regain) high compliance are used.

(Continued)

Table 4.38 (Continued) QC checklist. PRECIS: A tool to help trial designers—Pragmatic and explanatory approaches to each domain

Domain	Pragmatic trial	Explanatory trial
Practitioner adherence to study protocol.	There is unobtrusive (or no) measurement of practitioner adherence and no special strategies to maintain or improve it are used.	There is close monitoring of how well the participating clinicians and centers are adhering to even the minute details in the trial protocol and "manual of procedures."
Analysis. Analysis of primary outcome.	The analysis includes all patients, regardless of compliance, eligibility, and others (the intention-to-treat analysis). In other words, the analysis attempts to see if the treatment works under the usual conditions, with all the "noise" inherent therein.	An intention-to-treat analysis is usually performed; however, this may be supplemented by a per-protocol analysis or an analysis restricted to "compliers" or other subgroups to estimate maximum achievable treatment effect. Analyses are conducted that attempt to answer the narrowest, "mechanistic" question (whether biological, educational, or organizational).

Source: Reprinted from J Clin Epidemiol, Thorpe KE, Zwarenstein M, Oxman AD et al. A pragmatic-explanatory continuum indicator summary (PRECIS): a tool to help trial designers. vol 62, pages 464–75. Copyright ©2009, with permission from Elsevier.[46]

Table 4.39 QC checklist. Rethinking pragmatic randomized controlled trials (RCTs): Introducing the cohort multiple RCT (cmRCT)

The cmRCT is most suited to:	The cmRCT is least suited to:
Settings.	**Settings.**
• Open trials with usual care as the comparator.	• Closed trial designs with masking or a placebo arm.
• Studies whose aim is to inform health-care decisions in routine practice (pragmatic trials).	• Studies whose aim is to further knowledge as to how and why a treatment works (efficacy trials).
• Research questions that address easily measured and collected outcomes.	• Research questions that address hard-to-collect outcomes.
Populations.	**Populations.**
• Stable patient populations.	• Populations with high attrition.
• Easily identified populations.	• Unstable patient populations.
Clinical conditions.	• Difficult-to-identify populations.
• Clinical conditions for which many trials are conducted, e.g., obesity, diabetes, chronic pain.	**Clinical conditions.**
• Chronic conditions.	• Acute or short-term conditions.
• Conditions for which previous studies have struggled with recruitment.	
Treatments.	**Treatments.**
• Treatments highly desired by patients.	• Treatments not highly desired by patients.
• Expensive treatments.	

Source: Reproduced from *BMJ*, Relton C, Torgerson D, O'Cathain A et al. Rethinking pragmatic randomised controlled trials: introducing the "cohort multiple randomised controlled trial" design. vol. 340, pages 963–7. Copyright ©2010 with permission from BMJ Publishing Group Ltd.[47]

Table 4.40 QC checklist. CONSORT—Pragmatic trials

Section	Item	Standard CONSORT description	Extension for pragmatic trials
Title and abstract.	1	How participants were allocated to interventions (e.g., "random allocation," "randomized," or "randomly assigned").	–
Introduction.			
Background.	2	Scientific background and explanation of rationale.	Describe the health or health service problem that the intervention is intended to address and other interventions that may commonly be aimed at this problem.
Methods.			
Participants.	3	Eligibility criteria for participants; settings and locations where the data were collected.	Eligibility criteria should be explicitly framed to show the degree to which they include typical participants and/or, where applicable, typical providers (e.g., nurses), institutions (e.g., hospitals), communities (or localities, e.g., towns) and settings of care (e.g., different health-care financing systems).
Interventions.	4	Precise details of the interventions intended for each group and how and when they were actually administered.	Describe: (a) Extra resources added to (or resources removed from) usual settings to implement intervention. Indicate if efforts were made to standardize the intervention or if the intervention and its delivery were allowed to vary between participants, practitioners, or study sites. (b) The comparator in similar detail to the intervention.
Objectives.	5	Specific objectives and hypotheses.	–
Outcomes.	6	Clearly defined primary and secondary outcome measures and, when applicable, any methods used to enhance the quality of measurements (e.g., multiple observations, training of assessors).	Explain why the chosen outcomes and, when relevant, the length of follow-up, are considered important to those who will use the results of the trial.

(Continued)

Table 4.40 (Continued) QC checklist. CONSORT—Pragmatic trials

Section	Item	Standard CONSORT description	Extension for pragmatic trials
Methods.			
Sample size.	7	How sample size was determined; explanation of any interim analyses and stopping rules when applicable.	If calculated using the smallest difference considered important by the target decision-maker audience (the minimally important difference), then report where this difference was obtained.
Randomization—sequence generation.	8	Method used to generate the random allocation sequence, including details of any restriction (e.g., blocking, stratification).	–
Randomization—allocation concealment.	9	Method used to implement the random allocation sequence (e.g., numbered containers or central telephone), clarifying whether the sequence was concealed until interventions were assigned.	
Randomization—implementation.	10	Who generated the allocation sequence, who enrolled participants, and who assigned participants to their groups.	–
Blinding (masking).	11	Whether participants, those administering the interventions, and those assessing the outcomes were blinded to group assignment.	If blinding was not done, or was not possible, explain why.
Statistical methods.	12	Statistical methods used to compare groups for primary outcomes; methods for additional analyses, such as subgroup analyses and adjusted analyses.	–

(*Continued*)

Table 4.40 (Continued) QC checklist. CONSORT—Pragmatic trials

Section	Item	Standard CONSORT description	Extension for pragmatic trials
Results.			
Participant flow.	13	Flow of participants through each stage (a diagram is strongly recommended)—specifically, for each group, report the numbers of participants randomly assigned, receiving intended treatment, completing the study protocol, and analyzed for the primary outcome; describe deviations from planned study protocol, together with reasons.	The number of participants or units approached to take part in the trial, the number who were eligible, and reasons for non-participation should be reported.
Recruitment.	14	Dates defining the periods of recruitment and follow-up.	–
Baseline data.	15	Baseline demographic and clinical characteristics of each group.	–
Numbers analyzed.	16	Number of participants (denominator) in each group included in each analysis and whether analysis was by "intention-to-treat"; state the results in absolute numbers when feasible (e.g., 10/20, not 50%).	–
Outcomes and estimation.	17	For each primary and secondary outcome, a summary of results for each group and the estimated effect size and its precision (e.g., 95% confidence interval).	–
Ancillary analyses.	18	Address multiplicity by reporting any other analyses performed, including subgroup analyses and adjusted analyses, indicating which are prespecified and which are exploratory.	–
Adverse events.	19	All important adverse events or side effects in each intervention group.	–

(Continued)

Table 4.40 (Continued) QC checklist. CONSORT—Pragmatic trials

Section	Item	Standard CONSORT description	Extension for pragmatic trials
Discussion. Interpretation.	20	Interpretation of the results, taking into account study hypotheses, sources of potential bias or imprecision, and the dangers associated with multiplicity of analyses and outcomes.	–
Generalizability.	**21**	Generalizability (external validity) of the trial findings.	Describe key aspects of the setting which determined the trial results. Discuss possible differences in other settings where clinical traditions, health service organization, staffing, or resources may vary from those of the trial.
Overall evidence.	**22**	General interpretation of the results in the context of current evidence.	

Source: Reproduced from *BMJ*, Zwarenstein M, Treweek S, Gagnier JJ et al. Improving the reporting of pragmatic trials: an extension of the CONSORT statement. vol. 337, page a2390. Copyright ©2008 with permission from BMJ Publishing Group Ltd.[48]

Table 4.41 QC checklist. COREQ

Item	No.	Guide questions/descriptions
Domain 1: Research Team and Reflexivity. Personal characteristics.		
Interviewer/facilitator.	1	Which authors conducted the interview or focus group?
Credentials.	2	What were the researcher's credentials? For example, PhD, MD?
Occupation.	3	What was their occupation at the time of the study?
Gender.	4	Was the researcher male, or female?
Experience and training.	5	What experience or training did the researcher have?
Relationship with participants: Relationship established.	6	Was a relationship established before study commencement?
Participant knowledge of the interviewer.	7	What did the participants know about the researcher? *For example, personal goals, reasons for doing the research.*
Interviewer characteristics.	8	What characteristics were reported about the interviewer/facilitator? *For example, bias, assumptions, reasons, and interests in the research topic.*
Domain 2: Study Design. Theoretical framework.		
Methodological orientation and theory. Participant selection.	9	What methodological orientation was stated to underpin the study? *For example, grounded theory, discourse analysis, ethnography, phenomenology, content analysis.*
Sampling.	10	How were participants selected? *For example, purposive, convenience, consecutive, snowball.*
Method of approach.	11	How were participants approached? *For example, face-to-face, telephone, mail, email.*
Sample size.	12	How many participants were in the study?
Nonparticipation setting.	13	How many people refused to participate or dropped out? Reasons?
Setting of data collection.	14	Where were the data collected? *For example, home, clinic, workplace.*
Presence of nonparticipants.	15	Was anyone else present besides the participants and researchers?
Description of sample.	16	What are the important characteristics of the sample? *For example, demographic data, date.*
Data collection. Interview guide.	17	Were questions, prompts, or guides provided by the authors? Were they pilot tested?
Repeat interviews.	18	Were repeat interviews carried out? If yes, how many?

(Continued)

Table 4.41 (Continued) QC checklist. COREQ

Item	No.	Guide questions/descriptions
Audio/visual recording.	19	Did the research use audio or visual recording to collect the data?
Field notes.	20	Were field notes made during and/or after the interview or focus group?
Duration.	21	What was the duration of the interview or focus group?
Data saturation.	22	Was data saturation discussed?
Transcripts returned.	23	Were transcripts returned to participants for comment and/or correction?
Domain 3: Analysis and Findings.		
Data analysis.		
Number of data coders.	24	How many data coders coded the data?
Description of the coding tree.	25	Did authors provide a description of the coding tree?
Derivation of themes.	26	Were themes identified in advance, or derived from the data?
Software.	27	What software, if applicable, was used to manage the data?
Participant checking.	28	Did participants provide feedback on the findings?
Reporting: quotations presented.	29	Were participant quotations presented to illustrate the themes/findings? Was each quotation identified? *For example, participant number.*
Data and findings consistent.	30	Was there consistency between the data presented and the findings?
Clarity of major themes.	31	Were major themes clearly presented in the findings?
Clarity of minor themes.	32	Is there a description of diverse cases or discussion of minor themes?

Source: Reprinted from Tong A, Sainsbury P, Craig J, Consolidated criteria for reporting qualitative research (COREQ): a 32-item checklist for interviews and focus groups. *Int J Qual Health Care*, 2007, vol. 19, pages 349–57, by permission of the International Society for Quality in Health Care.[49]

Table 4.42 QC checklist. Guidelines for submitting adverse-event (AE) reports for publication

Information to include			
Category	Required	Highly Desirable	If Relevant
Title.	Consistent with content of the report.	–	–
Patient demographics.	–	–	–
	Age group.	Exact age.	Height.
	Sex.	Body weight.	Race and ethnicity.
	–	–	Obstetrical status.
	–	–	Body mass index.
	–	–	Occupation.
Current health status.	Disease or symptoms being treated with suspect drug.	Duration of illness.	Severity of disease/ symptoms.
Medical history.	Medical history relevant to AE.	Prior exposure to drug product or class.	Previous therapy of active disease.
	–	–	Alcohol, tobacco, and substance abuse history.
	–	Underlying risk factors.	Relevant social circumstances.
	–	–	Family history.
	–	–	Drugs taken by household members.
	–	–	–
Physical examination.	Abnormal physical or laboratory findings.	Baseline laboratory findings with normal range of values of the laboratory.	Pertinent negative physical findings.
	For off-label use, documentation of the reason.		–
Patient disposition.	Presence or absence of death, life-threatening circumstances, hospitalization or prolonged hospitalization, or significant disability.	Status several months after AE.	–

(Continued)

Table 4.42 (Continued) QC checklist. Guidelines for submitting adverse-event (AE) reports for publication

Information to include			
Category	Required	Highly Desirable	If Relevant
Drug identification.	Suspected drug identified by generic name.	Suspected brand name with strength/dosage unit.	Product formulation.
	Herbal products can be described by Latin binomial of herbal ingredients, plants part(s) and type of preparation (e.g., crude herb or extract).	For herbal extracts, type and concentration of extraction solvent used.	For manufactured herbal products, whether the product was standardized for which constituent(s) and concentration(s), and, for extracts, the drug: extract ratio.
	Proprietary name and name of producer for manufactured products.	For herbal products, state whether the product(s) implicated are authorized or licensed, and whether or not sample(s) have been retained for analysis, and any results.	–
Dosage.	Approximate dosage.	Exact dosage.	Serum or other fluid drug concentrations.
	Duration of therapy.	Start and stop dates.	Restart dates.
	–	Route.	Patient adherence.
Administration/ Drug-reaction interface.	Therapy duration before the AE.	First dose–event interval.	Last dose–resolution interval.
	–	Last dose–event interval.	–
Concomitant therapies.	Assessment of potential contribution of concomitant therapies.	Description of concomitant therapies, including nonprescription, herbal, or complementary medicines.	Start and stop doses of concomitant therapies.
AE	Description of AE and its severity compared to established definitions.*	Description of AE and its severity.	Case definition if more than one patient involved.
	Outcome of AE.	Onset date.	Specific treatment of AE.
	–	Duration of AE.	–

(Continued)

Table 4.42 (Continued) QC checklist. Guidelines for submitting adverse-event (AE) reports for publication

Information to include			
Category	**Required**	**Highly Desirable**	**If Relevant**
Discussion.	Include presence or absence of evidence supporting a causal link, including timing, dechallenge and rechallenge (or state why these were not possible).	• Diagnostic procedures performed to confirm the final diagnosis. • Biological plausibility.	For case series reports, follow recommendations of Edwards et al.[50]
	Discussion of previous reports of the AE in biomedical journals, and on product labeling.	• Assessment of competing explanations. • Discussion of prior reports to regulatory agencies.	Discussion of progress or planned clinical trials of the AE.

Source: Reproduced from Kelly WN, Arellano FM, Barnes J et al. Guidelines for submitting adverse event reports for publication. *Pharmacoepidemiol Drug Saf* 2007;16:581–7, with permission from John Wiley. Copyright ©2007 John Wiley & Sons, Inc.[51]

*Use consensus conference criteria whenever possible.

Table 4.43 QC checklist. SPIRIT 2013 statement

Section/Item	No.	Description
Administrative information.		
Title.	1	Descriptive title identifying the study design, population, interventions, and, if applicable, trial acronym.
Trial registration.	2a	Trial identifier and registry name. If not yet registered, name of intended registry.
	2b	All items from the World Health Organization Trial Registration Data Set.
Protocol version.	3	Date and version identifier.
Funding.	4	Sources and types of financial, material, and other support.
Roles and responsibilities.	5a	Names, affiliations, and roles of protocol contributors.
	5b	Name and contact information for the trial sponsor.
	5c	Role of study sponsor and funders, if any, in study design; collection, management, analysis, and interpretation of data; writing of the report; and the decision to submit the report for publication, including whether they will have ultimate authority over any of these activities.
	5d	Composition, roles, and responsibilities of the coordinating center, steering committee, endpoint adjudication committee, data management team, and other individuals or groups overseeing the trial, if applicable (see item 21a for data monitoring committee [DMC]).
Introduction.	6	
Background and rationale.	6a	Description of research question and justification for undertaking the trial, including summary of relevant studies (published and unpublished) examining benefits and harms for each intervention.
	6b	Explanation for choice of comparators.
Objectives.	7	Specific objectives or hypotheses.
Trial design.	8	Description of trial design, including type of trial (e.g., parallel-group, crossover, factorial, single group), allocation ratio, and framework (e.g., superiority, equivalence, noninferiority, exploratory).
Methods: Participants, Interventions, and Outcomes.		
Study setting.	9	Description of study settings (e.g., community clinic, academic hospital) and list of countries where data will be collected. Reference to where list of study sites can be obtained.
Eligibility criteria.	10	Inclusion and exclusion criteria for participants. If applicable, eligibility criteria for study centers and individuals who will perform the interventions (e.g., surgeons, psychotherapists).
Interventions.	11a	Interventions for each group, with sufficient detail to allow replication, including how and when they will be administered.

(Continued)

Table 4.43 (Continued) QC checklist. SPIRIT 2013 statement

Section/Item	No.	Description
Methods.		
	11b	Criteria for discontinuing or modifying allocated interventions for a given trial participant (e.g., drug dose change in response to harms, participant request, or improving/worsening disease).
	11c	Strategies to improve adherence to intervention protocols, and any procedures for monitoring adherence (e.g., drug tablet return, laboratory tests).
	11d	Relevant concomitant care and interventions that are permitted or prohibited during the trial.
Outcomes.	**12**	Primary, secondary, and other outcomes, including the specific measurement variable (e.g., systolic blood pressure), analysis metric (e.g., change from baseline, final value, time to event), method of aggregation (e.g., median, proportion), and time point for each outcome. Explanation of the clinical relevance of chosen efficacy and harm outcomes is strongly recommended.
Participant timeline.	**13**	Schedule of enrollment, interventions (including any run-ins and washouts), assessments, and visits for participants. A schematic diagram is highly recommended.
Sample size.	**14**	Estimated number of participants needed to achieve study objectives and how it was determined, including clinical and statistical assumptions supporting any sample size calculations.
Recruitment.	**15**	Strategies for achieving adequate participant enrollment to reach target sample size.
Methods: Assignment of Interventions (for Controlled Trials).		
Sequence generation.	**16a**	Method of generating the allocation sequence (e.g., computer-generated random numbers), and list of any factors for stratification. To reduce predictability of a random sequence, details of any planned restriction (e.g., blocking) should be provided in a separate document that is unavailable to those who enroll participants or assign interventions.
Allocation. Allocation concealment mechanism.	**16b**	Mechanism of implementing the allocation sequence (e.g., central telephone; sequentially numbered, opaque, sealed envelopes), describing any steps to conceal the sequence until interventions are assigned.
Implementation.	**16c**	Who will generate the allocation sequence, who will enroll participants, and who will assign participants to interventions.
Blinding (masking).	**17a**	Who will be blinded after assignment to interventions (e.g., trial participants, care providers, outcome assessors, data analysts), and how.

(Continued)

Table 4.43 (Continued) QC checklist. SPIRIT 2013 statement

Section/Item	No.	Description
	17b	If blinded, circumstances under which unblinding is permissible and procedure for revealing a participant's allocated intervention during the trial.
Methods: Data Collection, Management, and Analysis.		
Data collection methods.	18a	Plans for assessment and collection of outcome, baseline, and other trial data, including any related processes to promote data quality (e.g., duplicate measurements, training of assessors) and a description of study instruments (e.g., questionnaires, laboratory tests) along with their reliability and validity, if known. Reference to where data collection forms can be found, if not in the protocol.
	18b	Plans to promote participant retention and complete follow-up, including list of any outcome data to be collected for participants who discontinue or deviate from intervention protocols.
Data management.	19	Plans for data entry, coding, security, and storage, including any related processes to promote data quality (e.g., double data entry; range checks for data values). Reference to where details of data management procedures can be found, if not in the protocol.
Statistical methods.	20a	Statistical methods for analyzing primary and secondary outcomes. Reference to where other details of the statistical analysis plan can be found, if not in the protocol.
	20b	Methods for any additional analyses (e.g., subgroup and adjusted analyses).
	20c	Definition of analysis population relating to protocol nonadherence (e.g., as randomized analysis), and any statistical methods to handle missing data (e.g., multiple imputation).
Methods: Monitoring.		
Data monitoring.	21a	Composition of DMC; summary of its role and reporting structure; statement of whether it is independent from the sponsor and competing interests; and reference to where further details about its charter can be found, if not in the protocol. Alternatively, an explanation of why a DMC is not needed.
	21b	Description of any interim analyses and stopping guidelines, including who will have access to these interim results and make the final decision to terminate the trial.
Harms.	22	Plans for collecting, assessing, reporting, and managing solicited and spontaneously reported adverse events and other unintended effects of trial interventions or trial conduct.

(Continued)

Table 4.43 (Continued) QC checklist. SPIRIT 2013 statement

Section/Item	No.	Description
Auditing.	23	Frequency and procedures for auditing trial conduct, if any, and whether the process will be independent from investigators and the sponsor.
Ethics and dissemination.		
Research ethics approval.	24	Plans for seeking research ethics committee/institutional review board (REC/IRB) approval.
Protocol amendments.	25	Plans for communicating important protocol modifications (e.g., changes to eligibility criteria, outcomes, analyses) to relevant parties (e.g., investigators, REC/IRBs, trial participants, trial registries, journals, regulators).
Consent/assent.	26a	Who will obtain informed consent or assent from potential trial participants or authorized surrogates, and how (see item 32).
	26b	Additional consent provisions for collection and use of participant data and biological specimens in ancillary studies, if applicable.
Confidentiality.	27	How personal information about potential and enrolled participants will be collected, shared, and maintained to protect confidentiality before, during, and after the trial.
Declaration of interests.	28	Financial and other competing interests for principal investigators for the overall trial and each study site.
Access to data.	29	Statement of who will have access to the final trial dataset, and disclosure of contractual agreements that limit such access for investigators.
Ancillary/post-trial care.	30	Provisions, if any, for ancillary and post-trial care, and for compensation to those who suffer harm from trial participation.
Dissemination policy.	31a	Plans for investigators and sponsor to communicate trial results to participants, health-care professionals, the public, and other relevant groups (e.g., via publication, reporting in results databases, or other data-sharing arrangements), including any publication restrictions.
	31b	Authorship eligibility guidelines and any intended use of professional writers.
	31c	Plans, if any, for granting public access to the full protocol, participant-level dataset, and statistical code.
Appendices.		
Informed-consent materials.	32	Model consent form and other related documentation given to participants and authorized surrogates.
Biological specimens.	33	Plans for collection, laboratory evaluation, and storage of biological specimens for genetic or molecular analysis in the current trial and for future use in ancillary studies, if applicable.

Source: Reproduced from *BMJ*, Chan AW, Tetzlaff JM, Gøtzsche PC et al. SPIRIT 2013 explanation and elaboration guidance for protocols of clinical trials. vol. 346, page e7586. Copyright ©2013 with permission from BMJ Publishing Group Ltd.[52]

*It is strongly recommended that this checklist be read in conjunction with the SPIRIT 2013 Explanation & Elaboration for important clarification on the items. Amendments to the protocol should be tracked and dated.

Table 4.44 QC checklist. Qualitative research review guidelines; RATS: Relevance, Appropriateness, Transparency, Soundness

	Ask this of the manuscript:	This should be included in the manuscript:
R	**Relevance of study question**	
	Is the research question interesting?	Research question explicitly stated.
	Is the research question relevant to clinical practice, public health, or policy?	Research question justified and linked to the existing knowledge base (empirical research, theory, policy).
A	**Appropriateness of qualitative method**	
	Is qualitative methodology the best approach for the study aims?	Study design described and justified, i.e., why was a particular method (e.g., interviews) chosen?
	Interviews: Experience, perceptions, behavior, practice, process.	
	Focus groups: Group dynamics, convenience, nonsensitive topics.	
	Ethnography: Culture, organizational behavior, interaction.	
	Textual analysis: Documents, art, representations, conversations.	
T	**Transparency of procedures**	
	Sampling:	
	Are the participants selected the most appropriate to provide access to type of knowledge sought by the study?	Criteria for selecting the study sample justified and explained.
	Is the sampling strategy appropriate?	*theoretical:* based on preconceived or emergent theory.
		purposive: diversity of opinion.
		volunteer: feasibility, hard-to-reach groups.
	Recruitment:	
	Was recruitment conducted using appropriate methods?	Details of how recruitment was conducted and by whom.
	Is the sampling strategy appropriate?	
	Could there be selection bias?	Details of who chose not to participate and why.
	Data collection:	
	Was collection of data systematic and comprehensive?	Method(s) outlined and examples given (e.g., interview questions).
	Are characteristics of the study group and setting clear?	Study group and setting clearly described.
	Why and when was data collection stopped, and was this reasonable?	End of data collection justified and described.
	Role of researchers:	
	Is/are the researcher(s) appropriate? How might they bias (good and bad) the conduct of the study and results?	Do the researchers occupy dual roles (clinician and researcher)? Are the ethics of this discussed? Do the researcher(s) critically examine their own influence on the formulation of the research question, data collection, and interpretation?

(Continued)

Table 4.44 (Continued) QC checklist. Qualitative research review guidelines; RATS: Relevance, Appropriateness, Transparency, Soundness

Ask this of the manuscript:	This should be included in the manuscript:
Ethics:	
Was informed consent sought and granted?	Informed-consent process explicitly and clearly detailed.
Were participants' anonymity and confidentiality ensured?	Anonymity and confidentiality discussed.
Was approval from an appropriate ethics committee received?	Ethics approval cited.
S **Soundness of interpretive approach**	
Analysis:	
Is the type of analysis appropriate for the type of study?	Analytic approach described in depth and justified.
thematic: exploratory, descriptive, hypothesis generating	*Indicators of quality:* Description of how themes were derived from the data (inductive or deductive).
framework: e.g., policy.	
constant comparison/grounded theory: theory generating, analytical.	Evidence of alternative explanations being sought.
	Analysis and presentation of negative or deviant cases.
Are the interpretations clearly presented and adequately supported by the evidence?	Description of the basis on which quotes were chosen.
Are quotations used, and are these appropriate and effective?	Semiquantification when appropriate.
	Illumination of context and/or meaning, richly detailed.
Were trustworthiness and reliability of the data and interpretations checked?	Method of reliability check described and justified, e.g., was an audit trail, triangulation, or member checking employed? Did an independent analyst review data and contest themes? How were disagreements resolved?
Discussion and presentation:	
Are findings sufficiently grounded in a theoretical or conceptual framework?	Findings presented with reference to existing theoretical and empirical literature, and how they contribute.
Is adequate account taken of previous knowledge and how the findings add?	
Are the limitations thoughtfully considered?	Strengths and limitations explicitly described and discussed.
Is the manuscript well written and accessible?	Evidence of following guidelines (format, word count). Detail of methods or additional quotes contained in appendix. Written for a health sciences audience.

(Continued)

Table 4.44 (Continued) QC checklist. Qualitative research review guidelines; RATS: Relevance, Appropriateness, Transparency, Soundness

Ask this of the manuscript:	This should be included in the manuscript:
Are red flags present? These are common features of ill-conceived or poorly executed qualitative studies, are a cause for concern, and must be viewed critically. They might be fatal flaws, or they may result from lack of detail or clarity.	*Grounded theory:* Not a simple content analysis but a complex, sociological, theory-generating approach. *Jargon:* Descriptions that are trite, pat, or jargon filled should be viewed skeptically. *Overinterpretation:* Interpretation must be grounded in "accounts" and semiquantified if possible or appropriate. *Seems anecdotal, self-evident:* May be a superficial analysis, not rooted in conceptual framework or linked to previous knowledge, and lacking depth. *Consent process thinly discussed:* May not have met ethics requirements. *Doctor-researcher:* Consider the ethical implications for patients and the bias in data collection and interpretation.

Table 4.45 QC checklist. STARD

Section and topic	No.	Item	On pg. no
Title or abstract.	1	Identification as a study of diagnostic accuracy, using at least one measure of accuracy (e.g., sensitivity, specificity, predictive values, AUC).	
Abstract.	2	Structured summary of study design, methods, results, and conclusions (may include study aims such as estimating diagnostic accuracy or comparing accuracy between tests or across participant groups).	
Introduction.	3	Scientific and clinical background, including the intended use and clinical role of the index test.	
	4	Study objectives and hypotheses.	
Methods: Study design.	5	Whether data collection was planned before the index test and reference standard were performed (prospective study) or after (retrospective study).	
Participants.	6	Eligibility criteria.	
	7	On what basis were potentially eligible participants identified (e.g., symptoms, results from previous tests, inclusion in registry).	
	8	Where and when potentially eligible participants identified (setting, location, dates).	
	9	Whether participants formed a consecutive, random, or convenience series.	
Test methods.	10a	Index test, in sufficient detail to allow replication.	
	10b	Reference standard, in sufficient detail to allow replication.	
	11	Rationale for choosing the reference standard (if alternatives exist).	
	12a	Definition of and rationale for test positivity cutoffs or result categories of the index test, distinguishing prespecified from exploratory.	
	12b	Definition of and rationale for test positivity cutoffs or result categories of the reference standard, distinguishing prespecified from exploratory.	
	13a	Whether clinical information and reference standard results were available to the performers/readers of the index test.	
	13b	Whether clinical information and index test results were available to the assessors of the reference standard.	
Analysis.	14	Methods for estimating or comparing measures of diagnostic accuracy.	
	15	How indeterminate index test or reference standard results were handled.	
	16	How missing data on the index test and reference standard were handled.	
	17	Any analyses of variability in diagnostic accuracy, distinguishing prespecified from exploratory.	
	18	Intended sample size and how it was determined.	

(Continued)

Table 4.45 (Continued) QC checklist. STARD

Section and topic	No.	Item	On pg. no
Results.	**19**		
Participants.		Flow of participants, using a flow diagram.	
	20	Baseline demographic and clinical characteristics of participants.	
	21a	Distribution of severity of disease in those with the target condition.	
	21b	Distribution of alternative diagnosis in those without the target condition.	
	22	Interval and any clinical interventions between index test and reference standard.	
Test results.	**23**	Cross-tabulation of the index test results (or their distribution) by the results of the reference standard.	
	24	Estimates of diagnostic accuracy and their precision (e.g., 95% confidence intervals).	
	25	Any adverse events from performing the index test or the reference standard.	
Discussion.	**26**	Study limitations, including sources of potential bias, statistical uncertainty, and generalizability.	
	27	Implications for practice, including the intended use and clinical role of the index test.	
Other information.	**28**	Registration number and name of registry.	
	29	Where the full study protocol can be accessed.	
	30	Sources of funding and other support; role of funders.	

Source: Reproduced from *BMJ*, Bossuyt PM, Reitsma JB, Bruns DE et al. STARD 2015: an updated list of essential items for reporting diagnostic accuracy studies. vol. 351, page h5527. Copyright ©2015, with permission from BMJ Publishing Group Ltd.[53]

Abbreviation: AUC, area under curve (e.g., the receiver-operating characteristics [ROC] curve plotting sensitivity on the *y*-axis and 1 − specificity on the *x*-axis).

Table 4.46 QC checklist. TRIPOD initiative: Prediction model development and validation

Section/Topic	No.	D, V, or D;V*	Checklist item	On pg. no.
Title.	1	**D;V**	Identify the study as developing and/or validating a multivariable prediction model, the target population, and the outcome to be predicted.	
Abstract.	2	**D;V**	Provide a summary of objectives, study design, setting, participants, sample size, predictors, outcome, statistical analysis, results, and conclusions.	
Introduction. Background.	3a	**D;V**	Explain the medical context (including whether diagnostic or prognostic) and rationale for developing or validating the multivariable prediction model, including references to existing models.	
Objectives.	3b	**D;V**	Specify the objectives, including whether the study describes the development or validation of the model or both.	
Methods. Source of data.	4a	**D;V**	Describe the study design or source of data (e.g., randomized trial, cohort, or registry data), separately for the development and validation data sets, if applicable.	
	4b	**D;V**	Specify the key study dates, including start of accrual; end of accrual; and, if applicable, end of follow-up.	
Participants.	5a	**D;V**	Specify key elements of the study setting (e.g., primary care, secondary care, general population), including number and location of centers.	
	5b	**D;V**	Describe eligibility criteria for participants.	
	5c	**D;V**	Give details of treatments received, if relevant.	
Outcomes.	6a	**D;V**	Clearly define the outcome that is predicted by the prediction model, including how and when assessed.	
	6b	**D;V**	Report any actions to blind assessment of the outcome to be predicted.	
Predictors.	7a	**D;V**	Clearly define all predictors used in developing or validating the multivariable prediction model, including how and when they were measured.	
	7b	**D;V**	Report any actions to blind assessment of predictors for the outcome and other predictors.	
Sample size.	8	**D;V**	Explain how the study size was arrived at.	

(Continued)

Table 4.46 (Continued) QC checklist. TRIPOD initiative: Prediction model development and validation

Section/topic	No.	D, V, or D;V*	Checklist item	On pg. no.
Methods.				
Missing data.	9	D;V	Describe how missing data were handled (e.g., complete-case analysis, single imputation, multiple imputation), with details of any imputation method.	
Statistical analysis methods.	10a	D	Describe how predictors were handled in the analyses.	
	10b	D	Specify type of model, all model-building procedures (including any predictor selection), and method for internal validation.	
	10c	V	For validation, describe how the predictions were calculated.	
	10d	D;V	Specify all measures used to assess model performance and, if relevant, to compare multiple models.	
	10e	V	Describe any model updating (e.g., recalibration) arising from the validation, if done.	
Risk groups.	11	D;V	Provide details on how risk groups were created, if done.	
Development vs. validation.	12	V	For validation, identify any differences from the development data in setting, eligibility criteria, outcome, and predictors.	
Results. Participants.	13a	D;V	Describe the flow of participants through the study, including the number of participants with and without the outcome and, if applicable, a summary of the follow-up time. A diagram may be helpful.	
	13b	D;V	Describe the characteristics of the participants (basic demographics, clinical features, available predictors), including the number of participants with missing data for predictors, and outcome.	
	13c	V	For validation, show a comparison with the development data of the distribution of important variables (demographics, predictors, and outcome).	
Model development.	14a	D	Specify the number of participants and outcome events in each analysis.	
	14b	D	If done, report the unadjusted association between each candidate predictor and outcome.	

(Continued)

Table 4.46 (Continued) QC checklist. TRIPOD initiative: Prediction model development and validation

Section/topic	No.	D, V, or D;V*	Checklist item	On pg. no.
Results.				
Model specification.	15a	D	Present the full prediction model to allow predictions for individuals (i.e., all regression coefficients, and model intercept or baseline survival at a given time point).	
	15b	D	Explain how to use the prediction model.	
Model performance.	16	D;V	Report performance measures (with confidence intervals) for the prediction model.	
Model updating.	17	V	If done, report the results from any model updating (i.e., model specification, model performance).	
Discussion. Limitations.	18	D;V	Discuss any limitations of the study (such as nonrepresentative sample, few events per predictor, missing data).	
Interpretation.	19a	V	For validation, discuss the results with reference to performance in the development data, and any other validation data.	
	19b	D;V	Give an overall interpretation of the results, considering objectives, limitations, results from similar studies, and other relevant evidence.	
Implications.	20	D;V	Discuss the potential clinical use of the model and implications for future research.	
Other information. Supplementary information.	21	D;V	Provide information about the availability of supplementary resources, such as study protocol, Web calculator, and datasets.	
Funding.	22	D;V	Give the source of funding and the role of the funders for the present study.	

Source: Reproduced from *BMJ*, Collins GS, Reitsma JB, Altman DG et al. Transparent Reporting of a multivariable prediction model for Individual Prognosis or Diagnosis (TRIPOD): the TRIPOD statement. vol. 350, page g7594. Copyright ©2015 with permission from BMJ Publishing Group Ltd.[54]
*Items relevant only to the development of a prediction model are denoted by D, items relating solely to a validation of a prediction model are denoted by V, and items relating to both are denoted by D;V. Use the TRIPOD Checklist in conjunction with the TRIPOD Explanation and Elaboration document.

Table 4.47 QC checklist. GRRAS

Component	Item	Guideline
Title and abstract.	1	Identify in title or abstract that inter-rater/intrarater reliability or agreement was investigated.
Introduction.	2	Name and describe the diagnostic or measurement of interest explicitly.
	3	Specify the subject population of interest.
	4	Specify the rater population of interest (if applicable).
	5	Describe what is already known about reliability and agreement and provide a rationale for the study (if applicable).
Methods.	6	Explain how the sample size was chosen. State the determined number of raters, subjects/objects, and replicate observations.
	7	Describe the sampling method.
Results.	8	Describe the measurement/rating process (e.g., interval between repeated measurements, availability of clinical information, blinding).
	9	State whether measurements/ratings were conducted independently.
	10	Describe the statistical analysis.
	11	State the actual number of raters and subjects/objects who were included and the number of replicate observations that were conducted.
	12	Describe the sample characteristics of raters and subjects (e.g., training, experience).
	13	Report estimates of reliability and agreement, including measures of statistical uncertainty.
Discussion.	14	Discuss the practical relevance of the results.
Auxiliary material.	15	Provide detailed results if possible (e.g., online).

Source: Reprinted from *Int J Nurs Studies*, vol. 48, Kottner J, Audige L, Brorson S et al. Guidelines for Reporting Reliability and Agreement Studies (GRRAS) were proposed, pages 661–71. Copyright ©2011 with permission from Elsevier.[55]

Table 4.48 QC checklist. CARE guidelines for clinical case reporting

Topic	Item	Checklist item description	Reported on pg. no
Title.	1	The words "case report" or "case study" should be in the title along with the phenomenon of greatest interest (e.g., symptom, diagnosis, test, intervention).	
Key words.	2	Two to five key words that identify areas covered in the case report.	
Abstract.	3a	**Introduction:** What does this case report add to the medical literature?	
	3b	Case Presentation: —The main symptoms of the patient. —The main clinical findings. —The main diagnoses and interventions. —The main outcomes.	
	3c	**Conclusion:** What were the main "takeaway" lessons from this case?	
Introduction.	4	Brief background summary of the case, referencing the relevant medical literature.	
Patient information.	5a	Demographic information (e.g., age, gender, ethnicity, occupation).	
	5b	Main symptoms of the patient (chief complaints).	
	5c	Medical, family, and psychosocial history, including diet, lifestyle, and genetic information whenever possible, and details about relevant comorbidities, including past interventions and their outcomes.	
Clinical findings.	6	Describe the relevant physical examination (PE).	
Timeline.	7	Depict important dates and times in the case (table or figure).	
Diagnostic assessment.	8a	Diagnostic methods (e.g., PE, laboratory testing, imaging, questionnaires).	
	8b	Diagnostic challenges (e.g., financial/cultural).	
	8c	Diagnostic reasoning, including other diagnoses considered.	
	8d	Prognostic characteristics (e.g., staging) where applicable.	
Therapeutic intervention.	9	Types of intervention (e.g., pharmacologic, surgical, preventive, self-care). —Administration of intervention (e.g., dosage, strength, duration). —Changes in intervention (with rationale).	
Follow-up and outcomes.	10a	Clinician- and patient-assessed outcomes. Summarize the clinical course of all follow-up visits, including:	
	10b	—Important follow-up test results (positive or negative).	
	10c	—Intervention adherence and tolerability. (How was this assessed?) —Adverse and unanticipated events.	

(Continued)

Table 4.48 (Continued) QC checklist. CARE guidelines for clinical case reporting

Topic	Item	Checklist item description	Reported on pg. no
Discussion.	11a	The strengths and limitations of the management of this case.	
	11b	The relevant medical literature.	
	11c	The rationale for conclusions (including assessment of cause and effect).	
	11d	The main "takeaway" lessons of this case report.	
Patient perspective.	12	Patients should share their perspective or experiences whenever possible.	
Informed consent.	13	Did the patient give informed consent? Please provide if requested.	

Source: Reprinted from *J Diet Suppl*, vol. 10, Gagnier JJ, Kienle G, Altman DG et al, The CARE guidelines: consensus-based clinical case report guideline development, pages 381–90. Copyright ©2013 with permission from Elsevier.[56]

Table 4.49 QC checklist. Case series

1. Explicitly state the hypothesis/hypotheses under consideration.
2. Explicitly provide eligibility criteria for subjects in the report.
3. Precisely describe how treatments were administered or potential risk factors defined.
4. Compare observed results to those in an appropriate external comparison group; discuss potential biases arising from such comparison.
5. Perform appropriate statistics, ensuring that assumptions of the statistical methods are reasonable in this setting.
6. Discuss the biological plausibility of the hypothesis in light of the report's observations.
7. Explicitly discuss the report's limitations and how these limitations could be overcome in future studies.

Source: Reprinted from *Am J Ophthalmol*, vol. 151, Kempen JH, Appropriate use and reporting of uncontrolled case series in the medical literature, pages 7–10. Copyright ©2011 with permission from Elsevier.[57]

Table 4.50 QC checklist. The ARRIVE guidelines

Item	No.	Recommendation
Title.	1	Provide as accurate and concise a description of the content of the article as possible.
Abstract.	2	Provide an accurate summary of the background and research objectives, including details of the species or strain of animal used, key methods, principal findings, and conclusions of the study.
Introduction.		
Background.	3	(a) Include sufficient scientific background (including relevant references to previous work) to understand the motivation and context of the study, and explain the experimental approach and rationale.
		(b) Explain how and why the animal species and model being used can address the scientific objectives and, where appropriate, the study's relevance to human biology.
Objectives.	4	Clearly describe the primary and any secondary objectives of the study or specific hypotheses being tested.
Methods.		
Ethical statement.	5	Indicate the nature of the ethical review process, relevant licenses (e.g., Animal [Scientific Procedures] Act of 1986), and national or institutional guidelines for the care and use of animals, that cover the research.
Study design.	6	For each experiment, give brief details of the study design, including:
		(a) The number of experimental and control groups.
		(b) Any steps taken to minimize the effects of subjective bias when allocating animals to treatment (e.g., randomization procedure) and when assessing results (e.g., if done, describe who was blinded and when).
		(c) The experimental unit (e.g., a single animal, group, or cage of animals).
		A timeline diagram or flowchart can be useful to illustrate how complex study designs were carried out.
Experimental procedures.	7	For each experiment and each experimental group, including controls, provide precise details of all procedures carried out. For example:
		(a) How (e.g., drug formulation and dose, site, and route of administration, anesthesia and analgesia used [including monitoring], surgical procedure, method of euthanasia)? Provide details of any specialist equipment used, including supplier(s).
		(b) When (i.e., time of day)?
		(c) Where (e.g., home cage, laboratory, water maze)?
		(d) Why (e.g., rationale for choice of specific anesthetic, route of administration, drug dose used)?
Experimental animals.	8	(a) Provide details of the animals used, including species, strain, sex, developmental stage (e.g., mean or median age plus age range) and weight (e.g., mean or median weight plus weight ranges).
		(b) Provide further relevant information such as the source of animals, international strain nomenclature, genetic modification status, (e.g., knockout or transgenic), genotype, health/immune status, drug or test naïve, previous procedures.

(Continued)

Table 4.50 (Continued) QC checklist. The ARRIVE guidelines

Item	No.	Recommendation
Methods.		
Housing and husbandry.	9	**Provide details of:** (a) Housing (type of facility, e.g., specific-pathogen–free [SPF]; type of cage or housing; bedding material; number of cage companions; tank shape and material, etc., for fish). (b) Husbandry conditions (e.g., breeding program, light/dark cycle, temperature, quality of water; for fish, type of food, access to food and water, environmental enrichment). (c) Welfare-related assessments and interventions that were carried out before, during, or after the experiment.
Sample size.	10	(a) Specify the total number of animals used in each experiment, and the number of animals in each experimental group. (b) Explain how the number of animals was arrived at. Provide details of any sample size calculation used. (c) Indicate the number of independent replications of each experiment, if relevant.
Allocating animals to experimental groups.	11	(a) Give full details of how animals were allocated to experimental groups, including randomization or matching if done. (b) Describe the order in which the animals in the different experimental groups were treated and assessed.
Experimental outcomes.	12	Clearly define the primary and secondary experimental outcomes assessed (e.g., cell death, molecular markers, behavioral changes).
Statistical methods.	13	(a) Provide details of the statistical methods used for each analysis. (b) Specify the unit of analysis for each dataset (e.g., single animal, group of animals, single neuron). (c) Describe any methods used to assess whether the data met the assumptions of the statistical approach.
Results. Baseline data.	14	For each experimental group, report relevant characteristics and health status of animals (e.g., weight, microbiological status, drug or test naïve) before treatment or testing (this information can often be tabulated).
Numbers analyzed.	15	(a) Report the number of animals in each group included in each analysis. Report absolute numbers (e.g., 10/20, not 50%). (b) If any animals or data were not included in the analysis, explain why.
Outcomes and estimation.	16	Report the results for each analysis carried out, with a measure of precision (e.g., standard error or confidence interval).
Adverse events.	17	(a) Give details of all important adverse events in each experimental group. (b) Describe any modifications to the experimental protocols made to reduce adverse events.

(Continued)

Table 4.50 (Continued) QC checklist. The ARRIVE guidelines

Item	No.	Recommendation
Discussion. Interpretation/ scientific implications.	**18**	(a) Interpret the results, taking into account the study objectives and hypotheses, current theory, and other relevant studies in the literature.
		(b) Comment on the study limitations, including any potential sources of bias, any limitations of the animal model, and imprecision associated with the results.
		(c) Describe any implications of your experimental methods or findings for the replacement, refinement, or reduction (the 3Rs) of the use of animals in research.
Generalizability and translation.	**19**	Comment on whether, and how, the findings of this study are likely to translate to other species or systems, including any relevance to human biology.
Funding.	**20**	List all funding sources (including grant number) and the role of the funder(s) in the study.

Table 4.51 QC checklist. Overview of research, publication planning, and journal selection

Item	Step
Gap analysis/ Research.	When reviewing recent literature, consider whether a new intervention described in your manuscript might meet an emerging treatment need. Does your study report offer an improved methodology? Examples include an observational study if real-world evidence is scarce; a meta-analysis or other pooled-data study if existing conclusions are constrained by limited statistical power; or a propensity-score-matched (or other statistically advanced) analysis or modeling if existing literature suffers from biases or other issues.
	The first objective is to determine how the study advances the science on a topic and the report's unique or incremental value in meeting educational needs. Next, determine which journal's (or journals') readers might benefit from reading the paper. If your study and report are not entirely unique, which journal readers might find it of interest anyway?
	To acquaint yourself with the disease state, including definition, etiology, pathogenesis, natural history, epidemiology, diagnosis, and consensus management, seek consensus guidelines at a major society's website and/or a recent review in a high-quality journal (e.g., *Ann Intern Med, BMJ, Cochrane Database of Systematic Reviews [CDSR], JAMA, Lancet, NEJM*). Be a "source snob," but not to the exclusion of potentially relevant reviews or similar articles in a lower-tier journal being targeted. To extend your search scope and enrich the manuscript, seek government (e.g., WHO) statistics on disease epidemiology and regulatory guidance on study design (e.g., FDA, EMA) and pharmacovigilance (e.g., FDA Adverse Event Reporting System [FAERS]).
	Search PubMed/MEDLINE/EMBASE/CDSR (cochrane.org). Use relevant MeSH or other key words and/or title terms, and search the last 3 to 5 years. Search for types of studies and publications similar to your own [e.g., RCTs or meta-analyses of RCTs if you are reporting an RCT]).
	Search for evidence-based consensus clinical practice guidelines (CPGs), which can be found at major professional-society websites (and/or the societies' flagship journal publications) and the US Agency for Healthcare Research and Quality (www.guidelines.gov).
	If you have already targeted a small number of potential journals, review their online content from the last 3 to 5 years, to ensure that a similar study/report has not been published recently. Also consider articles/manuscripts posted ahead of print.
	Gap analysis is particularly consequential if your study findings result from analysis of a common, frequently shared database (e.g., an administrative claims database or patient registry). How does your study/report stand out from the others?
	Considering §801 of the Food and Drug Administration Amendments Act (FDAAA) of 2007, review the www.clinicaltrials.gov website for other similar studies involving the disease as well as the pharmacologic class and/or individual therapy assessed by your study. www.clinicaltrials.gov also includes URLs to publications concerning therapies evaluated. Other registry URLs are listed in the Introduction to this chapter.
	Try to determine when other, related studies are planned to be reported.

(Continued)

Table 4.51 (Continued) QC checklist. Overview of research, publication planning, and journal selection

Item	Step
Selecting a journal.	Seek to understand the educational needs of your reader, including primary-care physicians vs. specialists, surgeons vs. internists, basic vs. applied (clinical) scientists, policymakers/third-party payers, and dwellers of different regions (and/or non-English speakers) of the world.
	Determine the media via which you wish to reach these professionals, including print, electronic, or some combination of both.
	Be realistic and proactively "manage expectations" concerning publication prospects (e.g., at the kickoff meeting).
	Prepare a "long list" of potential journal publishers (see Table 4.52 immediately below). One way to winnow the long list is my own very "old-school" statistical mode approach. Which three journals are cited most frequently in either your outline or final manuscript? Consider submitting your manuscript to one of these, especially if these options meet other requirements (see below).
	Aggregate and share with your author team pivotal publication data, including circulation (e.g., open-access if available; see the Directory of Open Access Journals), impact factor, rejection rate, geographical distribution, individual and/or institutional subscriptions, time from submission to acceptance/posting/publication (i.e., "T sub to pub"), including any expedited publication options and potential per-page charges for these. Review and share any other potential journal charges, including for color illustrations and open access.
	Consider the benefit: risk calculus and wider-ranging and longer-term implications of journal selection, including the potential consequences of publishing a paper rapidly, via a costly per-page expedited process, in a lower-impact factor journal (compared to, say, a society journal with a higher impact factor that rejects a higher proportion of papers and may require several months, rather than weeks, to publish).
	What are the potential implications of a journal's being a professional society publication? Can your paper be disseminated to a desired, influential readership (e.g., a "vanguard" of KOL clinician/educators)? If you are submitting your manuscript to a society journal, should you consider "syncing" publication and dissemination at an upcoming (e.g., annual, international, regional) congress of the society?
	Does the journal publish "theme issues," supplements (e.g., single-sponsored satellite symposia proceedings), and supplementary online appendices to accommodate findings that cannot be included in the main report?
	Carefully review the Aims and Scope and Author Guidelines (as well as online content) of the journal to determine if it publishes papers similar to yours. Be particularly mindful of your study's design. Some journals will not publish (or will publish much less frequently) certain types of studies, including those with open-label or *post hoc* subgroup-analysis designs.

(Continued)

Table 4.51 (Continued) QC checklist. Overview of research, publication planning, and journal selection

Item	Step
Selecting a journal.	Review and share with your author team or publication committee any journal processes that might influence manuscript preparation, including the need for independent statistical review; receptivity to transparently disclosed industry sponsorship; receptivity to transparently and disclosed assistance of medical writers and other supportive professionals; and receptivity to "preview" a blinded abstract of your work (see below).
	Carefully review and distribute to your author team or publication committee the journal's Author Guidelines and recent online content related to your paper, including any QC requirement checklist, needed author disclosures, and limits on numbers of words, figures/tables, and references.
	Presubmission inquiry to gauge potential journal interest in a blinded manner: Contact the journal's managing or other production editor to "preview" a blinded abstract of your paper, which may derive from a congress presentation (i.e., without author, sponsor, or medication names; substitute "NAME OF DRUG" for the actual name). Consult the Author Guidelines first, to ensure that the journal allows presubmission inquiries (some do not).
	Be mindful of regulatory and other requirements and make sure that they have been met. Potentially include in your cover letter the fact that the study was conducted in a manner consistent with Good Clinical Practices and ethical tenets originating in the Declaration of Helsinki, has been registered on www.clinicaltrials.gov (include the NCT ID #), and that all authors met ICMJE criteria. (See below, **Form 1**, Example of a cover letter for manuscript submission.)

Source: Selected data from Chipperfield L, Citrome L, Clark J et al. Authors' Submission Toolkit: a practical guide to getting your research published. *Curr Med Res Opin* 2010;26:1967–82.[12]

Abbreviations: *Ann Intern Med, Annals of Internal Medicine*; BMJ, *British Medical Journal*; EMA, European Medicines Agency; FDA, Food and Drug Administration; ICMJE, International Committee of Medical Journal Editors; *JAMA, Journal of the American Medical Association*; KOL, key opinion leader; MeSH, Medical Subject Heading; *NEJM, New England Journal of Medicine*; RCT, randomized controlled trial; WHO, World Health Organization.

Table 4.52 Example of a publication/journal options grid ("long list"): Brief report manuscript on adherence to an oral antidiabetic drug

Journal	Impact factor	Circulation	Acceptance %	$T_{Sub \rightarrow Pub}$,* wk	Brief reports (data provided if yes)?
Acta Diabetologica.	3.34	1,000 (print) 118,247 (downloads)	25	5–12	Max words text = 1,000 No abstract Max. refs = 5 Max. tables/figures = 2
Clinical Endocrinology.	3.327	191 (print)	43	14	No brief reports.
Diabetes.	8.684	1,600 (print)	18	12–26	Max. words text = 2,000 Max. refs = 25 Max. tables/figures = 4
Diabetes and Vascular Disease Research.	3.417	923 (print)	25	7–10	Max. words text = 1,500 Max. refs = 10–12 Max. tables/figures = 1
Diabetes Care.	11.857	6,600 (print)	13	9–24	No brief communications.
Diabetes Research and Clinical Practice.	3.639	23 (print)	39	7–17	Max. words text = 1,000 (w/summary ≤50 words) Max. refs = 20
Diabetic Medicine.	3.054	854 (print) 16,047 (monthly downloads)	67	18	Max. words text = 1,500 (w/structured abstract) Max. refs = 20 Max. tables/figures = 2
Diabetes, Obesity and Metabolism.	6.715	11,000 (print)	20	4–13	Max. words = 1,200 (w/180-word unstructured abstract) Max. refs = 12 Max. tables/figures = 2
Endocrine Practice.	2.347	4,400 (print)	35	13–16	Commentaries. Max. words text = 1,500 Max. refs = 15 Max. tables/figures = 1

(Continued)

Table 4.52 (Continued) Example of a publication/journal options grid ("long list"): Brief report manuscript on adherence to an oral antidiabetic drug

Journal	Impact factor	Circulation	Acceptance %	$T_{Sub \to Pub}$* wk	Brief reports (data provided if yes)?
Endocrine Reviews.	15.745	763 (print)	30	12–24	Commentaries Max. words text = 1,000 Max. refs = 8 0 tables/figures
Endocrinology.	4.286	1,398 (print)	30	24–28	Max. words text = 2,400
European Journal of Endocrinology.	4.101	800 (print)	25	16–18	No brief reports
International Journal of Endocrinology.	2.510	N/A	25	15	No brief reports
Journal of Clinical Endocrinology and Metabolism.	5.455	6,925 (print)	25	20	Commentaries Max. words text = 1,000 Max. refs = 8 0 tables/figures
Journal of Diabetes and Its Complications.	2.056	9,199 (average monthly visits)	40	4–18	Max. words text = 1,000 (w/summary ≤50 words) Max. refs = 20
Journal of Endocrinology.	4.706	850 (print)	20	13	No brief reports
Metabolism.	5.777	38 (print) 17,225 (average monthly visits)	39	5–16	Max. words text = 1,500 (w/structured abstract) Max. refs = 20 Max. tables/figures = 2
Pancreas.	2.967	12,815 (average monthly visits)	50	9–25	Yes, but no posted max. words (except summary of ≤50 words)
Primary Care Diabetes.	1.381	2,757 (average monthly visits) 850 (print) 40,000 (average monthly users worldwide)	43	11–41	Max. words text = 1000 Max. refs = 20

Source: Data available from PubsHub, an ICON plc Company. Available by subscription at: https://journalsandcongresses.pubshub.com. Last accessed February 9, 2018.

Note: "Author Team: Journal aims/scope, free recent on-line content, and editorial contact information are provided under separate cover."

Abbreviation: N/A, not applicable.

*$T_{Sub \to Pub}$, time from manuscript submission to publication or posting ahead of print, including under assumptions of expedited publication.

Table 4.53 Committee on Publication Ethics (COPE): How to spot authorship problems

- Corresponding author seems unable to respond to reviewer's comments.
- Changes are made by someone not on the author list. (Check Word document properties to determine who made the changes, but bear in mind that there may be an innocent explanation for this, such as using a shared PC or an assistant making changes.)
- Document properties show that the manuscript was drafted by someone not on the author list or not properly acknowledged.
- "Impossibly prolific" author, e.g., of review articles/opinion pieces (check also for redundant/overlapping publication; this may be detected by a MEDLINE or Google search using the author's name).
- Several similar review articles/editorials/opinion pieces have been published under different author names. (This may be detected by a MEDLINE or Google Scholar search using the author's name.)
- Roles missing from list of contributors (e.g., it appears that none of the named authors were responsible for analyzing the data or drafting the paper).
- Unfeasibly long or short author list (e.g., a simple case report with a dozen authors or a randomized trial with a single author).
- Industry-funded study with no authors from the sponsor company. (This may be legitimate but may also mean that deserving authors have been omitted; reviewing the protocol may help to determine roles of employees.)

Source: Reproduced with permission from COPE and Wager E. Authors, ghosts, damned lies, and statisticians. *PLoS Med* 2007;4:e34.[59] Gøtzsche PC, Hrobjartsson A, Johansen HK et al. Ghost authorship in industry-initiated randomised trials. *PLoS Med* 2007;4:e19.[60] Available at www.publicationethics.org.

Note: This is an open-access article distributed under the terms of the Creative Commons Attribution License, which permits unrestricted use, distribution, and reproduction in any medium, provided that the original author and source are credited.

Table 4.54 Summary of key elements for peer-reviewed medical journals' conflict of interests policies

Element	Key aspect	Comments
Definition and scope.	A clear definition the journal uses as to what is conflict of interest and who is captured in the definition.	Sample definition: Conflict of interests exist when a participant in the publication process (author, peer reviewer, or editor) has a competing interest that could unduly influence (or be reasonably seen to do so) his or her responsibilities in the publication process (submission of manuscripts, peer review, editorial decisions, and communication between authors, reviewers, and editors).
Types of competing interests.	A clear statement of examples of the types of competing interests (and their definitions) the journal says must be declared. Should include the following as examples, but there could be others: (a) Financial ties. (b) Academic commitments. (c) Personal relationships. (d) Political or religious beliefs. (e) Institutional affiliations.	There is a need to consider a wide range of competing interests (and a recognition that they can coexist) that the individual assesses as to whether they unduly influence (or can be reasonably seen to do so) his or her responsibilities in the publication process. Examples and definitions of what competing interests should be declared need to be articulated with journals moving beyond just financial conflict of interest.
Declaring conflict of interests.	Clear statements on (a) what is to be declared, when, and to whom; (b) format for declaration; (c) a journal's role in asking additional questions or seeking clarification about disclosures; and (d) consequences for failing to disclose before or after publication.	Journals rely on disclosure about the facts because routine monitoring or investigation is not possible. This creates a particular onus on the declarer to report carefully and comprehensively. It also means that journals should ask about conflict of interest in such a way that there will be a high likelihood of reporting relevant conflict of interest.
Managing conflict of interests.	A clear statement on how conflict of interest will be managed by the journal, including the position that all relevant conflict of interests disclosures (or the declaration of no conflict of interests) will be published with the article and clarity about what conflict of interest situations will result in a manuscript not being considered.	Journals use various rules about how they will deal with conflict of interest and conflict of interest disclosures, and these need to be made known to all those involved in the publication process.

Source: Reproduced with permission from Ferris LE, Fletcher RH. World Association of Medical Editors (WAME) editorial on conflicts of interests. Conflict of interest in peer-reviewed medical journals: the WAME position on a challenging problem. Copyright ©2016 WAME. Available at: http://www.wame.org/about/wame-editorial-on-coi. Last accessed February 28, 2018.

PART 2: FORMS RELATED TO TRANSPARENT AND ETHICAL DISCLOSURES

Form 1

Example/Template of a Cover Letter to Submit a Manuscript to a Peer-Reviewed Journal.

DATE

A.A. Bashmachkin, MD, PhD
Editor-in-Chief
Journal of Publishable Data (JPD)
2100 Yoghurt Prospect
Old Tbilisi, Georgia 4090912

SUBMITTED ELECTRONICALLY VIA *JPD* AUTHOR CENTER PORTAL

Re: Eric Tate. Evaluation of involuntary noisome hiccup syndrome in a busy Hungarian eatery.

Dear Dr. Bashmachkin:

On behalf of my coauthors, I am pleased to submit herewith the above-referenced manuscript for publication in the *Journal of Publishable Data (JPD)*.

[[BUILD TO CLINICAL OR OTHER PROBLEM/OBJECTIVE ADDRESSED BY YOUR STUDY/ REPORT:]]

Malodorous hiccupping, also known as involuntary noisome hiccup syndrome (INHS), is a major cause of distress that erodes quality of life for many Eastern European adults, particularly those who frequently consume garlic-laden Hungarian goulashes. Because of embarrassment and halitosis, these patients have been difficult to recruit and treat in controlled clinical trials. A recent Cochrane Collaboration review[1] identified only five high-quality studies, and none was actively controlled (i.e., vs. placebo + usual care). These and other methodological challenges have impeded development and testing of potential medications for INHS. We project that *JPD* readers will be interested in our work because our review of papers published in the past 3 years by *JPD* found no study reports on medications for INHS, which also has no standard of care.

[[CLOSE INTRODUCTION WITH THE UNIQUE/INCREMENTAL VALUE OF YOUR STUDY/ REPORT:]]

For the first time (to our knowledge), we report findings from a randomized controlled trial evaluating the effects of an investigational anticholinergic agent (spastex HCl) on signs and symptoms of INHS in large numbers of Hungarian adults. Also unprecedented are our study's findings that spastex significantly reduced (i.e., improved) the primary efficacy outcome measure (the Belching Uniform Reflux Plan Index [BURPI]) and increased (improved) scores on disease-related and generic quality of life indices. Long-term safety could not be assessed in our 12-week study but is the object of consideration in an ongoing 52-week extension trial involving more vulnerable patients, including those with congenital high-frequency diaphragmatic spasm [CHFDS]).

[[ETHICS:]]

The study was conducted in accordance with Good Clinical Practices and ethical tenets originating in the Declaration of Helsinki. All study participants provided written informed consent before any study assessment or treatment, and both the informed-consent document and study protocol were reviewed and approved by local institutional review boards. As per §801 of the Food and Drug Administration Amendments Act (FDAAA) of 2007, the study was registered at www.clinicaltrials.gov (NCT # 10μ8508λ). All authors had access to study data and protocols, and take full responsibility for the integrity of both the analysis and report, which were supported financially by ABC Pharma (as disclosed on the title page of manuscript). Authors' financial disclosures are also summarized on the title page. I am a major stockholder (>$10,000 equity) in ABC Pharma.

[[ICMJE AUTHORSHIP:]]

All authors met criteria for authorship as set forth by the ICMJE, including having read and approved the final manuscript submitted herewith. ABC provided funding for professional-writing support by Boris Ilivič, MPH, who did not meet ICMJE authorship criteria and is named in the Acknowledgments section of the manuscript. The contents of the manuscript represent original work and have not been published, in whole or in part, before or concomitant with, this submission to the *JPD*. Selected data were presented at the 33rd Annual Congress of the International Eructation Society, November 4, 2016, Brașov, Transylvania. However, the findings were not published in congress proceedings or transactions of meetings or symposium volumes. The present manuscript has not been simultaneously submitted to any other journal and hence is not under consideration for publication by another journal and does not infringe existing copyright or third-party rights.

[[PEER REVIEWERS RECOMMENDED AND RECOMMENDED AGAINST:]]

My coauthors and I recommend the following independent and unbiased individuals as peer reviewers of our work:

1. Gevalt O MD, Professor of Gastroenterology, University of Pécs School of Medicine, Budapest, Hungary, gevaltoy@pecs.edu.
2. Gottenyu O MD, PhD, Professor of Internal Medicine, University of Debrecen (Hungary) Medical School, gottenyuoy@debrecen.edu.

Professor Dr. Hans Onpoopick, Professor of Anthropometric Studies, Semmelweiss Medical School, is conducting research on a competing therapy and, in our opinion, would not be a disinterested reviewer.

[[EXPRESS INTEREST IN MANUSCRIPT REVIEW/DISPOSITION AND PROVIDE CONTACT INFO.]]

My coauthors and I are keenly interested in the journal's review of our manuscript and its disposition. Kindly direct notifications about the manuscript to me (contact information below).

Thank you in advance to the editors and referees for reviewing our work. We hope that our manuscript meets the needs of the *JPD* and its readers.

Sincerely yours,

Eric Tate, MD
Hungary Professor of Gastroenterology
Szekszard Prospect School of Medicine
100 Szekszard Prospect
Szekszard, Hungary 04044
Tel: +36 00 000 000
Fax: +36 00 000 000
Email: etate@szekszardmail.edu

REFERENCE

1. Gevalt O, Gottenyu O. To belch, or not to belch? Is that a question? Meta-analysis of published studies on noisome involuntary hiccup syndrome (INHS). *Cochr Collab Rev* 2015;101:18–38.

Form 2

Author Disclosure Form to Facilitate Submission of Manuscript to Journal.
Dear Author/Contributor: Kindly complete and return the form below before the kickoff meeting.

Your name:	Academic affiliation	Hospital affiliation (or indicate "private practice")	Other info. to ease submission
	University:	Hospital/Medical Center/ Clinic/VAMC	
Your academic degrees:	Your title:	Your title:	Log-in information for Journal Author Center:
"Honorifics" (e.g., FACP, FACS)	Department(s):	Department(s):	User ID:
	Postal address:	Postal address:	P/W:
Office assistant's information			Recommended peer reviewers (include name, institution, and email address):
E-mail:	Street:	Street:	1:
Tel:	City:	City:	2:
Fax:	State/Province:	State/Province:	3:
Your office #:	Postal code:	Postal code:	
Your cell #:	Country:	Country:	
Best time(s) of day to reach you			
AM; PM			
If possible, insert jpeg of your signature in one of the following columns:			

Form 3

Author Intellectual Contributions.

Dear Prospective Author: To qualify for authorship, you need to check at least one box in each category and thus make some definitive intellectual contribution to the paper. It is not sufficient to merely approve each manuscript draft; reviewing and approving the manuscript is a necessary but not sufficient criterion of authorship. Please complete this form after the manuscript has been completed (but before it is submitted to the journal).

Category	Your contribution	Page #
Category I.		
Conceived/designed study	☐Date(s):	N/A
Acquired, analyzed, or interpreted data	☐Date(s):	N/A
Acquired data	☐Date(s):	N/A
Category II.		
Drafted the manuscript	☐Date(s):	Page(s):
Revised the manuscript for intellectual content	☐Date(s):	Page(s):
Category III.		
Reviewed and approved final manuscript	☐Date(s):	
Category IV.		
	☐Had access to all data and take responsibility for the study and manuscript.	N/A
Agree to be responsible for the work and answer any questions about the accuracy and integrity of any part of the study and its report.		

Source: Forms 3 and 4 are derived from documents authored by the International Committee of Medical Journal Editors (ICME), which are available at www.icmje.org.

Form 4A

Author Financial Disclosures.

Your name:	Relationship with study/ MS sponsor	Relationship with relevant competing or associated entity* (name)	USG or other government support (include grant #)	I.P. (Patents with USPTO numbers)
Employee of sponsor				
Otherwise compensated by study sponsor to coauthor paper				
Other compensation for coauthoring manuscript				
Equity (major ≥$10,000 or minor) holder in sponsor				
Options (major ≥$10,000 or minor) holder in sponsor				
Principal investigator				
Personal monies†				
Grant support (include only entities that could be affected financially by the published work, not public-funding sources)				
Academic support (last 36 mo.)				
Royalties (e.g., from patent)				
Expert testimony				

Source: Forms 3 and 4 are derived from documents authored by the International Committee of Medical Journal Editors (ICME), which are available at www.icmje.org. An electronic form that can be filled out by each author ("fillable pdf") is Available at: http://www.icmje.org/conflicts-of-interest. Last accessed October 28, 2017.

Abbreviations: I.P. Intellectual Property; USG, United States government; USPTO, United States Patent and Trademark Office.

*Any commercial or other organization researching/pursuing diagnostic or treatment modalities for the overall therapeutic category (not just the narrow topic) researched by you/your study.

†Personal monies include fees for services rendered, generally honoraria, royalties, or fees for consulting, lectures, speakers' bureaus, expert testimony, employment, or other affiliations.

Form 4B

Author Financial Disclosures [Hypothetical completed example].

Your name: H. Onpoopick, MD	Relationship with study/ MS sponsor	Relationship with relevant competing or associated entity (name)	USG or other government support (include grant #)	I.P. (Patents with numbers)
Employee of sponsor	No	No	–	–
Otherwise compensated by study sponsor to coauthor paper.	Yes	–	–	–
Other compensation for coauthoring manuscript	No	–	–	–
Equity (major ≥$10,000 or minor) holder in sponsor	Minor	Minor: Apex Pharma, Coracoid Diagnostics	–	–
Options (major ≥$10,000 or minor) holder in sponsor	No	No	–	–
Principal investigator	Yes	Apex Pharma	–	–
Personal monies‡	Yes	Apex Pharma, Nadir Pharma	–	–
Grant support (include only entities that could be affected financially by the published work, not public-funding sources)	No	–	NHLBI # 22,189	
Academic support (last 36 mo.) related to project	–	I was also supported by my institution, under a $1.5 million educational grant from The Scapula Society.	–	–
Royalties (e.g., from patent)		Apex Pharma licensed patented technology.	–	Yes. USPTO #118,879.
Expert testimony	No	Median Diagnostics	–	–

Abbreviations: I.P. Intellectual Property; USG, United States government; USPTO, United States Patent and Trademark Office.

REFERENCES

1. Dal-Ré R, Ioannidis JP, Bracken MB et al. Making prospective registration of observational research a reality. *Sci Transl Med* 2014;6:224cm1.

2. Kearsley-Fleet L, Zavada J, Hetland ML et al. The EULAR Study Group for Registers and Observational Drug Studies: comparability of the patient case mix in the European biologic disease modifying antirheumatic drug registers. *Rheumatology (Oxford)* 2015;54:1074–9.

3. Suresh K. An overview of randomization techniques: An unbiased assessment of outcome in clinical research. *J Hum Reprod Sci* 2011;4:8–11.

4. Weir JP. Quantifying test-retest reliability using the intraclass correlation coefficient and the SEM. *J Strength Cond Res* 2005;19:231–40.

5. Allison PD. *Missing Data*. Safe University Papers Series on Quantitative Applications in the Social Sciences, series no. 07-136. ed. Thousand Oaks, CA: Sage Publications Inc., 2002.

6. Shults J, Sun W, Tu X et al. A comparison of several approaches for choosing between working correlation structures in generalized estimating equation analysis of longitudinal binary data. *Stat Med* 2009;28:2338–55.

7. Moher D, Schulz KF, Altman D. The CONSORT statement: revised recommendations for improving the quality of reports of parallel-group randomized trials. *JAMA* 2001;285:1987–91.

8. Taichman DB, Backus J, Baethge C et al. Sharing clinical trial data: a proposal from the International Committee of Medical Journal Editors. *N Engl J Med* 2016;374:384–6.

9. Battisti WP, Wager E, Baltzer L et al. Good Publication Practice for Communicating Company-Sponsored Medical Research: GPP3. *Ann Intern Med* 2015;163:461–4.

10. International Committee of Medical Journal Editors. Recommendations for the conduct, reporting, editing, and publication of scholarly work in medical journals. Updated December 2014. Available at: www.icmje.

org/recommendations. Last accessed April 16, 2017.

11. *AMA Manual of Style: A Guide for Authors and Editors*. 10th ed. New York: Oxford University Press, 2007: 128–31.

12. Chipperfield L, Citrome L, Clark J et al. Authors' Submission Toolkit: a practical guide to getting your research published. *Curr Med Res Opin* 2010;26:1967–82.

13. Brown P, Brunnhuber K, Chalkidou K et al. How to formulate research recommendations. *BMJ* 2006;333:804–6.

14. Schünemann HJ, Oxman AD, Vist G. In: Higgins JPT, Green S eds. *Cochrane Handbook for Systematic Reviews of Interventions*. Version 5.1.0 of the Cochrane Handbook. West Sussex, UK: The Cochrane Collaboration and Wiley-Blackwell, 2011: 12.1–12.24.

15. Moher D, Liberati A, Tetzlaff J et al. Preferred Reporting Items for Systematic Reviews and Meta-Analyses: the PRISMA statement. *PLoS Med* 2009;6:e1000097.

16. Shamseer L, Moher D, Clarke M et al. Preferred Reporting Items for Systematic Review and Meta-Analysis protocols (PRISMA-P) 2015: elaboration and explanation. *BMJ* 2015;349:g7647.

17. Booth A. A brimful of "STARLITE": toward standards for reporting literature searches. *J Med Libr Assoc* 2006;94:421–9, e205.

18. Stroup DF, Berlin JA, Morton SC et al. Meta-analysis of observational studies in epidemiology: a proposal for reporting. Meta-analysis of Observational Studies in Epidemiology (MOOSE) group. *JAMA* 2000;283:2008–12.

19. Tramér MR, Reynolds DJ, Moore RA et al. Impact of covert duplicate publication on meta-analysis: a case study. *BMJ* 1997;315:635–40.

20. Egger M, Zellweger-Zahner T, Schneider M et al. Language bias in randomised controlled trials published in English and German. *Lancet* 1997;350:326–9.

21. Khan KS, Daya S, Collins JA et al. Empirical evidence of bias in infertility research: overestimation of treatment effect in crossover trials using pregnancy as the outcome measure. *Fertil Steril* 1996;65:939–45.

22. Schulz KF, Chalmers I, Hayes RJ et al. Empirical evidence of bias. Dimensions of methodological quality associated with estimates of treatment effects in controlled trials. *JAMA* 1995;273:408–12.

23. Moher D, Pham B, Jones A et al. Does quality of reports of randomised trials affect estimates of intervention efficacy reported in meta-analyses? *Lancet* 1998;352:609–13.

24. Jadad AR, Moore RA, Carroll D et al. Assessing the quality of reports of randomized clinical trials: is blinding necessary? *Control Clin Trials* 1996;17:1–12.

25. Berlin JA. Does blinding of readers affect the results of meta-analyses? University of Pennsylvania Meta-analysis Blinding Study Group. *Lancet* 1997;350:185–6.

26. Thompson SG. Why sources of heterogeneity in meta-analysis should be investigated. *BMJ* 1994;309:1351–5.

27. Marusic A, Bates T, Anic A et al. How the structure of contribution disclosure statements affects validity of authorship: a randomized study in a general medical journal. *Curr Med Res Opin* 2006;22:1035–44.

28. Simes RJ. Publication bias: the case for an international registry of clinical trials. *J Clin Oncol.* 1986;4:1529–41.

29. Moher D, Cook DJ, Eastwood S et al. Improving the quality of reports of meta-analyses of randomised controlled trials: the QUOROM statement. Quality of Reporting of Meta-analyses. *Lancet* 1999;354:1896–900.

30. Moher D, Hopewell S, Schulz KF et al. CONSORT 2010 Explanation and Elaboration: Updated guidelines for reporting parallel group randomised trials. *J Clin Epidemiol* 2010;63:e1–37.

31. Campbell MK, Elbourne DR, Altman DG. CONSORT statement: extension to cluster randomised trials. *BMJ* 2004;328:702–8.

32. Ioannidis JPA, Evans SJ, Gøtzsche PC et al. Better reporting of harms in randomized trials: an extension of the CONSORT statement. *Ann Intern Med* 2004;141:781–8.

33. Hopewell S, Clarke M, Moher D et al. CONSORT for reporting randomised trials in journal and conference abstracts. *Lancet* 2008;371:281–3.

34. von Elm E, Altman DG, Egger M et al. The Strengthening the Reporting of Observational Studies in Epidemiology (STROBE) statement: guidelines for reporting observational studies. *Lancet* 2007;370:1453–7.

35. Benchimol EI, Smeeth L, Guttmann A et al. The REporting of studies Conducted using Observational Routinely collected health Data (RECORD) Statement. *PLoS Med* 2015;12:e1001885.

36. Gallo V, Egger M, McCormack V et al. STrengthening the Reporting of OBservational studies in Epidemiology—Molecular Epidemiology (STROBE–ME): an extension of the STROBE Statement. *PLoS Med* 2011;8:e1001117.

37. Field N, Cohen T, Struelens MJ et al. Strengthening the Reporting of Molecular Epidemiology for Infectious Diseases (STROME–ID): an extension of the STROBE statement. *Lancet Infect Dis* 2014;14:341–52.

38. Stone SP, Cooper BS, Kibbler CC et al. The ORION statement: guidelines for transparent reporting of outbreak reports and intervention studies of nosocomial infection. *J Antimicrob Chemother* 2007;59:833–40.

39. Little J, Higgins JP, Ioannidis JPA et al. STrengthening the REporting of Genetic Association Studies (STREGA): an extension of the STROBE statement. *PLoS Med* 2009;6:e1000022.

40. Hollenbach JA, Mack SJ, Gourraud PA et al. A community standard for immunogenomic data reporting and analysis: proposal for a STrengthening the REporting of Immunogenomic Studies statement. *Tissue Antigens* 2011;78:333–44.

41. Janssens ACJW, Ioannidis JPA, van Duijn CM et al. Strengthening the reporting of Genetic RIsk Prediction Studies: the GRIPS Statement. *PLoS Med* 2011;8:e1000420.

42. Husereau D, Drummond M, Petrou S et al. Consolidated Health Economic Evaluation Reporting Standards (CHEERS) statement. *BMJ* 2013;346:f1049.

43. Des Jarlais DC, Lyles C, Crepaz N. Improving the reporting quality of nonrandomized evaluations of behavioral and public health interventions: the TREND statement. *Am J Public Health* 2004;94:361–6.

44. Berger ML, Mamdani M, Atkins D et al. Good research practices for comparative effectiveness research: defining, reporting and interpreting nonrandomized studies of treatment effects using secondary data sources: the ISPOR Good Research Practices for Retrospective Database Analysis Task Force Report—Part I. *Value Health* 2009;12:1044–52.

45. Davidoff F, Batalden P, Stevens D et al. Publication guidelines for improvement studies in health care: evolution of the SQUIRE Project. *BMJ* 2009;338:a3152.

46. Thorpe KE, Zwarenstein M, Oxman AD et al. A pragmatic-explanatory continuum indicator summary (PRECIS): a tool to help trial designers. *J Clin Epidemiol* 2009;62:464–75.

47. Relton C, Torgerson D, O'Cathain A et al. Rethinking pragmatic randomised controlled trials: introducing the "cohort multiple randomised controlled trial" design. *BMJ* 2010;340:963–7.

48. Zwarenstein M, Treweek S, Gagnier JJ et al. Improving the reporting of pragmatic trials: an extension of the CONSORT statement. *BMJ* 2008;337:a2390.

49. Tong A, Sainsbury P, Craig J. Consolidated criteria for reporting qualitative research (COREQ): a 32-item checklist for interviews and focus groups. *Int J Qual Health Care* 2007;19:349–57.

50. Edwards IR, Lindquist M, Wiholm BE et al. Quality criteria for early signals of possible adverse drug reactions. *Lancet* 1990;336:156–8.

51. Kelly WN, Arellano FM, Barnes J et al. Guidelines for submitting adverse event reports for publication. *Pharmacoepidemiol Drug Saf* 2007;16:581–7.

52. Chan AW, Tetzlaff JM, Gøtzsche PC et al. SPIRIT 2013 explanation and elaboration: guidance for protocols of clinical trials. *BMJ* 2013;346:e7586.

53. Bossuyt PM, Reitsma JB, Bruns DE et al. STARD 2015: an updated list of essential items for reporting diagnostic accuracy studies. *BMJ* 2015;351:h5527.

54. Collins GS, Reitsma JB, Altman DG et al. Transparent Reporting of a multivariable prediction model for Individual Prognosis or Diagnosis (TRIPOD): the TRIPOD statement. *BMJ* 2015;350:g7594.

55. Kottner J, Audige L, Brorson S et al. Guidelines for Reporting Reliability and Agreement Studies (GRRAS) were proposed. *Int J Nurs Studies* 2011;48:661–71.

56. Gagnier JJ, Kienle G, Altman DG et al. The CARE guidelines: consensus-based clinical case report guideline development. *J Diet Suppl* 2013;10:381–90.

57. Kempen JH. Appropriate use and reporting of uncontrolled case series in the medical literature. *Am J Ophthalmol* 2011;151:7–10.

58. Kilkenny C, Browne WJ, Cuthill IC et al. Improving bioscience research reporting: the ARRIVE guidelines for reporting animal research. *PLoS Biol* 2010;8:e1000412.

59. Wager E. Authors, ghosts, damned lies, and statisticians. *PLoS Med* 2007;4:e34.

60. Gøtzsche PC, Hrobjartsson A, Johansen HK et al. Ghost authorship in industry-initiated randomised trials. *PLoS Med* 2007;4:e19.

Appendix 1: Minimum clinically important differences (MCIDs) in patient-reported outcomes (PROs)

Suppose that you or your colleagues administer a patient quality of life (QOL) questionnaire scored from 0 (worst) to 80 (best). You observe an 8-point difference from baseline to endpoint. What does it mean to the patient and how does it inform your (or your colleagues') decision making in disease management? Certain surrogate biologic variables are tightly associated with (and/or predictive of) "hard" clinical endpoints such as hospitalization, progression-free survival, and overall longevity. These include lipid levels and blood pressure in cardiovascular diseases; CD4 T-cell counts and viral loads in HIV; liver enzymes in hepatic diseases; and protein expression by tumor cells in cancer. However, the consequences to patients of changes in their scores on QOL instruments are typically much less clear.

The concept of the minimum clinically important difference (MCID) was introduced by Jaeschke and colleagues in 1989.[1] The research team defined MCID as "the smallest difference in score in the domain of interest which patients perceive as beneficial and which would mandate, in the absence of troublesome side effects and excessive cost, a change in the patient's management." The definition hence comprises two constructs related to change: (1) the minimum change discerned (and reported) by the patient and (2) the minimum variation on a patient-reported outcome (PRO) that alters disease management.[2]

There are four approaches to determine MCID: one informal and three, more formal. The informal approach is to designate as clinically meaningful a ≥10% change of the total score on an instrument/index/questionnaire.

The three, more formal strategies include anchor- and distribution-based approaches, as well as the Delphi method. The anchor approach compares changes on a questionnaire with some reference ("anchor") that patients consider meaningful.

The anchor can be elicited prospectively by asking a patient or population of patients, "What change (improvement) in QOL as measured by the instrument would you require to agree to receive an intervention?" The population distribution-based strategy is to use some measure of population dispersion, for instance 1 standard error[3] or one-half of the standard deviation (SD). The Delphi method is an iterative process that is based on average scores of ratings by experts.

If an intervention improves QOL in the vast majority of individuals while leaving test scores unchanged in very few, the anchor method may need to be adjusted by using a higher threshold of "substantial (rather than minimal) clinically important difference." This threshold segregates patients who improve greatly compared to those who merely improve. If possible, the MCID should be computed via more than one approach.

The most common generic health-related QOL measures are the Medical Outcomes Study/RAND 36-Item Short Form Health Survey (SF-36; US) and the EuroQol 5D (EQ-5D).[4–8] The SF-36 includes eight domains: four each map to a Physical Component Summary (PCS; Physical Functioning, Role Physical, Bodily Pain, and General Health) and a Mental Component Summary (MCS; Energy/Vitality, Social Functioning, Role Emotional, and Mental Health). Scores on the PCS and MCS are linearly transformed to a T-score metric with a US population mean equal to 50 and an SD of 10.[8] Higher scores indicate better function: scores on each of the eight scales range from 0 to 100, where 0 is consistent with maximum disability (worst possible health) and 100, no disability (best possible health).

A standardized preference-based instrument, the EQ-5D evaluates five dimensions across three or five levels of problems and also includes a 20-cm visual analog scale (EQ-VAS) scored from

0 to 100, where 0 signifies the worst imaginable health and 100, the best. The five dimensions are Self-Care, Usual Activities, Mobility, Pain/Discomfort, and Anxiety/Depression. Each can be scored as "no problems," "slight problems," "moderate problems," "severe problems," and "extreme problems." A weighted EQ-5D index score is anchored at 0 for death to 1.0 for perfect health. Minimum clinically important differences on both the SF-36 and EQ-5D vary across different disease states.

Table A.1 presents MCIDs for representative chronic conditions with adverse effects on patient QOL and well-being. Some ranges presented in the table encompass values computed using both anchor- and distribution-based methods. Apart from the 6-minute walk test (6MWT), most of the measures are PROs.

Table A.1 Thresholds for minimum clinically important differences related to selected chronic medical conditions with adverse effects on health-related quality of life (HRQOL) and other patient-reported outcomes (PROs)

Clinical category	Representative questionnaire/test/endpoint	MCID (point or unit)
Autoimmune/allergic (selected).		
Angioedema.[9]	• AE-QoL.	• 6.
Systemic lupus erythematosus.[10]	➢ SLEDAI-2000.	➢ ≥1 decrease (improvement).
		➢ ≥3 increase (worsening).
Cardiovascular.		
Coronary heart disease. (CHD; cardiac rehabilitation).[11]	• 6MWT.	• 25 meters (m).
Depression and anxiety in CHD.	• HADS-A.	• 3.80.
	• HADS-D.	• 3.99.
	• HADS-T.	• 5.68.
Heart failure.	• 6MWT.[12]	• 45 m.
	❖ MLHFQ.	❖ 5 to 7 (overall score).
Peripheral arterial disease[13] (CLI).	• VascuQoL.	• 0.36 to 0.48 (total score).
Acne.[14]	• Acne-QoL.	• 0.50 to 10.3 mean change per item.
General[15,16] (thresholds for severely impaired HRQOL).	• Skindex-29.	• Symptoms scale: ≥52 points.
		• Emotions scale: ≥39.
		• Functioning scale: ≥37.
		• ≥44 (overall).
Hyperhidrosis.[17]	• HidroQOL©.	• 3 points (overall MCID).
		➢ 1.94 to 3.07 (generalized).
		➢ 2.16 to 4.36 (axillary).
		➢ 2.15 to 3.39 (palmoplantar).
Psoriasis.[18]	➢ DLQI.	➢ 3.2.
	❖ PASI.	❖ >75%.
Urticaria.[19,20]	• DLQI.	• 2.24 to 3.10.
	➢ CU-Q$_2$oL.	➢ 15 (for Thai version).
Endocrine.		
Cushing's disease.[21]	• CushingQoL.	• 10.1.

(Continued)

Table A.1 (Continued) Thresholds for minimum clinically important differences related to selected chronic medical conditions with adverse effects on health-related quality of life (HRQOL) and other patient-reported outcomes (PROs)

Clinical category	Representative questionnaire/test/endpoint	MCID (point or unit)
Endocrine.		
Diabetes mellitus.	• HFS-II Worry scale.[22] • DHP-18.[23]	• 2.0 to 5.8. • Psychological distress domain 6.99 to 10.59. • Barriers to activity domain 6.48 to 9.89. • Disinhibited eating domain 7.52 to 11.39.
Gout.[24]	• GIS (0–100).	• 5 to 8.
Thyroid disorders. Graves orbitopathy.[25,26]	• GO-QOL.	• ≥6 (minor treatment). • ≥10 (orbital decompression/ major treatment).
Various.[27,28]	• ThyPRO.	• 0.2 = no change.
Genitourinary.		
Benign prostatic hyperplasia.[29,30]	• IPSS.	MCID = 3 points or >25% reduction (on total IPSS). • 3 = slight symptom improvement. • 5 = moderate improvement. • 8 = marked improvement.[29]
	➢ Urinary flow rate.	➢ 2 mL/s.
Erectile dysfunction (ED).[31]	• IIEF.	Overall = 4. • 2 for mild ED. • 5 moderate ED. • 7 severe ED.
Female pelvic floor disorders.[32]	• UDI. • UDI Stress. ➢ UIQ.	• 6.4 to 22.4. • 4.6 to 16.5. ➢ 6.5 to 17.0.
Stress urinary incontinence.[33]	• I-QOL.	• 2.5 to 6.3.
Gastrointestinal.		
Gastroesophageal reflux.[34]	• NDI.	• 10.
Inflammatory bowel disease. ➢ Crohn's disease.[35–37]	• SIBDQ. • CDAI. ➢ SF-36 PCS. ➢ SF-36 MCS. ❖ EQ-5D VAS.	• 16. • 50. ➢ 1.6 to 7.0. ➢ 2.3 to 8.7. ❖ 4.2 to 14.8.

(*Continued*)

Table A.1 (Continued) Thresholds for minimum clinically important differences related to selected chronic medical conditions with adverse effects on health-related quality of life (HRQOL) and other patient-reported outcomes (PROs)

Clinical category	Representative questionnaire/test/endpoint	MCID (point or unit)
Gastrointestinal.		
➢ Ulcerative colitis.[37–39]	• Mayo Score.	• 2.5.
Irritable bowel syndrome.[40,41]	• SIP.	• 2.8.
	➢ IBS-QOL.	➢ 10 to 14.
	❖ IBS pain severity.	❖ 50%.
Musculoskeletal.		
Ankylosing spondylitis.[42]	• BASFI.	• 7 mm or 17.5%.
	• BASDAI.	• 10 mm or 22.5%.
	• BASG.	• 15 mm or 27.5%.
Fibromyalgia.[43]	• BPI Pain (average).	• 2.1 (32.3% reduction from baseline [BL]).
	• BPI Severity.	• 2.2 (34.2% reduction from BL).
Pain/disability[44] after anterior cervical discectomy.	• VAS.	• VAS-NP 2.6.
		• VAS-AP 4.1.
	➢ NDI.	➢ 17.3%.
	❖ SF-12 PCS.	❖ 8.1.
	❖ SF-12 MCS.	❖ 4.7.
Pain/disability after lumbar-spine surgery.[45]	• ODI.	• 12.8.
	➢ SF-36 PCS.	➢ 4.9.
Duchenne muscular dystrophy.[46]	• 6MWT.	• 20 to 30 m.
Osteoarthritis (and other chronic musculoskeletal pain, including rheumatoid arthritis [RA]).[47]	• PI-NRS.	• 1 point or 15%.
RA.[48]	• CDAI.	• 12 for patients with high RA activity.
		• 6 for moderate RA activity.
		• 1 to 2 for low RA activity.
Fatigue in RA.[49]	• FSS.	• 20.2.
	➢ Vitality scale of SF-36.	➢ 14.8.
	❖ MAF.	❖ 18.7.
	• MFI.	• 16.6.
	○ FACIT-F.	○ 15.9.
	• CFS.	• 9.9.
	➢ 10-point numerical rating scale.	➢ 19.7 for normalized scores (0–100).
Neurologic.		
Alzheimer's disease.[50,51]	• MMSE.	• 1.40 to 3.72.
	➢ BADLS.	➢ 3.5.
	❖ NPI.	❖ 8.

(Continued)

Table A.1 (Continued) Thresholds for minimum clinically important differences related to selected chronic medical conditions with adverse effects on health-related quality of life (HRQOL) and other patient-reported outcomes (PROs)

Clinical category	Representative questionnaire/test/endpoint	MCID (point or unit)
Neurologic.		
Generalized anxiety disorder.[52]	• HAM-A.	• 50%.
	➢ CGI scale.	➢ 1 to 2.
CBVD (stroke). Upper-extremity motor function.[53]	• ARAT.	• 12 and 17 (nondominant and dominant hand/arm, respectively).
	➢ WMFT.	➢ 1.0 and 1.2.
	❖ MAL.	❖ 1.0 and 1.1.
Depression in acute stroke.	• HADS.	• >8 indicates depression.
Fibromyalgia.	• BPI Pain.	• 2.1 (32.3%).
	• BPI Severity.	• 2.2 (34.2%).
Major depressive disorder.[54]	• MADRS.	• 1.6 to 1.9.
Multiple sclerosis.[55–65]	• FSS.	• 0.6.
	➢ EQ-5D.	➢ 0.050 to 0.084.
	❖ 6MWT.	❖ 53.35 to 55.06 meters.
	• BBT (dominant hand).	• 3.48 to 5.23 blocks.
	❖ GAS.	❖ 10 for mean GAS.
	• GNDS.	• 3.
	➢ MSFC.	➢ 15% to 20%.
	• MSIS-29.	• 8.
Parkinson's disease; EPD, APD.[66]	• UPDRS.	EPD.
		• UPDRS II = 1.8 to 2.0.
		• UPDRS III = 6.1 to 6.2.
		• UPDRS II + III = 8.0 to 8.1.
		APD.
		• UPDRS II = 1.8 to 2.3.
		• UPDRS III = 5.2 to 6.5.
		• UPDRS II + III = 7.1 to 8.8.
	• Off-time.	• 1.0 to 1.3 hours.
PTSD.[67]	• EQ-5D.	• 0.04 to 0.10.
	➢ QWB-SA.	➢ 0.02 to 0.05.
Schizophrenia.[68,69]	• PANSS.	• 20.2.
	➢ Lenert utility score.	➢ 0.15.
	❖ HCQLS.	❖ 1.13.
	• QWB.	• 0.17.

(Continued)

Table A.1 (Continued) Thresholds for minimum clinically important differences related to selected chronic medical conditions with adverse effects on health-related quality of life (HRQOL) and other patient-reported outcomes (PROs)

Clinical category	Representative questionnaire/test/endpoint	MCID (point or unit)
Oncology.		
Oropharyngeal cancer.[70]	• UW-QOLQ.	• 13.07 (global QOL).
	➢ EORTC C-30.	➢ 9.43 (global QOL).
Gynecologic cancers.[71,72]	• FACT-G.	• Positive MCID = 4.37 (4.0%) to 5.48 (4.9%).
		• Negative MCID = 8.28 (7.7%) to 9.87 (8.8%).
	➢ PROMIS.®	➢ 3 to 5 (fatigue, anxiety, and depression).
		➢ 4 to 6 (pain and physical function).
Prostate cancer.[73]	• PCI.	• Urinary function = 8.
		• Bowel function = 7.
		• Sexual function = 8.
		• Urinary bother = 9.
		• Bowel bother = 8.
		• Sexual bother = 11.
	➢ SF-36 domains.	➢ Physical = 7.
		➢ Role physical = 14.
		➢ Bodily pain = 9.
		➢ General health = 8.
		➢ Mental health = 6.
		➢ Role emotional = 12.
		➢ Energy/Vitality = 9.
		➢ Social function = 9.
Respiratory.		
Asthma.[74]	• AQLQ.	• Total score = 0.52.
Cystic fibrosis.[75]	➢ CFQ-R.	➢ 4 (stable disease) to 8.5 (exacerbation).
COPD.[76,77]	• TDI.	• 1.
	➢ SGRQ.	➢ 4.
	❖ CCQ.	❖ 0.4.
Chronic heart failure and chronic lung disease.[1]	• CRQ.	• Overall = approximately 0.50:
		➢ Dyspnea = 0.43.
		➢ Fatigue = 0.64.
		➢ Emotional function = 0.49.

(Continued)

Table A.1 (Continued) Thresholds for minimum clinically important differences related to selected chronic medical conditions with adverse effects on health-related quality of life (HRQOL) and other patient-reported outcomes (PROs)

Clinical category	Representative questionnaire/test/endpoint	MCID (point or unit)
Obstructive sleep apnea.[78]	• SAQLI.	• 1.0.
Rhinoconjunctivitis.[79,80]	• RQLQ.	• 0.5.
	➢ Mini-RQLQ.	• 0.4.
	❖ TNSS.	• 0.55.

Abbreviations: Acne-QoL, Acne-Specific Quality of Life questionnaire; AE-QoL, Angioedema Quality of Life questionnaire; APD, advanced Parkinson's disease; AQLQ, Asthma Quality of Life Questionnaire; ARAT, Action Research Arm Test; BADLS, Bristol Activities of Daily Living Scale; BASDAI, Bath Ankylosing Spondylitis Disease Activity Index; BASFI, Bath Ankylosing Spondylitis Function Index; BAS-G, Bath Ankylosing Spondylitis Patient Global score; BBT, Box and Block Test; BPI, Brief Pain Inventory; CBVD, cerebrovascular disease; CCQ, Clinical COPD Questionnaire; CDAI, either Crohn's Disease Activity Index or Clinical Disease Activity Index (in RA); CFQ-R, Cystic Fibrosis Questionnaire-Revised; CFS, Chalder Fatigue Scale; CGI, Clinical Global Impression scale; CLI, chronic critical limb ischemia; COPD, chronic obstructive pulmonary disease; CRQ, Chronic Respiratory Disease Questionnaire; CU-Q$_2$oL, Chronic Urticaria Quality of Life Questionnaire; DHP, Diabetes Health Profile; DLQI, Dermatology Life Quality Index; EORTC C30, European Organisation for Research and Treatment of Cancer Quality of Life Questionnaire Core 30; EPD, early Parkinson's disease; FACIT-F, Functional Assessment of Chronic Illness Therapy–Fatigue; FACT-G, Functional Assessment of Cancer Therapy-General measurement scale; FSS, Fatigue Severity Scale; GAS, Goal Attainment Scale; GIS, Gout Impact Scale; GNDS, Guy's Neurological Disability Scale; GO-QOL, Graves Ophthalmology Quality of Life; HADS, Hospital Anxiety and Depression Scale (HADS-A [Anxiety], HADS-D [Depression], HADS-T [Total]); HAM-A, Hamilton Anxiety Rating Scale; HCQLS, Heinrichs–Carpenter Quality of Life Scale; HFS-II, Hypoglycaemia Fear Survey; HidroQOL©, Hyperhidrosis Quality of Life index; IBS-QOL, Irritable Bowel Syndrome Quality of Life; IIEF, International Index of Erectile Function; IPSS, International Prostate Symptom Score; I-QOL, Incontinence Quality of Life; MADRS, Montgomery–Åsberg Depression Rating Scale; MAF, Multidimensional Assessment of Fatigue; MAL, Motor Activity Log; MFI, Multidimensional Fatigue Inventory; MLHFQ, Minnesota Living with Heart Failure questionnaire; MMSE, Mini-Mental State Examination; MSFC, Multiple Sclerosis Functional Composite; MSIS-29, Multiple Sclerosis Impact Scale; NDI, Neck Disability Index or Nepean Dyspepsia Index; NPI, Neuropsychiatric Inventory; NRS, Numerical Rating Scale; ODI, Oswestry Disability Index; PANSS, Positive and Negative Syndrome Scale; PASI, Psoriasis Area and Severity Index; PCI, Prostate Cancer Index; PFS, Patient-specific Functional Scale; PI-NRS, Pain Intensity Numerical Rating Scale; PROMIS, PROMIS® Patient-Reported Outcomes Measurement Information System; PTSD, post-traumatic stress disorder; QWB-SA, Quality of Well-Being Scale-Self-Administered; RQLQ, Rhinoconjunctivitis Quality of Life Questionnaire; SAQLI, Sleep Apnea Quality of Life Index; SGRQ, St. George's Respiratory Questionnaire; SIBDQ, Short Inflammatory Bowel Disease Questionnaire (Short Quality of Life in Inflammatory Bowel Disease Questionnaire); SIP, Sickness Impact Profile; SLEDAI-2000, Systemic Lupus Erythematosus Disease Activity Index 2000; TDI, Transition Dyspnoea Index 2; ThyPRO, Thyroid-Related Patient-Reported Outcome; TNSS, Total Nasal Symptom Score; UDI, Urinary Distress Inventory; UIQ, Urinary Impact Questionnaire; UPDRS, Unified Parkinson's Disease Rating Scale; UW-QOL, University of Washington Quality of Life Questionnaire; VAS, visual analog scale; VAS-AP, visual analog scale arm pain; VascuQoL, Vascular Quality of Life questionnaire; VAS-NP, visual analog scale neck pain; WMFT, Wolf Motor Function Test.

REFERENCES

1. Jaeschke R, Singer J, Guyatt GH. Measurement of health status: ascertaining the minimal clinically important difference. *Control Clin Trials* 1989;10:407–15.

2. Cook CE. Clinimetrics Corner: The Minimal Clinically Important Change Score (MCID): a necessary pretense. *J Man Manip Ther* 2008;16:E82–E83.

3. Wyrwich KW, Tierney WM, Wolinsky FD. Further evidence supporting an SEM-based criterion for identifying meaningful intra-individual changes in health-related quality of life. *J Clin Epidemiol* 1999;52:861–73.

4. EuroQol Group. EQ-5D: A standardized instrument for use as a measure of health outcomes. Available at: https://www.euroqol.org/Last accessed February 24, 2018; Copyright © 2017 EuroQol Research Foundation.

5. SF-36. Available at: https://www.rand.org/health/surveys_tools/mos/36-item-short-form.html. Last accessed April 28, 2018.

6. Luo N, Johnson J, Coons SJ. Using instrument-defined health state transitions to estimate minimally important differences for four preference-based health-related quality of life instruments. *Med Care* 2010;48:365–71.

7. Wyrwich KW, Tierney WM, Babu AN, Kroenke K, Wolinsky FD. A comparison of clinically important differences in health-related quality of life for patients with chronic lung disease, asthma, or heart disease. *Health Serv Res* 2005;40:577–91.

8. Laucis NC, Hays RD, Bhattacharyya T. Scoring the SF-36 in orthopaedics: a brief guide. *J Bone Joint Surg Am* 2015;97:1628–34.

9. Weller K, Magerl M, Peveling-Oberhag A, Martus P, Staubach P, Maurer M. The Angioedema Quality of Life Questionnaire (AE-QoL): assessment of sensitivity to change and minimal clinically important difference. *Allergy* 2016;71:1203–9.

10. Yee CS, Farewell VT, Isenberg DA et al. The use of Systemic Lupus Erythematosus Disease Activity Index-2000 to define active disease and minimal clinically meaningful change based on data from a large cohort of systemic lupus erythematosus patients. *Rheumatology (Oxford)* 2011;50:982–8.

11. Gremeaux V, Troisgros O, Benaim S et al. Determining the minimal clinically important difference for the six-minute walk test and the 200-meter fast-walk test during cardiac rehabilitation program in coronary artery disease patients after acute coronary syndrome. *Arch Phys Med Rehabil* 2011;92:611–9.

12. Shoemaker MJ, Curtis AB, Vangsnes E, Dickinson MG. Triangulating clinically meaningful change in the six-minute walk test in individuals with chronic heart failure: A Systematic Review. *Cardiopulm Phys Ther J* 2012;23:5–15.

13. Frans FA, Nieuwkerk PT, Met R et al. Statistical or clinical improvement? Determining the minimally important difference for the vascular quality of life questionnaire in patients with critical limb ischemia. *Eur J Vasc Endovasc Surg* 2014;47:180–6.

14. McLeod LD, Fehnel SE, Brandman J, Symonds T. Evaluating minimal clinically important differences for the Acne-Specific Quality of Life Questionnaire. *Pharmacoeconomics* 2003;21:1069–79.

15. Nijsten T, Sampogna F, Abeni D. Categorization of Skindex-29 scores using mixture analysis. *Dermatology* 2009;218:151–4.

16. Prinsen CA, Lindeboom R, Sprangers MA, Legierse CM, de Korte J. Health-related quality of life assessment in dermatology: Interpretation of Skindex-29 scores using patient-based anchors. *J Invest Dermatol* 2010;130:1318–22.

17. Kamudoni P. Development, validation and clinical application of a patient-reported outcome measure in hyperhidrosis: The Hyperhidrosis Quality of Life Index (HidroQoL©). Cardiff (Wales, UK) University, 2014.

18. Mattei PL, Corey KC, Kimball AB. Psoriasis Area Severity Index (PASI) and the Dermatology Life Quality Index (DLQI): the correlation between disease severity and

psychological burden in patients treated with biological therapies. *J Eur Acad Dermatol Venereol* 2014;28:333–7.

19. Kulthanan K, Chularojanamontri L, Tuchinda P, Rujitharanawong C, Baiardini I, Braido F. Minimal clinical important difference (MCID) of the Thai Chronic Urticaria Quality of Life Questionnaire (CU-Q$_2$oL). *Asian Pac J Allergy Immunol* 2016;14:61.

20. Shikiar R, Harding G, Leahy M, Lennox RD. Minimal important difference (MID) of the Dermatology Life Quality Index (DLQI): Results from patients with chronic idiopathic urticaria. *Health Qual Life Outcomes* 2005;3:36.

21. Webb SM, Ware JE, Forsythe A et al. Treatment effectiveness of pasireotide on health-related quality of life in patients with Cushing's disease. *Eur J Endocrinol* 2014;171:89–98.

22. Stargardt T, Gonder-Frederick L, Krobot KJ, Alexander CM. Fear of hypoglycaemia: Defining a minimum clinically important difference in patients with type 2 diabetes. *Health Qual Life Outcomes* 2009;7:91.

23. Mulhern B, Meadows K. Investigating the minimally important difference of the Diabetes Health Profile (DHP-18) and the EQ-5D and SF-6D in a UK diabetes mellitus population. *Health* 2013;5:1045–54.

24. Khanna D, Sarkin AJ, Khanna PP et al. Minimally important differences of the Gout Impact Scale in a randomized controlled trial. *Rheumatology (Oxford)* 2011;50:1331–6.

25. Kashkouli MB, Heidari I, Pakdel F, Jam S, Honarbakhsh Y, Mirarmandehi B. Change in quality of life after medical and surgical treatment of Graves' ophthalmopathy. *Middle East Afr J Ophthalmol* 2011;18:42–7.

26. Terwee CB, Dekker FW, Mourits MP et al. Interpretation and validity of changes in scores on the Graves' ophthalmopathy quality of life questionnaire (GO-QOL) after different treatments. *Clin Endocrinol (Oxf)* 2001;54:391–8.

27. Watt T, Bjorner JB, Groenvold M et al. Development of a short version of the Thyroid-Related Patient-Reported Outcome ThyPRO. *Thyroid* 2015;25:1069–79.

28. Watt T, Cramon P, Hegedus L et al. The thyroid-related quality of life measure ThyPRO has good responsiveness and ability to detect relevant treatment effects. *J Clin Endocrinol Metab* 2014;99:3708–17.

29. Barry MJ, Williford WO, Chang Y et al. Benign prostatic hyperplasia specific health status measures in clinical research: how much change in the American Urological Association symptom index and the Benign Prostatic Hyperplasia Impact Index is perceptible to patients? *J Urol* 1995;154:1770–4.

30. Nickel JC, Brock GB, Herschorn S et al. Proportion of tadalafil-treated patients with clinically meaningful improvement in lower urinary tract symptoms associated with benign prostatic hyperplasia: integrated data from 1,499 study participants. *BJU Int* 2014;115:815–21.

31. Rosen RC, Allen KR, Ni X, Araujo AB. Minimal clinically important differences in the erectile function domain of the International Index of Erectile Function scale. *Eur Urol* 2011;60:1010–6.

32. Barber MD, Spino C, Janz NK et al. The minimum important differences for the urinary scales of the Pelvic Floor Distress Inventory and Pelvic Floor Impact Questionnaire. *Am J Obstet Gynecol* 2009;200:580–7.

33. Yalcin I, Patrick DL, Summers K, Kinchen K, Bump RC. Minimal clinically important differences in Incontinence Quality-of-Life scores in stress urinary incontinence. *Urology* 2006;67:1304–8.

34. Jones M, Talley NJ. Minimum clinically important difference for the Nepean Dyspepsia Index, a validated quality of life scale for functional dyspepsia. *Am J Gastroenterol* 2009;104:1483–8.

35. Coteur G, Feagan B, Keininger DL, Kosinski M. Evaluation of the meaningfulness of health-related quality of life improvements as assessed by the SF-36 and the EQ-5D VAS in patients with active Crohn's disease. *Aliment Pharmacol Ther* 2009;29:1032–41.

36. Feagan BG, McDonald JWD. Crohn's disease. In: Feagan BG, Burroughs AK, McDonald JWD, eds. *Evidence-Based Gastroenterology and Child Health.* Malden, MA: Blackwell Publishing Ltd.; 2004:179–96.

37. Guyatt G, Mitchell A, Irvine EJ et al. A new measure of health status for clinical trials in inflammatory bowel disease. *Gastroenterology* 1989;96:804–10.

38. Bewtra M, Brensinger CM, Tomov VT et al. An optimized patient-reported ulcerative colitis disease activity measure derived from the Mayo score and the Simple Clinical Colitis Activity Index. *Inflamm Bowel Dis* 2014;20:1070–8.

39. Lewis JD, Chuai S, Nessel L, Lichtenstein GR, Aberra FN, Ellenberg JH. Use of the noninvasive components of the Mayo score to assess clinical response in ulcerative colitis. *Inflamm Bowel Dis* 2008;14:1660–6.

40. Spiegel B, Camilleri M, Bolus R et al. Psychometric evaluation of patient-reported outcomes in irritable bowel syndrome randomized controlled trials: a Rome Foundation report. *Gastroenterology* 2009;137:1944–53.

41. Drossman D, Morris CB, Hu Y et al. Characterization of health related quality of life (HRQOL) for patients with functional bowel disorder (FBD) and its response to treatment. *Am J Gastroenterol* 2007;102:1442–53.

42. Pavy S, Brophy S, Calin A. Establishment of the minimum clinically important difference for the Bath Ankylosing Spondylitis Indices: a prospective study. *J Rheumatol* 2005;32:80–5.

43 Mease PJ, Spaeth J, Clauw DJ et al. Estimation of minimum clinically important difference for pain in fibromyalgia. *Arth Care Res* 2011;6:821–6.

44. Parker SL, Godil SS, Zuckerman SL et al. Comprehensive assessment of 1-year outcomes and determination of minimum clinically important difference in pain, disability, and quality of life after suboccipital decompression for Chiari malformation I in adults. *Neurosurgery* 2013;73:569–81.

45. Copay AG, Glassman SD, Subach BR, Berven S, Schuler TC, Carreon LY. Minimum clinically important difference in lumbar spine surgery patients: a choice of methods using the Oswestry Disability Index, Medical Outcomes Study questionnaire Short Form 36, and pain scales. *Spine J* 2008;8:968–74.

46. McDonald CM, Henricson EK, Abresch RT et al. The 6-minute walk test and other clinical endpoints in Duchenne muscular dystrophy: Reliability, concurrent validity, and minimal clinically important differences from a multicenter study. *Muscle Nerve* 2013;48:357–68.

47. Salaffi F, Stancati A, Silvestri CA, Ciapetti A, Grassi W. Minimal clinically important changes in chronic musculoskeletal pain intensity measured on a numerical rating scale. *Eur J Pain* 2004;8:283–91.

48. Curtis JR, Yang S, Chen L et al. Determining the minimally important difference in the Clinical Disease Activity Index for improvement and worsening in early rheumatoid arthritis patients. *Arthritis Care Res (Hoboken)* 2015;67:1345–53.

49. Pouchot J, Kherani RB, Brant R et al. Determination of the minimal clinically important difference for seven fatigue measures in rheumatoid arthritis. *J Clin Epidemiol* 2008;61:705–13.

50. Burback D, Molnar FJ, St John P, Man-Son-Hing M. Key methodological features of randomized controlled trials of Alzheimer's disease therapy: minimal clinically important difference, sample size and trial duration. *Dement Geriatr Cogn Disord* 1999;10:534–40.

51. Muayqil T, Camicioli R. Systematic review and meta-analysis of combination therapy with cholinesterase inhibitors and memantine in Alzheimer's disease and other dementias. *Dement Geriatr Cogn Dis Extra* 2012;2:546–72.

52. Roseman AS, Cully JA, Kunik ME et al. Treatment response for late-life generalized anxiety disorder: moving beyond symptom-based measures. *J Nerv Ment Dis* 2011;199:811–4.

53. Lang CE, Edwards DF, Birkenmeier RL, Dromerick AW. Estimating minimal clinically important differences of upper-extremity measures early after stroke. *Arch Phys Med Rehabil* 2008;89:1693–1700.

54. Duru G, Fantino B. The clinical relevance of changes in the Montgomery–Asberg Depression Rating Scale using the minimum clinically important difference approach. *Curr Med Res Opin* 2008;24:1329–35.

55. Kohn CG, Sidovar MF, Kaur K, Zhu Y, Coleman CI. Estimating a minimal clinically important difference for the EuroQol 5-Dimension health status index in persons with multiple sclerosis. *Health Qual Life Outcomes* 2014;12:66.

56. Goldman MD, Marrie RA, Cohen JA. Evaluation of the six-minute walk in multiple sclerosis subjects and healthy controls. *Mult Scler* 2008;14:383–90.

57. Goodkin DE, Hertsgaard D, Seminary J. Upper extremity function in multiple sclerosis: improving assessment sensitivity with Box-and-Block and Nine-Hole Peg tests. *Arch Phys Med Rehabil* 1988;69:850–4.

58. Lord SE, Wade DT, Halligan PW. A comparison of two physiotherapy treatment approaches to improve walking in multiple sclerosis: a pilot randomized controlled study. *Clin Rehabil* 1998;12:477–86.

59. Mathiowetz V, Volland G, Kashman N, Weber K. Adult norms for the Box and Block Test of manual dexterity. *Am J Occup Ther* 1985;39:386–91.

60. Jacobson GP, Newman CW. The development of the Dizziness Handicap Inventory. *Arch Otolaryngol Head Neck Surg* 1990;116:424–7.

61. Khan F, Pallant JF, Turner-Stokes L. Use of goal attainment scaling in inpatient rehabilitation for persons with multiple sclerosis. *Arch Phys Med Rehabil* 2008;89:652–9.

62. Sharrack B, Hughes RA. The Guy's Neurological Disability Scale (GNDS): A new disability measure for multiple sclerosis. *Mult Scler* 1999;5:223–33.

63. Rudick RA, Polman CH, Cohen JA et al. Assessing disability progression with the Multiple Sclerosis Functional Composite. *Mult Scler* 2009;15:984–97.

64. Costelloe L, O'Rourke K, Kearney H et al. The patient knows best: significant change in the physical component of the Multiple Sclerosis Impact Scale (MSIS-29 physical). *J Neurol Neurosurg Psychiatry* 2007;78:841–4.

65. Paltamaa J, Sarasoja T, Leskinen E et al. Measuring deterioration in interventional classification of functioning domains of people with multiple sclerosis who are ambulatory. *Phys Ther* 2008;88:176–90.

66. Hauser RA, Gordon MF, Mizuno Y et al. Minimal clinically important difference in Parkinson's disease as assessed in pivotal trials of pramipexole extended release. *Parkinson's Dis* 2014;2014:Article ID 467131.

67. Le QA, Doctor JN, Zoellner LA, Feeny NC. Minimal clinically important differences for the EQ-5D and QWB-SA in Post-traumatic Stress Disorder (PTSD): results from a doubly randomized preference trial (DRPT). *Health Qual Life Outcomes* 2013;11:59.

68. Thwin SS, Hermes E, Lew R et al. Assessment of the minimum clinically important difference in quality of life in schizophrenia measured by the Quality of Well-Being Scale and disease-specific measures. *Psychiatry Res* 2013;209:291–6.

69. Falissard B, Sapin C, Loze JY, Landsberg W, Hansen K. Defining the minimal clinically important difference (MCID) of the Heinrichs-carpenter quality of life scale (QLS). *Int J Methods Psychiatr Res* 2016;25:101–11.

70. Binenbaum Y, Amit M, Billan S, Cohen JT, Gil Z. Minimal clinically important differences in quality of life scores of oral cavity and oropharynx cancer patients. *Ann Surg Oncol* 2014;21:2773–81.

71. Ringash J, O'Sullivan B, Bezjak A, Redelmeier DA. Interpreting clinically significant changes in patient-reported outcomes. *Cancer* 2007;110:196–202.

72. Yost KJ, Eton DT, Garcia SF, Cella D. Minimally important differences were estimated for six Patient-Reported Outcomes Measurement Information System-Cancer scales in advanced-stage cancer patients. *J Clin Epidemiol* 2011;64:507–16.

73. Jayadevappa R, Malkowicz SB, Wittink M, Wein AJ, Chhatre S. Comparison of distribution- and anchor-based approaches to infer changes in health-related quality of life of prostate cancer survivors. *Health Serv Res* 2012;47:1902–25.

74. Jones PW. Interpreting thresholds for a clinically significant change in health status in asthma and COPD. *Eur Respir J* 2002;19:398–404.

75. Quittner AL, Modi AC, Wainwright C, Otto K, Kirihara J, Montgomery AB. Determination of the minimal clinically important difference scores for the Cystic Fibrosis

Questionnaire-Revised respiratory symptom scale in two populations of patients with cystic fibrosis and chronic *Pseudomonas aeruginosa* airway infection. *Chest* 2009;135:1610–18.

76. Jones PW, Mahler DA, Gale R, Owen R, Kramer B. Profiling the effects of indacaterol on dyspnoea and health status in patients with COPD. *Respir Med* 2011;105:892–9.

77. Kocks JW, Tuinenga MG, Uil SM, van den Berg JW, Stahl E, van der Molen T. Health status measurement in COPD: the minimal clinically important difference of the clinical COPD questionnaire. *Respir Res* 2006;7:62.

78. Flemons WW, Reimer MA. Measurement properties of the Calgary Sleep Apnea Quality of Life Index. *Am J Respir Crit Care Med* 2002;165:159–64.

79. Juniper EF, Guyatt GH, Griffith LE, Ferrie PJ. Interpretation of rhinoconjunctivitis quality of life questionnaire data. *J Allergy Clin Immunol* 1996;98:843–5.

80. Barnes ML, Vaidyanathan S, Williamson PA, Lipworth BJ. The minimal clinically important difference in allergic rhinitis. *Clin Exp Allergy* 2010;40:242–50.

Appendix 2: Probability distribution data tables to compute p values

The following tables enable the user to compute p values and complete the "pencil-and-paper" exercises in Chapter 3 (Biostatistics).

Table A2.1 Normal distribution

Z (No. of SDs to right of mean)	One-tailed applications		Two-tailed applications	
	One-tailed α (area in right tail)	1–α (area except right tail)	Two-tailed α (area in both tails)	1– α (area except both tails)
0	0.500	0.500	1.00	0
0.10	0.460	0.540	0.920	0.080
0.20	0.421	0.579	0.842	0.158
0.30	0.382	0.618	0.764	0.236
0.40	0.345	0.655	0.690	0.310
0.50	0.308	0.692	0.619	0.381
0.60	0.274	0.726	0.548	0.452
0.70	0.242	0.758	0.484	0.516
0.80	0.212	0.788	0.424	0.576
0.90	0.184	0.816	0.368	0.632
1.00	0.159	0.841	0.318	0.682
1.10	0.136	0.864	0.272	0.728
1.20	0.115	0.885	0.230	0.770
1.281	0.100	0.900	0.200	0.800
1.30	0.097	0.903	0.194	0.806
1.40	0.081	0.919	0.162	0.838
1.50	0.067	0.933	0.134	0.866
1.60	0.055	0.945	0.110	0.890
1.645	0.050	0.950	0.100	0.900
1.70	0.045	0.955	0.090	0.910
1.80	0.036	0.964	0.072	0.928
1.90	0.029	0.971	0.054	0.946
1.960	0.025	0.975	0.050	0.950
2.00	0.023	0.977	0.046	0.954
2.10	0.018	0.982	0.036	0.964
2.20	0.014	0.986	0.028	0.972
2.30	0.011	0.989	0.022	0.978
2.326	0.010	0.990	0.020	0.980
2.40	0.008	0.992	0.016	0.984
2.50	0.006	0.994	0.012	0.988
2.576	0.005	0.995	0.010	0.990
2.60	0.0047	0.9953	0.0094	0.9906
2.70	0.0035	0.9965	0.0070	0.9930
2.80	0.0026	0.9974	0.0052	0.9948
2.90	0.0019	0.9981	0.0038	0.9962
3.00	0.0013	0.9987	0.0026	0.9974
3.100	0.0010	0.9990	0.0020	0.9980
3.20	0.0007	0.9996	0.0014	0.9986
3.300	0.0005	0.9995	0.0010	0.9990
3.40	0.0003	0.9997	0.0006	0.9994
3.50	0.0002	0.9998	0.0004	0.9996

Source: Data as presented by Robert H. Riffenburgh in Statistics in Medicine. 3rd ed. Amsterdam: Academic Press (an imprint of Elsevier); 2012.
Abbreviation: SD, standard deviation.

Table A2.2 *t* Distribution

One-tailed α (area in right tail)	0.1000	0.0500	0.0250	0.0100	0.0050	0.0010	0.0005
One-tailed 1–α (area except right tail)	0.9000	0.9500	0.9750	0.9900	0.9950	0.9990	0.9995
Two-tailed α (area in both tails)	0.2000	0.1000	0.0500	0.0200	0.0100	0.0020	0.0010
Two-tailed 1–α (area except both tails)	0.8000	0.9000	0.9500	0.9800	0.9900	0.9980	0.9990
df = 2	1.886	2.920	4.303	6.965	9.925	22.327	31.598
3	1.638	2.353	3.182	4.541	5.841	10.215	12.941
4	1.533	2.132	2.776	3.747	4.604	7.173	8.610
5	1.476	2.015	2.571	3.365	4.032	5.893	6.859
6	1.440	1.943	2.447	3.143	3.707	5.208	5.959
7	1.415	1.895	2.365	2.998	3.499	4.785	5.405
8	1.397	1.860	2.306	2.896	3.355	4.501	5.041
9	1.383	1.833	2.262	2.821	3.250	4.297	4.781
10	1.372	1.812	2.228	2.764	3.169	4.144	4.587
11	1.363	1.796	2.201	2.718	3.106	4.025	4.437
12	1.356	1.782	2.179	2.681	3.055	3.930	4.318
13	1.350	1.771	2.160	2.650	3.012	3.852	4.221
14	1.345	1.761	2.145	2.624	2.977	3.787	4.140
15	1.341	1.753	2.131	2.602	2.947	3.733	4.073
16	1.337	1.746	2.120	2.583	2.921	3.686	4.015
17	1.333	1.740	2.110	2.567	2.898	3.646	3.965
18	1.330	1.734	2.101	2.552	2.878	3.610	3.922
19	1.328	1.729	2.093	2.539	2.861	3.579	3.883
20	1.325	1.725	2.086	2.528	2.845	3.552	3.850
21	1.323	1.721	2.080	2.518	2.831	3.527	3.819
22	1.321	1.717	2.074	2.508	2.819	3.505	3.792
23	1.319	1.714	2.069	2.500	2.807	3.485	3.767
24	1.318	1.711	2.064	2.492	2.797	3.467	3.745
25	1.316	1.708	2.060	2.485	2.787	3.450	3.725
26	1.315	1.706	2.056	2.479	2.779	3.435	3.707
27	1.314	1.703	2.052	2.473	2.771	3.421	3.690
28	1.313	1.701	2.048	2.467	2.763	3.408	3.674
29	1.311	1.699	2.045	2.462	2.756	3.396	3.659
30	1.310	1.697	2.042	2.457	2.750	3.385	3.646
40	1.303	1.684	2.021	2.423	2.704	3.307	3.551
60	1.296	1.671	2.000	2.390	2.660	3.232	3.460
100	1.290	1.660	1.984	2.364	2.626	3.174	3.390
∞	1.282	1.645	1.960	2.326	2.576	3.090	3.291

Source: Data as presented by Robert H. Riffenburgh in *Statistics in Medicine.* 3rd ed. Amsterdam: Academic Press (an imprint of Elsevier); 2012.

Table A2.3 χ^2 Distribution (right tail)

α (area in right tail)	0.1000	0.0500	0.0250	0.0100	0.0050	0.0010	0.0005
1–α (area except right tail)	0.9000	0.9500	0.9750	0.9900	0.9950	0.9990	0.9995
df =1	2.71	3.84	5.02	6.63	7.88	10.81	12.13
2	4.61	5.99	7.38	9.21	10.60	13.80	15.21
3	6.25	7.81	9.35	11.34	12.84	16.26	17.75
4	7.78	9.49	11.14	13.28	14.86	18.46	20.04
5	9.24	11.07	12.83	15.08	16.75	20.52	22.15
6	10.64	12.59	14.45	16.81	18.54	22.46	24.08
7	12.02	14.07	16.01	18.47	20.28	24.35	26.02
8	13.36	15.51	17.53	20.09	21.95	26.10	27.86
9	14.68	16.92	19.02	21.67	23.59	27.86	29.71
10	15.99	18.31	20.48	23.21	25.19	29.58	31.46
11	17.28	19.68	21.92	24.72	26.75	31.29	33.13
12	18.55	21.03	23.34	26.22	28.30	32.92	34.80
13	19.81	22.36	24.74	27.69	29.82	34.54	36.47
14	21.05	23.69	26.12	29.14	31.32	36.12	38.14
15	22.31	25.00	27.49	30.57	32.81	37.71	39.73
16	23.54	26.30	28.84	32.00	34.27	39.24	41.31
17	24.77	27.59	30.19	33.41	35.72	40.78	42.89
18	25.99	28.87	31.53	34.80	37.16	42.32	44.47
19	27.20	30.14	32.85	36.19	38.58	43.81	45.97
20	28.41	31.41	34.17	37.57	39.99	45.31	47.46
21	29.62	32.67	35.48	38.94	41.40	46.80	49.04
22	30.81	33.92	36.78	40.29	42.80	48.25	50.45
23	32.01	35.17	38.08	41.64	44.19	49.75	52.03
24	33.20	36.41	39.36	42.97	45.56	51.15	53.44
25	34.38	37.65	40.65	44.31	46.93	52.65	51.93
26	35.56	38.88	41.92	45.64	48.30	54.05	56.43
27	36.74	40.11	43.20	46.97	49.65	55.46	57.83
28	37.92	41.34	44.46	48.28	51.00	56.87	59.24
29	39.09	42.56	45.72	49.59	52.34	58.27	60.73
30	40.26	43.77	46.98	50.89	53.68	59.68	62.23
35	46.06	49.80	53.20	57.34	60.27	66.62	69.26
40	51.80	55.76	59.34	63.69	66.76	73.39	76.11
50	63.17	67.51	71.42	76.16	79.50	86.66	89.56
60	74.40	79.08	83.30	88.38	91.96	99.58	102.66
70	85.53	90.53	95.02	100.43	104.22	112.32	115.66
80	96.58	101.88	106.63	112.32	116.32	124.80	128.32
100	118.50	124.34	129.56	135.81	140.16	149.41	153.11

Source: Data as presented by Robert H. Riffenburgh in *Statistics in Medicine.* 3rd ed. Amsterdam: Academic Press (an imprint of Elsevier); 2012.

Table A2.4 χ^2 Distribution (left tail)

α (area in left tail)	0.0005	0.0010	0.0050	0.0100	0.0250	0.0500	0.1000
1−α (area except left tail)	0.9995	0.9990	0.9950	0.9900	0.9750	0.9500	0.9000
df = 1	0.0000004	0.0000016	0.0000390	0.0001600	0.0009800	0.0039000	0.0160000
2	0.0009900	0.0020000	0.0100000	0.0200000	0.0510000	0.1000000	0.2100000
3	0.0150000	0.0240000	0.0720000	0.1200000	0.2200000	0.3500000	0.5800000
4	0.0650000	0.0910000	0.21000000	0.3000000	0.4800000	0.7100000	1.0600000
5	0.1600000	0.2100000	0.41000000	0.5500000	0.8300000	1.1500000	1.6100000
6	0.3000000	0.3800000	0.6800000	0.8700000	1.2400000	1.6400000	2.2000000
7	0.4800000	0.6000000	0.9900000	1.2400000	1.6900000	2.1700000	2.8300000
8	0.7100000	0.8600000	1.3400000	1.6500000	2.1800000	2.7300000	3.4900000
9	0.9700000	1.1500000	1.7300000	2.0900000	2.7000000	3.3300000	4.1700000
10	1.2600000	1.4800000	2.1600000	2.5600000	3.2500000	3.9400000	4.8700000
11	1.5800000	1.8300000	2.6000000	3.0500000	3.8200000	4.5700000	5.5800000
12	1.9300000	2.2100000	3.0700000	3.5700000	4.4000000	5.2300000	6.3000000
13	2.3100000	2.6100000	3.5700000	4.1100000	5.0100000	5.8900000	7.0400000
14	2.7000000	3.0400000	4.0700000	4.6600000	5.6300000	6.5700000	7.7900000
15	3.1000000	3.4800000	4.6000000	5.2300000	6.260000	7.2600000	8.5500000
16	3.5400000	3.9400000	5.1400000	5.81000000	6.9100000	7.9600000	9.3100000
17	3.9800000	4.4200000	5.7000000	6.4100000	7.5600000	8.6700000	10.090000
18	4.4400000	4.9000000	6.2600000	7.0100000	8.2300000	9.3900000	10.8600000
19	4.9200000	5.4100000	6.8400000	7.6300000	8.9100000	10.1200000	11.6500000
20	5.4100000	5.9200000	7.4300000	8.2600000	9.590000	10.8500000	12.4400000

(Continued)

Table A2.4 (Continued) χ^2 Distribution (left tail)

| α (area in left tail) | 0.0005 | 0.0010 | 0.0050 | 0.0100 | 0.0250 | 0.0500 | 0.1000 |
1−α (area except left tail)	0.9995	0.9990	0.9950	0.9900	0.9750	0.9500	0.9000
21	5.8900000	6.4500000	8.0300000	8.9000000	10.2800000	11.5900000	13.2400000
22	6.4200000	6.9900000	8.6400000	9.5400000	10.9800000	12.3400000	14.0400000
23	6.9200000	7.5400000	9.2600000	10.2000000	11.6900000	13.0900000	14.8500000
24	7.4500000	8.0900000	9.8900000	10.8600000	12.4000000	13.8500000	15.6600000
25	8.0000000	8.6600000	10.5200000	11.5200000	13.1200000	14.6100000	16.4700000
26	8.5300000	9.2300000	11.1600000	12.2000000	13.8400000	15.3800000	17.2900000
27	9.1000000	9.8000000	11.8100000	12.8800000	14.5700000	16.1500000	18.1100000
28	9.6800000	10.3900000	12.4600000	13.5700000	15.3100000	16.9300000	18.9400000
29	10.2400000	10.9900000	13.1200000	14.2500000	16.0500000	17.7100000	19.7700000
30	10.8100000	11.5800000	13.7900000	14.9500000	16.7900000	18.4900000	20.6000000
35	13.8000000	14.6800000	17.1900000	18.5100000	20.5700000	22.4600000	24.8000000
40	16.9200000	17.9300000	20.7100000	22.1600000	24.4300000	26.5100000	29.0500000
50	23.4700000	24.6800000	27.9900000	29.7100000	32.3600000	34.7600000	37.6900000
60	30.3200000	31.7300000	35.5300000	37.4900000	40.4800000	43.1900000	46.4600000
70	37.4400000	39.0200000	43.2800000	45.4400000	48.7600000	51.7400000	55.3300000
80	44.8200000	46.4900000	51.1700000	53.5400000	57.1500000	60.3900000	64.2800000
100	59.9400000	61.9200000	67.3200000	70.0700000	74.2200000	77.9300000	82.3600000

Source: Data as presented by Robert H. Riffenburgh in Statistics in Medicine. 3rd ed. Amsterdam: Academic Press (an imprint of Elsevier); 2012.

Table A2.5 F Distribution

Denominator df	Numerator df																		
	1	2	3	4	5	6	7	8	9	10	12	15	20	25	30	40	60	100	∞
2	18.51	19.00	19.16	19.25	19.30	19.33	19.35	19.37	19.38	19.40	19.41	19.43	19.45	19.46	19.46	19.47	19.48	19.49	19.50
3	10.13	9.55	9.28	9.12	9.01	8.94	8.89	8.85	8.81	8.79	8.74	8.70	8.66	8.63	8.62	8.59	8.57	8.55	8.53
4	7.71	6.94	6.59	6.39	6.26	6.16	6.09	6.04	6.00	5.96	5.91	5.86	5.80	5.77	5.75	5.72	5.69	5.66	5.63
5	6.61	5.79	5.41	5.19	5.05	4.95	4.88	4.82	4.77	4.74	4.68	4.62	4.56	4.52	4.50	4.46	4.43	4.41	4.36
6	5.99	5.14	4.76	4.53	4.39	4.28	4.21	4.15	4.10	4.06	4.00	3.94	3.87	3.83	3.81	3.77	3.74	3.71	3.67
7	5.59	4.74	4.35	4.12	3.97	3.87	3.79	3.73	3.68	3.64	3.57	3.51	3.44	3.40	3.38	3.34	3.30	3.27	3.23
8	5.32	4.46	4.07	3.84	3.69	3.58	3.50	3.44	3.39	3.35	3.28	3.22	3.15	3.11	3.08	3.04	3.01	2.97	2.93
9	5.12	4.26	3.86	3.63	3.48	3.37	3.29	3.23	3.18	3.14	3.07	3.01	2.94	2.89	2.86	2.83	2.79	2.76	2.71
10	4.96	4.10	3.71	3.48	3.33	3.22	3.14	3.07	3.02	2.98	2.91	2.85	2.77	2.73	2.70	2.66	2.62	2.59	2.54
11	4.84	3.98	3.59	3.36	3.20	3.09	3.01	2.95	2.90	2.85	2.79	2.72	2.65	2.60	2.57	2.53	2.49	2.46	2.40
12	4.75	3.89	3.49	3.26	3.11	3.00	2.91	2.85	2.80	2.75	2.69	2.62	2.54	2.50	2.47	2.43	2.38	2.35	2.30
13	4.67	3.81	3.41	3.18	3.03	2.92	2.83	2.77	2.71	2.67	2.60	2.53	2.46	2.41	2.38	2.34	2.30	2.26	2.21
14	4.60	3.74	3.34	3.11	2.96	2.85	2.76	2.70	2.65	2.60	2.53	2.46	2.39	2.34	2.31	2.27	2.22	2.19	2.13
15	4.54	3.68	3.29	3.06	2.90	2.79	2.71	2.64	2.59	2.54	2.48	2.40	2.33	2.28	2.25	2.20	2.16	2.12	2.07
16	4.49	3.63	3.24	3.01	2.85	2.74	2.66	2.59	2.54	2.49	2.42	2.35	2.28	2.23	2.19	2.15	2.11	2.07	2.01
17	4.45	3.59	3.20	2.96	2.81	2.70	2.61	2.55	2.49	2.45	2.38	2.31	2.23	2.18	2.15	2.10	2.06	2.02	1.96
18	4.41	3.55	3.16	2.93	2.77	2.66	2.58	2.51	2.46	2.41	2.34	2.27	2.19	2.14	2.11	2.06	2.02	1.98	1.92
19	4.38	3.52	3.13	2.90	2.74	2.63	2.54	2.48	2.42	2.38	2.31	2.23	2.16	2.11	2.07	2.03	1.98	1.94	1.88
20	4.35	3.49	3.10	2.87	2.71	2.60	2.51	2.45	2.39	2.35	2.28	2.20	2.12	2.07	2.04	1.99	1.95	1.91	1.84
22	4.30	3.44	3.05	2.82	2.66	2.55	2.46	2.40	2.34	2.30	2.23	2.15	2.07	2.02	1.98	1.94	1.89	1.85	1.78
25	4.24	3.39	2.99	2.76	2.60	2.49	2.40	2.34	2.28	2.24	2.16	2.09	2.01	1.96	1.92	1.87	1.82	1.78	1.71
30	4.17	3.32	2.92	2.69	2.53	2.42	2.33	2.27	2.21	2.16	2.09	2.01	1.93	1.88	1.84	1.79	1.74	1.70	1.62
40	4.08	3.23	2.84	2.61	2.45	2.34	2.25	2.18	2.12	2.08	2.00	1.92	1.84	1.78	1.74	1.69	1.64	1.59	1.51
50	4.03	3.18	2.79	2.56	2.40	2.29	2.20	2.13	2.07	2.03	1.95	1.87	1.78	1.73	1.69	1.63	1.57	1.52	1.44
60	4.00	3.15	2.76	2.53	2.37	2.25	2.17	2.10	2.04	1.99	1.92	1.83	1.75	1.69	1.65	1.59	1.53	1.48	1.39
80	3.96	3.11	2.72	2.49	2.33	2.21	2.13	2.06	2.00	1.95	1.88	1.79	1.70	1.64	1.60	1.54	1.48	1.43	1.32
100	3.94	3.09	2.70	2.46	2.31	2.19	2.10	2.03	1.97	1.93	1.85	1.77	1.68	1.62	1.57	1.52	1.45	1.39	1.28
150	3.90	3.06	2.66	2.43	2.27	2.16	2.07	2.00	1.94	1.89	1.82	1.73	1.64	1.58	1.54	1.48	1.41	1.34	1.22
∞	3.84	3.00	2.60	2.37	2.21	2.10	2.01	1.94	1.88	1.83	1.75	1.67	1.57	1.51	1.46	1.39	1.32	1.24	1.00

Source: Data as presented by Robert H. Riffenburgh in Statistics in Medicine. 3rd ed. Amsterdam: Academic Press (an imprint of Elsevier); 2012.

Table A2.6 Critical values for the Wilcoxon signed-rank test of matched pairs

N*	One-tailed p value					N	One-tailed p value			
	0.050	0.025	0.010	0.005			0.050	0.025	0.010	0.005
	Two-tailed p value						Two-tailed p value			
	0.100	0.050	0.020	0.010			0.100	0.050	0.020	0.010
5	1					28	130	117	102	92
6	2	1				29	141	127	111	100
7	4	2	0			30	152	137	120	109
8	6	4	2	0		31	163	148	130	118
9	8	6	3	2		32	175	159	141	128
10	11	8	5	3		33	188	171	151	138
11	14	11	7	5		34	201	183	162	149
12	17	14	10	7		35	214	195	174	160
13	21	17	13	10		36	228	208	186	171
14	26	21	16	13		37	242	222	198	183
15	30	25	20	16		38	256	235	211	195
16	36	30	24	19		39	271	250	224	208
17	41	35	28	23		40	287	264	238	221
18	47	40	33	28		41	303	279	252	234
19	54	46	38	32		42	319	295	267	248
20	60	52	43	37		43	336	311	281	262
21	68	59	49	43		44	353	327	297	277
22	75	66	56	49		45	371	344	313	292
23	83	73	62	55		46	389	361	329	307
24	92	81	69	61		47	408	397	345	323
25	101	90	77	68		48	427	397	362	339
26	110	98	85	76		49	446	415	380	356
27	120	107	93	84		50	466	434	398	373

Source: Data as presented by Kirkwood BR and Sterne JAC. *Essential Medical Statistics.* 2nd ed. Malden, MA: Blackwell Science; 2007.

*N is the number of nonzero differences.

Appendix 3: Common abbreviations[a] in clinical and pharmaceutical sciences

Abbreviation	Definition
AAA	Abdominal aortic aneurysm
AAAAI (also known as "quad AI")	American Academy of Allergy, Asthma, and Immunology
AAAS	American Association for the Advancement of Science
AAD	Antibiotic-associated diarrhea
AADA	Abbreviated antibiotic drug application
AAI	Acute arterial insufficiency
A-a gradient	Alveolar: arterial gradient
AAL	Anterior axillary line
AAOx3	Awake, alert, and oriented ×3 (to place, person, and time)
AAP	Accelerated assessment procedure
AAPMC	Antibiotic-associated pseudomembranous colitis
AAPS	American Association of Pharmaceutical Scientists
AAS	Acute abdominal series; atomic absorption spectroscopy
AAT	Activity as tolerated; atypical antibody test
A/B	Acid-base ratio
Ab	Antibody
ABC	Airway, breathing, circulation; aspiration, biopsy, cytology; avidin biotin complex
ABCD	Airway, breathing, circulation disability; asymmetry, borders, color, diameter (malignant melanoma); ABCD rating (prostate cancer staging)
Abd	Abdomen
ABG	Arterial blood gas
ABHI	Association of British Healthcare Industries (Medical Devices Sector)
ABPI	Association of the British Pharmaceutical Industry
Abx	Antibiotics
AC	Before eating (Latin *ante cibum*)
ACA	Affordable Care Act (Patient Protection and Affordable Care Act); acinic cell carcinoma
A-CASI	Audio computer-assisted self-interviewing
ACC	American College of Cardiology; anterior cingulate cortex
ACCU	Acute coronary care unit
ACD	Anemia of chronic disease
ACDF	Anterior cervical discectomy and fusion
Ace	Acetone
ACE	Angiotensin-converting enzyme
ACh	Acetylcholine
AChE	Acetylcholinesterase

(*Continued*)

Abbreviation	Definition
ACKD	Anemia of chronic kidney disease
ACL	Anterior cruciate ligament
ACLS	Advanced cardiac life support
ACO	Addendum to clinical overview
ACP	American College of Physicians; advanced-care planning
ACPA	Anti-cyclic citrullinated peptide (protein) autoantibody
ACPO	Acute colonic pseudo-obstruction
ACRP	Association of Clinical Research Professionals
ACS	Acute coronary syndromes; acute chest syndrome; altered conscious state
ACTD	ASEAN common technical dossier (see ASEAN)
ACTH	Adrenocorticotropic hormone (i.e., corticotropin)
ACU	Ambulatory-care unit ad. Right ear (Latin *auris dexter*)
ACVM	Agricultural Compounds and Veterinary Medicines (New Zealand)
AD	Alzheimer's disease; autonomic dysreflexia; affective disorder; acute distress
ADA	Adenosine deaminase; American Dental Association; American Diabetes Association
ADC	Automated data collection; antibody-drug conjugate; AIDS dementia complex
ADCC	Antibody-dependent cell-mediated cytotoxicity
ADE	Adverse device event /effect (AE judged to be related to the medical device)
ADEC	Australian Drug Evaluation Committee
ADH	Antidiuretic hormone (vasopressin)
ADHD	Attention-deficit/hyperactivity disorder
ADHF	Acute decompensated heart failure
ADHR	Autosomal dominant hypophosphatemic rickets
ADI	Acceptable daily intake
Ad lib	*Ad libitum* (as much as needed)
ADLs	Activities of daily living
adm	Admission
ADME	Absorption, distribution, metabolism and excretion/elimination (also AME absorption, metabolism, excretion/elimination). Key processes of pharmacokinetics
Adn	Adnexae
aDNA	Ancient DNA
ADP	Adenosine diphosphate
ADPase	Adenosine diphosphatase
ad. part. dolent.	To the painful parts (Latin *ad partes dolentes*)
ADR	Adverse drug reaction
ADROIT	Adverse Drug Reactions On-Line Information Tracking System
AE	Adverse event
AEB	As evidenced by
AED	Automated external defibrillator
AEFI	Adverse event following immunization
AEGIS	Adverse Experience Gathering Information System
AEM	Ambulatory electrocardiographic monitoring
AEMPS	*Agencia Española de Medicamentos y Productos Sanitarios* (Spain)

(*Continued*)

Abbreviation	Definition
AEPAR	*Associación Española de Profesionales de Actividades de Registro* (Spanish Regulatory Affairs Association)
AERS	Adverse event reporting system (US FDA)
AESGP	*Association Européenne des Spécialitiés Pharmaceutiques* Grand Public (Association of the European Self-Medication Industry)
AF	Atrial fibrillation; atrial flutter; amniotic fluid
AF-AFP	Amniotic-fluid alpha fetoprotein
AFAR	*Association Française des Affaires Reglémentaires* (French Regulatory Affairs Association)
AFB	Acid-fast bacteria (bacilli)
AFDO	Association of Food and Drug Officials (US)
AFI	Amniotic-fluid index
AFib	Atrial fibrillation
AFl	Atrial flutter
AFMPS	*Agence Fédérale des Médicaments et des Produits de Santé* (Belgian regulatory body)
AFNTR	Acute febrile nonhemolytic transfusion reaction
AFO	Ankle foot orthosis
AFP	Alpha-Fetoprotein
AFSOF	Anterior fontanelle soft, open, flat
Afssaps	Former French regulatory agency (*Agence Française de Sécurité Sanitaire des Produits de Santé*) replaced by ANSM in 2012 (see below)
A/G	Albumin: globulin (ratio)
Ag	Antigen
AGES	Age, grade, extent, size (tumor)
AGN	acute glomerulonephritis
AH	Auditory hallucinations
a.h.	Every other hour (Latin *alternis horis*)
AHD	Atherosclerotic heart disease
AHF	Antihemophilic factor
AHFS	American Hospital Formulary Service
AHG	Antihemophilic globulin
AHH	Aryl hydrocarbon hydroxylase
AHR	Airway hyper-reactivity
AHRQ	Agency of Healthcare Research and Quality (US)
AHSC	Academic Health Science Centre (UK)
AHT	Antihyaluronic acid test
AI	Autonomic insufficiency; aortic insufficiency; artificial insemination; aromatase inhibitor
AICD	Automated implantable cardioverter defibrillator
AID	Artificial insemination by donor
AIDS	Acquired immunodeficiency syndrome
AIFA	*Agenzia Italiana del Farmaco* (Italy's health authority)
AIH	Artificial insemination by husband
AIHD	Artificial insemination by pooled husband and donor semen

(Continued)

Abbreviation	Definition
AIM	Active ingredient manufacturer
AIMD	Active implantable medical device
AIN	Allergic/acute interstitial nephritis
AIPD	Acute infectious and parasitic diseases; acute inflammatory demyelinating polyneuropathy; autoimmune progesterone dermatitis
AIR	Anterior interval release; acute inpatient rehabilitation
AIS	Adenocarcinoma in situ; androgen insensitivity syndrome
AITS	Adverse Incident Tracking System (medical devices sector)
AK	*Acanthamoeba keratitis*
AKA	Above-the-knee amputation
AKP (or ALP)	Alkaline phosphatase
ALA	Aminolevulinic acid
ALARP	As low as reasonably practical
ALATF	As low as technically feasible
ALCAPA	Anomalous left coronary artery from the pulmonary artery
ALDH	Aldehyde dehydrogenase
ALF	Assisted-living facility
ALG	Antilymphocytic globulin
ALI	Acute lung (or limb) injury
ALL	Acute lymphoblastic leukemia
allo-SCT	Allogeneic stem cell transplantation
ALP	Alkaline phosphatase
ALPS	Autoimmune lymphoproliferative syndrome
ALS	Amyotrophic lateral sclerosis (Lou Gehrig's disease); advanced life support
ALT	Alanine aminotransferase (SGPT)
altern. d.	Every other day (Latin *alterno die*)
AM	*Agence du Medicament* (France)
AMA	American Medical Association; antimitochondrial antibody; against medical advice; advanced maternal age (often ≥35)
amb	Ambulate
AMC	Arthrogryposis multiplex congenita
AMCP	Academy of Managed Care Pharmacy
AMI	Acute myocardial infarction; acute mesenteric ischemia
AML	Acute myeloid leukemia
AMM	*Autorisation de mise sur le marché* (France) = Product licence
AMO	Advanced medical optics
AMP	Adenosine monophosphate; authorized medicinal product; auxiliary medicinal product
AMR	Antimicrobial resistance
AMRH	African Medicines Regulatory Harmonization
AMS	Acute mountain sickness; atypical measles syndrome; altered mental status
AMWA	American Medical Writers Association; American Medical Women's Association
ANA	Antinuclear antibody
ANADA	Abbreviated New Animal Drug Application (US)

(Continued)

Abbreviation	Definition
ANCA	Antineutrophil cytoplasmic antibody
ANCOVA	Analysis of covariance
ANDA	Abbreviated New Drug Application
ANDS	Abbreviated New Drug Submission (Canada)
ANF	Atrial natriuretic factor
ANLL	Acute nonlymphocytic leukemia
ANMV	*Agence Nationale du Médicament Vétérinaire* (French Veterinary Medicines Agency)
ANOVA	Analysis of variance
ANP	Atrial natriuretic peptide
ANS	Autonomic nervous system
ANSES	*Agence Nationale de Securite Sanitaire*
ANSM	French regulatory agency (*Agence Nationale de Sécurité du Médicament et des Produits de Santé* [formerly Afssaps])
ANTR	Asymmetrical tonic reflex
ANUG	Acute necrotizing ulcerative gingivitis
A&O or A/O	Aware and oriented or alert and oriented
A&Ox3	Alert and oriented times three (person, place, and time)
A&Ox4	Alert and oriented times four (person, place, time, and circumstances)
ANVISA	*Agência Nacional de Vigilância Sanitária* (Brazilian regulatory agency)
ANZTPA	Australia New Zealand Therapeutic Products Agency
AOAC	Association of Official Analytical Chemists (US)
AOB	Alcohol on breath
AODM	Adult-onset diabetes mellitus (type 2 diabetes mellitus)
AOM	Acute otitis media
AOR	Adjusted odds ratio
a.p.	Before a meal (Latin *ante prandium*)
AP	Anteroposterior; abdominal-perineal; action potential; adaptive pathways; alkaline phosphatase; angina pectoris; area postrema
A/P	Anatomy and physiology; assessment and plan
APACHE	Acute Physiology and Chronic Health Evaluation
APAP	*N*-Acetyl-para-aminophenol (paracetamol; acetaminophen)
APB	Atrial premature beat
APC	Atrial premature contraction; antigen-presenting cell; activated protein C
APD	Adult polycystic disease; automated peritoneal dialysis; autoimmune progesterone dermatitis
APEC	Asia–Pacific Economic Cooperation
APECED	Autoimmune polyendocrinopathy-candidiasis-ectodermal dystrophy
APGAR	Appearance, pulse, grimace, activity, respiration
APH	Antepartum hemorrhage
APHIS	Animal and Plant Health Inspection Service (US)
API	Active pharmaceutical ingredient
APKD	Adult polycystic kidney disease
APLS	Antiphospholipid syndrome
APMA	Australian Pharmaceutical Manufacturers Association

(*Continued*)

Abbreviation	Definition
APMPPE	Acute posterior multifocal placoid pigment epitheliopathy
APR	Abdominoperineal resection
APS	Autoimmune polyendocrine/polyglandular syndrome; antiphospholipid syndrome
APSAC	Anisoylated plasminogen streptokinase activator complex
aPTT	Activated partial thromboplastin time
APVMA	Australian Pesticides and Veterinary Medicines Authority (Australia)
AQL	Acceptable quality level
AR	Absolute risk; adverse reaction; aortic regurgitation; assessment report (EU); attributable risk
ARB	Angiotensin$_{II}$ receptor blocker
ARBI	Alcohol-related brain injury
ARC	AIDS-related complex
ARD	Absolute risk difference; alcohol-related dementia
ARDS	Acute respiratory distress syndrome
ARF	Acute renal failure
ARfD	Acute reference dose (veterinary)
Arg	Arginine
ARM	Artificial rupture of membranes; active range of motion
ARMD	Age-related macular degeneration
ARMS	Alveolar rhabdomyosarcoma
AROM	Active range of motion; artificial rupture of membranes
ARR	Absolute risk reduction
ART	Antiretroviral therapy; assisted reproductive technology
ARVC	Arrhythmogenic right-ventricular cardiomyopathy
ARVD	Arrhythmogenic right-ventricular dysplasia
AS	Aortic stenosis; ankylosing spondylitis
ASA	Acetylsalicylic acid (aspirin); American Society of Anesthesiologists
ASAP	Accelerated Stability Assessment Program
ASB	Asymptomatic bacteriuria
ASC	Adult stem cell; atypical squamous cells; ambulatory surgical center
ASCA	Anti-*Saccharomyces cerevisiae* antibodies
ASC-H	Atypical squamous cells, cannot exclude high-grade squamous intraepithelial lesion [HSIL]
ASCII	American Standard Code for Information Interchange
ASCO	American Society of Clinical Oncology
ASC-US	Atypical squamous cells of undetermined significance
ASCVD	Atherosclerotic cardiovascular disease
ASD	Atrial septal defect; autistic spectrum disorder
ASDI	Acceptable single-dose intake
ASEAN	Association of Southeast Asian Nations
ASG-US/AGUS	Atypical squamous glandular cells of undetermined significance
ASH	American Society of Hematology; alcoholic steatohepatitis
ASHD	Atherosclerotic heart disease
ASIA	American Spinal Injury Association

(Continued)

Abbreviation	Definition
ASIS	Anterior superior iliac spine
ASMA	Anti–smooth-muscle antibody
ASMF	Active Substance Master File
ASO	Antistreptolysin-O
ASOT	Antistreptolysin-O titer
ASPECTS	Alberta Stroke Program Early CT (computed tomography) Score
ASPR	Anonymized single patient report (formerly ASPP – anonymized single patient printout)
AST	Aspartate aminotransferase (SGOT)
ASX	Asymptomatic
A-T	Ataxia-telangiectasia
AT-III	Antithrombin III
ATA	Antitransglutaminase antibodies
ATB	Antibiotic
ATC	Anatomical therapeutic chemical (WHO); Animal Test Certificate (UK)
ATCC	Anatomical Therapeutic Chemical Code (or American Type Culture Collection)
ATD	Access to documents (EMA policy)
ATG	Anti-thymocyte globulin
ATLS	Advanced trauma life support
ATMPs	Advanced therapy medicinal products (aka "advanced therapies")
ATN	Acute tubular necrosis
ATNR	Asymmetrical tonic neck reflex
ATP	Adenosine triphosphate; acute thrombocytopenic purpura; anti-tachycardia pacing
ATPase	Adenosine triphosphatase
ATRA	All-*trans* retinoic acid
ATS	American Thoracic Society antitetanus serum
ATU	Authorisation for temporary use
AUC	Area-under-the-curve. In pharmacokinetics, area under the drug concentration (y-axis) versus time (x-axis; typically 0 to 24 hours or 0 to infinity) plot is equivalent to drug "exposure." In prognostic modeling, the AUC of the receiver operating characteristics (ROC) curve plotting sensitivity (y-axis) versus 1 – specificity (x-axis) is a measure of the discriminative performance of the model. Values exceeding 0.70 signify acceptable model performance.
aur.	Ear (Latin *auris*)
aur. dextro	To the right ear (Latin *auris dextrae*)
aur. laev	To the left ear (Latin *auris laevae*)
aurist.	Ear drops (Latin *auristillae*)
AUROC	Area under the receiver operating characteristic curve (also known as the C-statistic, a measure of prognostic model performance)
AV	Atrioventricular; arteriovenous
AVEG	AIDS Vaccine Evaluation Group
AVF	Arteriovenous fistula
AVN	Atrioventricular node; avascular necrosis

(Continued)

Abbreviation	Definition
AVR	Aortic valve replacement
AVSS	Afebrile, vital signs stable
A-VO$_2$	Arteriovenous oxygen
Ax	Axilllary
AXR	Abdominal x-ray
AXREM	Association of X-ray Equipment Manufacturers
AYA	Adolescents and young adults
AZT	Azidothymidine
Ba	Barium
BA	Bioavailability
BAC	Blood alcohol concentration
BACPAC	Bulk active chemical post approval changes (US)
BAD	Bipolar affective disorder
BADL	Basic activities of daily living
BAER	Brainstem auditory evoked response
BAI	Breath actuated inhaler
BAID	Batch identifier
BAL	Bronchoalveolar lavage; blood alcohol level
BAN	British Approved Name
BAO	Basic acid output
BAP	Biotechnology Action Programme
BARQA	British Association of Research Quality Assurance
BAT	Brown adipose tissue
BAV	Bicuspid aortic valve
BBA	Bilateral breast augmentation
BBB	Bundle branch block; blood-brain barrier
BBT	Basal body temperature
BC	Bowel care; bone conduction; blood culture
BCAA	Branched-chain amino acids
BCC	Basal-cell carcinoma
BCG	Bacille Calmette–Guérin
BCP	Birth control pill; blood chemistry profile
BCS	Biopharmaceutics Classification System
BCx	Blood culture
BD	Bipolar disorder
bd/bid	Twice a day (Latin *bis in die*)
BDA	Bulgarian Drug Agency
BDD	Body dysmorphic disorder
BDI	Beck Depression Inventory
BDR	Background diabetic retinopathy
BE	Barium enema; bioequivalence
BEE	Basal energy expenditure
BEP	Bleomycin, etoposide, cisplatin

(Continued)

Abbreviation	Definition
BfArM	*Bundesinstituts für Arzneimittel und Medizinprodukte* (German Federal Institute for Drugs and Medica Devices)
BFP	Bundle-forming pilus
BG	Blood glucose
BGAT	Blood glucose awareness training
BGMA	British Generic Manufacturers Association
BIBRA	British Industrial Biological Research Association
bilat	Bilateral
BIM	Budget impact model
BIND	Biological Investigational New Drug
BIO	Biotechnology Innovation Organization (US)
BiPAP	Bilevel positive airway pressure
BIS	Bispectral index
BiVAD	Bilateral ventricular assist device
BK	Bradykinin
BKA	Below-the-knee amputation
BL	Burkitt's lymphoma
BLA	Biologics License Application (US); bilateral amygdala
BLE	Bilateral lower extremity
BLS	Basic life support
BLAST	Bilateral alternating stimulation-tactile
BMA	British Medical Association
BMBx	Bone marrow biopsy
BMC	Bone mineral content
BMD	Bone mineral density
BMG	*Bundesministerium für Gesundheit* = Federal Ministry of Health (Germany)
BMGF	*Bundesministerium für Gesundheit und Frauen* (Austria)
BMI	Body mass index
BMP	Basic metabolic panel
BMR	Basal metabolic rate
BMS	Bare-metal stent
BNF	British National Formulary
BNO	Bowel not open
BNP	Brain natriuretic peptide
BO	Bowel open
BOA	Born out of asepsis
BoH	Board of Health
BOM	Bilateral otitis media
BOOP	Bronchiolitis obliterans–organizing pneumonia
BOS	Break-out session
BP	Blood pressure; British Pharmacopoeia
BPAD	Bipolar affective disorder
BPC	Bulk pharmaceutical chemicals; British Pharmacopoeia Commission
BPCA	Best Pharmaceuticals for Children Act (US)

(Continued)

Abbreviation	Definition
BPD	Biparietal diameter; borderline personality disorder; bronchopulmonary dysplasia
BPH	Benign prostatic hyperplasia/hypertrophy
BPI	*Bundesverband der Pharmazeutischen Industrie* (German pharmaceutical industry association)
BPM	Beats per minute
BPP	Biophysical profile
BPPV	Benign paroxysmal positional vertigo
BPR	Biocidal Products Regulation
BPWP	Blood Products Working Party (EMA)
BR	Bed rest
BRA	Bilateral renal agenesis
BRAS	Belgian Regulatory Affairs Society
BRAT	Benefit–Risk Action Team; BRAT diet (bananas, rice, applesauce, toast)
BRATY	Bananas, rice applesauce, toast, and yogurt
BRB	Bright red blood
BRBPR	Bright red blood per rectum
BRCA1/BRCA2	Breast cancer genes
BRCA1/BRCA2	Breast cancer proteins
BRIC	Brazil, Russia, India, & China
BRICK	Brazil, Russia, India, China, & (South) Korea
BRICS	Brazil, Russia, India, China, & South Africa
BROMI	Better Regulation of Over the Counter Medicines Initiative
BRTO	Balloon-occluded retrograde transvenous obliteration
BRVO	Branch retinal vein occlusion
BSA	Body surface area; bovine serum albumin
BS x 4	Bowel signs in all 4 quadrants
BSE	Bovine spongiform encephalopathy; breast self-examination
BSO	Bilateral salpingo-oophorectomy
BSP	Bromsulphthalein
BSU	Bartholin, Skene and urethra
BT	Bleeding time; brachytherapy
BTB	Breakthrough bleeding
BTD	Breakthrough therapy designation (US)
BTL	Bilateral tubal ligation
BTP	Breakthrough pain
BUN	Blood urea nitrogen
BV	Bacterial vaginosis
BVM	Bag valve mask
BVP	Biventricular pacing; bleomycin, vincristine, and cisplatin
BW	Birth weight; blood work; body weight
BWP	Biologics Working Party (EMA)
Bx	Biopsy
BZDs	Benzodiazepines
C1	Atlas (first cervical vertebra)

(*Continued*)

Abbreviation	Definition
C2	Axis (second cervical vertebra)
C&P	Chemistry and Pharmacy
C&S	Culture and sensitivity
CA	Cancer/carcinoma; commercial appraisal; competent authority
Ca	Calcium
CAA	Crystalline amino acids; coronary artery aneurysm
CABG	Coronary artery bypass graft
CAC	Codex Alimentarius Commission (veterinary sector)
CAD	Coronary artery disease
CADASIL	Cerebral autosomal dominant arteriopathy with subcortical infarcts and leukoencephalopathy
CADREAC	Collaboration agreement between drug regulatory authorities of European Union associated countries (also nCADREAC – new Collaboration Agreement)
CADTH	Canadian Agency for Drugs and Technologies in Health (formerly CCOHTA)
CAGE	Cut down, annoyed, guilty, eye opener (alcoholism screening)
CAH	Chronic active hepatitis; congenital adrenal hyperplasia
CALLA	Common acute lymphocytic leukemia antigen
CAM	Cellular adhesion molecule; complementary and alternative medicine
CAMD	Competent Authorities for Medical Devices
CAMS	Chinese Academy of Medical Sciences
cAMP	Cyclic adenosine monophosphate
CANDA	Computer Assisted New Drug Application
CAO	Central Agricultural Office (Hungary); conscious, alert, and oriented
CAP	Centrally authorized product; community-acquired pneumonia
CAPA	Corrective and preventive action
CAPD	Continuous ambulatory peritoneal dialysis
CAPLA	Computer Assisted Product License Application
CAPRA	Canadian Association of Pharmaceutical Regulatory Affairs
CAS	Central alerting system (UK); chemical abstract systems
CAT	Computerized axial tomography; Committee for Advance Therapies (EMA)
CATMP	Combined Advanced Therapy Medicinal Product
CAVDRI	Collaboration agreement between veterinary drug registration institutions
CAVOMP	Clinical added value orphan medicinal product
CBA	Cost-benefit analysis
CBC	Complete blood count
CBD	Common bile duct
CBE	Clinical breast examination
CBER	Center for Biologics Evaluation and Research (US FDA)
CBF	Cerebral blood flow
CBG	Capillary blood gas
CBG/MEB	*College ter Beoordeling van Geneesmiddelin* Medicines Evaluation Board (The Netherlands)
CBP	Corticoid binding protein
CC	Candidate country (EU); chief complaint; cardiac catheter/catheterization

(Continued)

Abbreviation	Definition
CCA	Clear-cell adenocarcinoma
CCB	Calcium channel blocker
CCCU	Critical coronary care unit
CCDS	Company core data sheet
CCE	[C/C/E] Clubbing, cyanosis, and edema
CCG	Clinical Commissioning Group (UK NHS)
CCG IAC	Clinical Commissioning Group Indicator Advisory Committee
CCK	Cholecystokinin
CCK-PZ	Cholecystokinin-pancreozymin
CCNS	Cell cycle-nonspecific [chemotherapeutic drug]
CCOC	Clear-cell odontogenic carcinoma
CCOT	Calcifying cystic odontogenic tumor
CCP	Cyclic citrullinated peptide
CCR	Cardiocerebral resuscitation
CCSI	Company core safety information
CCU	Clean catch urine; cardiac care unit; critical care unit
CCV	Critical closing volume
CD	Cesarean derived; chemical dependency; controlled delivery; controlled drug; Crohn's disease
CDAD	*Clostridium difficile*–associated diarrhea
CDAI	Clinical disease activity index; Crohn's disease activity index
CDC	Centers for Disease Control and Prevention (US)
CDDD	Clinical Dossier of Drug Development (Brazil)
CDEC	Canadian Drug Expert Committee (Canada)
CDER	Center for Drug Evaluation and Research (US FDA)
CDH	Congenital dislocated hip
CDI	Central diabetes insipidus; *Clostridium difficile* infection; cool, dry, intact
CDMA	Canadian Drug Manufacturers Association
CDR	Common Drug Review (Canada); cutaneous drug reaction
CDRH	Center for Devices and Radiological Health (US FDA)
CDSCO	Central Drug Standard Organization (India's clinical trials licensing authority)
CDSM	Committee on Dental and Surgical Materials (UK)
CDx	Companion Diagnostic
CE	*Conformité Européenne* (mark)
CEA	Carcinoembryonic antigen; carotid endarterectomy; cost-effectiveness analysis
CEE	Central and Eastern Europe
CEEC	Central and Eastern European Countries
CEFTA	Central Europe Free Trade Agreement
CEN	*Comité Européen de Normalisation* European Committee for Standardization
CER	Comparative effectiveness research
CESP	Common European Submissions Platform
CF	Cystic fibrosis
CFA	Complement-fixing antibody; colonization factor antigen

(Continued)

Abbreviation	Definition
CFC	Chlorofluorocarbons
CFDA	China Food and Drug Administration (formerly State FDA SFDA)
CFIDS	Chronic fatigue immune dysfunction syndrome
CFR	Case fatality rate; Code of Federal Regulations (US)
CFS	Certificate of Free Sale; chronic fatigue syndrome
CFSAN	Center for Food Safety and Applied Nutrition (US)
CFT	Capillary filling time; complement fixation test
CFTR	Cystic fibrosis transmembrane conductance regulator
CFU	Colony-forming unit
CGD	Chronic granulomatous disease
CGI	Clinical Global Impression
CGL	Chronic granulocytic leukemia
cGLP	Current Good Laboratory Practice
cGMP	Current Good Manufacturing Practice; cyclic guanosine monophosphate
CGN	Chronic glomerulonephritis
CGP	Clinical Guidance Panel (Canada)
CH	Clinical hold; congenital hypothyroidism
CHAI	Commission for Healthcare Audit and Inspection (UK)
CHD	Coronary heart disease; congenital heart defect
ChE	Cholinesterase
CHEERS	Consolidated Health Economic Evaluation Reporting Standards (see Chapter 4)
CHF	Congestive heart failure
CHO	Carbohydrate; Chinese hamster ovary cells
CHF	Congestive heart failure
CHMP	Committee for Medicinal Products for Human Use (EMA)
CHOP	Cyclophosphamide, hydroxydaunorubicin (doxorubicin) Oncovin (vincristine) prednisone
CHPA	Consumer Healthcare Products Association
CHS	Cannulated hip screw
CHT	Congenital hyporthyroidism
CI	Cardiac index; contraindication; confidence interval
CIA	Corporate Integrity Agreement (US)
CICU	Cardiac intensive care unit
CIDP	Chronic inflammatory demyelinating polyneuropathy
CIMF	Chronic idiopathic myelofibrosis
CIN	Cervical intraepithelial neoplasia
CINV	Chemotherapy-induced nausea and vomiting
CIOMS	Council for International Organizations of Medical Sciences (WHO)
CIRS	Centre for Innovation in Regulatory Science
CIS	Carcinoma in situ; Commonwealth of Independent States (members are former Soviet Republic countries)
CIVI	Continuous intravenous infusion
CIWA	Clinical Institute Withdrawal Assessment for Alcohol
CJD	Creutzfeldt–Jakob disease

(Continued)

Abbreviation	Definition
CK	Creatine kinase
CK-BB	Creatine kinase BB (BB isoenzyme)
CKD	Chronic kidney disease
CK-MB	Creatine kinase MB (MB isoenzyme)
CK-MM	Creatine kinase MM (MM isoenzyme)
CL	Confidence limit
CLARE	Contact lens acute red eye
CLIA	Clinical Laboratory Improvement Amendments
CLL	Chronic lymphocytic leukemia
CLN	Cervical lymph node
CLND	Cervical (or complete) lymph node dissection
CLO	Clinical overview
CLP	Classification, labelling and packaging (medical devices); cleft lip and palate
CLS	Clinical summary; capillary leak syndrome
CM	Chirurgiae Magister, Master of Surgery (UK and Commonwealth countries' medical degree)
Cm or Cmax	Maximum plasma concentration at steady state
CMA	Conditional marketing authorization (US)
CMC	Chemistry, manufacturing, and controls
CMD	Cystic medial degeneration
CMDh	Coordination Group for Mutual Recognition and Decentralized Procedures Human (European Medicine Agency [EMA])
CMDv	Co-ordination Group for Mutual Recognition and Decentralized Procedures Veterinary (European Medicine Agency [EMA])
CME	Continuing medical education
CMI	Cell-mediated immunity
CML	Chronic myelogenous (myeloid) leukemia
CMN	*Comiteé de Moléculas Nuevas* (New Molecules Committee) (Mexico)
CMP	Certificate of Medicinal Product; common product model; complete metabolic profile; cytosine monophosphate
CMR	Carcinogenic, mutagenic or reprotoxic [toxic to reproduction]; Centre for Medicines Research
CMS	Centers for Medicare and Medicaid Services; chronic mountain sickness; concerned member state (EU)
CMT	Cervical motion tenderness; convergent medical technologies
CMV	Cytomegalovirus
CN	Cranial nerve
CNS	Central nervous system; clinical nurse specialist; Crigler–Najjar syndrome
C/O	Complaining of
CO	Cardiac output; carbon monoxide
CO_2	Carbon dioxide
COA/CofA	Certificate of analysis
COAD	Chronic obstructive airways disease
COCP	Combined oral contraceptive pill
COE	Council of Europe

(Continued)

Abbreviation	Definition
COH	Controlled ovarian hyperstimulation
COLD	Chronic obstructive lung disease
COMP	Committee for Orphan Medicinal Products (EMA)
CONSORT	Consolidated Standards of Reporting Trials (see Chapter 4)
COPD	Chronic obstructive pulmonary disease
COPE	Committee on Publication Ethics
COREPER	Committee of Permanent Representatives (i.e., Ambassadors) to the Community
COSHH	Control of Substances Hazardous to Health
COSTART	Coding Symbols for a Thesaurus of Adverse Reaction Terms
COX-2	Cyclooxygenase-2
CP	Centralised procedure (EU); cerebral palsy; chest pain; comparability protocol (US); constrictive pericarditis
CPAC	Central Pharmaceutical Affairs Council (Japan)
CPAP	Continuous positive airway pressure
CPCR	Cardiopulmonary-cerebral resuscitation
CPD	Continuing professional development; cephalopelvic disproportion
CPE	Carbapenemase-producing Enterobacteriaceae; cardiogenic pulmonary edema; *Clostridium perfringens* enterotoxin
CPI	Critical Path Initiative (US)
CPK	Creatine phosphokinase
CPMP	Committee for Proprietary Medicinal Products (EMA)
CPP	Certificate of pharmaceutical product; cerebral perfusion pressure; critical process parameter
CPPD	Calcium pyrophosphate deposition disease; cyclic perimenstrual pain and discomfort
CPQ	Costs per quality-adjusted life year
CPR	Cardiopulmonary resuscitation; Cosmetic Products Regulation
CPRD	Clinical Practice Research Datalink
CPS	Chemistry Pharmacy and Standards Subcommittee of the CSM (UK)
CPT	Current Procedural Terminology
CPU	Clinical pharmacology unit
CPWP	Cell-based Products Working Party (EMA)
CQA	Clinical quality assurance; critical quality attribute
CQI	Continuous quality improvement
CR	Computed radiology; controlled release; complete remission
CRC	Colorectal cancer
CrCl	Creatinine clearance
CRD	Chronic renal disease; circadian rhythm disorder
CRE	Carbapenem-resistant Enterobacteriaceae
CREST	Calcinosis, Raynaud's phenomenon esophageal dysmotility, sclerodactyly, telangiectasia
CRF	Case report form; chronic renal failure; corticotropin-releasing factor
CRG	Clinical reference group (UK)
CrGN	Crescentic glomerulonephritis

(Continued)

Abbreviation	Definition
CRH	Corticotropin-releasing hormone
CRI	Chronic renal insufficiency
CRISPR	Clustered regularly interspaced short palindromic repeats
CRL	Crown-rump length
CRNA	Certified registered nurse anesthetist
CRO	Contract Research Organization
CRP	C-reactive protein
CRPC	Castration-resistant prostate cancer
CRPS	Complex regional pain syndrome
CRRT	Continuous renal replacement therapy
CRS	Congenital rubella syndrome
CRSD	Circadian rhythm sleep disorder
CRT	Capillary refill time; cardiac resynchronization therapy; central retinal thickness; certified respiratory therapist; conformal radiotherapy
CRTS	Certified recreational therapy specialist
CS	Cesarean section (now termed cesarean birth or delivery); Churg-Strauss (syndrome); clinically significant; compartment syndrome
C&S	Culture and sensitivity
CsA	Cyclosporin A
CSA	Controlled Substances Act
CSF	Cerebrospinal fluid; colony-stimulating factor
CSI	Core safety information
CSM	Centralized statistical monitoring
CSME	Clinically significant macular edema
CSO	Consumer Safety Officer (US)
CSOM	Chronic suppurative otitis media
CSP	Core safety profile
CSPC	Community specialist palliative care
CSR	Clinical study report; cumulative survival rate
C-SSR	Columbia Suicide Severity Rating Scale
CST	Contraction stress test
CSU	Catheter specimen of urine
CSW	Certified social worker
CT	Clinical trial; computed tomography/tomographic
CTA	Clear to auscultation; clinical trial application; clinical trial assay; clinical trial authorization
CTAG	Clinical Trials Action Group (Australia); Clinical Trials Coordination and Advisory Group
CTAP	CT during arterial portography
CTC	Clinical trial certificate (Hong Kong, Singapore)
CTCAE	Common Terminology Criteria for Adverse Events
CTD	Clinical Trials Directive; common technical document; connective-tissue disease
CTE	Chronic traumatic encephalopathy; coefficient of thermal expansion
CTFG	Clinical Trials Facilitation Group

(Continued)

Abbreviation	Definition
CTMS	Clinical trial management system
CTN	Clinical trial notification (Australia)
CTO	Chronic total occlusion; community treatment order
CTOC	Comprehensive Table of Contents Headings and Hierarchy
CTP	Child-Turcotte-Pugh score; clear to percussion; cytidine triphosphate; cytosine triphosphate
CTPA	Computed tomographic pulmonary angiography
CTPE	CT scan for pulmonary emboli
CTR	Carpal tunnel release
CTS	Carpal tunnel syndrome; common technical specification; Communication Tracking System (formerly Eudratrack)
CTU	Cancer treatment unit
CTX	Clinical trial exemption (UK)
CTZ	Chemoreceptor trigger zone
CUA	Cost-utility analysis; chronic ulcerative colitis
CV	Controlled vocabulary
CVA	Cerebrovascular accident (stroke; arguably, stroke is preventable and hence not an "incident"); costovertebral angle
CVAD	Central venous access device
CVAT	Costovertebral angle tenderness
CVC	Central venous catheter; chronic venous congestion
CVD	Cardiovascular disease
CVI	Cerebrovascular incident
CVID	Common variable immunodeficiency
CVL	Central venous line
CVM	Center for Veterinary Medicine (US)
CVMP	Committee for Medicinal Products for Veterinary Use (EMA)
CVO	Chief Veterinary Officer
CVP	Central venous pressure
CVS	Cardiovascular system; chorionic villus sampling
CVZ	*College voor zorgverzekeringen* (Dutch Health Care Insurance Board)
CWP	Coal worker's pneumoconiosis
CXR	Chest X-ray (roentgenogram is preferred term)
CZ	Climatic zone
D&C	Dilation and curettage
D5W	5% dextrose in water
D25	25% dextrose in water
DA	Dopamine
DAB	*Deutsches Arzneibuch* (German Pharmacopoeia)
DACS	Detailed and critical summary
DAE	Discontinuation due to an adverse event
DAEC	Diffusely adherent *Escherichia coli*
DAL	Defect action level (US)
DALY	Disability-adjusted life-year
DAMOS	Drug application methodology with optical storage

(Continued)

Abbreviation	Definition
dAMP	Deoxyadenosine monophosphate (deoxyadenylate)
DAPT	Dual antiplatelet therapy
DAS-28-CRP	Disease Activity Score in 28 joints C-reactive protein
DASH	Dietary Approaches to Stop Hypertension
DAT	Diet as tolerated
DAW	Dispense as written
DB	Device Bulletin (MHRA)
DBP	Diastolic blood pressure
DBS	Deep-brain stimulation; dried blood spots
DCBE	Double-contrast barium enema
DCCV	Direct-current cardioversion
DCD	Donation after cardiac death
DCIS	Ductal carcinoma in situ
DCGI	Drugs Controller General of India; India's regulatory authority (Directorate General of Health Services in the Ministry of Health and Family Welfare)
DCM	Dilated cardiomyopathy
DCP	Decentralised procedure (EU)
DD	District director (US); differential diagnosis
DDAVP	Desmopressin acetate/deamino-delta-D-arginine vasopressin
DDC	Dideoxycytidine
DDD	Defined daily dose; degenerative disc disease
DDH	Developmental dysplasia of the hip
DDMAC	Division of Drug Marketing, Advertising and Communications (CDER)
DDPS	Detailed description of pharmacovigilance system
DDT	Dichlorodiphenyltrichloroethane (chlorophenothane)
DDx	Differential diagnosis
DDX	Doctors and dentists exemption (UK)
DE	Designated examination; dose equivalent
D&E	Dilation and evacuation
DEA	Drug Enforcement Agency (US)
DEREK	Deductive estimation of risk from existing knowledge
DES	Data exchange standard (EU); diethylstilbestrol; drug-eluting stent (vs. BMS, bare-metal stent)
DESI	Drug efficacy study implementation (US)
DEV	Duck embryo vaccine
DEXA	Dual-energy x-ray absorptiometry
DFA	Direct fluorescence assay
DG	Directorate-General (at the European Commission)
dGMP	Deoxyguanosine monophosphate (deoxyguanylate)
DH	Department of Health (UK)
DHE	Dihydroergotamine
DHEAS	Dehydroepiandrosterone sulfate
DHF	Decompensated heart failure
DHHS	Department of Health and Human Services (US)
DI	Diabetes insipidus

(Continued)

Abbreviation	Definition
DIA	Drug Information Association (US)
DIC	Disseminated intravascular coagulation
DID	Design inputs document
Di-Di	Dichorionic diamniotic (twins)
DIMDI	*Deutsches Institut für Medizinische Dokumentation und Information* (Germany)
DIL	Drug-induced lupus
DILI	Drug-induced liver injury
DIP	Distal interphalangeal joint; diffuse interstitial pneumonitis
DiTe	Diphtheria-tetanus (vaccine)
DIU	Death *in utero*
DJD	Degenerative joint disease
DKA	Diabetic ketoacidosis
DKMA	*Lægemiddelstyrelsen*/Danish Medicines Agency
DLB	Dementia with Lewy bodies
DLCO	Diffusing capacity of the lung for carbon monoxide
DLE	Disseminated lupus erythematosus
DLI	Donor lymphocyte infusion
DLP	Data lock point
DM	Diabetes mellitus
DMARD	Disease-modifying antirheumatic drug
DMD	Duchenne muscular dystrophy; *Dentariae Medicinae* Doctor (Doctor of Dental Medicine)
DME	Durable medical equipment
DMF	Drug master file
DMPA	Depot medroxyprogesterone acetate
DMPK	Drug metabolism and pharmacokinetics
DMRC	Defective Medicines Report Centre (MHRA)
DMS	Document management system
DM2	Type 2 diabetes mellitus
DNA	Deoxyribonucleic acid
DNACPR	Do not attempt cardiopulmonary resuscitation
DNAR/DNR	Do not attempt resuscitation; do not resuscitate
DNH	Do not hospitalize
DNI	Do not intubate
DO	Doctor of Osteopathic Medicine
DOA	Dead on arrival
DOB	Difficulty of breathing; date of birth
DOE	Design of experiments; dyspnea on exertion
DOH	Department of Health; Declaration of Helsinki
DOL	Day of life
DOS	Date of service
DOSS	Dioctyl sulfosuccinate sodium salt
DOT	Directly observed therapy
DOTS	Directly observed therapy, short course

(Continued)

Abbreviation	Definition
DP	Drug product; *dorsalis pedis*
DPI	Dry powder inhaler
DPL	Diagnostic peritoneal lavage
DPLD	Diffuse parenchymal lung disease
DPT	Diphtheria-pertussis-tetanus
DR	Deliberate release; digital radiology
DRA	Drug Regulatory Authority (non–EU)
DRE	Digital rectal examination
DRF(S)	Dose range finding (study)
DRG	Diagnosis-related group
DRMP	Developmental risk management plan
DS	Down syndrome; drug substance; duplex sonography
DSA	Digital subtraction angiography; donor-specific antibody
DSC	Differential scanning calorimetry
DSD	Dry sterile dressing
DSM	*Diagnostic and Statistical Manual of Mental Disorders*
DSMB	Data and Safety Monitoring Board
dsRNA	Double-stranded RNA
DSRU	Drug Safety Research Unit (EMA)
DSUR	Development safety update report
DT	Delirium tremens
DTA	Descending thoracic aorta
DTaP	Diphtheria and tetanus toxoids and acellular pertussis [vaccine]
DTC	Direct-to-consumer
DTR	Deep tendon reflex
DU	Duodenal ulcer
DUB	Dysfunctional uterine bleeding
DUS	Drug utilization study
DVPHNFS	Department for Veterinary Public Health, Nutrition and Food Safety (Italy)
DVT	Deep venous (vein) thrombosis
EA	Environmental assessment
EAA	Essential amino acids
eAF	Electronic Application Form
EAI	Estimated acute intake
EAMS	Early access to medicines scheme (UK)
EBE	European Biopharmaceutical Enterprises
EBL	Estimated blood loss
EBM	Evidence-based medicine
EBV	Epstein-Barr virus
EC	Ethics committee; European Commission
ECA	Epidemiologic catchment area
ECD	External continence device
ECDC	European Centre for Disease Prevention and Control
ECG	Electrocardiogram

(Continued)

Abbreviation	Definition
ECHAMP	European Coalition on Homoeopathic & Anthroposophic Medicinal Products
ECHR	European Court of Human Rights
ECJ	European Court of Justice
ECMO	Extracorporeal membrane oxygenation
ECPHIN	European Community Pharmaceutical Information Network
ECRAB	European Committee on Regulatory Aspects of Biotechnology
eCRF	Electronic case report form
ECT	Electroconvulsive therapy
eCTD	Electronic common technical document
ED	Effective dose; emergency department; erectile dysfunction
ED_{50}	Median effective dose
EDA	Egyptian Drug Authority
EDC	Electronic data capture
EDD	Estimated date of delivery/discharge
EDF	End-diastolic flow
EDH	Epidural hematoma
EDM	Esophageal Doppler monitor
EDMF	European drug master file
eDMS	Electronic document management system
EDQM	European Directorate for the Quality of Medicines & HealthCare
EDRF	Endothelium-derived relaxing factor (nitric oxide)
EDS	Ehlers-Danlos Syndrome
EDT	Electronic data transfer
EDTA	Ethylenediaminetetraacetic acid
EDV	End-diastolic volume
EEA	European Economic Area (comprising the EU countries, with Iceland, Liechtenstein, and Norway)
EEC	European Economic Community
EEE	Eastern equine encephalomyelitis (encephalitis)
EEG	Electroencephalogram
EENT	Ears, eyes, nose, and throat
EF	Ejection fraction
EFA	European Federation of Allergy and Airways Diseases Patients' Associations; Editorial Freelancers Association
EFAD	Essential fatty acid deficiency
EFM	Electronic fetal monitoring
EFPIA	European Federation of Pharmaceutical Industries and Associations
EFQM	European Foundation for Quality Management
EFS	Event-free survival
EFTA	European Free Trade Association
EFW	Estimated fetal weight
EGA	European Generic medicines Association
EGD	Esophagogastroduodenoscopy
EGF	Epidermal growth factor

(Continued)

Abbreviation	Definition
EGGVP	European Group for Generic Veterinary Products
EGP	Economic Guidance Panel (Canada)
EGPA	Eosinophilic granulomatosis with polyangiitis (Churg-Strauss syndrome)
EHEC	Enterohemorrhagic *Escherichia coli*
EHR	Electronic health-care record
EIA	Environmental Impact Assessment; enzyme immunoassay; external iliac artery
EIEC	Enteroinvasive *Escherichia coli*
EINECS	European Inventory of Existing Chemical Substances
EKG	Electrocardiogram (typically now abbreviated "ECG")
EJ	Elbow-jerk (triceps reflex)
ELA	Establishment license application (US)
ELISA	Enzyme-linked immunosorbent assay
EM	Electron microscope; electron microscopic; electron microscopy
EMA	European Medicines Agency
EMB	Endometrial biopsy; endomyocardial biopsy
EMC	Encephalomyocarditis
EMCDDA	European Monitoring Centre for Drugs and Drug Addiction
EMD	Early-morning discovery; electromechanical dissociation
EMDEX	Essential Medicines Index
EMDR	Eye Movement Desensitization and Reprocessing
EMEA	Europe, Middle East & Africa
EMEAA	Europe, Middle East, Africa & Asia
EMF	Endomyocardial fibrosis
EMG	Electromyogram; electromyographic
EMIT	Enzyme-multiplied immunoassay technique
EMLSCS	Emergency lower-segment cesarian section (birth/delivery)
EMRC	European Medical Research Councils
EMS	Electrical muscle stimulation; emergency medical services
EMT	Emergency medical technician
EMU	Early-morning urine
EMV	Eyes, motor, verbal response (Glasgow coma scale)
EMVS	European Medicines Verification System
ENCePP	European Network of Centres for Pharmacoepidemiology and Pharmacovigilance
ENG	Electronystagmogram; electronystagmographic
ENP	European Neighborhood Policy
Enpr-EMA	European Network of Pediatric Research at the European Medicines Agency
ENS	Early notification system
ENT	Ears, nose, and throat
EOB	Edge of bed; end of business
EOF	*Ethnikos Organismos Farmakon* or National Organization for Medicines (Greece's regulatory agency)
EOG	Electrooculogram; electro-oculographic
EOM	Extraocular muscles; end of massage

(Continued)

Abbreviation	Definition
EOP	End of Phase (US Regulatory Phases 1 through 4)
EOQ	European Organization for Quality
EP	European Parliament
EP/Ph Eur	European Pharmacopoeia (Pharm Eur)
EPA	Environmental Protection Agency (US)
EPAA	European Partnership for Alternative Approaches to Animal testing
EPAD	European Prevention of Alzheimer's Dementia
EPAR	European Public Assessment Report
EPC	European Pharmacopoeia Commission
EPCT	Estrogen-progesterone challenge test
EPEC	Enteropathogenic *E. coli*
EPH	Edema-proteinuria-hypertension
EPHA	European Public Health Alliance
EPI	Essential Program for Immunization
EPID	Extended (also Expanded) Public Information Document
EPITT	European Pharmacovigilance Issues Tracking Tool
EPL	Effective patent life
EPO	European Patent Office; erythropoietin
EPPOSI	European Platform for Patients' Organization Science and Industry
EPPV	Early post-marketing phase vigilance (e.g., in Japan)
EPRG	European Pharmacovigilance Research Group
EPRUMA	European Platform for the Responsible Use of Medicines in Agriculture
EPS	Electrophysiology; extrapyramidal symptoms
ePSUR	Electronic periodic safety update report
EQ-5D	Euroqol-5D (generic health-related quality of life index)
EQUATOR	Enhancing the Quality and Transparency of Health Research
ER	Emergency room (increasingly referred to as emergency department)
ERA	European regulatory affairs
ERB	Ethical review board
ERCP	Endoscopic retrograde cholangiopancreatography
ERG	Electroretinogram; electroretinographic
ERM	Epiretinal membrane
eRMR	Electronic Reaction Monitoring Report
ERMS	Embryonal rhabdomyosarcoma; European risk management strategy
ESA	Erythropoiesis-stimulating agent
ESBL	Extended-spectrum β-lactamase
ESC	Embryonic stem cell
ESF	European Science Foundation
ESHAP	**E**toposide, methylprednisolone (**s**olu medrol), **h**igh-dose cytarabine (**a**ra-C) and cisplatin (**p**latinum)
ESL	Extracorporeal shockwave lithotripsy (also ESWL; treatment for kidney stones/calculi)
ESM	Ejection systolic murmur; European stakeholder model
ESMO	European Society for Medical Oncology

(Continued)

Abbreviation	Definition
ESPAR	Executive Summary Pharmacovigilance Assessment Report (EU)
ESR	Erythrocyte sedimentation rate
ESRA	European Society of Regulatory Affairs
ESRD	End-stage renal disease (also ESRF, end-stage renal failure)
ESS	Empty-sella syndrome; enhanced support service
EST	Endodermal sinus tumor
ESTRI	Electronic Standards for the Transfer of Regulatory Information
ESV	End-systolic volume
ESWL	Extracorporeal shock wave lithotripsy
ETASU	Elements to ensure safe use (US)
ETEC	Enterotoxigenic *E. coli*
eTMF	Electronic Trial Master File
EtOH	Ethanol (alcohol)
ETOMEP	European Technical Office for Medical Products (within EMA)
ETS	Endoscopic thoracic sympathectomy
ETT	Endotracheal tube
EU	European Union
EU5	Group of five countries: Germany, France, Italy, Spain, and the UK
EUA	Examination under anesthesia
EU-ADR	Exploring and Understanding Adverse Drug Reactions by Integrative Mining of Clinical Records and Biomedical Knowledge (formerly known as ALERT) (EU)
EUCERD	EU Committee of Experts on Rare Diseases (now replaced by EC Expert Group on Rare Diseases)
EUCOMED	European Confederation of Medical Devices Associations
EUDAMED	European Databank on Medical Devices
EUDRA	European Union Drug Regulating Authorities
EudraCT	European Union Drug Regulating Authorities Clinical Trials database
EudraNet	European Union Drug Regulating Authorities Network
EUnetHTA	European Network for Health Technology Assessment
EUPATI	European Patients' Academy on Therapeutic Innovation
EuPFI	European Pediatric Formulation Initiative
EURD	European Union reference date
EUREC	European Network of Research Ethics Committees
EUS	Endoscopic ultrasonography
EUTCT	European Union Telematics Controlled Terms
EVAR	Endovascular aneurysm repair
EVCTM	EudraVigilance Clinical Trial Module
EV EudraVigilance	European Union Drug Regulating Authorities Pharmacovigilance
EV-EWG	EudraVigilance Expert Working Group
EVF	Erythrocyte volume fraction
EVIDENT	Evidence Database on New Technologies
EVM	European Vaccine Manufacturers
EVMPD	EudraVigilance medicinal products dictionary
EVPM	EudraVigilance post-authorization module
EVPRM	EudraVigilance product report message

(Continued)

Abbreviation	Definition
EWG	Expert Working Group
EWP	Efficacy Working Party (EMA)
F	French (gauge; e.g., add the word *catheter*; use only with a number, e.g., 12F catheter)
FA	Fanconi anemia
FACC	Fellow of the American College of Cardiology; Food Additives and Contaminants Committee (UK)
FACP	Fellow of the American College of Physicians
FACS	Fellow of the American College of Surgeons
FAGG	*Federaal Agentschap voor Geneesmiddelen en Gezondheidsproducten* (Belgium)
FAMHP	Federal Agency for Medicines and Healthcare Products (Belgium)
FAMMM	Familial atypical multiple mole melanoma (syndrome)
FANA	Fluorescent antinuclear antibody test
FAR	Final assessment report
FBC	Full blood count
FBE	Full-blood examination
FBG	Fasting blood glucose
FBS	Fasting blood sugar/failed-back syndrome
FCC	Food Chemical Codex
FCS	Faciocutaneoskeletal syndrome
FDA	Food and Drug Administration
FDAAA	FDA Amendments Act
FDAMA	FDA Modernization Act
FDASIA	Food and Drug Administration Safety and Innovation Act
FDC	Fixed-dose combination; follicular dendritic cells
FDC Act	Food, Drug, and Cosmetic Act (US)
FDG	Fluorodeoxyglucose
FDIU	Fetal death in utero
FDP	Fibrin degradation product
$FEF_{25\%-75\%}$	Forced expiratory flow, midexpiratory phase at 25%–75% of forced vital capacity (FVC)
FEN	Fluids, electrolytes, nutrition
FEP	Free erythrocyte protoporphyrin; fibroepithelial polyp
FES	Functional electrical stimulation
FESS	Functional endoscopic sinus surgery
FET	Frozen embryo transfer
FEV	Forced expiratory volume
FEV_1	Forced expiratory volume in the first second of expiration
FF	Free fluids
FFA	Free fatty acids
FFP	Fresh frozen plasma
5-HIAA	5-Hydroxyindoleacetic acid (terminal metabolite of 5-HT)
FHR	Fetal heart rate
FHS	Fetal heart sound

(Continued)

Abbreviation	Definition
FHT	Fetal heart tones
5-HT	5-Hydroxytryptamine (serotonin)
FIH	First-in-human (FIM first-in-man; and FTIM first-time-in-human)
FIM-A	Federal Institute for Medicines (Austria)
FIMEA	Finnish Medicines Agency (Finland)
FIO_2	Fraction of inspired oxygen
FISH	Fluorescence in situ hybridization
FL	Femur length
FLAIR	Fluid-attenuated inversion recovery
510(k)	Medical device premarket notification (US FDA)
FLAIR	Fluid-attenuated inversion recovery
FM	Fetal movements (FMF, fetal movements felt)
FMD	Falsified Medicines Directive (EU)
FMEA	Failure modes and effects analysis
FMECA	Failure Modes Effects and Criticality Assessment
FMP	First menstrual period (menarche)
FMPP	Familial male-limited precocious puberty
fMRI	Functional magnetic resonance imaging
FMS	Fibromyalgia syndrome
FNA	Fine-needle aspiration
FNOM-CeO	*Federazione Nazionale degli Ordini dei Medici-Chirurghi e degli Odontoiatri* (Italy)
FOB	Fecal occult blood test; follow-on biologic
FOFI	*Federazione Ordini Farmacisti Italiani* (IT) = Italian Organization of Pharmacists
FOM	Francophone Overseas Markets
FONSI	Finding of no significant impact
FOP	Follow-on protein
FP	Family physician; family planning
FPG	Fasting plasma glucose
FPIF	Finnish Pharmaceutical Industry Association (Pharmacy Industry Finland)
FPP	Finished pharmaceutical product
FPRC	Final product release control
FPRR	Final product release responsibility
FQA	Full quality assurance
FR	Federal Register (US)
FRC	Functional residual capacity
FRDA	Friedreich's ataxia
FROM	Full range of motion
FrP	French Pharmacopoeia
FSBG	Finger-stick blood glucose
FSCA	Field safety corrective action (medical devices sector)
FSE	Fetal-scalp electrode
FSGS	Focal segmental glomerulosclerosis
FSH	Follicle-stimulating hormone

(Continued)

Abbreviation	Definition
FSIS	Food Safety and Inspection Service (US)
FSN	Field safety notice (medical devices)
FTA	Fault tree analysis; fluorescent treponemal antibody
FTA-ABS	Fluorescent treponemal antibody absorption
FTC	Federal Trade Commission (US)
FTE	Full-time equivalent (employee)
FTIM	First-time-in-human
FTIR	Fourier transform infrared
FtT	Failure to thrive
FU (f/u)	Follow-up; *Farmacopea Ufficiale* (Italian Pharmacopoeia)
FUE/FUT	Follicular unit extraction/transplantation
FUM	Follow-up measure
FUO	Fever of unknown origin
FWB	Full-weight-bearing
FVAR	Final Variation Assessment Report
FVC	Forced vital capacity
GA	General anesthesia; gestational age
GABA	γ-Aminobutyric acid
GABHS	Group A beta (or β)-hemolytic streptococcus
GAD	Generalized anxiety disorder
GAF	Global Assessment of Functioning [Scale]
GAIN Act	Generating Antibiotic Incentives Now Act (US)
GATT	General Agreement on Tariffs and Trade
GBC	Gallbladder carcinoma
GBM	Glioblastoma multiforme; glomerular basement membrane
GBS	Group B streptococcus; Guillain-Barré Syndrome
GC	(GC-MS) Gas chromatography with mass spectrometry
GCA	Giant-cell arteritis
GCC (region)	Gulf Cooperation Council (region)
GCC-DR	Gulf Central Committee for Drug Registration
GCG	Global Cooperation Group (ICH)
G6PD	Glucose-6-phosphate dehydrogenase
GCP	Good Clinical Practice
GCPv	Good Clinical Practice (Veterinary)
GCS	Glasgow Coma Scale
G-CSF	Granulocyte colony-stimulating factor
GCT	Germ-cell tumor; giant-cell tumor; glucose challenge test
GDA	Gastroduodenal artery
GDLH	Glutamate dehydrogenase
GDM	Gestational diabetes mellitus
GDP	Good distribution practice; guanosine diphosphate
GDS	Geriatric Depression Scale
GED	General Education Development
GERD	Gastroesophageal reflux disease
GETT	General (anesthesia) by endotracheal tube

(Continued)

Abbreviation	Definition
GFR	Glomerular filtration rate
GGP	Good guidance practice
GGT	γ (or gamma) glutamyl transferase
GGTP	γ (or gamma) glutamyl transpeptidase
GH	Growth hormone
GHRF/GHRH	Growth hormone–releasing factor (hormone)
GHTF	Global Harmonization Task Force
GI	Gastrointestinal
GIB/H	Gastrointestinal bleeding (hemorrhage)
GIFT	Gamete intrafallopian transfer
GIP	Gastric inhibitory polypeptide
GIST	Gastrointestinal stromal tumor
GIT	Gastrointestinal tract
GLC	Gas-liquid chromatography
GLP	Good Laboratory Practice; glucagon-like peptide
GLPMA	Good Laboratory Practice Monitoring Authority (UK)
GMA	Global marketing authorization
GMC	General Medical Council (UK); general medical condition
GM-CSF	Granulocyte-macrophage colony-stimulating factor
GMDN	Global medical device nomenclature (medical devices sector)
GMiA	Generic Medicines industry Association (Australia)
GMO	Genetically modified organism
GMP	Good Manufacturing Practice; guanosine monophosphate
GMRI	Gated magnetic resonance imaging
GMT	Geometric mean titer
GN	Glomerulonephritis
GNA	Grounds for nonacceptance
GnRH	Gonadotropin-releasing hormone
GOAT	Galveston Orientation and Amnesia Test
GOD	Glucose oxidase
GOT	Glutamic oxaloacetic transaminase
GP	General practitioner; Goodpasture's syndrome
GPA	Granulomatosis with polyangiitis (Wegener's granulomatosis); Generic Pharmaceutical Association (US)
GPCL	Gas-permeable contact lens
GPMSP	Good Postmarketing Surveillance Practice (Japan)
GPP	Good Pharmacoepidemiology Practice; Good Publication Practice
GPSP	Good Post-marketing Study Practice
GPT	Glutamic-pyruvic transaminase
GpvP	Good pharmacovigilance practice
GQCLP	Good Quality Control Laboratory Practice
GQP	Good quality practice
gr	Grain (1 grain = 65 mg)
GRAS	Generally Recognized as Safe (US)
GRB	Global Regulatory Board

(Continued)

Abbreviation	Definition
GRP	Good regulatory practice; good review practice (US)
GSL	General sales list
GSP	Good statistics practice
GSW	Gunshot wound
GTI	Genotoxic impurity
GTN	Glyceryl trinitrate; gestational trophoblastic neoplasia
GTP	Gene therapy product
GTT	Gestational trophoblastic tumor; glucose tolerance test
GTWP	Gene Therapy Working Party
GU	Gastric ulcer; genitourinary; graphical user (interface)
GUM	Genitourinary medicine
GVHD	Graft-vs-host disease
GVP	Good pharmacovigilance practice
GXT	Graded exercise tolerance (stress test)
HA	Headache; health authority; hydroxyapatite (calcium hydroxyapatite); hypertonia arterialis
HAA	Hepatitis-associated antigen
HAART	Highly active antiretroviral therapy
HACA	Human anti-chimeric antibody
HACCP	Hazard analysis critical control point (inspection technique) (US)
HACE	High-altitude cerebral edema
HACEK	Haemophilus spp., *Aggregatibacter actinomycetemcomitans*, *Cardiobacterium hominis*, *Eikenella corrodens*, and *Kingella kingae* (pathogens that can cause endocarditis in children)
HAD	HIV–associated dementia
HADS	Hospital Anxiety and Depression Scale
HAE	Hereditary angioedema
HAI	Health Action International
HALE	Health-adjusted life expectancy
HAPE	High-altitude pulmonary edema
HAQ	Health Assessment Questionnaire
HAS	*Haute Autorité de santé* (French Health Authority)
HAV	Hepatitis A virus
Hb	Hemoglobin
HB	Heart block
HbA1c	Hemoglobin A1c
HbCO	Carboxyhemoglobin
HBD	Harmonized Birth Date
HbF	Fetal hemoglobin
HBO	Hyperbaric oxygen
HbO_2	Oxyhemoglobin; oxygenated hemoglobin
HBP	High blood pressure (hypertension)
HbS	Sickle cell hemoglobin
Hb_sAg	Hepatitis B surface antigen
HBSS	Hanks balanced salt solution

(*Continued*)

Abbreviation	Definition
HBV	Hepatitis B virus
HC	Head circumference; hemorrhagic colitis
HCC	Hepatocellular carcinoma
HCF	Health-care facility
hCG	Human chorionic gonadotropin
HCL	Hairy-cell leukemia
HCM	Health-care maintenance
HCP	Health-care professional (provider)
HCPWP	Healthcare Professionals Working Party (EMA)
HCR	Holder of certificate of registration (South Africa)
HCRP	Hospital Cornea Retrieval Program
HCS	Human chorionic somatomammotropin
Hct	Hematocrit
HCT	Hematopoietic cell transplantation
HCTZ	Hydrochlorothiazide
HCV	Hepatitis C virus
HD	Hodgkin's disease; Huntington's disease
HDE	Humanitarian Device Exemption
HDI	Human development index
HDL	High-density lipoprotein
HDL-C	HDL-cholesterol
HDN	Hemolytic disease of the newborn
HDRS	Hamilton Depression Rating Scale
HDU	High-dependency unit
HDV	Hepatitis D virus
HDW	Hemoglobin distribution width
HE	Hepatic encephalopathy
H&E	Hematoxylin and eosin
HECOR	Health economics and clinical outcomes research
HEENT	Head, eyes, ears, nose, and throat
HELLP	Hemolysis, elevated liver enzymes, and low platelets in pregnancy
HEOR	Health economics and outcomes research
HETE	Hydroxyeicosatetraenoic acid
HEV	Hepatitis E virus
HF	Heart failure
HFM/HFMD	Hand, foot, and mouth (disease)
HFpEF/HFrEF	Heart failure with preserved (or reduced) ejection fraction
HFRS	Hemorrhagic fever with renal syndrome
HGAC	Human Genetics Advisory Committee
Hgb	Hemoglobin
hGH	Human growth hormone
HGPRT	Hypoxanthine-guanine-phosphoribosyltransferase (also HGPRTase)
HGSIL	High-grade squamous intraepithelial lesion
HGV	Hepatitis G virus
H/H	Henderson-Hasselbach equation or hemoglobin/hematocrit

(Continued)

Abbreviation	Definition
HH	Hiatal hernia
HHEC	Highly emetogenic chemotherapy
HHS	(US Department of) Health and Human Services
HHT	Hereditary hemorrhagic telangiectasia (Osler–Weber–Rendu disease/syndrome)
HHV	Human herpesvirus
HI	Homicidal ideation
Hib	*Haemophilus influenzae* type b
HIDA	Hepatobiliary iminodiacetic acid
HIDS	Hyperimmunoglobulinemia D (with periodic fever) syndrome
HIMA	Health Industry Manufacturers Association (US)
HIPAA	Health Insurance Portability and Accountability Act
HIT	Heparin-induced thrombocytopenia
HIV	Human immunodeficiency virus
HJR	Hepatojugular reflux
HL	Hearing level; hepatic lipase; Hodgkin's lymphoma
HL7	Health Level Seven
H&M	Hematemesis and melena
HLA	Histocompatibility locus antigen; human leukocyte antigen
HLHS	Hypoplastic left-heart syndrome
HLT	High-level term
HMA	Heads of Medicines Agencies (Human and Veterinary) (EU)
HMG	Human menopausal gonadotropin
HMG-CoA	3-Hydroxy-3-methylglutaryl coenzyme A (rate-limiting step in endogenous cholesterol biosynthesis)
HMO	Health-maintenance organization (US)
HMS	Hyperreactive malarial splenomegaly
HMSN	Hereditary motor sensory neuropathy
HN	Hemagglutinin-neuraminidase
HNC	Head and neck cancer
HNP	Herniated nucleus pulposus (herniated spinal disc)
HNPCC	Hereditary nonpolyposis colorectal cancer
HO	History of
HoA	Heads of Agencies
HoB	Head of bed
HOCM	Hypertrophic obstructive cardiomyopathy
HOPI	History of present illness
HPA	Hypothalamic-pituitary-adrenal
HPB	Health Protection Board (Canada)
HPETE	Hydroperoxyeicosatetraenoic acid
HPF	High-power field
HPI	History of present illness
hPL	Human placental lactogen
HPLC	High-performance liquid chromatography
HPOA	Hypertrophic pulmonary osteoarthropathy (clubbing)

(Continued)

Abbreviation	Definition
HPRA	Health Products Regulatory Authority (formerly Irish Medicines Board)
HPS	Hantavirus pulmonary syndrome
HPV	Human papillomavirus
HR	Hazard ratio; heart rate
HRA	Health Research Authority (UK)
HRAS	Harvey rat sarcoma viral oncogene homolog
HRCT	High-resolution computed tomography
HREC	Human Research Ethics Committee
HRQOL	Health-related quality of life
h.s./hs	At bedtime (Latin *hora somni*); hours of sleep
HSA	Human serum albumin
HSC	Hematopoietic stem cell
HSIL	High-grade squamous intraepithelial lesion
HSM	Hepatosplenomegaly
HSP	Henoch–Schönlein purpura
HST	Highly specialized technologies
HSV	Herpes simplex virus
HT	Hormone therapy
HTA	Health technology assessment (appraisal)
HTLV	Human T-lymphotropic virus
Htn	Hypertension
HTPA/HTPAA	Hypothalamic-pituitary-adrenal (axis)
HTS	High-throughput screening
HTVD	Hypertensive vascular disease
HUS	Hemolytic uremic syndrome
HV	Healthy volunteer
HVA	Homovanillic acid
Hx	History
H&P	History and physical (examination)
I&AC	Imaging and acute care (medical devices sector)
I&D	Incision and drainage
I&O	Intake and output
IA	Intra-arterial
IAA	Insulin autoantibody
IABP	Intra-aortic balloon pump
IADL	Instrumental activities of daily living (1 IADL, 6 IADLs)
IAI	Intra-amniotic infection
IAPO	International Alliance of Patients' Organizations
IB	Investigator's brochure
IBC	Inflammatory breast cancer
IBD	Inflammatory bowel disorder; International Birth Date
IBMS	Institute of Basic Medical Sciences (China)
IBS	Irritable bowel syndrome
IC	Informed consent; ileocecal; immunocompromised; intensive care; insular cortex; interstitial cystitis; immune complex; intracardiac

(Continued)

Abbreviation	Definition
ICACT	International Congress on Anti-Cancer Treatment
ICCU	Intensive cardiac care unit
ICD	Implantable cardioverter-defibrillator; informed-consent document; *International Classification of Diseases*
ICDRA	International Conference of Drug Regulatory Authorities
ICDS	Integrated Child Development Services
ICF	Intracellular fluid
ICG	Impedance cardiography
ICH	International Council for Harmonisation of Technical Requirements for Pharmaceuticals for Human Use; intracerebral hemorrhage
ICM	Ischemic cardiomyopathy
ICMJE	International Committee of Medical Journal Editors (see Chapter 4)
ICMRA	International Coalition of Medicines Regulatory Authorities
ICP	Intracranial pressure
ICP-MS	Inductively coupled plasma mass spectrometry
ICS	Inhaled corticosteroid; intercostal space; internal carotid-artery stenosis
ICSR	Individual case safety report
ICTRP	International Clinical Trials Registry Platform (WHO)
ICU	Intensive care unit
ICX	Inhibition concentration at X%
ID	Identifying data; infectious disease; infectious dose
IDA	Iron-deficiency anemia
IDC	Idiopathic dilated cardiomyopathy; indwelling catheter; infiltrating ductal carcinoma
IDDM	Insulin-dependent diabetes mellitus (type 1 diabetes)
IDE	Investigational Device Exemption
IDL	Intermediate-density lipoprotein
IDMP	Identification of medicinal products; infectious diseases management program (US)
IDP	Infectious disease precautions
IDR	Idiosyncratic drug reaction
IDRAC	International Drug Registration Assisted by Computer
IDU	Injecting/injection drug user
IE	Infective endocarditis
IEC	Independent ethics committee
IFAH	International Federation for Animal Health
IFG	Impaired fasting glucose
IFN	Interferon
IFPMA	International Federation of Pharmaceutical Manufacturers and Associations
IFU	Instructions for use
Ig	Immunoglobulin
IGDRP	International Generic Drug Regulators Programme
IGF-1	Insulin-like growth factor 1
IGPA	International Generic Pharmaceutical Alliance
IGT	Impaired glucose tolerance

(Continued)

Abbreviation	Definition
IHC	Immunohistochemistry
IHD	Ischemic heart disease
IHPS	Infantile hypertrophic pyloric stenosis
IHSS	Idiopathic hypertrophic subaortic stenosis
IIEF	International Index of Erectile Function
IIG	Inactive ingredient guide (US)
IL	Interleukin
ILD	Interstitial lung disease
IM	Intramuscular
IMA	Icelandic Medicines Agency; inferior mesenteric artery
IMB	Irish Medicines Board; intermenstrual bleeding (or hemorrhage)
IMCA	Inferior mesenteric artery
IMD	Implantable medical device
IMDA	Irish Medical Devices Association
IMDRF	International Medical Device Regulators Forum
IME	Important medical event
IMI	Innovative Medicines Initiative; intramuscular injection
IMID	Immune-mediated inflammatory disease
IMM	Irreversible morbidity or mortality; intramyometrial
IMN	Infectious mononucleosis
IMP	Investigational medicinal product
ImPACT	Imaging performance assessment of CT scanner
IMPD	Investigational medicinal product dossier
IMRT	Intensity-modulated radiotherapy
IMS	Information management strategy
IMT	Intima-media thickness (often carotid IMT; CIMT); inflammatory myofibroblastic tumor
IMV	Intermittent mandatory ventilation
IN	Intraepithelial neoplasia
INADA	Investigational new animal drug application
IND	Investigational new drug (US)
INDA	Investigational new drug application (US)
INFARMED	*Instituto Nacional da Farmácia e do Medicamento* (Portugal's regulatory agency)
INN	International nonproprietary name
INR	International normalized ratio
INT	Intermittent needle therapy
IODM	Infant of diabetic mother
IOL	Induction of labor; intraocular lens
IOP	Intraocular pressure; intraorifice pressure
IP	Intraperitoneal; intellectual property; investigational product
IPA	Intimate partner abuse; isopropyl alcohol (isopropanol)
IPAC	International Pharmaceutical Aerosol Consortium
IPEC	International Pharmaceutical Excipients Council
IPF	Idiopathic pulmonary fibrosis

(Continued)

Abbreviation	Definition
IPG	Implantable pulse generator
IPH	Intraparenchymal (or intraperitoneal) hemorrhage; idiopathic pulmonary hemosiderosis
IPMN	Intraductal papillary mucinous neoplasm
IPO	Intellectual Property Office
IPPB/IPPV	Intermittent positive pressure breathing (ventilation)
IPR	Intellectual property rights
IPRF	International Pharmaceutical Regulators Forum
IPU	Irish Pharmacy Union
IPV	Intimate partner violence
IQ	Intelligence quotient
IQM	Integrated quality management
IR	Immediate-release; infrared; insulin resistance
IRAS	Integrated Research Application System
IRB	Institutional review board
IRBBB	Incomplete right bundle branch block
IRC	Institutional Review Committee
IRDS	Infant respiratory distress syndrome
IRIDA	Iron-refractory iron deficiency anemia
IRIS	Immune reconstitution inflammatory syndrome
IRMA	Immunoradiometric assay
IR(ME)R	Ionising radiation (medical exposure) regulations
IRN	Incident Review Network
IRP	Independent review panel
IRR	Ionising radiation regulation
IRT	Interactive response technology; Interdisciplinary Review Team (US)
IS	Incentive spirometry; information science/systems; internal standard
ISA	Intrinsic sympathomimetic activity
ISBN	International Standard Book Number
ISE	Integrated summary of efficacy
ISG	Immune serum globulin
ISH	Isolated systolic hypertension (common in elderly patients)
ISMN	Isosorbide mononitrate
ISMPP	International Society for Medical Publication Professionals
ISO	International Standards Organization
ISPOR	International Society for Pharmacoeconomics and Outcomes Research
ISQ	No change (Latin *in status quo*)
ISRB	Integrated summary of risk benefit
ISS	Integrated summary of safety
ISSN	International Standard Serial Number
IT	Immature teratoma; information technology; intrathecal
ITF	Innovation Task Force (EMA)
ITI	Intratubal insemination
ITP	Idiopathic (or immune) thrombocytopenic purpura
ITT	Intention (intent)-to-treat

(Continued)

Abbreviation	Definition
IU	International unit
IUD	Intrauterine death; intrauterine device
IUGR	Intrauterine growth restriction
IUI	Intrauterine insemination
IUP	Intrauterine pregnancy
IUPAC	International Union of Pure and Applied Chemistry
IUPC	Intrauterine pressure catheter
IUS	Intrauterine system
IUT	Intrauterine transfusion
IV	Intravenous
IVC	Intravenous cholangiogram; inferior vena cava
IVD	In vitro diagnostics; In vitro (medical) device; intervertebral disc
IV-DSA	Intravenous digital subtraction angiography
IVDR	In vitro diagnostic device regulation
IVDU	Intravenous drug user
IVF	In vitro fertilization; intravenous fluids
IVIG	Intravenous immunoglobulin
IVIVC	In vitro in vivo correlation
IVMP	Immunological veterinary medicinal product
IVP	Intravenous pyelogram
IVPG	Intravenous pyogenic granuloma
IVR	Interactive voice response
IVRS	Interactive voice response system
IVU	Intravenous urogram
IVUS	Intravascular ultrasonography
IWG	Implementation working group
IWP	Immunologicals Working Party (EMA)
JAN	Japanese Approved Name
JAZMP	*Javna agencija Republike Slovenije za zdravila in medicinske pripomočke* (Slovenia's regulatory agency)
JEV	Japanese encephalitis virus
JFDA	Jordan Food & Drug Administration
JIA	Juvenile idiopathic arthritis
JIACRA	Joint Interagency Antimicrobial Consumption and Resistance Analysis
JNDA	Japanese New Drug Application
JODM	Juvenile-onset diabetes mellitus
JP	Japanese Pharmacopoeia; Jackson–Pratt (drain)
JPEG	Joint photographic experts group (computer file format for digital images)
JPMA	Japan Pharmaceutical Manufacturers Association
JRA	Juvenile rheumatoid arthritis (juvenile idiopathic arthritis)
J-RMP	Japanese risk management plan (template)
JVD	Jugular venous distention
JVP	Jugular venous pressure
K	Potassium (Latin *kalium*)
KA	Ketoacidosis

(*Continued*)

Abbreviation	Definition
KAFO	Knee ankle foot orthosis
KAS	Known active substance
KCCT	Kaolin cephalin clotting time
KELS	Kohlman Evaluation of Living Skills
KFDA	Korean Food and Drug Administration (now known as Ministry of Food and Drug Safety)
KIT	Key intelligence topic
KIV	Keep in view
KLS	Kidney, liver, spleen
KM	Knowledge management
KOH	Potassium hydroxide
KOL	Key opinion leader
KS	Kaposi's sarcoma; Kartagener syndrome
KSHV	Kaposi's sarcoma–associated herpesvirus
KT	Kinesiotherapy or kinesiotherapist
KUB	Kidneys, ureters, and bladder
KVO	Keep vein open
L&D	Labor and delivery
LA	Left atrium; local anesthetic
LAAM	L-alpha [α]-acetylmethadol
LABA	Long-acting beta [β] agonist
LAD	Left anterior descending (coronary artery); left axis deviation; leukocyte adhesion deficiency
LAE	Left atrial enlargement
LAH	Left anterior hemiblock
LAHB	Left anterior hemiblock
LAO	Left anterior oblique coronary artery
LAP	Left atrial pressure; leukocyte alkaline phosphatase
LAS	Lymphadenopathy syndrome
LASEK	Laser epithelial keratomileusis
Laser	Light amplification by stimulated emission of radiation
LASIK	Laser in situ keratomileusis
LAV	Lymphadenopathy-associated virus
LBBB	Left bundle branch block
LBO	Large-bowel obstruction
LBP	Low back pain
LBW	Low birth weight
LC	Locus coeruleus
LCA	Left coronary artery
LCHAD	Long-chain 3-hydroxyacyl-coenzyme A dehydrogenase
LCIS	Lobular carcinoma in situ
LCM	Lifecycle management; lymphocytic meningitis
LCMV	Lymphocytic choriomeningitis virus
LCP	Leukocytoclastic vasculitis
LCPD	Legg–Calvé–Perthes disease

(Continued)

Abbreviation	Definition
LCR	Locus control region
LCV	Leukocytoclastic vasculitis
LCx (Cx)	Left circumflex (coronary artery)
LD	Lethal dose
L-DOPA	*Levo*-dihydroxyphenylalanine
LD_{50}	Lethal dose required to kill 50% (median lethal dose)
LDH	Lactate dehydrogenase
LDL	Low-density lipoprotein
LDL-C	LDL-cholesterol
LE	Lupus erythematosus; lower extremity
LEEM	*Les Entreprises du Médicament* (French Pharmaceutical Industry Association)
LEEP	Loop electrosurgical excision procedure (US)
LES	Lower-esophageal sphincter
LFT	Liver function test
LGA	Large for gestational age
LGL	Lown–Ganong–Levine syndrome
LGM	Lymphogranulomatosis maligna
LGSIL	Low-grade squamous intraepithelial lesion
LGV	Lymphogranuloma venereum
LH	Luteinizing hormone
LHC	Left-heart catheterization
LHRH	Luteinizing hormone-releasing hormone
LiCT	Low-intervention clinical trial
LIF	*Läkemedelsindustriföreningen* (Swedish Pharmaceutical Industry Association)
LIH	Left inguinal hernia
LLD	Leg length discrepancy
LLE	Left lower extremity
LLETZ	Large loop excision of the transformation zone (ex-US)
LLL	Left lower lobe
LLQ	Left-lower quadrant
LM	Left main
LMA	Left mentoanterior; laryngeal mask airway
LMCA	Left main coronary artery
LMIC	Low- and middle-income countries
LMP	Last menstrual period; low malignant potential
LMW	Low molecular weight (e.g., LMW heparin)
LN	Lymph node
LND	Lymph-node dissection
LNI	Lymph-node involvement
LNMP	Last normal menstrual period
LOA	Left occiput anterior; lysis of adhesions
LOC	Loss (level) of consciousness
LOCF	Last observation carried forward

(Continued)

Abbreviation	Definition
LOD	Logarithm of odds; loss on drying
logMAR	Logarithm of the minimum angle of resolution
LOH	Loss of heterozygosity
LOI	Letter of intent (US); loss of imprinting
LOM	Loss of motion
LoOI	List of outstanding issues
LOP	Left occiput posterior
LoQ	List of questions
LORTA/LORA	Loss of resistance to air
LOS	Length of stay
LOT	Left occiput transverse
LP	Lumbar puncture
LPH	Left-posterior hemiblock
LPL	Lipoprotein lipase
LPN	Licensed practical nurse
LPP	Lichen planopilaris
LQTS	Long−QT syndrome
LR	Likelihood ratio
LRINEC	Laboratory Risk Indicator for Necrotizing Soft Tissue Infections
LRS	Lactated Ringer's solution
LRTI	Lower-respiratory-tract infection
L/S	Lecithin: sphingomyelin ratio
LS	Lichen sclerosis; Lynch syndrome
LSB	Left sternal border
LSCA	Lung sounds clear to auscultation
LSD	Lysergic acid diethylamide
LSIF	Life Sciences Innovation Forum
LSIL	Low-grade squamous intraepithelial lesion
LST	Laterally spreading tumor
LT	Long-term
LTAC	Long-term acute care
LTCF	Long-term care facility
LTCS	Low-transverse cesarean section (birth/delivery)
LTT	Lines to take [document usually not for publication] (EMA)
LUL	Left upper lobe
LUQ	Left upper quadrant
LUS	Lower uterine segment
LUTS	Lower-urinary-tract symptoms
LV	Left ventricle; left ventricular
LVAD	LV assist device
LVEDP	LV end-diastolic pressure
LVEDV	LV end-diastolic volume
LVEF	LV ejection fraction
LVH	LV hypertrophy
LVOT	LV outflow tract

(Continued)

Abbreviation	Definition
LVP	Large-volume parenterals (or paracentesis)
M&S	Modeling and simulation
MA	Marketing authorization
MAA	Marketing authorisation application (EU)
MABEL	Minimal anticipated biological effect level
MAC	Mycobacterium *avium* complex
MACE	Major adverse cardiovascular events
MAD	Multiple ascending dose (study)
MAE	Moves all extremities
MAFF	Ministry of Agriculture, Forestry and Fisheries (Japan)
MAH	Marketing authorization holder
MAHA	Microangiopathic hemolytic anemia
MAL	Midaxillary Line
MALAM	Medical Lobby for Appropriate Marketing
MALT	Mucosa-associated lymphoid tissue
MANOS	Minilaparoscopy-assisted natural orifice surgery
MAO	Monoamine oxidase
MAOI	MAO inhibitor
MAP	Mean arterial pressure; mitogen-activated protein (and MAP kinase)
MAPC	Multipotent adult progenitor cell
MAPPs	Medicines Adaptive Pathways to Patients
MAR	Medication administration record
MARSA	Methicillin- and aminoglycoside-resistant *Staphylococcus aureus*
MAS	Morgagni–Adams–Stokes syndrome; meconium-aspiration syndrome
MAT	Microscopic agglutination test; multifocal atrial tachycardia
MAUDE	Manufacturer and User Facility Device Experience (US)
MaxSPRT	Maximized sequential probability ratio test
MBC	Minimum bactericidal concentration
MBSS	Modified barium swallow study
MBT	Maternal blood type
MCA	Mucinous cystadenoma
MCAT	Medical college admission test
MCC	Medicines Control Council (South Africa)
MCD	Minimal-change disease
MCDA	Multicriteria decision analysis
MCH	Mean cell hemoglobin; mean corpuscular hemoglobin
MCHC	Mean corpuscular hemoglobin concentration
MCID	Minimum clinically important difference (see Appendix 1)
MCL	Mantle-cell lymphoma
MCO	Managed-care organization
MCP	Metacarpophalangeal
MC&S	Microscopy, culture, and sensitivity
MCTD	Mixed connective-tissue disease
MCV	Mean cell volume; mean corpuscular volume; Medical College of Virginia
MD	Medical device (doctor); muscular dystrophy

(Continued)

Abbreviation	Definition
MDA	Medical device alert
MDCG	Medical Device Coordination Group
MDCT	Multidetector row computed tomography
MDD	Major depressive disorder; Medical Device Directive
MDE	Major depressive episode
MDEG	Medical Devices Expert Group
MDEG-BC	Medical Devices Expert Group on Borderline and Classification
MDI	Metered dose inhaler
MDLO	Medical Device Liaison Officer
MDR	Medical Device Regulation; Medical device reporting; multidrug-resistant
MDS	Myelodysplastic syndrome
MDSAP	Medical Devices Single-Audit Programme (Canada)
MDV	Medical device vigilance
M/E	Microscopic examination
ME	Myalgic encephalopathy (chronic fatigue syndrome)
MEB	Medicines Evaluation Board (Netherlands)
MEC	Mean effective concentration; moderately emetogenic chemotherapy
MedDRA	Medical Dictionary for Regulatory Activities
MEDEV	Medicine Evaluation Committee (EU)
MEDLINE	Medical Literature Analysis and Retrieval System Online
MEDSAFE	New Zealand Medicines and Medical Devices Safety Authority
MEM	Minimum essential medium
MEN	Multiple endocrine neoplasia
MENA	Middle East and North Africa
MERS	Multiagency electronic regulatory system
MeSH	Medical Subject Heading
MET	Metabolic equivalent for task
MFM	Maternal and fetal medicine
MG	Myasthenia gravis
MGN	Membranous glomerulonephritis
MGUS	Monoclonal gammopathy of undetermined significance
MHA-TP	Microhemagglutination assay for *Treponema pallidum*
MHC	Major histocompatibility complex
MHRA	Medicines and Healthcare products Regulatory Agency
MHW	Ministry of Health, Labour and Welfare (Japan); mental health worker
MI	Myocardial infarction; mitral insufficiency
MIC	Minimum inhibitory concentration
MICU	Medical (mobile) intensive-care unit
MIF	Müllerian inhibitory factor
MIMS	Monthly Index of Medical Specialties (UK)
MIS	Minimally invasive surgery; Müllerian inhibiting substance
mL	Milliliter (cubic centimeter; cc; cm^3)
ML	Manufacturer's license (UK)
MLC	Mixed lymphocyte culture
MLD	Minimal lethal dose

(Continued)

Abbreviation	Definition
MLE	Midline episiotomy
MM	Middle meningeal; multiple myeloma; myeloid metaplasia
MMEF	Maximal midexpiratory flow
MMFR	Midmaximal flow rate
MMI	Maximum medical improvement
MMK	Marshall–Marchetti–Krantz procedure
mmol	Millimolar
MMPI	Minnesota Multiphasic Personality Inventory
MMR	Measles, mumps, rubella; mismatch repair
MMR-D	Mismatch repair deficiency syndrome
MMSE	Mini-Mental State Examination
MMT	Malignant mesenchymal tumor; mixed malignant Müllerian tumor
MN	Membranous nephropathy
MND	Motor neuron disease (e.g., amyotrophic lateral sclerosis; Charcot disease)
MOA	Mechanism of action; Ministry of Agriculture
MoCA	Mechanism of Coordinated Access
MODS	Multiple-organ dysfunction syndrome
MODY	Maturity onset diabetes of the young
Mono-Di (Mo-Di)	Monochorionic-diamniotic (twins)
Mono-Mono (Mo-Mo)	Monochorionic-monoamniotic (twins)
MOOSE	Meta-analysis of Observational Studies in Epidemiology (see Chapter 4)
MOPP	Mechlorethamine, vincristine (Oncovin), procarbazine, and prednisone (prednisolone)
MORE	Manufacturer's On-line Reporting Environment (MHRA) (medical devices sector)
MOU	Memorandum of Understanding
MPA	Medical Products Agency Sweden; medroxyprogesterone acetate
MPD	Medicinal Products Directive; main pancreatic duct; myeloproliferative disease
MPGN	Membranoproliferative glomerulonephritis
MPID	Medicinal product identifier
MPO	Myeloproliferative disease (disorder)
MPS	Mortality Probability Score
MPV	Mean platelet volume
MQAS	Model Quality Assurance System
MQSA	Mammography Quality Standards Act (US)
MR	Mental retardation; mitral regurgitation; modified-release
MRA	Magnetic resonance angiography; mutual recognition agreement
MRC	Medical Research Council
MRCP	Magnetic resonance cholangiopancreatography
MRD	Multiple rising dose
MRFG	Mutual Recognition Facilitation Group (EMA)
MRG	Murmurs, rubs, and gallops
MRI	Magnetic resonance imaging
MRL	Maximum residue limit

(Continued)

Abbreviation	Definition
mRNA	Messenger RNA
MRP	Mutual recognition procedure (EU)
MRSA	Methicillin-resistant *Staphylococcus aureus*
MS	Multiple sclerosis; mitral stenosis; morphine sulfate; member state(s) (EU); mass spectrometry; mental state
MSA	Metropolitan statistical area
MS-AFP	Maternal serum alpha[α]- fetoprotein
MSC	Mesenchymal stem cell
MSE	Mental status examination
MSET	Multistage exercise test
MSH	Melanocyte-stimulating hormone
MSK	Medullary sponge kidney; Memorial Sloan–Kettering; musculoskeletal
MSM	Men who have sex with men (WSW: women who have sex with women; objective medical terms related to behavior are preferred)
MSSA	Methicillin-sensitive *Staphylococcus aureus*
MSU	Midstream urine sample; monosodium urate
MSUC	Maple syrup urine disease
MTBI	Mild traumatic brain injury
MTD	Maximum tolerated dose
MTS	Medicines testing scheme (MHRA)
MTX	Methotrexate
mUC	Metastatic urothelial carcinoma
MUFA	Monounsaturated fatty acid
MUGA	Multiple gated acquisition (image)
MUMS	Minor use and minor species (veterinary)
MUSE	Medicated urethral system for erection
MVA	Motor vehicle accident
MVC	Motor vehicle crash
MVI	Multivitamin
MVO_2	Mixed-venous oxygen concentration
MVP	Mitral-valve prolapse
MVPS	Mitral-valve prolapse syndrome
MVR	Mitral-valve replacement
MVV	Maximum voluntary ventilation
Na/NA	Sodium (Latin *natrium*); negative appendectomy; nucleus accumbens
N-11	Next 11 (group of countries comprising Bangladesh, Egypt, Indonesia, Iran, Korea, Mexico, Nigeria, Pakistan, Philippines, Turkey, and Vietnam)
NAD	Nicotinamide adenine dinucleotide; no abnormality detected; no active disease; no apparent distress
NADA	New animal drug application (US)
NADP	Nicotinamide adenine dinucleotide phosphate
NAFDAC	National Agency for Food and Drug Administration and Control (Nigeria)
NAFLD	Nonalcoholic fatty liver disease
NAFTA	North American Free Trade Agreement
NAI	No action indicated

(Continued)

Abbreviation	Definition
NAO	National Audit Office (UK)
NAP	Nationally authorized product
NAS	New active substance; no added salt
NASH	Nonalcoholic steatohepatitis
NB	*Nota bene* (take special notice) Notified body (EU)
NBE	New biological entity
NBIA	Neurodegeneration with brain iron accumulation
NBN	Newborn nursery
NBT	Nitroblue tetrazolium
NBTE	Nonbacterial thrombotic endocarditis
NC	Nerve conduction
NCA	National competent authority
NCAS	New chemically active substance
NCC	Noncompaction cardiomyopathy
NCE	New chemical entity
NCEP	National Cholesterol Education Program
NC3Rs	National Centre for the Replacement, Refinement and Reduction of Animals in Research (UK)
NCI	National Cancer Institute (US)
NCO	Nonclinical overview
NCS	Nonclinical summary
NCT	Nerve conduction test (NCS = NC study)
NCTR	National Center for Toxicological Research (US)
NCV	Nerve conduction velocity
Nd:YAG	Neodymium-doped yttrium aluminium garnet ($Nd:Y_3Al_5O_{12}$) laser
NDA	New Drug Application (US)
NDAC	New Drug Advisory Committee (India)
NDS	New Drug Submission (Canada)
NDI	Nephrogenic diabetes insipidus
NE	Norepinephrine; not estimable (in survival/proportional-hazards analyses)
NEAP	Net endogenous acid production
NEC	Necrotizing enterocolitis; no evidence of disease
NED	No evidence of disease; noneffective dose
NeeS	Non eCTD electronic submission
NES	Not elsewhere specified
NETEC	Necrotizing enterocolitis
NETWG	New & Emerging Technologies Working Group
NF	National Formulary
NfG	Note for Guidance (EU)
ng	Nanogram
NG	Nasogastric (NGT = nasogastric tube)
NGT	Negative to date; no growth to date
NGU	Nongonococcal urethritis
NHL	Non-Hodgkin's lymphoma
NHS	National Health Service (UK)

(Continued)

Abbreviation	Definition
NIAID	National Institute of Allergy and Infectious Diseases (US)
NIBSC	National Institute for Biological Standards and Control (UK)
NICE	National Institute for Health and Care Excellence (UK)
NICHD	National Institute of Child Health and Human Development (US)
NICU	Neonatal intensive-care unit
NIDDK	National Institute of Diabetes and Digestive and Kidney Diseases (US)
NIDDM	Non–insulin-dependent diabetes mellitus (type 2 diabetes)
NIF	Negative inspiratory force
NIH	National Institutes of Health (US)
NIHR	National Institute for Health Research (UK)
NIMH	National Institute of Mental Health
NIMP	Noninvestigational medicinal product
NIR	Near infrared (spectroscopy)
NK	Natural killer
NKA	No known allergies
NKDA	No known drug allergies
NLEA	Nutrition Labeling and Education Act of 1990 (US)
NLN	Nordic Council on Medicines
NLP	No light perception (most severe blindness)
NMA	National Medicines Agency (Romania)
NMCA	Norwegian Medicines Control Agency
NME	New molecular entity
NMFS	National Marine Fisheries Service (US)
NMN	Nicotinamide mononucleotide
NMR	Nuclear magnetic resonance
NMVRVI	*Nacionalinis Maisto Ir Veterinarijos Rizikos Vertinimo Institutas* (National Food and Veterinary Risk Assessment Institute) (Lithuania)
NNH	Number needed to harm
NNS	Number needed to screen
NNT	Number needed to treat to benefit (NNT_B) or harm (NNT_H) (See Chapter 3)
NO	Nitric oxide (endothelial-derived relaxing factor)
NOAEL	No observable adverse effect level
NOAH	National Office of Animal Health (UK)
NOAL	No observed adverse effect level
NOC	Notice of Compliance (Canada)
NOC/c	Notice of Compliance with Conditions (Canada)
Nocte	Night
NOEL	No observed effect level
NOF	Neck of femur (hip) fracture
NoMA	Norwegian Medicines Agency
NOMI	Nonocclusive mesenteric ischemia
NOS	Not otherwise specified; nitric oxide synthase
NP	Nurse practitioner
NPA	Nasopharyngeal aspirate
NPCB	National Pharmaceutical Control Bureau (Malaysia)

(Continued)

Abbreviation	Definition
NPH	Normal-pressure hydrocephalus
NPO	Nothing by mouth (*nil per os*)
NPPV	Noninvasive positive pressure ventilation
NPT	Neuropsychological testing
NPTAC	No previous tracing available for comparison
NPV	Negative predictive value
NRB	Non-rebreather mask
NRBC	Nucleated red blood cells
NREM	Non–rapid-eye movement
NRM	No regular medications
NS	Normal saline
NSA	No significant abnormality
NSAID	Nonsteroidal anti-inflammatory drug
NSB	Nonsimilar biologic
NSBB	Nonselective beta[β] blocker
NSC	Neural stem cell
NSCC	Non–squamous-cell carcinoma
NSCLC	Non–small-cell lung cancer
NSD	Normal spontaneous delivery
NSE	Neuron-specific enolase
NSR	Normal sinus rhythm
NSSI	Nonsuicidal self-injury
NST	Nonstress test
NSTEMI	Non–ST-segment elevation
NSU	Nonspecific urethritis
NSVA	National Sanitary Veterinary Agency (Romania)
NSVD	Normal spontaneous vaginal delivery
NT	Nasotracheal; nontested
NTA	Notice to applicants (EC)
NTD	Neglected tropical disease; neural-tube defect
NTE	No toxic effect level
NTG	Nitroglycerin
NTI	Narrow therapeutic index
NUI	Non-urgent information ("Infofax") (EU)
NVD	Natural vaginal delivery; nausea, vomiting and diarrhea
NVDC	Nausea, vomiting, diarrhea, and constipation
NWB	Non–weight-bearing
NWIP	New work item proposal (EU)
NYD	Not yet diagnosed
NYHA	New York Heart Association
O/E	Observed versus expected [analysis]
oab	On anhydrous basis
OAI	Official action indicated
oasfb	On anhydrous and solvent-free basis
OBS	Organic brain syndrome

(Continued)

Abbreviation	Definition
OC	Office of the Commissioner (USFDA); oral contraceptive
OCA	Office of Consumer Affairs (US)
OCABR	Official Control Authority Batch Release
OCD	Obsessive-compulsive disorder
OCG	Oral cholecystogram
OCI	Office of Criminal Investigations (US)
OCP	Office of Combination Products (USFDA); oral-contraceptive pill
OCT	Optical coherence tomography
OD	*Oculus dexter* (right eye); overdose; once daily; orphan drug
ODA	Orphan Drug Act (US)
ODC	Optimal diagnostic concentration (used on allergy products); ornithine decarboxylase
ODD	Orphan drug designation; oppositional-defiant disorder
OE	Oral explanation; otitis externa
OECD	Organisation for Economic Co-operation and Development
OEI	Official establishment inventory (US)
OGTT	Oral glucose tolerance test
OHL	Oral hairy leukoplakia
OHS	Obesity hyoventilation syndrome
OJEC	Official Journal of the European Communities
OM	Otitis media
OMCL	Official Medicines Control Laboratories (part of EDQM)
OME	Otitis media with effusion
OMP	Orphan medicinal product
1-1-1	One dossier, one European scientific assessment, one decision for marketing authorization
O&P	Ova and parasites
OOB	Out of bed
OOO	Out of office
OOPD	Office of Orphan Products Development (US FDA)
OOS	Out of specification
OPA	Office of Public Affairs (US)
OPAE	Office of Planning, Analysis and Evaluation
OPD	Original pack dispensing; outpatient department
OPPT	Oriented to person, place, and time
OPV	Oral polio vaccine; outpatient visit
OR	Odds ratio; operating room
ORA	Office of Regulatory Affairs (US FDA)
ORIF	Open reduction internal fixation
ORSA	Oxacillin-resistant *S. aureus*
ORT	Oral rehydration therapy
OS	*Oculus sinister* (left eye)
OSA	Obstructive sleep apnea
OT	Occupational therapy/therapist
OTC	Over-the-counter

(Continued)

Abbreviation	Definition
OTPP	Oriented to time, place, and person
OTTR	Organ Transplant Tracking Record
OU	*Oculus unitas* (both eyes)
P to GSL	Pharmacy to General Sales List
PA	Physician assistant; posterior-anterior; primary aldosteronism psoriatic arthritis; pulmonary artery
P&A	Percussion and auscultation
P&L	Packaging and labeling
P&PD	Percussion and postural drainage
P&R	Pricing and reimbursement
PAC	Premature atrial contraction; pulmonary artery catheter
PAC-ATLS	Post Approval Change Analytical Testing Laboratory Site (US)
PACMP	Post-approval change management protocol
PaCO$_2$	Partial pressure of carbon dioxide (arterial)
PACU	Post-Anesthesia Care Unit
PAD	Peripheral artery disease; postadmission day; peripheral airspace disease
PAES	Post-authorization efficacy study
PAF	Pure autonomic failure; platelet-activating factor; paroxysmal atrial fibrillation
PAGB	Proprietary Association of Great Britain
PAH	Pulmonary arterial hypertension; phenylalanine hydroxylase
PAI	Pre-approval inspection
PAI-1	Plasminogen activator inhibitor 1
PAL	Pharmaceutical Affairs Law (Japan); posterior axillary line
PALS	Pediatric Advanced Life Support
PAN	Polyarteritis nodosa
PAO	Period after opening (cosmetic products); peak acid output
PAO$_2$	Partial pressure of oxygen (arterial)
PAP	Pulmonary arterial pressure; positive airway pressure; pulmonary alveolar proteinosis
Pap	Papanicolaou (stain)
PAPP-A	Pregnancy-associated plasma protein A
PAR	Public assessment report
PARENT	Patient Registries Initiative (EU)
PAS	Periodic acid–Schiff; Public Affairs Specialist (US)
PASS	Post authorization safety study
PAT	Paroxysmal atrial tachycardia; Pharmaceutical Industries and Associations (EFPIA); process analytical technology
PBAC	Pharmaceutical Benefits Advisory Committee (Australia)
PBC	Primary biliary cholangitis (formerly cirrhosis)
PBF	Peripheral blood film
PBI	Protein-bound iodine
PBPK	Physiologically based pharmacokinetic modeling
PBRER	Periodic benefit–risk evaluation report
PBS	Pharmaceutical Benefit Scheme (Australia); phosphate-buffered saline
PBSC	Peripheral blood stem cell

(Continued)

Abbreviation	Definition
PBT	Persistent, bioaccumulative and toxic (biocidal products)
p.c.	After eating (Latin *post-cibum*)
PCA	Patient-controlled anesthesia
PCa	Prostate cancer
PCD	Postconcussion disorder; primary ciliary dyskinesia
PCI	Percutaneous coronary intervention
PCID	Physical-chemical identifier
PCIOL	Posterior-chamber intraocular lens
PCL	Posterior cruciate ligament
PCNSL	Primary central nervous system [CNS] lymphoma
pCODR	pan-Canadian Oncology Drug Review
PCOS	Polycystic ovarian syndrome
PCP	Pneumocystis pneumonia; primary care provider (physician)
PCPA	Pan-Canadian Pricing Alliance
PCR	Polymerase chain reaction; patient care report
PCS	Postconcussion syndrome
PCT	Practical clinical trial; pragmatic clinical trial; primary care trust (UK); progesterone challenge test
PCV	Packed cell volume; polycythemia vera
PCWG	Prostate Cancer Working Group
PCWP	Patients' and Consumers' Working Party; pulmonary capillary wedge pressure
PD	Parkinson's disease; peritoneal dialysis; personality disorder; pharmacodynamics; physical diagnosis
PDA	Patent ductus arteriosus; posterior descending artery
PDCO	Paediatric Committee (EMA)
PDE	Permitted daily exposure; phosphodiesterase
PDF	Portable document format
PDG	Pharmacopoeial (Pharmacopoeial) discussion group
PDGF	Platelet-derived growth factor
PDMA	Prescription Drug Marketing Act (US)
PDP	Product development protocols (for medical devices) (US)
PDT	Photodynamic therapy
PDUFA	Prescription Drug User Fee Act (US)
PDVT	Postoperative deep-vein thrombosis
PE	Pulmonary embolism (embolus); pleural effusion; physical examination; pharmacoeconomics; pre-eclampsia
PEAE	Pulseless electrical activity
PEAG	Pharmacovigilance Expert Advisory Group (MHRA)
PEARL	Pupils equal and reactive to light
PEB	Cisplatin (platinum), etoposide, and bleomycin
PEEP	Positive end-expiratory pressure
PEFR	Peak expiratory flow rate
PEFRAS	Pan European Federation of Regulatory Affairs
PEG	Percutaneous endoscopic gastrostomy; pneumoencephalography; polyethylene glycol

(Continued)

Abbreviation	Definition
PEI	Paul–Ehrlich–Institut (Federal Institute for Vaccines and Biomedicines German regulatory agency)
PEM	Prescription-event monitoring (study); protein-energy malnutrition
PEP	Postexposure prophylaxis
PER	Pharmaceutical evaluation report
PeRC	Pediatric Review Committee (US)
PERF	Pan European Regulatory Forum
PERLA	Pupils equal and reactive to light and accommodation
PERRL	Pupils equal, round, and reactive to light
PERRLA	Pupils equal, round, and reactive to light and accommodation
PET	Positron emission tomography
PET/CT	Positron emission tomography and computerized tomography
pfa (or b)	Pure free acid (or base)
PFGE	Pulsed-field gel electrophoresis
PFI	Pediatric Formulations Initiative (US)
PFO	Patent foramen ovale
PFT	Pulmonary function test
PGCS	Paediatric Glasgow Coma Scale
PGD	Patient group direction (written instructions)
PGENI	Pharmacogenetics for Every Nation Initiative
PGE	Protein gel electrophoresis
PGF	Placental growth factor
PGI	Potentially genotoxic impurity
PgWP	Pharmacogenomics Working Party
PGx	Pharmacogenomics
PH	Pulmonary hypertension
pH	Negative (inverse) logarithm (p) of hydrogen ion (H^+) concentration
PHA	Preliminary hazard analysis
Ph Eur	European Pharmacopoeia
PHARE	Poland and Hungary: Assistance for Restructuring their Economies
PHARMO	Institute for Drug Outcomes Research (the Netherlands)
PHC	Personalized health care
PhI	Pharmacological intelligence
PHN	Postherpetic neuralgia
PHP	Partial Hospitalization Program
PhPID	Pharmaceutical product identifier (EU)
PHQ	Patient Health Questionnaire
PhRMA	Pharmaceutical Research and Manufacturers of America
PHS	Public Health Service (US)
PHTLS	Prehospital trauma life support
PhV/PV	Pharmacovigilance
PhVWP	Pharmacovigilance Working Party (EMA)
PI	Principal investigator; prescribing information; package insert; penile implant; personal injury; product information; protease inhibitor; present illness
PIA	Pharmaceutical Industry Association

(Continued)

Abbreviation	Definition
PIC	Pharmaceutical Inspection Convention (EU)
PICC	Peripherally inserted central catheter
PICO	Population, intervention, comparator, outcome(s)
PIC/S	Pharmaceutical Inspection Co-operation Scheme
PICU	Pediatric intensive care unit
PID	Pelvic inflammatory disease; pulmonary insufficiency disease; prolapsed intervertebral disc
PIG-A	Phosphatidylinositol glycan class A
PIIGS	Portugal, Ireland, Italy, Greece, and Spain
PIH	Pregnancy-induced hypertension
PIL	Patient information leaflet
PIM	Product information management (EMA); Promising Innovative Medicine
PIN	Patient identification number; pancreatic intraepithelial neoplasia
PIP	Paediatric investigation plan; poly implant prothèse (breast implant); proximal interphalangeal (joint)
PJS	Peutz–Jeghers syndrome
PK	Pharmacokinetics; protein kinase
pKa	Acid dissociation constant
PKD	Polycystic kidney disease
PKP	Penetrating keratoplasty
PKU	Phenylketonuria
PL	Package leaflet; product license (US)
PLIF	Posterior lumbar interbody fusion
PLR	Physician Labeling Rule (US); product license renewal (US)
PLT	Platelet (count)
PMA	Premarket approval (application for medical devices) (US)
PMB	Postmenopausal bleeding
PMCF	Postmarket clinical follow-up (studies)
PMDA	Japan's regulatory agency the Pharmaceutical and Medical Devices Agency (within the Ministry of Health, Labor and Welfare MHLW)
PMDD	Premenstrual dysphoric disorder
PMDI	Pressurized metered-dose inhaler
PMF	Plant master file (US and Canada)
PMH	Previous medical history; perimesencephalic subarachnoid hemorrhage
PMI	Point of maximal impulse; pharmacological, metabolic, and immunological
PML	Progressive multifocal leukoencephalopathy
PMN	Polymorphonuclear leukocyte (neutrophil)
PMOA	Primary mode of action
PMP	*Pseudomyxoma peritonei*
PMPRB	Patented Medicines Prices Review Board (Canada)
PMR	Percutaneous myocardial revascularization; polymyalgia rheumatica; proportional mortality rate
PM&R	Physical medicine and rehabilitation
PMS	Postmarket(ing) surveillance; premenstrual syndrome
PNA	Postnatal age

(Continued)

Abbreviation	Definition
PND	Paroxysmal nocturnal dyspnea; postnasal drip
PNET	Primitive neuroectodermal tumor
PNH	Paroxysmal nocturnal hemoglobinuria
PNM	Perinatal mortality
PNV	Prenatal vitamin
p.o.	By mouth/orally (Latin *per os*)
PO_2	Partial pressure of oxygen
POA	Power of attorney
POAG	Primary open-angle glaucoma
POC	Plan of care; postoperative care; products of conception; proof of concept
POD	Postoperative day
POM	Prescription-only medicine
POM to P	Prescription-only medicine to pharmacy
PONV	Postoperative nausea and vomiting
POP	Pain on palpation
POP db	Planned and Ongoing Projects database
POT	Plan of treatment
PP	Postprandial, pulsus paradoxus, postpartum
PPCS	Prolonged (persistent) postconcussion syndrome
PPD	Purified protein derivative; packs per day; postpartum depression
PPG	Postprandial glucose
PPH	Postpartum hemorrhage, primary pulmonary hypertension, procedure for prolapse and hemorrhoids
PPI	Patient and public involvement (UK); patient package insert (US); proton pump inhibitor
PPMS	Primary progressive multiple sclerosis
PPO	Preferred provider organization
PPP	Public–private partnership
PPROM	Preterm premature rupture of membranes
PPRREG	Pandemic Pharmacovigilance Rapid Response Expert Group (EU)
PPRS	Pharmaceutical Price Regulation Scheme
PPS	Post-polio syndrome
PPSR	Proposed Pediatric Study Request (US)
PPTCT	Prevention of parent-to-child transmission
PPTP	Pediatric preclinical testing program
PPV	Positive predictive value
p.r.	Per rectum
PR	Pulse rate
PRA	Plasma renin activity
PRAC	Pharmacovigilance Risk Assessment Committee (EMA)
PRBC	Packed red blood cells
PREA	Pediatric Research Equity Act (US)
PRES	Posterior reversible encephalopathy syndrome
PRISMA	Preferred Reporting Items for Systematic Reviews and Meta-Analyses
p.r.n.	*Pro re nata* (as needed)

(*Continued*)

Abbreviation	Definition
PRO	Patient-reported outcome; peer review organization; professional review organization
PRO-AE	Patient-reported outcomes in adverse event reporting
PROM	Patient-reported outcome measure; premature rupture of membranes
PROSPER	Patient-reported outcomes safety event reporting
PROSPERO	International Prospective Register of Systematic Reviews (UK)
PRP	Panretinal photocoagulation; progressive rubella panencephalitis
PRR	Proportional reporting ratio
PRS	PIM review system (EU); also see PIM
PRSPH	Potential serious risk to public health
PRV	Polycythemia rubra vera
PS	Pulmonic stenosis
PSA	Prostate-specific antigen; parallel scientific advice
PSBO	Partial small-bowel obstruction
PSC	Primary sclerosis cholangitis
PSGN	Poststreptococcal glomerulonephritis
PSH	Previous surgical history; psychosocial history
PSI	Pneumonia severity index
$PscO_2T$	Subcutaneous tissue oxygen tension
PSR	Product safety reference
PSRO	Professional standards review organization
PSS	Personal social services; progressive systemic sclerosis
PSUR	Periodic safety update report
PSVT	Paroxysmal supraventricular tachycardia
PT	Physical therapy; prothrombin time; preferred term (MedDRA AEs); patient
PTB	Pulmonary tuberculosis; preterm birth
PTC	Percutaneous transhepatic cholangiography
PtC	Points to consider
PTCA	Percutaneous transluminal coronary angioplasty
PTD	Protection of technical documentation; preterm delivery
PTE	Patent term extension
PTH	Parathyroid hormone
PTHC	Percutaneous transhepatic cholangiogram
PTL	Preterm labor
PTSD	Post-traumatic stress disorder
PTT	Partial thromboplastin time
PUBS	Percutaneous umbilical blood sample
PUD	Peptic ulcer disease
PUFA	Polyunsaturated fatty acid
PUMA	Paediatric-use marketing authorisation (UK)
PUO	Pyrexia of unknown origin
PUVA	Psoralen ultraviolet A (radiation/light)
PV	Pharmacovigilance
PVAR	Preliminary Variation Assessment Report
PVC	Premature ventricular contraction

(Continued)

Abbreviation	Definition
PVD	Peripheral vascular disease
PVFS	Postviral fatigue syndrome
PVI	Peripheral vascular insufficiency; pulmonary-vein isolation
PVR	Peripheral vascular resistance; postvoid residual; pulmonary vascular resistance
PVS	Persistent vegetative state; Plummer–Vinson syndrome; pulmonary-valve stenosis
PWP	Pulmonary-wedge pressure
PXRD	Powder X-ray diffraction
PY	Pack-years; person-years
q	Every (each; Latin *quaque*)
QA	Quality assurance
QALY	Quality-adjusted life-year
QbD	Quality by design
QC	Quality control
qd	Once a day (*quaque die*)
qds/qid	Four times a day (*quater in die*)
qh	Every hour
QI	Quality improvement
QIDP	Qualified infectious disease product (US)
QMS	Quality management system
QNS	Quantity not sufficient
qod	Every other day
QOF	Quality and Outcomes Framework (UK)
QOL	Quality of life
QP	Qualified person
QPPV	Qualified person responsible for pharmacovigilance
QR (code)	Quick response (code) (EU)
QRD	Quality review of documents [template]
(Q)SAR	Quantitative structure activity relationships
QSE	Quality, safety, and efficacy
QSIT	Quality System Inspection Technique (US FDA)
QTPP	Quality target product profile
QUAMED	Quality Medicines for All
QUOROM	Quality of Reporting of Meta-Analyses (see Chapter 4)
QWP	Quality Working Party (EMA)
R&D	Research and development
R4BP	Register for Biocidal Products
RA	Rheumatoid arthritis; right atrium; regulatory affairs (activities); rapid alert; refractory anemia
RAA/RAAS	Renin-angiotensin-aldosterone (renin-angiotensin-aldosterone axis)
RAD	Right axis deviation; reflex-anal dilatation; reactive-airway disease; radiation-absorbed dose; reactive attachment disorder
RADAR	Research on adverse drug events and reports; response adjusted for duration of antibiotic risk
RAE	Right-atrial enlargement

(Continued)

Abbreviation	Definition
RAI	Radioactive iodine
RAIU	Thyroid-reactive iodine uptake
RAMA	Remote access to marketing authorisations (MHRA)
RANKL	Receptor activator of nuclear factor kappa B ligand
RAP	Right atrial pressure
RAPD	Relative afferent pupillary defect
RAPS	Regulatory Affairs Professionals Society (US)
RAS	Rapid Alert System; renal artery stenosis
RAST	Radioallergosorbent test
RATLH	Robotic-assisted total laparoscopic hysterectomy
RAVH	Radical vaginal hysterectomy
RBBB	Right bundle branch block
RBC	Red blood cell (count)
RBE	Relative biological effectiveness
RBI	Risk-based inspection
RBLM	Recurrent benign lymphocytic meningitis
RBM	Risk-based monitoring
RBP	Retinol-binding protein
RBRVS	Resource-based relative value scale
RCA	Right coronary artery
RCB	Registered certification body (Japan)
RCC	Renal-cell carcinoma
RCH	Remove clinical hold
R-CHOP	Rituximab, cyclophosphamide, hydroxydaunorubicin (doxorubicin), Oncovin (vincristine), prednisone
RCM	Right costal margin; restrictive cardiomyopathy
RCP	Royal College of Physicians (UK)
RCR	Rotator-cuff repair
RCT	Randomized controlled trial
RD	Retinal detachment
RDA	Recommended daily allowance; recommended dietary allowance
RDC	Research Diagnostic Criteria
RDE	Remote data entry
rDNA	Ribosomal DNA
RDP	Regulatory data protection
RDS	Repeat (repeated) dose study; Respiratory distress syndrome
RDT	Rising-dose tolerance
RDW	Red cell distribution width
REA	Relative effectiveness assessment
REACH	Registration, evaluation, authorisation and restriction of chemicals
REC	Research Ethics Committee
REI	Reproductive endocrinology and infertility
REM	Rapid eye movement
REMS	Risk evaluation and mitigation strategy (US)
RF	Rheumatoid factor; rheumatic fever

(Continued)

Abbreviation	Definition
RFDD	Regional Food and Drug Director (US)
RFLP	Restriction fragment length polymorphism
RFT	Renal function test
rh	Recombinant human
RH	Relative humidity
Rh	Rhesus
rhNGF	Recombinant human nerve growth factor
RHSC	Regulatory Harmonization Steering Committee
RI	Regulatory intelligence
RIA	Radioimmunoassay
RIBA	Radio immunoblotting assay
RICE	Rest, ice, compression, and elevation
RIH	Right inguinal hernia
RIM	Regulatory information management
RIMA	Reversible inhibitor of monoamine oxidase A
RIND	Reversible ischemic neurologic deficit
RING	Regulatory Intelligence Network Group (EU)
rINN	Recommended international nonproprietary name
RiskMAP	Risk minimization action plan
RL	Ringer's lactate
RLD	Reference listed drug (US)
RLE	Right-lower extremity
RLL	Right lower lobe
RLN	Recurrent laryngeal nerve; regional lymph node
RLQ	Right lower quadrant
R&M	Routine and microscopic
RML	Right middle lobe
RMM	Risk minimisation measure (EU)
RMP	Reference medicinal product; risk management plan
RMR	Reaction monitoring report; resting metabolic rate; risk management report
RMS	Reference member state (Europe)
RMSF	Rocky Mountain spotted fever
rMS	Reporting member state (Europe)
RNA	Ribonucleic acid
RNAi	RNA interference
RNH	Roux-en-Y hepaticojejunostomy (anastomosis)
RNP	Ribonucleoprotein
RNV	Radionuclide ventriculography
r/o	Rule out
ROA	Right occiput anterior
ROC	Receiver operating characteristic curve (curve plotting sensitivity vs. 1 – specificity)
RoHS	Restriction of hazardous substances
ROI	Residue on ignition; return on investment
ROM	Range of motion; rupture of membranes

(Continued)

Abbreviation	Definition
ROP	Retinopathy of prematurity; right occiput posterior
ROS	Run-on sentence; review of systems
ROSC	Return of spontaneous circulation
ROW	Rest of (the) world
RP	Responsible person
RPG	Retrograde pyelogram
RPGN	Rapidly progressive glomerulonephritis
RPLND	Retroperitoneal lymph node dissection
RPMS	Relapsing-progressive multiple sclerosis
RPR	Rapid plasma reagin
RPS	Regulated product submission
RPSGB	Royal Pharmaceutical Society of Great Britain
RQA	Research quality assurance
RR	Relative risk; risk ratio; respiratory rate
RRMS	Relapsing-remitting multiple sclerosis
RRP	Recurrent respiratory papillomatosis
RRR	Regular rate and rhythm; relative risk reduction; replacement, reduction, and refinement (in research using animals)
RS	Reed–Sternberg (cell)
RSB	Right sternal border
RSI	Rapid sequence induction; reference safety information; request for supplementary information (EU)
RSV	Respiratory syncytial virus
RT	Respiratory or radiation therapy; reverse transcriptase
RTA	Renal tubular acidosis
RTC	Return to clinic
RTF	Refusal-to-file (US)
RTI	Respiratory tract infection
RT-PCR	Reverse transcriptase-polymerase chain reaction
RTRT	Real time release testing
RTS	Revised trauma score
RU	Resin uptake (T_3)
RUE	Right-upper extremity
RUG	Retrograde urethrogram
RUL	Right upper lobe
RUP	Repeat use procedure
RUO	Research use only
RUQ	Right upper quadrant
rUTI	Recurrent urinary-tract infection
RV	Right ventricle/ventricular; residual volume
RVAD	Right-ventricular assist device
RVEF	RV ejection fraction
RVF	RV failure; rectovaginal fistula
RVH	RV hypertrophy
RVOT	RV outflow tract

(Continued)

Abbreviation	Definition
RVR	Rapid ventricular rate
RVSP	RV systolic pressure
RVT	Renal-vein thrombosis
RWD	Real-world data
RWE	Real-word evidence
Rx	Prescription
S&E	Sugar and acetone
S&O	Salpingo-oophorectomy
S&T	Sampling and testing
SA	Scientific advice; sinoatrial
SAA	Synthetic amino acid
SAAG	Serum-ascites albumin gradient
SAARC	South Asia Association for Regional Cooperation
SAB	*S. aureus* bacteremia
SABS	Safety alert broadcast system
SAD	Single ascending dose (study); seasonal affective disorder; subacromial decompression
SADR	Serious adverse drug reaction
SADS	Schedule for Affective Disorders and Schizophrenia
SAE	Serious adverse event
SAG	Scientific Advisory Group
SAH	Subarachnoid hemorrhage
SAL	Sterility assurance level
SAM	Systolic anterior motion (of the mitral valve)
SaMD	Software as a Medical Device
SAMM	Safety assessment of marketed medicines (US)
SAN	Sinoatrial node
SAP	Statistical analysis plan
SAPS	Simplified Acute Physiology Score
SAR	Serious adverse reaction; seasonal allergic rhinitis
SARS	Severe acute respiratory syndrome
SAWP	Scientific Advice Working Party
SB	Small bowel
SBA/SBOA	Summary basis of approval (US)
SBE	Subacute bacterial endocarditis
SBFT	Small-bowel follow through
SBMA	Spinal and bulbar muscular atrophy
SBO	Small-bowel obstruction
SBP	Similar biotherapeutic product (WHO); systolic blood pressure; spontaneous bacterial peritonitis
SBRT	Split-beam radiation therapy
SBS	Short-bowel syndrome
Sc	Subcutaneous (sq; Latin *subcutis*)
SCA	Spinocerebellar ataxia
SCAT	Sex cord tumor with annular tubules

(Continued)

Abbreviation	Definition
SCB	Scientific Coordination Board
SCC	Squamous-cell carcinoma
SCCHN	Squamous-cell carcinoma of the head and neck
SCCS	Self-controlled case series
SCD	Sequential compression device; sickle-cell disease; sudden cardiac death
SCI/D	Spinal cord injury/disorder
SCID	Severe combined immunodeficiency; Structured Clinical Interview for *DSM*
SCIWORA	Spinal-cord injury without radiographic abnormality
SCLC	Small-cell lung cancer
SCOTT	Standing Committee on Therapeutic Trials (Australia/New Zealand)
SCr	Serum creatinine
SCT	Sacrococcygeal teratoma
SD	Sprague–Dawley (rats); standard deviation; subdermal
SDAI	Simplified Disease Activity Index
SDH	Subdural hematoma
SDTI	Suspected deep-tissue injury
SDTM	Study Data Tabulation Model (US)
SE	Standard error; side effect; substantially equivalent
SEAR	Safety, Efficacy and Adverse Reactions (Subcommittee of Committee on Safety of Medicines)
SEB	Subsequent entry biologic
SEE	Syphilis elimination effort
SEED	Shaping European Early Dialogues (for Health Technologies Consortium)
SEM	Standard error of the mean; scanning electron microscope; systolic ejection murmur
SERM	Selective estrogen receptor modulator
SFA	Superficial femoral artery; serum folic acid
SF-36	36-Item Short Form Health Survey
SFDA	Saudi Food and Drug Authority
SFFC	Spurious/falsely labeled/falsified/counterfeit (medicines; US)
SG	Swan–Ganz; specific gravity
SGA	Small for gestational age
SGB	Stellate ganglion block
SGGT	Serum gamma-glutamyl transferase
SGML	Standard generalized markup language
SGOT	Serum glutamic-oxaloacetic transaminase (AST)
SGPT	Serum glutamic pyruvic transaminase (ALT)
SHBG	Sex hormone–binding globulin
SHPT	Secondary hyperparathyroidism
SI	Statutory instrument
SIADH	Syndrome of inappropriate antidiuretic hormone/arginine vasopressin (SIAVP)
SIBO	Small-intestinal bacterial overgrowth
SICU	Surgical intensive care unit
SIDS	Sudden infant death syndrome
sig	Write on label

(Continued)

Abbreviation	Definition
SIL	Squamous intraepithelial lesion
SIMV	Synchronized intermittent mechanical ventilation
SIP	Sickness Impact Profile
siRNA	Small interfering RNA
SIRS	Systemic inflammatory response syndrome
SIT	Stress inoculation training (therapy)
SJS	Stevens–Johnson syndrome
SK	Streptokinase
SKU	Stock-keeping unit
sl	Sublingual
SLA	Service level agreement
SLE	St. Louis encephalitis; systemic lupus erythematosus
SLK	*Statens legemiddelverk* (Norwegian Medicines Agency)
SLL	Small lymphocytic lymphoma
SLN/SLNB/SLND	Sentinel lymph node (biopsy, dissection)
SLP	Speech-language pathologist
SLR	Straight-leg raise (Lasègue's sign)
SMA	Sequential multiple analysis; spinal-muscular atrophy; superior mesenteric artery
SMAC	Sequential multiple analyzer chemistry (now Comprehensive Metabolic Panel [CMP]; "chem")
SMDA	Safe Medical Devices Act (US)
SMEs	Small- and medium-sized enterprises
SMF	Site master file
SMN	Statement of medical necessity
SMO	Site management organization
SmPAR	Summary Pharmacovigilance Assessment Report (EU)
SmPC	Summary of product characteristics (EMA)
SMQ	Standardised MedDRA query
SMT	Spinal manipulative therapy
SMV	Superior mesenteric vein
SN	Substantia nigra
SNB	Sentinel node biopsy
SNDA	Supplemental new drug application (US)
SNDS	Supplemental new drug submission (US)
SNF	Skilled-nursing facility
SNP	Single-nucleotide polymorphism; sodium nitroprusside
SNRI	Serotonin-norepinephrine reuptake inhibitor
SNV	Sin Nombre virus (hantavirus)
SO	Salpingo-oophoritis
SOA	Swelling of ankles
SOAP	Subjective, Objective, Assessment, Plan (SOAP note)
SOB	Shortness of breath
SOBOE	Shortness of breath on exertion
SOC	Standard of care; system organ class (MedDRA)

(Continued)

Abbreviation	Definition
SOCMA	Society of Chemical Manufacturers and Affiliates
SOCRA	Society of Clinical Research Associates (US)
SOL	Space-occupying lesion
SOOB	Sitting out of bed
SOP	Standard operating procedure; sterile ophthalmic preparation
SPA	Special protocol assessment
SPC	Summary of product characteristics; supplementary protection certificate (EU)
Spe	Streptococcal pyrogenic exotoxin
SPECT	Single-photon emission computed tomography
SPEP	Serum protein electrophoresis
SPET	Single-photon emission tomography
SPF	Sun protection factor
SPIN	Special interest network
SPL	Structured product labeling (US)
SPMS	Secondary progressive multiple sclerosis
SPOR	Substance, Product, Organisational and Referential (data; EMA)
SPSS	Statistical Product and Service Solutions (formerly Statistical Package for the Social Sciences)
SQ	Subcutaneous
SR	Significant risk; slow-release
SRM	Specified risk materials
SRN	Stroke Research Network (UK)
SROM	Spontaneous rupture of membranes
SRS	Stereotactic radiosurgery; sex (gender) reassignment surgery
SRU	Shock resuscitation unit
SS	Sjögren's Syndrome; subserosal
SSC	Scientific Steering Committee; somatic stem cell; saline sodium citrate; secondary sex characteristics
SSE	Sterile-speculum exam
SSEP	Somatosensory evoked potential
SSI	Sliding-scale insulin
SSNRI	Selective serotonin-norepinephrine reuptake inhibitor
SSPE	Sodium chloride, sodium phosphate, EDTA [buffer]; subacute sclerosing panencephalitis
SSRI	Selective serotonin reuptake inhibitor
ssRNA	Single-stranded ribonucleic acid
SSI	Sick sinus syndrome
SSSI	Skin and skin structure infection
SSSS	Staphylococcal scalded-skin syndrome
SSU	Study start up
ST	Sore throat; speech therapy
STAMP	Safe and Timely Access to Medicines for Patients (SE)
STARD	Standards for Reporting of Diagnostic Accuracy Studies
Stat	Immediately (Latin *statim*)
STEC	Shiga toxin–producing (enterohemorrhagic) *E. coli*

(Continued)

Abbreviation	Definition
STED	Summary Technical Documentation (for Demonstrating Conformity to the Essential Principles of Safety and Performance of In Vitro Medical Devices)
StEM/STEM	Stakeholder engagement meeting UK; science, technology, engineering, and mathematics
STEMI	ST-segment elevation myocardial infarction
STH	Somatotropic hormone
STI	Sexually transmitted infection; structured treatment interruption; soft-tissue injury
STN	Subthalamic nucleus; soft tissue neck
STNR	Symmetrical tonic neck reflex
STROBE	Strengthening the Reporting of Observational Studies in Epidemiology (see Chapter 4)
STRPC	Scientific, Technical and Regulatory Policy Committee (EU)
STS	Serologic test for syphilis; soft-tissue sarcoma
SUD	Single-use device; sudden unexpected death
SUE	Serious undesirable effect
SUI	Stress urinary incontinence
SUKL	State Institute for Drug Control (Czech Republic)
SUN	Serum urea nitrogen
SUPAC	Scale-up and post-approval changes
SUPAC-IR	Scale up and post approval changes immediate release
SUPAC-MR	Scale up and post approval changes modified release
SUSAR	Suspected unexpected serious adverse reaction
SUV	Standardized uptake value
SV	Seminal vesicle; stroke volume
SVC	Superior vena cava
SVD	Spontaneous vaginal delivery
SVE	Sterile-vaginal examination
SVG	Saphenous vein graft
SVI	Systemic viral infection
SVN	Small-volume nebulizer
SVR	Systemic vascular resistance
SVT	Supraventricular tachycardia
SW	Social worker; Sturge–Weber (syndrome)
SWP	Safety Working Party (EU)
Sx	Symptoms
SXA	Single-energy x-ray absorptiometry
SXR	Skull x-ray
T&A	Tonsillectomy with adenoidectomy
TA	Temporal arteritis
T&C	Type and cross (-match)
T&H	Type and hold
$t_{1/2}$	Terminal half-life of elimination
T3	Triiodothyronine
T4	Thyroxine

(Continued)

Abbreviation	Definition
TABST	Target animal batch safety testing
TAG	Technical Advisory Group (UK); Therapeutic Advisory Group (Australia)
TAH	Total abdominal hysterectomy
TAH-BSO	Total abdominal hysterectomy with bilateral salpingo-oophorectomy
TAP	Trypsinogen activation peptide
TAPVR	Total anomalous pulmonary venous return
TAS	Target animal safety (studies)
TAT	Thematic Apperception Test
TATFAR	Transatlantic Task Force on Antimicrobial Resistance
TB	Tuberculosis
TBC	The Biomarker Consortium
TbEc	Tablet enteric coated
TBG	Thyroxine-binding globulin
TBI	Traumatic brain injury; total body irradiation
TBLC	Term-birth living child
TBSA	Total body surface area
TCA	Tricyclic antidepressant
TCC	Transitional-cell carcinoma
TCD_{50}	Median tissue culture dose
TCM	Traditional Chinese medicine
TCOM	Transcutaneous oxygen measurement
TD	Tardive dyskinesia
Td	Tetanus, diphtheria
TDaP	Tetanus, diphtheria, and acellular pertussis
TDD	Transdermal drug delivery
TdP	*Torsades de pointes*
TdT	Terminal deoxynucleotidyl transferase
TD-PRV	Tropical disease priority review voucher (US)
tds/tid	Three times a day (Latin *ter die sumendum/ter in die*)
TE	Echo time; therapeutic equivalence; tracheoesophageal
TEB	Thoracic electrical bioimpedance
TEC	Transient erythroblastopenia of childhood
TEE	Transesophageal echocardiogram (echocardiography)
TEF	Tracheoesophageal fistula
TEM	Transmission electron microscope (microscopy)
TEN	Toxic epidermal necrolysis
TENS	Transcutaneous electrical nerve stimulator (stimulation)
TFEU	Treaty on the Functioning of the European Union
TFR	Tumor volume to fetal weight ratio
TFT	Thyroid function test
TGA	Therapeutic Goods Administration (Australia's regulatory agency); transposition of the great arteries
TGA	Thermogravimetric analysis
TGF	Tumor (transforming) growth factor
TGV	Transposition of the great vessels

(Continued)

Abbreviation	Definition
THA	Total-hip arthroplasty
THMP	Traditional herbal medicinal product
THMPD	Traditional Herbal Medicinal Products Directive
THMRS	Traditional Herbal Medicines Registration Scheme
THR	Traditional herbal registration; total hip replacement
TI	Inversion time
TIA	Transient ischemic attack
TIBC	Total iron-binding capacity
tid	Three times a day (Latin *ter in die*)
TIFF	Tagged Image File Format
TIG	Tetanus immune globulin
TIGes	Telematics Implementation Group for electronic submissions
TIN	Tubulointerstitial nephritis
TIND	Treatment IND
TIPS	Transjugular intrahepatic portosystemic shunt
Tk	To come (in publishing)
TK	Thymidine kinase; toxicokinetics
T2DM	Type 2 diabetes mellitus
TKA	Total knee arthroplasty
TKO	To keep (vein) open (for intravenous therapy)
TKR	Total knee replacement
TLC	Thin-layer chromatography; total lung capacity; total lymphocyte count
TLH	Total laparoscopic hysterectomy
TLR	Tonic labyrinthine reflex
TLV	Threshold limit value
TM	Tympanic membrane; transcendental meditation
TME	Total mesorectal excision
TMF	Trial Master File
TMJ	Temporomandibular joint
TNF	Tumor necrosis factor
TNG	Trinitroglycerin
TNM	Tumor, node, metastasis
TNTC	Too numerous to count
TO	Telephone order
TOA	Tubo-ovarian abscess
TOC	Table of contents; test of cure
TOD	Table of decisions; transesophageal Doppler
TOF	Tetralogy of Fallot
TOP	Termination of pregnancy
TOPRA	The Organisation for Professionals in Regulatory Affairs
TOPS	The Over-volunteering Prevention System (database)
tOPV	Trivalent oral polio vaccine
TOT	Transobturator tape
TOV	Transfer of value
TP	Total protein

(Continued)

Abbreviation	Definition
tPA	Tissue plasminogen activator
TPN	Total parenteral nutrition
TPP	Target product profile
TPR	Temperature, pulse, respiration; total peripheral resistance
TR	Tricuspid regurgitation
TQM	Total quality management
TRAM	Transverse rectus abdominis myocutaneous (flap)
TRAP	Tartrate-resistant acid phosphatase
tRF/TRF	Transfer RNA fragment; tamper-resistant formulation
TRH	Thyrotropin-releasing hormone
TRIPS	Trade-Related Aspects of Intellectual Property Rights
TRL	Total residue level (veterinary)
tRNA	Transfer RNA
TRUS	Transrectal ultrasonography
TS	Tricuspid stenosis
TSA	Therapeutic Substances Act
TSE	Transmissible spongiform encephalopathy
TSH	Thyroid-stimulating hormone (thyrotropin)
TSHR-Ab	TSH receptor antibody
TSI	Thyroid-stimulating immunoglobulin
TSS	Toxic shock syndrome
TT	Thrombin time
TTN	Transient tachypnea of the newborn
TTC	Threshold of toxicological concern
TTE	Transthoracic echocardiogram (echocardiography)
tTG	Tissue transglutaminase
TTP	Thrombotic thrombocytopenic purpura
TTR	Transthyretin
TTS	Transdermal therapeutic system
TTTS	Twin-to-twin transfusion syndrome
TU	Tuberculin unit
TUBA	Transumbilical breast augmentation
TÜBITAK	*Türkiye Bilimsel ve Teknolojik Araştırma Kurumu* (Scientific and Technological Research Council of Turkey)
TUIP	Transurethral incision of the prostate
TUMT	Transurethral microwave thermotherapy
TUNA	Transurethral needle ablation (of the prostate)
TUR	Transurethral resection
TURBT	Transurethral of bladder tumor
TURP	Transurethral resection of prostate
TV	Tidal volume
TVC	True vocal cord
TVH	Transvaginal (total) hysterectomy
TVT	Tension-free vaginal tape

(Continued)

Abbreviation	Definition
tw	Twice a week
Tx	Treatment; transplant
UA	Urinalysis; uric acid; unstable angina; umbilical artery; upper airway; upper arm; urinary albumin
UAE	Uterine-artery embolization
UBT	Urea breath test
UC	Ulcerative colitis; uterine contraction; urine culture
UCTD	Undifferentiated connective-tissue disease
UDS	Urine drug screening; undifferentiated sarcoma
ud	As directed
UDI	Unique device identification
UE	Upper extremity
UFE	Uterine fibroid embolization
UGI	Upper gastrointestinal
UHF	Ultrahigh frequency
UIP	Usual interstitial pneumonia
ULN	Upper limit of normal
ULTRA	Unlocking Lifesaving Treatments for Rare-Diseases Act (US)
UMBRA	Unified Methodologies for Benefit-Risk Assessment
UMP	Beijing Union Medical and Pharmaceutical General Corp (the innovative arm of the Chinese Academy of Medical Sciences)
UOP	Urinary output
UPJ	Ureteropelvic junction
URA	Unilateral renal agenesis
URI	Upper-respiratory infection; uniform resource identifier
URL	Uniform resource locator
URN	Uniform resource name
URTI	Upper-respiratory-tract infection
us	Ultrasonography; ultrasound
USAN	United States Adopted Names [Council]; United States Approved Name
USC	United States Code
USDA	United States Department of Agriculture
U&E	Urea and electrolytes
USKVBL	*Ústav pro státní kontrolu veterinárních biopreparátů a léčiv* (Institute for State Control of Veterinary Biologicals and Medicines; Czech Republic); *Ústav štátnej kontroly veterinárnych biopreparátov a liečiv* (Institute of State Control of Veterinary Bioproducts and Medicines; Slovenia)
USO	Unilateral salpingo-oophorectomy
USP	United States Pharmacopeia
USP-DI	United States Pharmacopeia-Drug (Dispensing) Information
USPI	United States Package Insert (prescribing information)
USP-NF	United States Pharmacopeia and National Formulary
USR	Urgent safety restriction; unheated serum reagin
USSC	Unrestricted somatic stem cell
UTI	Urinary tract infection

(Continued)

Abbreviation	Definition
UUN	Urine urea nitrogen
UUP	Urgent Union procedure (European Commission)
UUS	Upper-uterine segment
UV-A	Ultraviolet A
UVAL	Ultraviolet argon laser
UV-B	Ultraviolet B
UV-C	Ultraviolet C
VA	Visual acuity
VAC	Vincristine, actinomycin D and cyclophosphamide
VAD	Ventricular assist device; vincristine, doxorubicin (Adriblastina®) dexamethasone
VAERS	Vaccine Adverse Event Reporting System (US)
VAESCO	Vaccine adverse event surveillance & communication
VAF	Virus antibody free
VAI	Voluntary action indicated; vincristine, actinomycin, and ifosfamide
VAIN	Vaginal intraepithelial neoplasia
VAMF	Vaccine antigen master file (EMA)
VAMP	Vesicle-associated membrane protein
VAR	Variation assessment report (EMA)
VAS	Visual analog scale; vibroacoustic stimulation
VBA	Value-based assessment (UK)
VBAC	Vaginal birth after cesarean delivery
VBC	Value-based contracting
VBG	Venous blood gas
VBP	Value-based pricing
VC	Vital capacity
vCJD	Variant Creutzfeldt–Jakob disease
VCTC	Voluntary counseling and testing centers
VCUG	Voiding cystourethrogram
VD	Vaginal delivery; volume of distribution (V_D)
VDRF	Ventilator-dependent respiratory failure
VE	Vaginal examination
VEB	Ventricular ectopic beat
VED	Vaccum erectile device
VEE	Venezuelan equine encephalitis (virus)
VEGF	Vascular endothelial growth factor
VEP	Visual evoked potential
VER	Visual evoked response
VF	Ventricular fibrillation
VH	Visual hallucination; vaginal hysterectomy
VHF	Very high frequency; viral hemorrhagic fever
VHL	Von Hippel–Lindau disease
VHP	Voluntary harmonisation procedure (EMA)
VICH	International Cooperation on Harmonisation of Technical Requirements for Registration of Veterinary Medicinal Products (US–EU–Japan)
VIN	Vulvar intraepithelial neoplasia

(Continued)

Abbreviation	Definition
VIP	Vasoactive intestinal peptide
VIPPs	Verified Internet Pharmacy Practice Site (US)
VIR	Vascular and interventional radiology
VLBW	Very low birth weight
VLDL	Very low density lipoprotein
VM	Valsalva maneuver
VMA	Vanillylmandelic acid; violent mechanical asphyxia
VNSI	Van Nuys scoring index (ductal carcinoma in situ)
VO	Verbal or voice order
VO_2	Oxygen consumption rate
VO_{2max}	Maximum oxygen consumption rate
VOC	Vaso-occlusive crisis
VPA	Valproic acid
VPAP	Variable positive airway pressure
VPB	Ventricular premature beat
VPC	Veterinary Products Committee (UK)
VPI	Velopharyngeal insufficiency
vPvB	Very persistent and very bioaccumulative (biocidal products; EU)
V/Q	Ventilation/(quantitative) perfusion (scan)
VRE	Vancomycin-resistant enterococcus
VRSA	Vancomycin-resistant *S. aureus*
VS	Vital signs
VSD	Ventricular septal defect
VSR	Ventricular septal rupture
VSS	Vital signs stable
VT	Ventricular tachycardia; verotoxin
VTE	Venous thromboembolism
VTEC	Verotoxin-producing *E. coli*
VUR	Vesicoureteral reflux
vWD	Von Willebrand disease; ventral (body) wall defect
vWF	Von Willebrand factor
VWP	Vaccines Working Party (EMA)
VZIG	Varicella zoster immune globulin
VZV	Varicella zoster virus
WAIS	Wechsler Adult Intelligence Scale
WAME	World Association of Medical Editors
WAP	Wandering atrial pacemaker
WAS	Wiskott–Aldrich syndrome
WASP	Wiskott–Aldrich syndrome protein
WAT	White adipose tissue
WBAT	Weight bearing as tolerated
WBC	White blood cell
WC	Written confirmation (issued by competent authority); wheelchair
WCBP	Woman of childbearing potential
WD	Well developed

(Continued)

Abbreviation	Definition
WDL	Within defined limits
WDWN	Well developed and well nourished
WEBAE	Web adverse events
WEE	Western equine encephalomyelitis
WF	White female
WG	Wegener's granulomatosis
WGEO	Working Group of Enforcement Officers (EU)
WHO	World Health Organization
WISC	Wechsler Intelligence Scale for Children
WL	Warning letter (FDA)
WLE	Wide local excision
WM	White male
WMA	World Medical Association
WN	Well nourished
WNL	Within normal limits
WOCBP	Woman of child-bearing potential
WOI	Without incident
WPW	Wolff–Parkinson–White (syndrome)
WRAC	Worldwide Regulatory Affairs Committee
WS	Waardenburg syndrome; Warkany syndrome; water soluble; Werner syndrome; West syndrome; Williams syndrome; Wolfram syndrome
WSW	Women who have sex with women
w/u	Work-up
WTO	World Trade Organization
XEVIMPD	Extended EudraVigilance investigational medicinal product dictionary (EMA)
XEVMPD	Extended EudraVigilance medicinal product dictionary (EMA)
XEVPRM	Extended EudraVigilance medicinal product report message (EMA)
XML	Extensible markup language
XR	Extended-release
XRF	X-ray fluorescence
XRT	X-ray (radiation) therapy
YLD	Years living with disability
yo	Years old (year-old)
YOLS	Year(s) of life saved
YPLL	Year(s) of potential life lost
YST	Yolk-sac tumor
ZE	Zollinger–Ellison (syndrome)
ZIP (code)	Zone Improvement Plan
ZVA	*Zāļu valsts aģentūra* (State Agency for Medicines in Latvia)

All acronyms are abbreviations, but all abbreviations are not acronyms. Only the latter spell words or other felicitous-sounding terms (e.g., "RANKL"). Being an abbreviation is a necessary but not sufficient condition of being an acronym.

a Compiled, organized, and typeset with assistance from Priscilla K. Gutkin. Selected data from the Wikipedia article "Medical abbreviations" (https://en.wikipedia.org/wiki/List_of_medical_abbreviations), which is released under the Creative Commons Attribution-ShareAlike 3.0 Unported License (https://creativecommons.org/licenses/by-sa/3.0/). Wikipedia® is a registered trademark of the Wikimedia Foundation, Inc., a non-profit organization.

Index

Page numbers followed by f and t indicate figures and tables, respectively.